Third Edition

Foundations of

AURAL REHABILITATION

Children, Adults, and Their Family Members

Nancy Tye-Murray, Ph.D.

Washington University School of Medicine
St. Louis, Missouri

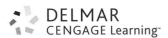

DELMAR
CENGAGE Learning™

Australia • Brazil • Japan • Korea • Mexico • Singapore • Spain • United Kingdom • United States

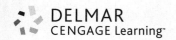

WB

DELMAR
CENGAGE Learning

**Foundations of Aural Rehabilitation:
Children, Adults, and Their Family
Members, 3rd edition**
Nancy Tye-Murray, Ph. D.

Vice President, Career and Professional
Editorial: Dave Garza

Director of Learning Solutions:
Matthew Kane

Senior Acquisitions Editor: Sherry Dickinson

Managing Editor: Marah Bellegarde

Product Manager: Laura Wood

Vice President, Career and Professional
Marketing: Jennifer McAvey

Marketing Director: Wendy Mapstone

Marketing Manager: Kristin McNary

Marketing Coordinator: Scott Chrysler

Production Director: Carolyn Miller

Production Manager: Andrew Crouth

Content Project Manager: Thomas Heffernan

Senior Art Director: David Arsenault

Senior Technology Product Manager:
Mary Colleen Liburdi

Technology Project Manager: Chris Catalina

© 2009, 2004, 1998 Delmar, Cengage Learning

ALL RIGHTS RESERVED. No part of this work covered by the copyright
herein may be reproduced, transmitted, stored, or used in any form or by
any means graphic, electronic, or mechanical, including but not limited to
photocopying, recording, scanning, digitizing, taping, Web distribution,
information networks, or information storage and retrieval systems, except
as permitted under Section 107 or 108 of the 1976 United States Copyright
Act, without the prior written permission of the publisher.

For product information and technology assistance, contact us at
Professional & Career Group Customer Support, 1-800-648-7450

For permission to use material from this text or product,
submit all requests online at **cengage.com/permissions**
Further permissions questions can be e-mailed to
permissionrequest@cengage.com

Library of Congress Control Number: 2008924605

ISBN-13: 978-1-4283-1215-9

ISBN-10: 1-4283-1215-3

Delmar
5 Maxwell Drive
Clifton Park, NY 12065-2919
USA

Cengage Learning is a leading provider of customized learning solutions with
office locations around the globe, including Singapore, the United Kingdom,
Australia, Mexico, Brazil, and Japan. Locate your local office at:
international.cengage.com/region

Cengage Learning products are represented in Canada by
Nelson Education, Ltd.

For your lifelong learning solutions, visit **delmar.cengage.com**

Visit our corporate website at **www.cengage.com**

Printed in the United States of America
2 3 4 5 6 7 12 11 10 09

5/25/10

CONTENTS

Preface vii

CHAPTER 1   Introduction 1

        The World Health Organization and hearing-related disability
        Services included in the aural rehabilitation plan
        Where does aural rehabilitation occur?
        Who provides aural rehabilitation?
        Hearing loss
        Service needs
        Cost-effectiveness and costs
        Evidence-based practice
        Case study: Evidence-based practice decision making

PART I   **SPEECH RECOGNITION AND PERSONS WHO HAVE HEARING LOSS** **39**

CHAPTER 2   Assessing Hearing Acuity and Speech Recognition 41

        Review of the audiological examination and the audiogram
        Purpose of speech recognition testing
        Patient variables
        Stimuli units
        Test procedures
        Difficulties associated with speech recognition assessment
        Multicultural issues
        Case study: Reason to go with a test battery approach

CHAPTER 3 Listening Devices and Related Technology 87

Hearing aids
Cochlear implants
Assistive listening devices (ALDs)
Case study: Listen to the music

CHAPTER 4 Auditory Training 139

Historical notes
Candidacy for auditory training
Four design principles
Developing analytic training objectives
Developing synthetic training objectives
Formal and informal auditory training
Interweaving auditory training with other components of aural
rehabilitation
Auditory training programs
Benefits of auditory training
Case studies: Listening with a new cochlear implant

CHAPTER 5 Speechreading 183

Speechreading for communication
Characteristics of a good lipreader
What happens when someone lipreads?
The difficulty of the lipreading task
What happens when someone speechreads?
Importance of residual hearing
Factors that affect the speechreading process
Oral interpreters
Case study: An exceptional lipreader

CHAPTER 6 Speechreading Training 219

Candidacy
Traditional methods of speechreading training
Developing speechreading skills
Analytic speechreading training objectives
Synthetic speechreading training objectives
Computerized instruction
Efficacy of speechreading training
Case study: Targeting training

PART II CONVERSATION AND COMMUNICATION BEHAVIORS 245

CHAPTER   7   Communication Strategies and Conversational Styles 247

Conversation

Facilitative communication strategies

Repair strategies

Research concerning repair strategies and communication breakdowns

Conversational styles and behaviors

Case study: A couple conversing

CHAPTER   8   Assessment of Conversational Fluency and Communication Difficulties . . .285

Conversational fluency

General considerations for evaluating conversational fluency and hearing-related disability

Interviews

Questionnaires

Daily logs

Group discussion

Structured communication interactions

Unstructured communication interactions

Case study: A school boy opens up

CHAPTER   9   Communication Strategies Training. 317

Self-efficacy

Issues to consider when developing a training program

Getting started

Model for training

Short-term training

Communication strategies training for frequent communication partners

Communication strategies training for children

Benefits of training

Case studies: An increased sense of self-efficacy

CHAPTER   10   Counseling, Psychosocial Support, and Assertiveness Training 349

Who provides counseling, psychosocial support, and assertiveness training?

Counseling

Psychosocial support

Assertiveness training

Related research

Case study: Solving challenging situations

PART **III** **AURAL REHABILITATION FOR ADULTS** **383**

CHAPTER **11** Adults Who Have Hearing Loss 385

Prevalence of hearing loss among adults

A patient-centered approach

Characteristics of adult-onset hearing loss

Who is this person?

Where is the person in terms of adjustment to hearing loss?

Case studies: One size doesn't fit all

CHAPTER **12** Aural Rehabilitation Plans for Adults 427

Assessment

Informational counseling

Development of an aural rehabilitation plan

Implementation

Outcomes assessment

Follow-up

Case study: A road map for success

CHAPTER **13** Aural Rehabilitation Plans for Older Adults 479

Activity limitations and participation restrictions

Audiological status and otologic health

Life-situation factors

Physical and cognitive variables

Aural rehabilitation intervention

Aural rehabilitation in the institutional setting

Case study: Staying active

PART **IV** **AURAL (RE)HABILITATION FOR CHILDREN** **529**

CHAPTER **14** Infants and Toddlers Who Have Hearing Loss 531

Detection of hearing loss

Identification and quantification of hearing loss

Health care follow-up

Parent counseling

Early-intervention overview and development of an aural rehabilitation strategy

Communication mode

Listening device

Early-intervention program

Parental support and parent instruction

Case study: A memorable journey

CHAPTER 15 School-Age Children Who Have Hearing Loss. 599

Creation of an Individualized Education Plan (IEP)

The multidisciplinary team

School and classroom placement

Amplification and assistive listening devices

Classroom acoustics

Speech, language, and literacy

Other services

Children who have mild or moderate hearing losses

Case studies: IDEA(s) for all

Appendix 666

Glossary 669

References 692

Author Index. 758

Subject Index 767

PREFACE

What exactly is aural/audiological rehabilitation? The answer to this question can conceivably include almost every aspect of audiology and education of children who are deaf and hard of hearing, and much of speech-language pathology. Under the rubric of aural rehabilitation may fall any of the following topics: identification and diagnosis of hearing loss and other hearing-related communication difficulties, patient and family counseling, selection and fitting of listening devices, follow-up services for the prescribed listening devices, communication strategies training, literacy promotion, speech and language therapy, classroom management, parent instruction, sign language instruction, and speechreading and auditory training. What is incontrovertible is that technology has come to play an increasingly important role in any aural rehabilitation service delivery model, whether it be in the provision of hearing aids or cochlear implants or in the administration of computerized tests and training activities. Nonetheless, the threads that run through the various services and that unify them into the discipline that we know as aural rehabilitation are an emphasis on understanding and addressing the needs of patients who have hearing loss and an emphasis on ensuring that patients achieve maximum communication success in their everyday environments.

For some readers, *Foundations of Aural Rehabilitation: Children, Adults, and Their Family Members* will be the only text they study that is entirely devoted to aural/audiological rehabilitation. A book of this nature must thus include materials that introduce students to the services just listed as well as more advanced materials that lead them to a level of understanding that is necessary for professional practice. In this third edition, I have made a concerted effort to improve the organization of the introductory materials and to include more advanced findings and more references.

My goal has been to offer a book that serves both as an introduction to aural rehabilitation and as a reference that can be revisited once students enter into professional practice.

Conversational fluency is the book's central theme. Almost every chapter to some extent either implicitly or explicitly concerns the impact of hearing loss on conversational fluency. Some chapters or sections are included primarily for the purpose of familiarizing readers with how reliance on speechreading and the need for communication strategies can affect everyday conversations. For instance, Chapter 5 provides an in-depth review of the speechreading process and Chapter 7 considers how hearing loss may affect conversations and conversational behaviors. I have learned through personal experience and through observation of first-class speech and hearing professionals that effective intervention plans are grounded in an in-depth understanding of conversational dynamics.

I have attempted to make the book both interesting to read and relevant to today's world. A number of case studies are included, and general demographic, medical, and pop-cultural trends are considered in parallel with corresponding developments in aural rehabilitation. Sidebars and chapter inserts provide lively additions to the text, and they include quotations by patients, professionals, and family members, bulleted "talking points," historical notes, and tangential asides.

New Features

The third edition has a different organization than previous editions. A review of assessment and listening devices now occurs before a review of conversation and communication behaviors, as opposed to vice versa. This reorganization was made in response to the recommendations of a number of professors who use the text. In addition to multiple-choice questions, the end of each chapter now includes a list of key terms. Every chapter concludes with a case study taken from the literature and a listing of key points. Key resources and appendixes accompany many chapters. Readers familiar with the second edition will find a new chapter devoted to infants and toddlers who have hearing loss (Chapter 14) and an expanded consideration of informational counseling in Chapter 10. They will also find models of intervention for adults (Chapter 12), older persons (Chapter 13), and school-age children (Chapter 15). More references are included, both historical and current, for readers who would like to learn more. Finally, the text is visually more interesting than previous editions, with contemporary graphics.

Organization

Chapter 1 provides an overview of aural rehabilitation, and introduces readers to the World Health Organization and its definitions of participation restrictions and disabilities and to the topic of *evidence-based practice*. The remaining chapters are divided into two halves. The first half primarily concerns the components of aural rehabilitation whereas the second half primarily concerns the patients themselves and the processes for putting an intervention plan into place. Each half has two parts, so the book has four parts. Part I concerns speech recognition: how to assess speech recognition, how to maximize speech listening through the use of technology, and how to develop listening and speechreading skills. Part II concerns conversation and communication breakdowns. It begins with a consideration of how hearing loss may affect a conversation and ends with a consideration of counseling techniques. Part III concerns the adult population with hearing loss whereas Part IV deals with children. Frameworks for developing aural rehabilitation plans are considered, along with example interventions.

Target Audience

The content is primarily targeted to undergraduate students who are in their junior or senior years in a university or to graduate students who are in their first year of graduate training. The book is appropriate as a primary source book for the disciplines of audiology, speech-language pathology, and education of children who are deaf and hard of hearing. In addition, it may serve as a supplemental text book for training programs in special education, medicine, nursing, occupational therapy, and vocational rehabilitation counseling.

ACKNOWLEDGMENTS

I thank all of the students and professors who have e-mailed me during the past few years with their suggestions, noting when a point was unclear or incomplete, or when a different presentation might have been more effective. Their input has had a tremendous impact on this revision. I also extend my thanks to Jill Premminger and her colleagues in Louisville, Kentucky, Maureen Valente, Lisa Davidson, and Cathy Schroy at Washington University School of Medicine, and the four Delmar reviewers who teach courses in aural rehabilitation for their comments and suggestions. Thanks are also extended to Geoff Plant with MED-EL Corp. and Don Schum with Oticon for providing photographs and for other assistance. I am also grateful to the staff at Delmar Cengage Learning for their support. Finally, I extend thanks to Elizabeth Mauzé at the Washington University School of Medicine for writing the instructor testbank questions that appear on the *Electronic Classroom Manager* to accompany *Foundations of Aural Rehabilitation: Children, Adults, and Their Family Members*.

I welcome any comments or suggestions from readers about future revisions and can be contacted with comments or questions at: *murrayn@ent.wustl.edu*. In the meantime, I wish you the very best with your efforts in aural rehabilitation.

REVIEWERS

We would like to thank the following reviewers for using their expertise to provide valuable feedback during the revision process:

Lou Echols-Chambers, M.S., CCC-A
University of Illinois at Urbana-Champaign
Champaign, IL

Colleen McAleer, PhD, CCC-SLP/A
Clarion University
Clarion, PA

Susan Naidu, PhD, CCC-A
University of Utah
Deer Mountain, UT

Keith S. Wolgemuth, PhD, CCC-A, F-AAA
University of Redlands
Redlands, CA

ABOUT THE AUTHOR

Nancy Tye-Murray is a research professor at the Washington University School of Medicine in St. Louis, Missouri, and the principal investigator of two RO1 grants from the National Institutes of Health and co-principal investigator of a third. Her research interests include the effects of aging on speech perception, conversational fluency, the efficacy of aural rehabilitation, and the speech production and perception of children who have hearing loss. Tye-Murray founded and ran both the aural rehabilitation program for adult cochlear implant users and the children's speech and language project at the University of Iowa Hospitals. At Central Institute for the Deaf, she taught the graduate level aural rehabilitation class at Washington University, helped assess the psychosocial therapy program for adult cochlear implant users, and for six years served as department head of the research program, which was composed of the Center for the Biology of Hearing and Deafness and the Center of Childhood Deafness and Adult Aural Rehabilitation. She has written six books, including, *Let's Converse! A How-To Guide to Expand the Conversational Skills of Children and Teenagers Who Have Hearing Loss* and *Cochlear Implants and Children: A Handbook for Parents, Teachers, and Speech and Hearing Professionals* (Alexander Graham Bell Association Publishing). Tye-Murray has published extensively in such peer-reviewed journals as *Ear and Hearing, Journal of Speech-Language-Hearing, Journal of the Acoustical Society of America,* and *Journal of the Academy of American Audiology.* She developed the CD-ROM aural rehabilitation series *Conversation Made Easy: Speechreading and Communication Training* (published by Central Institute for the Deaf). She is the former president of the Academy of Rehabilitative Audiology and the former chief editor of *Volta Review.*

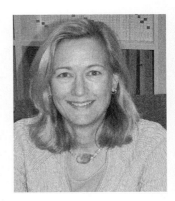

Nancy Tye-Murray

DEDICATION

To Ellen Thornber and Aubrey Fox Murray

CHAPTER 1

Introduction

OUTLINE

- The World Health Organization and hearing-related disability
- Services included in the aural rehabilitation plan
- Where does aural rehabilitation occur?
- Who provides aural rehabilitation?
- Hearing loss
- Service needs
- Cost-effectiveness and costs
- Evidence-based practice
- Case study: Evidence-based practice decision making
- Final remarks
- Key chapter points
- Terms and concepts to remember
- Multiple-choice questions
- Appendix 1-1
- Appendix 1-2
- Appendix 1-3

Hearing loss often has been called the "invisible condition," yet its impact may be anything but invisible. The consequences of hearing loss may be manifested in a broad spectrum of an individual's life. Everyday communication may be difficult and, for some persons, impossible without a great deal of effort. The adult may feel the ramifications of hearing loss at home, in the workplace, and in the community. The young child may share similar difficulties in everyday communication, and may also experience delays in speech, language, educational achievement, and social development.

One of the most deleterious effects of hearing loss is an impaired ability to converse with other people during everyday life activities. The person with hearing loss may miss out on casual conversations, on conversations that establish intimacy and friendship, and on conversations that convey important information or promote life goals. Everyday activities that persons with normal hearing take for granted, such as using the telephone or talking with a store clerk, may be effortful and frustrating. If the individual is a child, the difficulties may relate not only to hearing spoken messages, but also to formulating and expressing messages in light of limited speech and language skills. In the wake of a successful aural rehabilitation plan, persons with hearing loss are often able to converse more effectively with the people in their home, work, school, and social environments, and to achieve success in their communication efforts.

Aural rehabilitation is intervention aimed at minimizing and alleviating the communication difficulties associated with hearing loss.

Aural rehabilitation is aimed at restoring or optimizing a patient's participation in activities that have been limited as a result of hearing loss and also may be aimed at benefiting communication partners who engage in activities that include persons with hearing loss (Gagné, 2000). The goals of aural rehabilitation are to:

• Alleviate the difficulties related to hearing loss and
• Minimize its consequences

The concrete outcomes of achieving these goals are enhanced conversational fluency and reduced hearing-related disability.

Conversational fluency relates to how smoothly conversation unfolds.

Conversational fluency refers to how smoothly conversation flows (Chapter 7). Persons with hearing loss often experience reduced conversational fluency because they have difficulty in understanding the spoken messages of their communication partners. Children with hearing loss may also experience difficulty in formulating and expressing their own messages (Chapter 15).

A **hearing-related disability** is a loss of function imposed by hearing loss. The term denotes a multidimensional phenomenon.

Hearing-related disability is a loss of function imposed by hearing loss and is a multidimensional phenomenon. Disability is not an attribute of the individual per se. It arises from a complex collection of conditions, some of which stem from the individual's real-world environment. Following an effective aural rehabilitation plan, a patient will experience both enhanced conversational fluency and reduced hearing-related disability.

Those Whom We Serve

Children who receive aural rehabilitation services are often referred to as *students*, especially in the context of an educational setting. Terminology for adults who receive services is more variable, and includes *patients*, *clients*, and *consumers*. Hernandez and Amlani (2004) mailed out 1,428 surveys to a random sample of Fellows of the American Academy of Audiology. Thirty-two percent of the surveys were returned. The results showed that an overwhelming majority (90%) preferred the term *patient*, which is the term that is used in this text.

In this introductory chapter, we will consider a model of hearing-related disability in the context of formulating an aural rehabilitation intervention plan. General issues and terms associated with aural rehabilitation and hearing loss will be reviewed as well as locales where aural rehabilitation might occur, who might provide it, and who might receive it in terms of degree of hearing loss and age. The chapter will conclude with a discussion of how speech and hearing professionals go about selecting appropriate intervention services.

THE WORLD HEALTH ORGANIZATION AND HEARING-RELATED DISABILITY

Several years ago, the World Health Organization (WHO) considered that persons with hearing impairment had a disability and associated handicaps. In the original nomenclature, a disability was a loss of function imposed by an **impairment** of the auditory system, such as an inability to understand a conversation conducted at an office conference table. A **handicap** was the social or vocational consequence of a disability, such as having to change jobs because one can no longer perform the requisite responsibilities.

WHO (2001) now recognizes that the term *handicap* may sometimes convey pejorative and stigmatizing connotations and that the term *disability* denotes a multidimensional phenomenon. Disability arises from an individual's hearing

An **impairment** is a structural or functional impairment of the auditory system.

A **handicap** consists of the psychosocial disadvantages that result from a functional impairment. Use of this term is discouraged by the World Health Organization.

An **activity limitation** is a change at the level of the person brought about by an impairment at the levels of body structure (e.g., loss of hair cells in the cochlea) and function (e.g., loss of an ability to discriminate pitch); for example, a patient may no longer be able to engage easily in casual conversation.

A **participation restriction** is an effect of an activity limitation that results in a change in the broader scope of a patient's life; for example, a patient may avoid social gatherings.

impairment, physical and social environments, and individual qualities, such as personality and intelligence. The organization recommends that persons with hearing impairment be considered in terms of their **activity limitations** and their **participation restrictions**. An activity limitation is a change at the level of the patient, such as an inability to participate in a group conversation. A participation restriction is the effect of those limitations on the broader scope of life, such as a patient's tendency to avoid group interactions. Such a consideration takes into account the nature and extent of functioning and how it may be limited in quality or quantity and also takes into account the physical, social, and attitudinal environments in which a person lives.

Figure 1-1 presents a model of hearing-related disability that is based on the WHO's definitions. In this figure, the solid lines indicate an exacerbation and dotted lines indicate an alleviation. Four factors (i.e., limitations in communication activity, lifestyle, frequent communication partner, and psychosocial) contribute directly to a person's participation restrictions.

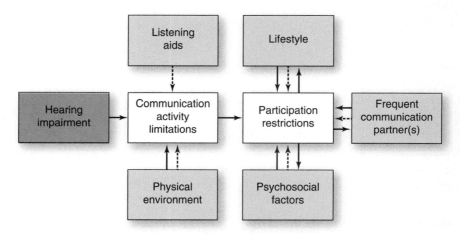

FIGURE 1-1. A model of hearing-related disability.

The impairment of hearing has a direct effect on the extent to which communication activity is limited. One goal of the aural rehabilitation plan is to minimize the impact of hearing loss through the provision of appropriate listening devices such as hearing aids or cochlear implants and through the provision of other listening aids such as assistive listening devices.

Limitations in communication activity can also be positively or negatively affected by the physical environment, as when the environment is either noisy or sound-treated. Another goal of the aural rehabilitation plan is to help patients and their communication partners tailor the listening situation to optimize conversation success and to use other strategies to lessen disability.

Lifestyle may have a major effect on participation restrictions. For instance, a male computer programmer and a salesman may have the same degree of hearing loss as measured audiometrically, yet the consequences for either one may differ. The programmer, who works alone at a computer monitor, may rarely experience conversational difficulties as a result of hearing loss. His typical day revolves around reading, problem solving at his desk, and working at the keyboard. On the other hand, the salesman must contact customers throughout the workday and may be devastated by a similar degree of hearing loss. He may frequently misunderstand an order, he may not be able to use the telephone effectively, and he may feel helpless to handle his communication difficulties at group meetings. The goal of the aural rehabilitation plan is to identify the effects of a patient's participation restrictions on lifestyle and to implement effective means to overcome them. To the extent that the restrictions cannot be overcome, the lifestyle may be adversely affected, as indicated by the reciprocal solid line leading from *participation restrictions* to *lifestyle* in Figure 1-1. If the restrictions experienced by an individual are great, the person may withdraw from lifestyle activities that formerly were found to be rewarding or pleasurable.

The behaviors and attitudes of **frequent communication partners** (the people the patient interacts with most often at home, in the workplace, in school, or during social activities) also affect participation restrictions and the degree of disability. For instance, a frequent communication partner who mumbles, who resents the patient's hearing loss, and who feels burdened and cheated out of a high quality of life may exacerbate the consequences of hearing loss. This relationship is a reciprocal one. Many times, the patient's participation restrictions impose an adverse effect on the quality of life experienced by the frequent communication partner. For instance, a man who refuses to attend parties or other social events because of his hearing loss may limit the social interactions of his wife by insisting that they stay home. Another common aim of an aural rehabilitation plan is to enhance the communication effectiveness between a patient and the communication partner, and to mollify the consequences of hearing loss for the frequent communication partner.

Frequent communication partners are persons with whom another often converses, such as a family member.

Psychological factors pertain to the patient's attitudes toward the hearing loss (e.g., to some persons a hearing loss might be a source of shame, whereas to others it may seem inconsequential in comparison to other life events), the patient's self-image, the patient's motivation to participate in aural rehabilitation, and the patient's assertiveness. For example, as will be noted in Chapter 7, an assertive person may effectively use communication strategies but a passive person may not, leading each to experience different degrees of participation restrictions. **Social factors** (also referred to as cultural factors) are the prevailing viewpoints of the society in which the patient lives and operates. If the prevailing view is that hearing loss is a negative state, as when it

Psychological factors pertain to an individual's attitudes, self-image, motivation, and assertiveness.

Social factors are the prevailing viewpoints of one's society.

is an indicant of aging in a youth-oriented society or a sign of inadequacy to maintain performance in the workforce, then the concomitant participation restrictions and other consequences may increase. The relationship between psychosocial factors and participation restrictions is reciprocal. For instance, just as a person's self-image may affect participation restrictions (e.g., "I'm a strong personality, I can handle this."), the restrictions experienced can affect self-image (e.g., "I'm not as valuable to my children because I can no longer interact with their friends and teachers like I once did."). An effective aural rehabilitation plan might focus on the patient's psychosocial issues and sometimes on those of the frequent communication partner.

Participation Restrictions: A Very Famous Case Study

Ludwig Van Beethoven, at the age of 28 years old, sent this letter to his two brothers, Carl and Johann. Despite his enormous success as a composer, Beethoven still suffered the participation restrictions imposed by significant hearing loss:

"Though born with a fiery, active temperament, even susceptible to the diversions of society, I was soon compelled to isolate myself, to live life alone. If at times I tried to forget all this, oh how harshly was I flung back by the doubly sad experience of my bad hearing. Yet it was impossible for me to say to people, 'Speak louder, shout, for I am deaf.' Ah, how could I possibly admit an infirmity in the one sense which ought to be more perfect in me than others, a sense which I once possessed in the highest perfection, a perfection such as few in my profession enjoy or ever have enjoyed. Oh I cannot do it; therefore, forgive me when you see me draw back when I would have gladly mingled with you. My misfortune is doubly painful to me because I am bound to be misunderstood; for me there can be no relaxation with my fellow men, no refined conversations, no mutual exchange of ideas. I must live almost alone, like one who has been banished; I can mix with society only as much as true necessity demands. If I approach near to people a hot terror seizes upon me, and I fear being exposed to the danger that my condition might be noticed."

(retrieved 8-1-07, *http://www.mumbai-central.com/nukkad/aug2001/ msg00001.html*)

SERVICES INCLUDED IN THE AURAL REHABILITATION PLAN

Table 1-1 presents components of several services often included in an aural rehabilitation plan and brief descriptions of each. These services help to alleviate hearing impairment, and hearing-related disability, and are described more fully in the remaining chapters of this textbook.

Table 1-1. Components of a typical aural rehabilitation program.

COMPONENT	DESCRIPTION
Diagnostics and quantification of hearing loss	Assessment of the hearing loss and speech-recognition skills
Provision of appropriate listening device	Provision of hearing aid(s) or tactile aid listening device or participation on a team that results in cochlear implantation and follow-up services
Provision of appropriate assistive listening devices (ALDs)	Explanation and dispensing of devices that supplement or replace a hearing aid or that serve to lessen hearing-related communication difficulties
Auditory training	Structured and unstructured listening practice
Communication strategies training	Teaching of strategies that enhance communication and minimize communication difficulties (facilitative strategies, repair strategies, environmental management)
Informational/educational counseling	Instruction about normal hearing, hearing loss, listening device technology, speech perception, available services
Personal adjustment counseling	Intervention to enhance the management and acceptance of hearing loss and communication difficulties
Psychosocial support	Addressing the psychological and social impact of hearing loss on the person with hearing loss, family, and friends (may include stress management and relaxation techniques)
Frequent communication partner training	Communication training for the spouse, partner, family, friends, or co-workers
Speechreading training	Training speech recognition via both auditory and visual channels
Speech-language therapy	For children primarily, training that emphasizes developing strategies to monitor one's own speech production and developing vocabulary, syntax, and pragmatics
In-service training	Specialized training for other professionals, such as teachers in the public school system or caretakers in senior citizen centers

Source: Adapted from Prendergast, S. G., and Kelley, L. A. (2002). Aural rehab services: Survey reports who offers which ones and how often. *The Hearing Journal, 55,* 30–35.

A typical aural rehabilitation plan may include diagnosis and quantification of the hearing loss and the provision of appropriate listening devices. In addition, aural rehabilitation for an adult may include communication strategies training, counseling related to hearing loss, assertiveness training, psychosocial support, and counseling and instruction for family members, colleagues, or caretakers. Less commonly, an aural rehabilitation program for an adult may also include auditory or speechreading training. For a child, aural rehabilitation may include diagnostics, provision of appropriate amplification and communication aids, auditory and speechreading training, and communication strategies training, as well as intervention related to speech, language, and academic achievement. Children's family members and teachers may also receive services under the umbrella of the aural rehabilitation plan.

Aural habilitation is intervention for persons who have not developed listening, speech, and language skills.

Other Terms Related to Aural Rehabilitation

Sometimes the terms aural habilitation or audiologic rehabilitation are used when discussing the provision of services related to alleviating the problems associated with hearing loss. The term **aural habilitation** instead of aural rehabilitation is used when the person receiving the services is a child rather than an adult. This is because in the strict sense, *rehabilitation* means to restore something that was lost. When we provide auditory training or speech and language therapy to children who have hearing loss, we are not aiming to restore lost function, but rather, to develop (that is, to habilitate or furnish) skills that were not present beforehand. Although this is a cogent distinction between the terms rehabilitation and habilitation, in this text, the two will be used synonymously for simplicity's sake.

The term audiologic rehabilitation closely parallels the term *aural rehabilitation*, but it usually encompasses a narrower breadth of services. The term **audiologic rehabilitation** implies an emphasis on the diagnosis of hearing loss and the provision of listening devices and a lesser emphasis on follow-up support services, such as communication strategies training.

Audiologic rehabilitation is a term often used synonymously with aural rehabilitation or aural habilitation; it may entail greater emphasis on the provision and follow-up of listening devices and less emphasis on communication strategies and auditory and speechreading training.

WHERE DOES AURAL REHABILITATION OCCUR?

Aural rehabilitation may occur in a variety of locales. For example, it may be provided in any of the following settings:

- A university speech and hearing clinic
- An audiology private practice

- A hearing aid dealer's private practice
- A hospital speech and hearing clinic
- A community center or nursing home
- A school (Figure 1-2)
- An otolaryngologist's office
- A speech-language pathologist's office
- Consumer organization meetings
- The home, sometimes with the aid of a computer

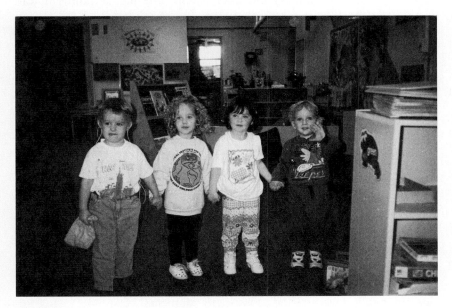

FIGURE 1-2. Aural rehabilitation in the educational setting. *Photograph by Julia Rottjakob, courtesy of the Central Institute for the Deaf.*

WHO PROVIDES AURAL REHABILITATION?

Aural rehabilitation might be provided by an audiologist, a speech-language pathologist, or a teacher for children who are deaf and hard of hearing. Typically, an audiologist takes a lead role in developing an individual's aural rehabilitation plan and coordinates the services provided by other professionals. Particularly with adults, the audiologist is the primary health-care professional in the management of the hearing loss.

In some cases, however, the speech-language pathologist may play the lead role for a child, especially in a school environment. For instance, the speech-language pathologist is most likely to provide speech and language therapy and often is the professional who provides auditory and speechreading training. Whereas the audiologist may fit and maintain a child's hearing aids and equip the classroom with appropriate assistive listening devices, the speech-language pathologist may be the person who has extended one-on-one contact with a child, and the one who knows the child well. The American Speech-Language-Hearing Association (ASHA) convened a working group on audiologic rehabilitation (ASHA, 2002). Its charge was to summarize the knowledge and skill sets that audiologists and speech-language pathologists should have if they are to provide aural rehabilitation. These outlines are presented in Appendix 1-1 (audiologists) and Appendix 1-2 (speech-language pathologists).

In addition to a general knowledge about basic communication processes, audiologists who provide aural rehabilitation are expected to understand the auditory system function and disorders, developmental status, cognition, sensory perception, audiologic assessment procedures, speech and language assessment procedures, evaluation and management of listening devices, effects of hearing impairment on functional communication, case management, interdisciplinary collaboration and public advocacy, and hearing conservation and acoustic environments.

In addition to general knowledge about the basic communication processes, speech-language pathologists are expected to have a broad knowledge of auditory system function and disorders, developmental status, cognition, sensory perception, audiologic assessment procedures, assessment of communication performance, listening devices, effects of hearing loss on psychosocial, educational, and vocational functioning, management, interdisciplinary collaboration and public advocacy, and acoustic environments.

HEARING LOSS

Individuals who have hearing loss represent a heterogeneous group, and they often vary in the nature of their hearing loss (Figure 1-3). The attributes of their hearing loss typically influence the design of the aural rehabilitation intervention plan.

Hearing loss may be categorized along four dimensions: degree, onset, causation, and time course. In terms of degree, hearing loss may be characterized as mild, moderate, moderate-to-severe, severe, or profound (Chapter 2).

The **pure-tone average (PTA)** is the average of the thresholds at 500, 1,000, and 2,000 Hz.

Degree of hearing impairment is often defined by the **pure-tone average (PTA)**, the average of the individual's pure-tone frequencies at 500, 1,000,

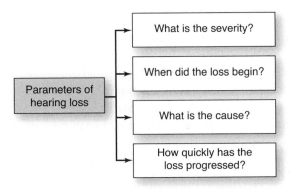

FIGURE 1-3. Parameterization of hearing loss along four dimensions: degree, onset, causation, and time course.

and 2,000 Hz obtained with headphones. In describing the degree of hearing loss, the speech and hearing professional takes into consideration the **configuration** of the loss. Configuration of hearing loss reflects the extent of hearing loss at each of the audiometric frequencies (audiograms measure hearing sensitivity at the frequencies of 250, 500, 1,000, 2,000, 4,000, and 8,000 Hz) and provides an overall picture of hearing sensitivity. For example, a person who has normal hearing for the frequencies 250–2,000 Hz and then reduced sensitivity for the frequencies 4,000–8,000 Hz may be described as having a "high-frequency hearing loss." A person who has equal sensitivity across the audiometric frequencies has a "flat hearing loss" (see Figure 1-4). Other descriptors associated with degree of hearing loss include the following:

> **Configuration** refers to the extent of the hearing loss at each frequency and gives an overall description of the hearing loss.

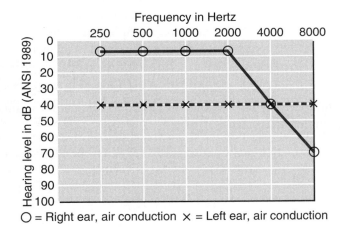

FIGURE 1-4. An audiogram that depicts an asymmetrical hearing loss. The left ear has a "flat" hearing loss; right ear has a "high-frequency" hearing loss.

An **asymmetrical** hearing loss is one in which the degree and/or configuration of loss in one ear differs from that in the other ear.

- *Bilateral versus unilateral.* Bilateral hearing loss means both ears have reduced sensitivity, whereas unilateral means only one ear is affected.
- *Symmetrical versus* **asymmetrical.** Symmetrical hearing loss means the degree and configuration of hearing loss are the same in each ear, whereas asymmetrical means the two ears differ.
- *Fluctuating versus stable.* Sometimes a person's hearing sensitivity may fluctuate (for example, if a child has fluid in the ear), whereas at other times sensitivity remains stable.

Hard of hearing means having a hearing loss; usually not used to refer to a profound hearing loss.

A person who has a mild, moderate, or moderate-to-severe hearing loss (i.e., a hearing loss between 26 and 70 dB) is often called **hard of hearing**. Sometimes the term *hearing-impaired* is used in lieu of the term hard of hearing. Many persons dislike it as it connotes that they may be exactly that, impaired, even though they may function effectively in their everyday lives. A person who has a profound hearing loss (and less often, severe) may sometimes be called **deaf**. People who belong to the Deaf community, often people who were born deaf or who grew up with deaf family members, may refer to themselves as *Deaf.* The capital "D" denotes their membership in the Deaf culture. As we will consider in Chapter 11, members of the Deaf culture share a similar sign language, culture, and often, educational experiences.

Deaf usually means having minimal or no hearing.

Prelingual refers to a hearing loss acquired before the acquisition of spoken language.

In terms of onset, a hearing loss may be described as prelingual, perilingual, or postlingual. A person who has a **prelingual** hearing loss incurred the loss before the acquisition of spoken language skills. Although there is no universally agreed cut-off time as to when the prelingual phase ends, generally, when a child incurs a hearing loss before the age of 2 years, he or she is said to have a prelingual loss. A **congenital** hearing loss is thought to be present at birth or associated with the birthing process. An **acquired** hearing loss is not present at birth but is incurred later, either as a child or as an adult. A child who lost his or her hearing after acquiring some spoken language but before acquisition was complete is said to have a **perilingual** hearing loss. Finally, a **postlingual** loss is one that occurred after the acquisition of speech and language. Again, there is no agreed-on age at which the perilingual stage ends and the postlingual stage begins, but it may be around the age of 5 years. The postlingual distinction may be further divided into four additional cohorts. These are:

A label of **congenital** implies the hearing loss was present at birth

A label of **acquired** implies the hearing loss was incurred after birth.

Perilingual refers to a hearing loss acquired during the stage of acquiring spoken language.

Postlingual refers to a hearing loss incurred after the acquisition of spoken language.

- Prevocational (around the ages 5–17 years)
- Early working age (18–44 years)
- Later working age (45–64 years)
- Retirement age (65 years and older)

Depending on a patient's membership in a cohort, his or her aural rehabilitation needs may vary. For instance, someone who is prevocational may benefit from having a special amplification system available in the classroom, and the child's family may benefit from communication strategies training. Another person of later working age, someone who before hearing loss may have been able and competent in every respect, may require personal adjustment counseling and even psychosocial support to accept his or her change in abilities.

The third dimension used to categorize hearing loss is causation. A hearing loss may be conductive, sensorineural, or a combination of both, a mix. The source of impairment determines the type.

A **conductive loss** stems from an obstruction in either the outer or middle ear that prevents sound from reaching the sensorineural structures in the inner ear. An obstruction might be congenital, such as **microtia** or **atresia**, or it might be acquired, such as **cerumen** accumulation in the ear canal or **otitis media** in the middle ear. Many conductive hearing losses are resolved with medical treatment or the passage of time. In instances when a loss in hearing sensitivity remains, effective amplification can minimize listening difficulties. Conductive losses result in speech being attenuated. If the speech can be amplified loud enough, the patient usually can recognize speech quite easily. Conductive losses typically are limited in degree as once the level of the sound rises above about 50 or 60 dBSPL, it is transmitted directly to the inner ear by bone conduction.

Sensorineural hearing loss stems from a disturbance in the inner ear, eighth nerve, brain stem, midbrain, or auditory cortex. Sensorineural losses are typically permanent. Prelingual sensorineural hearing losses might be caused by any number of factors, including genetic makeup, maternal infections, or postnatal infection such as **meningitis** or **encephalitis**. Postlingual sensorineural hearing losses might relate to noise exposure, the ingestion of **ototoxic drugs**, or aging. People who have sensorineural hearing loss often experience decreased ability to recognize speech, even if they are using appropriate amplification, because they have reduced or ablated neural capacity for conveying sound to the brain.

Sometimes an individual can have both a conductive and sensorineural hearing loss. For instance, a child who has a congenital sensorineural hearing loss may have **mixed hearing loss** if he or she suffers a bout of otitis media.

A **conductive loss** results from an obstruction within the outer or middle ear.

Microtia is a congenitally small external ear.

A congenital closure of the external auditory canal is called **atresia**.

Cerumen is ear wax.

Otitis media is an inflammation of the middle ear, often accompanied by the accumulation of fluid in the middle ear cavity.

Sensorineural hearing loss is a type of hearing loss that has a cochlear or retro cochlear origin.

Meningitis is a common cause of childhood sensorineural hearing loss caused by bacterial or viral inflammation of the meninges. The meninges are the membranous linings of the brain and spinal cord.

Encephalitis is an inflammation of the brain.

Ototoxic drugs are harmful to the structures of the inner ear and the auditory nerve.

A hearing loss that has both a conductive and a sensorineural component is called a **mixed hearing loss.**

"People with hearing loss are often embarrassed because they think they are different or that they have a rare condition . . . 31.5 million people report a hearing difficulty; that is around 10% of the U.S. population. So if you have a hearing loss, understand that you are not alone."

Sergei Kochkin, Executive Director of the Better Hearing Institute

(retrieved 8-1-07, http://www.org/hearing-loss/prevalence)

A **progressive hearing loss** is a hearing loss that increases over time.

A **sudden hearing loss** is a hearing loss that has an acute and rapid onset.

An **unserved** population refers to a group of patients in need of but not receiving services.

An **underserved** population is a group of patients receiving less than ideal services.

Finally, a hearing loss may be categorized as progressive or sudden. An individual who has a hearing loss that occurs over the course of several months or years has a **progressive hearing loss**. An individual who lost hearing suddenly, say as a result of head trauma, has a **sudden hearing loss**.

SERVICE NEEDS

Statistics underscore the fact that a significant number of persons have hearing loss. About 31.5 million people in the United States have some degree of reduced hearing sensitivity. By the year 2050, the number will top 40 million (Kochkin, 2005). Of this number, about 80% have an irreversible hearing loss. Hearing loss is on the rise around the world. For instance, in the Scandinavian countries of Denmark, Finland, Norway, and Sweden, and in the United Kingdom, hearing loss has an increasing incidence. In a review article of surveys performed on adult populations, Maki-Torkko et al. (2001) suggest that the incidence of hearing loss increases with age, and the proportion of people over the age of 65 years who have hearing loss may fall somewhere between 15% and 60%, depending on how one defines the age group and how one defines degree of hearing loss.

Many individuals who have hearing loss are unserved or underserved. **Unserved** means this population is a group that is not served as a result of policy, practice, or environmental barriers. **Underserved** denotes a population that is inadequately served, in part because of:

- A dearth of outreach and immediate or extended support services
- The attitudes of service delivery personnel
- The lack of reimbursement policies for aural rehabilitation
- Communication or environmental barriers

Increasingly, persons with hearing loss and their families are exerting pressure on lawmakers and policy makers to ensure that more services are provided to individuals who have hearing loss and deafness. There will be a need for speech and hearing professionals to provide these services. Patients range in age from infancy to old age (Figure 1-5).

Infants and Toddlers

Advances in neonatology and critical-care medicine have led to better survival rates of high-risk babies. Infants who might have died in earlier times now survive, often with a myriad of medical conditions that might include hearing loss. Families of babies who have hearing loss desire and expect assistance and support that will enable their children to grow up and achieve their full potential. Public policy reflects these trends. There is now a greater emphasis on earlier identification and service provision for young children who have hearing loss, under the auspices of Public Law 105-17 (Chapter 14).

School-Age Children

Once children enter school, they face the challenge of learning how to read and mastering academic material. They encounter new independence away form the home. Friends and classmates become increasingly important, and often, learning how to communicate effectively with their peer group becomes a high priority. Services for children and teenagers may include educational planning, accommodation in the classroom, including the use of assistive technology, and support in transitioning from elementary school to secondary school to postsecondary school settings (Chapter 15).

Adults

Individuals in the center of the life cycle also may desire aural rehabilitation services. They have learned that, with appropriate support, they can make meaningful contributions both in the workplace and in their communities. Indeed, this realization helped lead to the passage of the Americans with Disabilities Act (ADA, passed in 1990), which is landmark legislation that calls for equal access for all persons with disabilities (Chapter 12).

Older Persons

With the aging of the "baby boom" population, age-related hearing loss is affecting an increasing percentage of our citizens (Figure 1-6). These individuals often are unwilling to, nor should they be expected to, sit on the sidelines of life because they are unable to communicate with those around them. They have a demand for services that will enhance their ability to communicate with their families and friends, to participate in community activities and volunteer work, and to stay in touch with their world via multimedia technology. Some desire to continue in their professional careers and postpone retirement. With increased awareness of preventative medicine routines and a growing sophistication in medical practice, an ever-growing number of older persons are living longer, and many have few health problems other than hearing loss that restrict their day-to-day functioning (Chapter 13).

Family and Frequent Communication Partners

A primary goal of any aural rehabilitation plan is to develop and enhance communication between the person with hearing loss and his or her family

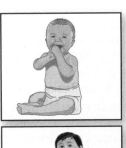
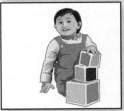
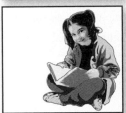
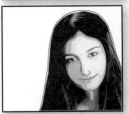
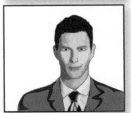
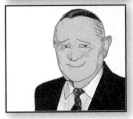

FIGURE 1-5. Demand for aural rehabilitation services across the life span.

> "Working adults and the elderly have been largely without services. Working adults often face not only the growing challenges to their hearing, communication, and linguistic abilities brought by the information society, but also the negative psycho-social effects of impaired hearing. . . . Preventive work with senior citizens can promote extended independent living and better quality of life."
>
> (Huttunen, 2001, p. 89)

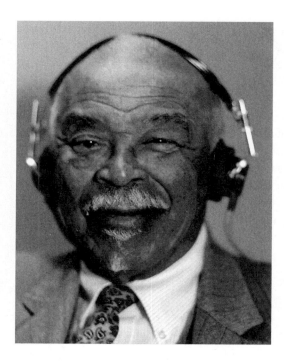

FIGURE 1-6. Aural rehabilitation and older persons. *Photograph by Marcus Kosa, courtesy of the Central Institute for the Deaf.*

and communication partners. Implicitly, this goal suggests that the plan must target not only the individual, but also the people with whom the individual interacts during everyday activities. For an adult patient, the aural rehabilitation might include those persons in the home, social/avocational settings, and the workplace. Figure 1-7 shows these communication realms as intersecting, because some communication partners may interact with the individual in both work and social environments. For a child, the plan might target the communication partners in the school system, social and extracurricular activities, and the home.

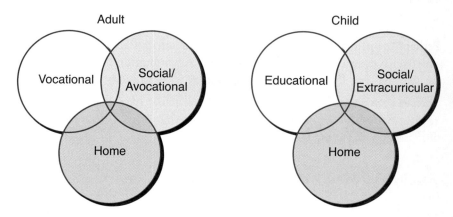

FIGURE 1-7. The aural rehabilitation plan and the individual's communication realms.

Communication partners of persons with hearing loss can acquire techniques for optimizing communication. For example, a wife may learn how to speak slowly and clearly so that her husband might better speechread her vocalizations (Chapter 9). A father might develop techniques for stimulating conversation between himself and his son (Chapter 14). In addition, communication partners sometimes need additional support from a speech and hearing professional. A mother may need personal adjustment counseling as she reconciles herself to her baby's hearing loss. A husband may need to adjust to the changed hearing status of his wife who may have just received a cochlear implant (Chapter 10).

COST-EFFECTIVENESS AND COSTS

Cost-effectiveness relates to the relevance of aural rehabilitation, whereas the costs of providing services relate to the reality of providing services in an environment where health care expenses are spiraling, and services are being cut for economic reasons.

Aural rehabilitation can promote an individual's quality of life and increase his or her conversational fluency in the home, workplace, and community. In the case of children, appropriate aural rehabilitation can promote success in school as well. For instance, children who receive cochlear implants and abundant aural rehabilitation, particularly auditory speech stimulation, are more likely to demonstrate benefit in terms of language, speech, and literacy development than those who do not receive such follow-up support (e.g., Geers, Nicholas, & Seedy, 2003). Research has shown that when counseling and follow-up programs are provided, adult patients are less likely to return their hearing aids to the audiologist than when they are not provided (Northern & Beyer, 1999) and that the benefits of an aural rehabilitation program justify the expense (Abrams, Chisolm, & McArdle, 2002).

Perhaps the primary obstacle to providing aural rehabilitation pertains to the short-term costs of service provision. Aural rehabilitation can be expensive for two reasons: Listening device technology is often costly, and providing services such as communication strategies training is labor-intensive. Often these kinds of costs are not covered by insurance companies and must be borne by the individual.

Coverage policies can be classified as private (e.g., health maintenance organizations [HMOs]), state (e.g., Blue Cross and Blue Shield), federal (e.g., **Medicare**), or a combination of state and federal (e.g., **Medicaid**). Policies vary in what they will cover in terms of costs. For instance, private

> "I believe it is important to train professionals to become highly proficient practitioners skilled at working with families. This is something that needs to be part of every training program."
> Warren Estabrooks, Director of the Learning to Listen Foundation
> (Scarola, 2005, p. 38)

Cost-effectiveness is the relationship between the money spent and the benefits accrued.

Medicare is a program under the United States Social Security Administration that reimburses hospitals and physicians for medical care they provide to qualified people who are 65 years or older.

Medicaid is a program in the United States authorized by Title XIX of the Social Security Act that is jointly funded by the federal government and state governments, which reimburses hospitals and physicians for providing health care to qualified people who cannot otherwise afford services.

insurance plans are governed by the terms of the individual policy. Sometimes when insurance plans provide coverage for services following receipt of a listening device, they do so only when the services are provided by a speech-language pathologist rather than an audiologist. If coverage is provided for a hearing aid or cochlear implant, follow-up services may not be included. Medicaid permits flexibility to the states in implementing their programs, but typically, hearing aids are covered if they are deemed medically necessary for a patient and the patient qualifies for Medicaid. Some states offer low-cost loans to individuals with hearing loss, with hearing aids being one of the common devices purchased with the loan funds (Hager, 2007).

EVIDENCE-BASED PRACTICE

In the following chapters, we will consider the services that may be included in an aural rehabilitation plan and how they might be customized for both adult and pediatric populations. To the extent possible, the focus will be on services that are based on an **evidence-based practice (EBP)** approach. This introductory chapter will conclude with a brief overview of EBP and how a speech and hearing professional might implement EBP in everyday practice.

Evidence-based practice (EBP) is clinical decision making that is based on a review of the scientific evidence of benefits and costs of alternative forms of diagnosis or treatment, and a critical examination of current and past practices.

Many aural rehabilitation services that are routinely provided to patients, and the techniques for providing them, have been well-researched and shown to work. Some, however, are supported more by tradition and expert opinion than scientific evidence. Historically, there has been a paucity of well-controlled experiments for such reasons as the following:

- The heterogeneity of patient populations, which makes generalization of research results problematic and sometimes makes definitions of success patient-specific
- The role played by the skill of the clinician in determining outcome
- The lack of agreement among researchers and clinicians about **outcome measures**
- The tendency for journals not to publish nonsignificant result studies (Elman, 2006)

An **outcome measure** indicates the amount or type of benefit experienced by either an individual or a group of individuals to a treatment or series of treatments, and/or indicates a response.

Nonetheless, in this age of managed care and accountability, increasingly the services included in an aural rehabilitation plan will have to be supported by empirical evidence. ASHA now encourages that whenever possible, services be based on EBP approaches (ASHA, 2005). EBP is "the integration of best research evidence with clinical expertise and patient values" (Sackett et al., 2000, p. 1). In such an approach, a speech and hearing professional judiciously integrates scientific evidence into clinical decision making, along with his or her own clinical expertise and knowledge about the particular preferences, environment, needs, culture, and values of the patient (ASHA, 2004) (Figure 1-8). Services should not be provided just because "that is what we have always done" and "this is the way we have always done it." Rather, selection of services should be driven by relevant and valid data obtained from clinically oriented studies (Johnson, 2006).

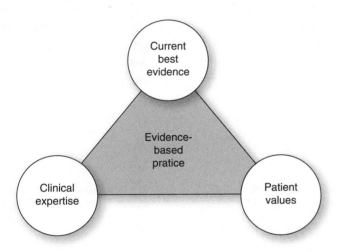

FIGURE 1-8. An evidence-based practice approach, which takes into account quality research evidence, clinical experience, and patient values and needs. Modeled after ASHA (2004).

The most compelling evidence for selecting services, sometimes referred to as "Level 1" evidence, results from a meta-analysis of more than one randomized controlled trial. **A randomized controlled trial** entails comparing participants who have been randomly assigned to receive a test treatment to participants who receive no such treatment (Figure 1-9). A **dependent variable** is measured, which is the variable that depends on the treatment or the manipulated or influential factor of the experiment, or the **independent variable**. Because it is unlikely that a single study will provide a definitive answer to a single scientific question, meta-analysis of the existing studies, where results from several studies are synthesized, provides the optimum basis for choosing treatment. This kind of evidence is not always available, so other levels of evidence might have to suffice. Table 1-2 presents the levels of evidence in order of quality and credibility, from optimal to least optimal, that can support EBP services.

In a **randomized controlled trial,** investigators randomly assign eligible people into treatment and control groups and then compare outcomes. The chance assignment reduces the likelihood that differences stem from preexisting differences between the two groups.

The **dependent variable** is the factor or item measured in an experiment.

The **independent variable** is the experimental factor that is manipulated or influential.

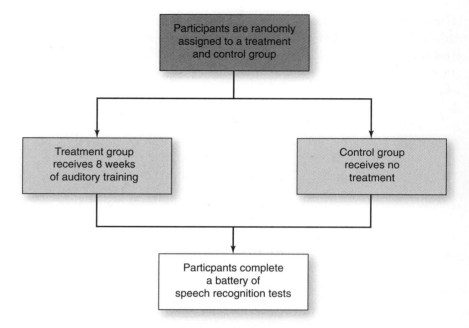

FIGURE 1-9. A randomized controlled trial designed to assess the benefits of auditory training. The independent variable is 8 weeks of auditory training. The dependent variable is participants' ability to recognize speech.

Table 1-2. Levels of evidence to support EBP treatment interventions, ranked in order of highest/most credible (Ia) to lowest/least credible (IV) (adapted from ASHA, 2004, p. 2).

LEVEL	DESCRIPTION
Ia	*Systematic meta-analysis of more than one randomized controlled trial.* A meta-analysis is a synthesis of the major findings of a group of studies.
Ib	*Well-designed randomized controlled trials.* In a randomized controlled trial, participants are assigned randomly to either a treatment or a control group. One reason that a researcher may opt not to conduct a randomized trial pertains to the ethical issue of withholding treatment.
IIa	*Well-designed controlled trials without randomization.* These are less reliable than randomized trials because the participant groups might differ in unanticipated or unrecognized ways.
IIb	*Well-designed quasi-experimental studies; e.g., cohort studies.* A cohort study is one in which a group of patients exposed to a particular treatment is followed over time and is compared to an unexposed group. It is not as reliable as a randomized controlled trial because the two groups may differ in ways that are not readily apparent.
III	*Well-designed nonexperimental studies, e.g., correlational and case studies.* A correlation study determines the relationships (correlations) between variables but does not permit causal interpretations. A case study is an uncontrolled study of a single individual or a series of individuals for the purpose of observing the outcome of an intervention. Neither one includes a control group.
IV	*Expert committee report, consensus conference, and expert opinion.* A committee report might define required procedures and practices, based on scientific data and/or expert opinion. Consensus is an agreement among experts about an issue, whereas an expert opinion reflects the scholarly knowledge and clinical experience of recognized leaders in the field.

When engaging in EBP, many clinicians follow a five-step approach (adapted from Canadian Cochrane Network/Centre Affiliate Representatives, 2003, p. 5):

1. *Ask a straightforward question.* For instance, in developing an aural rehabilitation plan for a white-collar executive who is experiencing communication difficulties despite having received appropriate amplification, you might pose the question: Does group communication strategies training, as compared with individual training, result in better adjustment to hearing loss in adults who have hearing loss? Your purpose is to determine whether you should recommend group communication strategies training for this patient, individualized training, or even, neither one.

2. *Find the best evidence to answer the question.* You might consult a journal or textbook, conduct a database search with an electronic bibliographic database, or engage in a citation search, where you determine if an article has been included in a review article bibliography (see Appendix 1-3 at the end of this chapter). You might perform an Internet search using specific terminology (in our example here, search terms might be "communication strategies training" and "hard-of-hearing") or contact professional organizations such as ASHA or the American Academy of Audiology (AAA) or government agencies such as the National Institutes of Health (NIH) National Institute on Deafness and Other Communication Disorders (NIDCD) for information.

3. *Critically assess the evidence and decide if the results pertain to your patient.* You might consult with Table 1-2 and determine the level of evidence available for EBP. You may also want to consider effect size, or the magnitude of benefit provided by a particular intervention, and consider whether this effect is of **clinical significance**. For example, a treatment might be shown to have a significant effect on a test group of patients, but the effect might be inconsequential to everyday communication or might not justify the time and effort entailed in providing the service.

4. *Integrate the evidence with your clinical judgment and the patient values and needs.* In considering the applicability and feasibility of an aural rehabilitation plan, you might talk to the patient and/or to the patient's family about possible options and weigh the potential benefits and disadvantages of each; for instance: Can the patient afford individualized communication strategies training and is there time in your workday to provide it?

"Good doctors [and clinicians] use both individual clinical expertise and the best available external evidence, and neither alone is enough. Without clinical expertise, practice risks becoming tyrannized by evidence, for even excellent external evidence may be inapplicable to or inappropriate for an individual patient. Without current best evidence, practice risks becoming rapidly out of date, to the detriment of patients."

(Sackett, Rosenberg, Gray, Haynes, & Richardson, 1996, p. 71)

Clinical significance relates to whether an experimental result has practical meaning to either the patient or the clinician.

5. *Evaluate the performance after having implemented your plan.* For this, you will choose measures to monitor progress and adjust your decisions if the desired outcomes are not being achieved.

Selecting the components to include in an aural rehabilitation plan is not always a straightforward proposition, and many variables will factor into the decision-making process. These variables will include the needs and desires of the patient, the availability of services within an aural rehabilitation practice and the surrounding community, and the cost-effectiveness of providing a particular intervention or treatment. An EBP approach is a means to ensure that the services that are included in the plan will likely result in the desired and predicted outcomes.

CASE STUDY

Evidence-Based Practice Decision Making

Cox (2005) describes a 75-year-old woman who lives alone on a fixed income. The woman has a bilateral, moderate, sensorineural hearing loss. She does not socialize often, but does visit her children for lunch every Sunday. She has difficulty in understanding their conversations around the dining table. Her daughter has accompanied her to today's audiology appointment. She is interested in purchasing one of the fancy "digital" hearing aids for her mother. Here are the steps that the audiologist pursues in practicing EBP:

Step 1: Generates the question. "Will an older woman with moderate bilateral presbycusis obtain better speech understanding in noise with digital processing hearing aids than with . . . analog devices . . . ?" (p. 422). Note that the key elements in this question are *the person* (i.e., an older woman with some social contacts), *the problem* (difficulty understanding conversation in social situations), *the proposed treatment* (digital hearing aids), *a comparison treatment* (analog hearing aids), and an *outcome measure* (how well the woman will recognize speech using a hearing aid in the presence of background noise).

Step 2: Finds the best available evidence. The audiologist conducts an Internet search of an online database. She enters into the search field the items: "hearing aid AND digital AND analog OR analogue" (p. 423). The database that she uses, PubMed (see Appendix 1-3), allows her to limit her search from 1995 to the present. The search yields 13 English-language articles. A quick reading of the articles' abstracts eliminates five as irrelevant to the question posed in Step 1.

Step 3: Evaluates the evidence. Beginning with the most recent article and working backward in time, the audiologist selects a subset of the remaining eight articles for a careful review. She assesses the strengths and weaknesses of the evidence.

Step 4: Makes a recommendation. The audiologist considers the similarities and differences between her patient and the participants included in the research studies that she has just

continues

CASE STUDY, *continued*

Evidence-Based Practice Decision Making, *continued*

read (e.g., tread (e.g.,heir ages, health, gender, education, and so forth) to determine the extent to which the evidence applies to her patient. She synthesizes this information with her own clinical judgment and what she knows about her patient, and decides on an appropriate course of action. She shares her recommendation with the patient and her daughter. A hearing aid is ordered for the patient.

Step 5. Follows up. After the patient is fitted with her new hearing aid, the audiologist schedules a follow-up clinic visit in case the recommendation is not successful and needs to be modified.

FINAL REMARKS

In the following chapters, both traditional and cutting-edge practices in aural rehabilitation will be reviewed. In the first half of the text (Parts I and II), we will consider some of the components of an aural rehabilitation service delivery model, including diagnostics and assessment, provision of listening devices, auditory and speechreading training, and communication strategies training. In the second half (Parts III and IV), we will consider specific populations and how an aural rehabilitation plan can be customized to meet the needs of individual patients.

A number of professional journals deal with aural rehabilitation. These journals are listed in Appendix 1-3 at the end of this chapter. They can provide interested readers with additional and timely information about the topics covered in this text. They are also a source for EBP.

KEY CHAPTER POINTS

- Hearing impairment may limit communication activity and impose participation restrictions on everyday activities.
- The impact of hearing loss on an individual may be mediated by that person's use of listening aids, by his or her physical environment, lifestyle, and frequent communication partners, and by individual characteristics such as personality.
- Aural rehabilitation for the adult may include diagnosis and quantification of hearing loss, provision of appropriate listening devices, training in communication strategies, counseling related to hearing loss, vocational counseling, noise protection, and counseling and instruction for family members. It may or may not include auditory and speechreading training.

- Aural rehabilitation for the child may include diagnostics, provision of appropriate amplification, auditory and speechreading training, communication strategies training, family training, and intervention related to speech, language, and educational development.

- Aural rehabilitation may occur in a variety of locales, including schools, hospitals, university speech and hearing clinics, and audiology private practices.

- Aural rehabilitation may be provided by an audiologist, speech-language pathologist, or educator.

- Hearing loss may be categorized by degree, onset, causation, and time course.

- The aural rehabilitation plan includes the communication realms of the person who has hearing loss.

- Aural rehabilitation is relevant for two general reasons: demographics and cost-effectiveness.

- Evidence-based practice (EBP) approaches reflect best research evidence, clinical expertise, and patient values.

- When engaging in EBP, clinicians ask a question, find evidence to answer it, assess the evidence, integrate the evidence with their judgment and patient values, and then evaluate performance.

TERMS AND CONCEPTS TO REMEMBER

Conversational fluency
Hearing-related disability
Ecological interpretation of aural rehabilitation
Communication activity limitations
Participation restrictions
Parameterization of hearing loss
Unserved and underserved
Evidence-based practice (EBP)
Levels of evidence
EBP five-step approach
Clinical significance

MULTIPLE-CHOICE QUESTIONS

1. In the World Health Organization nomenclature, a disability is:
   a. An abnormality of a body function or structure
   b. A psychosocial consequence of hearing loss

    c. A functional consequence of an impairment

    d. A handicap

2. A person has lost hearing in the right ear, presumably as a result of exposure to gun blasts during duck-hunting season. This person may best be described as:

    a. Deaf

    b. Hard of hearing with a flat hearing loss

    c. Hearing-impaired

    d. Unilaterally hard of hearing

3. A teacher and school speech-language pathologist wish to develop an aural rehabilitation plan for a 6-year-old child. They might search the audiological records for information concerning:

    a. Hearing loss degree, onset, causation, and progression

    b. Hearing configuration, handicap, and function

    c. Activity, participation, and context

    d. Disability, impairment, and handicap

4. If someone says to a speech and hearing professional, "The aural rehabilitation plan will address the patient's communication realms," the professional might interpret this statement as:

    a. The plan must optimize communication in the workplace through provision of hearing aids, assistive listening devices, and other technology.

    b. The family and the patient's frequent communication partners will be included in the aural rehabilitation plan.

    c. The patient will participate in communication strategies training, auditory and speechreading training, and psychosocial therapy.

    d. Counseling will be provided to family members.

5. A patient who has hearing loss asks her audiologist to fit her with an inexpensive hearing aid that she has read about in the newspaper. The audiologist performs a literature review and learns that three randomized controlled trials have shown this hearing aid to be less effective than a more expensive hearing aid. EBP would suggest the following course of action for the audiologist:

    a. The audiologist fits the inexpensive aid because the patient is the consumer and this is her choice.

b. The audiologist recommends another hearing aid (which is neither the inexpensive nor expensive hearing aid) that he typically fits for patients who have this degree and configuration of hearing loss, and explains his reasons for doing so.

c. The audiologist chooses the expensive, more effective hearing aid to provide optimal listening to the patient.

d. The audiologist integrates patient preference, scientific evidence, and his past clinical experience with various aids and makes a recommendation.

6. An example of Level III evidence is:

a. An ASHA position paper about auditory training.

b. A cohort study that includes individuals who have unilateral hearing loss and individuals who do not have unilateral hearing loss.

c. A case study describing two individuals who experienced sudden hearing loss.

d. A randomized controlled study that includes individuals who receive auditory training and individuals who do not.

APPENDIX 1-1

Knowledge and skills for audiologists providing aural rehabilitation (AR) services (From ASHA, Supplement No. 22, April 16, 2002, pp. 90–92. Copyright © by the American Speech-Language Hearing Association. Reprinted with permission.)

Basic Areas of Knowledge and Skills

Audiologists who provide AR services demonstrate knowledge in the basic areas that are the underpinnings of communication sciences and disorders. These include the following:

I. General Knowledge

    A. General psychology; human growth and development; psychosocial behavior; cultural and linguistic diversity; biological, physical, and social sciences; mathematics; and qualitative and quantitative research methodologies

II. Basic Communication Processes

    A. Anatomic and physiologic bases for the normal development and use of speech, language, and hearing (including anatomy, neurology, and physiology of speech, language, and hearing mechanisms)

B. Physical bases and process of the production and perception of speech and hearing (including acoustics or physics of sound, phonology, physiologic and acoustic phonetics, sensory perceptual processes, and psychoacoustics)

C. Linguistic and psycholinguistic variables related to the normal development and use of speech, language, and hearing (including linguistics [historical, descriptive, sociolinguistics, sign language, second-language usage], psychology of language, psycholinguistics, language and speech acquisition, verbal learning and verbal behavior, and gestural communication)

D. Dynamics of interpersonal skills, communication effectiveness, and group theory

Special Areas of Knowledge and Skills

Audiologists who provide AR have knowledge in the following special areas and demonstrate the itemized requisite skills in those areas:

III. Auditory System Function and Disorders

    A. Identify, describe, and differentiate among disorders of auditory function (including disorders of the outer, middle, and inner ear; the vestibular system; the auditory nerve and the associated neural and central auditory system pathways and processes)

IV. Developmental Status, Cognition, and Sensory Perception

    A. Provide for the administration of assessment measures in the client's preferred mode of communication

    B. Verify adequate visual acuity for communication purposes

    C. Identify the need and provide for assessment of cognitive skills, sensory perceptual and motor skills, developmental delays, academic achievement, and literacy

    D. Determine the need for referral to other medical and nonmedical specialists for appropriate professional services

    E. Provide for ongoing assessments of developmental progress

V. Audiologic Assessment Procedures

    A. Conduct interview and obtain case history

    B. Perform otoscopic examinations and ensure that the external auditory canal is free of obstruction, including cerumen

C. Conduct and interpret behavioral, physiologic, or electro-physiologic evaluations of the peripheral and central auditory systems

D. Conduct and interpret assessments for auditory processing disorders

E. Administer and interpret standardized self-report measures of communication difficulties and of psychosocial and behavioral adjustment to auditory dysfunction

F. Identify the need for referral to medical and nonmedical specialists for appropriate professional services

VI. Speech and Language Assessment Procedures

A. Identify the need for and perform screenings for effects of hearing impairment on speech and language

B. Describe the effects of hearing impairment on the development of semantic, syntactic, pragmatic, and phonologic aspects of communication, in terms of both comprehension and production

C. Provide for appropriate measures of speech and voice production

D. Provide for appropriate measures of language comprehension and production skills and/or alternate communication skills (e.g., signing)

E. Administer and interpret appropriate measures of communication skills in auditory, visual, auditory-visual, and tactile modalities

VII. Evaluation and Management of Devices and Technologies for Individuals with Hearing Impairment (e.g., hearing aids, cochlear implants, middle ear implants, implantable hearing aids, tinnitus maskers, hearing assistive technologies, and other sensory prosthetic devices)

A. Perform and interpret measures of electroacoustic characteristics of devices and technologies

B. Describe, perform, and interpret behavioral/psychophysical measures of performance with these devices and technologies

C. Conduct appropriate fittings with and adjustments of these devices and technologies

D. Monitor fitting of and adjustment to these devices and technologies to ensure comfort, safety, and device performance

E. Perform routine visual, listening, and electroacoustic checks of clients' hearing devices and sensory aids to troubleshoot common causes of malfunction

F. Evaluate and describe the effects of use of devices and technologies on communication and psychosocial functioning

G. Plan and implement a program of orientation to these devices and technologies to ensure realistic expectations; to improve acceptance of, adjustment to, and benefit from these systems; and to enhance communication performance

H. Conduct routine assessments of adjustment to and effective use of amplification devices to ensure optimal communication function

I. Monitor outcomes to ensure professional accountability

VIII. Effects of Hearing Impairment on Functional Communication

    A. Identify the individual's situational expressive and receptive communication needs

    B. Evaluate the individual's expressive and receptive communication performance

    C. Identify environmental factors that affect the individual's situational communication needs and performance

    D. Identify the effects of interpersonal relations on communication function

IX. Effects of Hearing Impairment on Psychosocial, Educational, and Occupational Functioning

    A. Describe and evaluate the impact of hearing impairment on psychosocial development and psychosocial functioning

    B. Describe systems and methods of educational programming (e.g., mainstream, residential) and facilitate selection of appropriate educational options

    C. Describe and evaluate the effects of hearing impairment on occupational status and performance (e.g., communication, localization, safety)

    D. Identify the effects of hearing problems on marital dyads, family dynamics, and other interpersonal communication functioning

    E. Identify the need and provide the psychosocial, educational, family, and occupational/vocational counseling in relation to hearing impairment and subsequent communication difficulties

    F. Provide assessment of family members' perception of and reactions to communication difficulties

X. AR Case Management

    A. Use effective interpersonal communication in interviewing and interacting with individuals with hearing impairment and their families

    B. Describe client-centered, behavioral, cognitive, and integrative theories and methods of counseling and their relevance in AR

    C. Provide appropriate individual and group adjustment counseling related to hearing loss for individuals with hearing impairment and their families

    D. Provide auditory, visual, and auditory-visual communication training (e.g., speechreading, auditory training, listening skills) to enhance receptive communication

    E. Provide training in effective communication strategies to individuals with hearing impairment, family members, and other relevant individuals

    F. Provide for appropriate expressive communication training

    G. Provide appropriate technological and counseling intervention to facilitate adjustment to tinnitus

    H. Provide appropriate intervention for management of vestibular disorders

    I. Develop and implement an intervention plan based on the individual's situational/environmental communication needs and performance and related adjustment difficulties

    J. Develop and implement a system for measuring and monitoring outcomes and the appropriateness and efficacy of intervention

XI. Interdisciplinary Collaboration and Public Advocacy

    A. Collaborate effectively as part of multidisciplinary teams and communicate relevant information to allied professionals and other appropriate individuals

    B. Plan and implement in-service and public-information programs for allied professionals and other interested individuals

    C. Plan and implement parent-education programs concerning the management of hearing impairment and subsequent communication difficulties

    D. Advocate implementation of public law in educational, occupational, and public settings

    E. Make appropriate referrals to consumer-based organizations

XII. Hearing Conservation/Acoustic Environments

    A. Plan and implement programs for prevention of hearing impairment to promote identification and evaluation of individuals exposed to hazardous noise and periodic monitoring of communication performance and auditory abilities (e.g., speech recognition in noise, localization)

    B. Identify need for and provide appropriate hearing protection devices and noise abatement procedures

    C. Monitor the effects of environmental influences, amplification, and sources of trauma on residual auditory function

    D. Measure and evaluate the environmental acoustic conditions and relate them to effects on communication performance and hearing protection

APPENDIX 1-2

Basic Areas of Knowledge and Skills

Speech-language pathologists who provide AR services demonstrate knowledge in the basic areas that are the underpinnings of communication sciences and disorders. These include the following:

I. General Knowledge

    A. General psychology; human growth and development; psychosocial behavior; cultural and linguistic diversity; biological, physical, and social sciences; mathematics; and qualitative and quantitative research methodologies

Knowledge and skills for speech-language pathologists providing aural rehabilitation (AR) services (From ASHA, Supplement No. 22, April 16, 2002, pp. 92–95. Copyright © by the American Speech-Language Hearing Association. Reprinted with permission.)

II. Basic Communication Processes

   A. Anatomic and physiologic bases for the normal development and use of speech, language, and hearing (including anatomy, neurology, and physiology of speech, language, and hearing mechanisms)

   B. Physical bases and process of the production and perception of speech and hearing (including acoustics or physics of sound, phonology, physiologic and acoustic phonetics, sensory perceptual processes, and psychoacoustics)

   C. Linguistic and psycholinguistic variables related to the normal development and use of speech, language, and hearing (including linguistics [historical, descriptive, sociolinguistics, sign language, second-language usage], psychology of language, psycholinguistics, language and speech acquisition, verbal learning and verbal behavior, and gestural communication)

   D. Dynamics of interpersonal skills, communication effectiveness, and group theory

Special Areas of Knowledge and Skills

Speech-language pathologists who provide AR have knowledge in the following special areas and demonstrate the itemized requisite skills in those areas:

III. Auditory System Function and Disorders

   A. Identify, describe, and differentiate among disorders of auditory function (including disorders of the outer, middle, and inner ear; the vestibular system; the auditory nerve and the associated neural and central auditory system pathways and processes)

IV. Developmental Status, Cognition, and Sensory Perception

   A. Provide for the administration of assessment measures in the client's preferred mode of communication

   B. Verify adequate visual acuity for communication purposes

   C. Identify the need and provide for assessment of cognitive skills, sensory perceptual and motor skills, developmental delays, academic achievement, and literacy

   D. Determine the need for referral to other medical and nonmedical specialists for appropriate professional services

   E. Provide for ongoing assessments of developmental progress

V. Audiologic Assessment Procedures

    A. Conduct audiologic screening as appropriate for initial identification and/or referral purposes

    B. Describe type and degree of hearing loss from audiometric test results (including pure-tone thresholds, immittance testing, and speech audiometry)

    C. Refer to and consult with an audiologist for administration and interpretation of differential diagnostic procedures (including behavioral, physiological, and electrophysiological measures)

VI. Assessment of Communication Performance

    A. Provide for assessment measures in the client's preferred mode of communication

    B. Identify and perform screening examinations for speech, language, hearing, auditory processing disorders, and reading and academic achievement problems

    C. Identify and perform diagnostic evaluations for the comprehension and production of speech and language in oral, signed, written, or augmented form

    D. Provide diagnostic evaluations of speech perception in auditory, visual, auditory-visual, or tactile modalities

    E. Identify the effects of hearing loss on speech perception, communication performance, listening skills, speechreading, communication strategies, and personal adjustment

    F. Provide for clients' self-assessment of communication difficulties and adjustment of hearing loss

    G. Monitor developmental progress in relation to communication competence

VII. Devices and Technologies for Individuals with Hearing Loss (e.g., hearing aids, cochlear implants, middle ear implants, implantable hearing aids, hearing assistive technologies, and other sensory prosthetic devices)

    A. Describe candidacy criteria for amplification or sensory-prosthetic devices (e.g., hearing aids, cochlear implants)

    B. Monitor clients' prescribed use of personal and group amplification systems

    C. Describe options and applications of sensory aids (e.g., assistive listening devices) and telephone/telecommunication devices

D. Identify the need and refer to an audiologist for evaluation and fitting of personal and group amplification systems and sensory aids

E. Implement a protocol, in consultation with an audiologist, to promote adjustment to amplification

F. Perform routine visual inspection and listening checks of clients' hearing devices and sensory aids to troubleshoot common causes of malfunctioning (e.g., dead or corroded batteries, obstruction or damage to visible parts of the system)

G. Refer on a regularly scheduled basis clients' personal and group amplification systems, other sensory aids, and assistive listening devices for comprehensive evaluations to ensure that instruments conform to audiologists' prescribed settings and manufacturers' specifications

H. Describe the effects of amplification on communication function

I. Describe and monitor the effects of environmental factors on communication function

VIII. Effects of Hearing Loss on Psychosocial, Educational, and Vocational Functioning

A. Describe the effects of hearing loss on psychosocial development

B. Describe the effects of hearing loss on learning and literacy

C. Describe systems and methods of educational programming (e.g., mainstream, residential) and facilitate selection of appropriate educational options

D. Identify the need for and availability of psychological, social, educational, and vocational counseling

E. Identify and appropriately plan for addressing affective issues confronting the person with hearing loss

F. Identify appropriate consumer organizations and parent support groups

IX. Intervention and Case Management

A. Develop and implement a rehabilitative intervention plan based on communication skills and needs of the individual and family or caregivers of the individual

B. Provide for communication and counseling intervention in the client's preferred mode of communication

C. Develop expressive and receptive competencies in the client's preferred mode of communication

D. Provide speech, language, and auditory intervention (including but not limited to voice quality and control, resonance, phonologic and phonetic processes, oral motor skills, articulation, pronunciation, prosody, syntax/morphology, semantics, pragmatics)

E. Facilitate appropriate multimodal forms of communication (e.g., auditory, visual, tactile, speechreading, spoken language, Cued Speech, simultaneous communication, total communication, communication technologies) for the client and family

F. Conduct interviews and interact effectively with individuals and their families

G. Develop and implement a system to measure and monitor outcomes and the efficacy of intervention

X. Interdisciplinary Collaboration and Public Advocacy

A. Collaborate effectively as part of multidisciplinary teams and communicate relevant information to allied professionals and other appropriate individuals

B. Plan and implement in-service and public-information programs for allied professionals and other interested individuals

C. Plan and implement parent-education programs concerning the management of hearing impairment and subsequent communication difficulties

D. Plan and implement interdisciplinary service programs with allied professionals

E. Advocate implementation of public law in educational, occupational, and public settings

F. Refer to consumer-based organizations

XI. Acoustic Environments

A. Provide for appropriate environmental acoustic conditions for effective communication

B. Describe the effects of environmental influences, amplification systems, and sources of trauma on residual auditory function

C. Provide for periodic hearing screening for individuals exposed to hazardous noise

APPENDIX 1-3

Professional Journals That Might Be Consulted for Evidence-Based Practice

Advance for Audiologists

Advance for Speech-Language Pathologists and Audiologists

American Annals of the Deaf

American Journal of Audiology: A Journal of Clinical Practice

American Journal of Speech-Language Pathology: A Journal of Clinical Practice

ASHA (American Speech-Language Hearing Association)

Audiology and Neuro-otology

Australian and New Zealand Journal of Audiology

Contact

Deafness and Education

Ear and Hearing

Educational Audiology

Hearing Journal

Hearing Review

International Journal of Audiology (formerly Audiology, British Journal of Audiology, & Scandinavian Audiology)

International Tinnitus Journal

Journal of the Academy of Rehabilitative Audiology

Journal of the American Academy of Audiology

Journal of Child Language

Journal of Communication Disorders

Journal of Deaf Studies and Deaf Education

Journal of Speech, Language, and Hearing Research

Language and Speech

Language, Speech, and Hearing Services in the School

Noise and Health

Noise Regulation Report

Seminars in Hearing

Seminars in Speech and Language

Speech Communication
Tinnitus Today
Topics in Language Disorders
Trends in Amplification
Volta Review
Volta Voices

Electronic Databases That Might Be Consulted for Evidence-Based Practice

Medline, described at http://www.ncbi.hlm.gov/, spotlights medical and health-related research.

PsychINFO, described at http://apa.org/psycinfo/, spotlights the psychological literature.

Educational Resource Information Center (ERIC), described at http://www.eric .ed.gov/, spotlights educational research.

ComDisDome, described at http://www.comdisdome.com/, lists dissertations and monographs that are peer-reviewed.

CINAHL, described at http://www.cinahl.com, lists trade journals.

Citation Indexes That Might Be Consulted for Evidence-Based Practice

Science Citation Index (SCI)
Social Science Citation Index (SSCI)

PART 1

Speech Recognition and Persons Who Have Hearing Loss

CHAPTER 2

Assessing Hearing Acuity and Speech Recognition

OUTLINE

- Review of the audiological examination and the audiogram

- Purpose of speech recognition testing

- Patient variables

- Stimuli units

- Test procedures

- Difficulties associated with speech recognition assessment

- Multicultural issues

- Case study: Reason to go with a test battery approach

- Final remarks

- Key chapter points

- Terms and concepts to remember

- Multiple-choice questions

- Key resources

Speech recognition is the ability to perceive a spoken message and make decisions about its lexical composition using auditory and sometimes visual information.

Speech recognition testing is performed in order to determine how well an individual can recognize speech units.

A key element in promoting conversational fluency and reducing hearing-related disability is to optimize an individual's ability to recognize speech. The reason that conversational fluency is often degraded is that persons with hearing loss cannot recognize the spoken messages of their communication partners. **Speech recognition**, also called speech perception, refers to how well people use auditory and/or visual information to understand spoken messages. **Speech recognition testing** involves assessing how well an individual can recognize speech units such as phonemes, words, and sentences. The first phase of most aural rehabilitation plans is to assess a patient's hearing acuity and assess how well the individual can recognize speech. Depending upon a person's hearing status and communication needs, he or she may then go on to receive a listening device such as a hearing aid or a cochlear implant and may engage in auditory or speechreading training or both. To the extent that speech recognition performance can be optimized, there will be a concomitant enhancement of conversational fluency and a reduction of hearing-related disability.

The audiogram provides a general description of the magnitude of a person's hearing loss. However, the audiogram does not adequately portray the communication difficulties an individual may experience or the person's aural rehabilitation needs. Speech recognition measurement is an important element in assessing how hearing loss affects an individual's life and communication interactions.

In this chapter, we will focus on four considerations underlying the assessment of speech recognition. The focus will be on children of about 3 years of age and older and on adults. We will consider means for assessing infants and very young children in Chapter 14. The four considerations are (Figure 2-1):

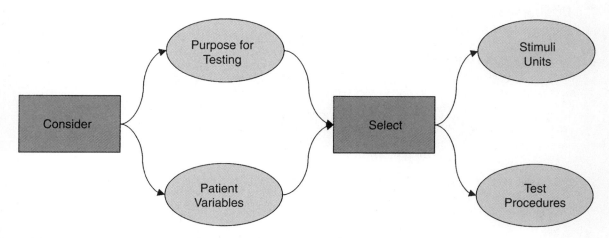

FIGURE 2-1. Four variables to consider when assessing speech recognition.

- Purpose
- Patient variables
- Stimuli units
- Test procedures

Before a consideration of these topics, a brief review of the audiogram and other components of the audiological examination is presented.

REVIEW OF THE AUDIOLOGICAL EXAMINATION AND THE AUDIOGRAM

A typical audiological assessment includes an **audiogram**, a determination of speech recognition threshold, and an assessment of speech recognition. Sometimes the examination might entail a determination of most comfortable loudness and uncomfortable loudness levels for speech as well.

An **audiogram** is a graphic representation of hearing thresholds as a function of stimulus frequency.

Pure-Tone Audiometry

The audiogram provides a quantitative assessment of an individual's ability to detect sounds. The test typically is performed by an audiologist, with the use of an **audiometer**. The audiometer presents tones, and the individual indicates when he or she hears them. The goal is to determine the softest sound level at which the tones can be detected, or the threshold. A **threshold** is the level of sound so faint that it can be detected only 50% of the time.

An **audiometer** is an instrument for measuring hearing sensitivity for a range of frequencies.

The level at which sound can be detected only 50% of the time is called a **threshold**.

Mr. Bell's Other Invention

Alexander Graham Bell, who was married to a woman with significant hearing loss (Chapter 15), invented the first audiometer in 1879. It consisted of a pair of induction coils and a telephone receiver. Calibrated frequencies of calibrated intensity could be generated to measure the hearing abilities of individuals. Bell's audiometer revealed "unsuspected vestiges of hearing in many previously classed as totally deaf. Once recognized, even a slight hearing capacity was useful in developing articulation and speechreading. The device also detected hearing impairment in many public school children whose handicap had been taken for stupidity or inattention. In exhibiting his audiometer to the National Academy of Sciences in 1885, Bell reported that of seven hundred pupils whom he and an assistant [Watson?] had tested with it, more than ten percent had some hearing impairment" (p. 394, Bruce, 1978).

"Mr. Watson, come here, I want you."

Alexander Graham Bell, inventor of the telephone, to his assistant on March 10, 1876, the day of the first successful telephone trial.

(Kricos & McCarthy, 2007)

Air conduction refers to when sound travels through the air into the external auditory canal and stimulation progresses through the middle ear, inner ear, and to the brain.

An **insert earphone** is an earphone whose receiver is attached to a tube that leads to an expandable cuff. It can be inserted into the external auditory canal.

Bone conduction refers to the transmission of sound through the bones in the body, particularly the skull.

An **air-bone gap** is the difference between air- and bone-conduction thresholds; a difference may indicate a conductive component in the hearing loss.

Sound level is the intensity of sound expressed in decibels.

Frequency is the number of regularly repeated events in a given unit of time; usually measured in cycles per second and expressed in Hertz (Hz).

The tones may be presented by **air conduction**, either through **insert earphones** (or headphones) or sound field, or by **bone conduction**, through a vibrator placed behind the ear against the mastoid. Air conduction test results indicate hearing losses that might be either conductive hearing loss (involving the outer or middle ear) or sensorineural hearing loss (involving the inner ear, eighth nerve, brain stem, midbrain, or auditory cortex) in nature. Bone conduction test results reflect only the sensorineural component. By comparing the air and bone conduction results, the audiologist can determine whether there is hearing loss stemming from a problem in either the outer or middle ear. The difference between the two sets of thresholds is termed the **air-bone gap**.

Audiological thresholds are plotted on an audiogram, where the Y-axis indicates **sound level** (loudness) and the X-axis indicates **frequency** (pitch). As shown in Figure 2-2, an X on the audiogram represents the left-ear and an O represents the right-ear thresholds when the test signals are presented via air conduction. A less-than sign (<) indicates an unmasked bone conduction threshold for the right ear and a left bracket ([) indicates a masked bone conduction threshold. A greater-than sign (>) indicates an unmasked bone conduction threshold for the left ear and a right bracket (]) indicates a masked bone conduction threshold. The capital letter *A* typically denotes an aided threshold or how the patient hears when wearing a hearing aid. An *R* subscript below the *A* is used to refer to testing with the right

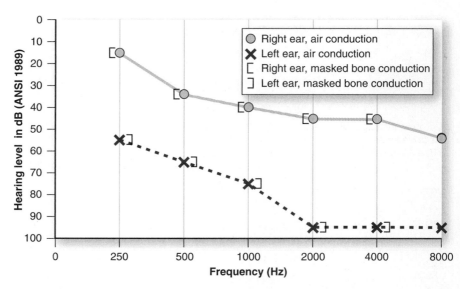

FIGURE 2-2. An audiogram for someone who has a PTA of 35 dB HL in the right ear (a mild hearing loss) and 73 dB HL in the left ear (a severe hearing loss).

hearing aid worn and an *L* subscript is used to refer to testing with the left hearing aid worn. The capital letter *C* denotes a threshold when the patient is wearing a cochlear implant. In this figure, the patient's audiogram indicates that her threshold for 250 Hz is 20 dB HL in the right ear and 60 dB HL in the left ear. The pure-tone average (PTA) is a means to summarize someone's hearing status. As noted in Chapter 1, the pure-tone average is an average of the hearing thresholds for the frequencies of 500, 1,000, and 2,000 Hz (Figure 2-2).

The pure-tone average often is used to assign a label to indicate the degree of hearing loss. The following descriptors are used to denote degree:

Normal: The PTA is 25 dB HL or better in adults or 20 dB HL or better in children.

Mild: The PTA is between 26 and 40 dB HL.

Moderate: The PTA is between 41 and 55 dB HL.

Moderate-to-severe: The PTA is between 56 and 70 dB HL.

Severe: The PTA is between 71 and 90 dB HL.

Profound: The PTA is poorer than 90 dB HL.

Table 2-1 indicates the relationship between degree of hearing loss and speech recognition, as a function of the descriptors outlined previously. Another class of descriptor often assigned to a patient's audiogram is the configuration of the hearing loss. Four common configurations of

Table 2-1. How degree of hearing loss affects speech recognition (Flexer, 1999).

HEARING LOSS	EFFECT ON WORD RECOGNITION
Mild (PTA = 26–40 dB HL)	In quiet situations, speech recognition will be fairly unaffected. In the presence of noise, speech recognition may decrease to 50% words correct if the PTA is 40 dB HL. Consonants are most likely to be missed, especially if the hearing loss involves primarily the high frequencies.
Mild-to-Moderate (PTA = 41–55 dB HL)	The patient will understand much of the speech signal if it is presented in a quiet environment face-to-face, and if the topic of conversation is known and the vocabulary is constrained. If a hearing aid is not used, the individual may miss up to 50–75% of a spoken message if the PTA is 40 dB HL and 80–100% if the PTA is 50 dB HL.
Moderate (PTA = 56–70 dB HL)	If the individual does not use a hearing aid, he or she may miss most or all of the message, even if talking face-to-face. He or she will have great difficulty conversing in group situations.
Severe (PTA = 71–90 dB HL)	The patient may not even hear voices, unless speech is loud. Without amplification, the individual probably will not recognize any speech in an audition-only condition. With amplification, he or she may recognize some speech and detect environmental sounds.
Profound (PTA = 90 dB HL or greater)	The patient may perceive sound as vibrations. An individual will rely on vision as the primary sense for speech recognition. He or she may not be able to detect the presence of even loud sound without amplification.

hearing loss appear in Figures 2-3, 2-4, 2-5, and 2-6, which illustrate a flat configuration of hearing loss, a high-frequency configuration, a low-frequency configuration, and a saucer-shaped configuration of hearing loss, respectively. These configurations may be defined as follows:

- **Flat:** Thresholds are within a 20-dB range of each other across the span of frequencies tested.

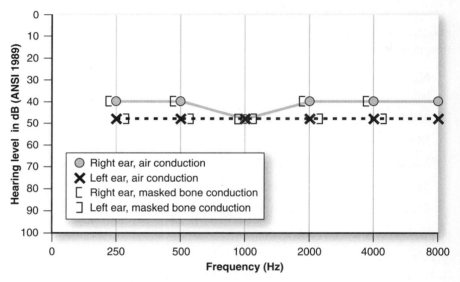

FIGURE 2-3. An audiogram for someone who has a flat configuration of hearing loss.

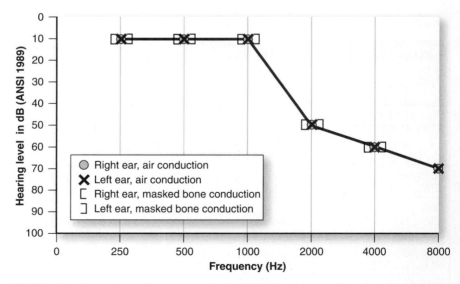

FIGURE 2-4. An audiogram for someone who has a high-frequency configuration of hearing loss.

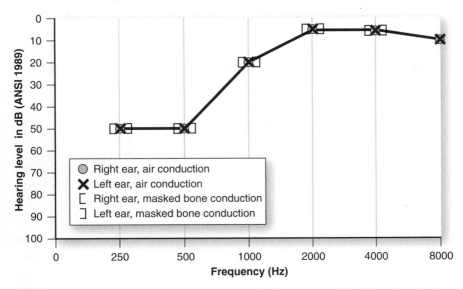

FIGURE 2-5. An audiogram for someone who has a low-frequency configuration of hearing loss.

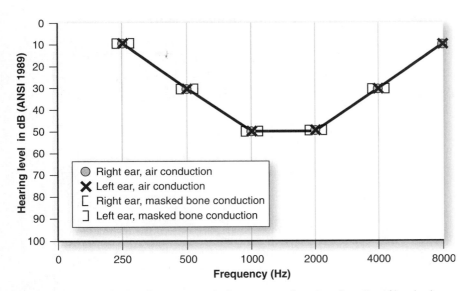

FIGURE 2-6. An audiogram for someone who has a saucer-shaped configuration of hearing loss.

- **High-frequency:** Thresholds are within normal range for the low and mid frequencies, but decline for the higher frequencies. A high-frequency loss may be described as *precipitous* if the loss at each of the higher frequencies is at least 20 dB greater with each ascending frequency. It may be described as *sloping* if thresholds for the higher frequencies are 20 dB or poorer than for the lower frequencies.

- **Low-frequency:** Thresholds are lowered for the low frequencies but are within normal range for the mid- and higher frequencies.
- **Saucer-shaped:** The loss is confined to the mid-frequencies.

The configuration of hearing loss, as well as the degree, affects how well the patient may recognize speech. Most of the acoustic information that contributes to speech recognition lies within the frequency band of 1,000 Hz to 3,000 Hz, as shown in Figure 2-7, which shows the approximate intensity and frequency of the speech sounds. For this reason, someone who has a low-frequency configuration (Figure 2-5) may likely receive more speech information and hence recognize more speech than someone who has a high-frequency configuration (Figure 2-4), even if they have similar PTAs. The person with the audiogram shown in Figure 2-4 will likely not hear such high-frequency consonant sounds as [s, ʃ, t, p, k, f] while

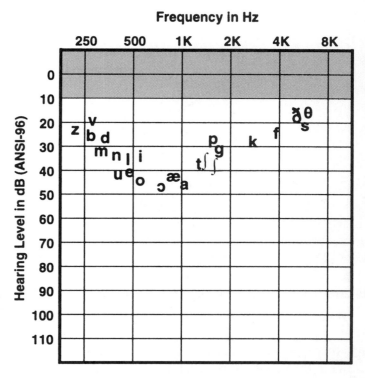

FIGURE 2-7. Generalized phonetic representations of speech sounds occurring at normal conversational levels plotted on an audiogram.

listening to everyday conversation, and he or she may not receive enough information to distinguish from one another consonants such as [d, b, g, v, ʒ, l, r, w].

Speech Audiometry

The audiological examination usually includes speech testing in addition to the audiogram. Results will indicate how hearing loss affects a patient's ability to detect and recognize speech and the level of sound necessary for comfortable listening.

When determining the **speech reception threshold (SRT)**, the audiologist determines the softest level at which a patient can understand simple words. In one procedure, an audiologist might ask the patient to repeat **spondees**. These are bisyllabic words that have equal stress on both words, such as *baseball, ice cream, hotdog,* and *sidewalk.* The words are presented through the audiometer, and the level is varied until the patient is able to repeat just 50% of the words correctly. This level is recorded as the SRT.

The audiological examination usually includes a test of speech recognition, in addition to the audiogram and SRT testing. For instance, the clinician might present monosyllabic words at a comfortable listening level and expect the patient to repeat each word. Historically, when word recognition scores were referred to in a clinical setting, they were often called **speech discrimination scores**. The term *speech recognition* is preferred increasingly, to avoid confusion with the term *discrimination* when it is used in an auditory or speechreading training context, to indicate discriminating one stimulus from the next.

Sometimes the audiologist might want to determine the hearing level at which speech is most comfortable to listen to and the level at which it becomes too loud. The **most comfortable loudness level (MCL)** typically is determined by asking the individual to listen to running speech. The initial presentation level may be just above the level of the SRT, and then it is gradually increased. The individual indicates when it is at a comfortable level, when it is too soft, and when it is too loud. The **uncomfortable loudness level (UCL)**, sometimes called the *threshold of discomfort,* is the threshold level at which the speech changes from being comfortably loud to being uncomfortably loud. A **dynamic range** for speech may be computed by subtracting the decibel value of the patient's SRT from the decibel value of the patient's UCL. The dynamic range will often influence the selection and programming of an individual's listening device and sometimes, the design of the individual's auditory training program.

Speech reception threshold (SRT) is the lowest presentation level for spondee words at which 50% can be identified correctly.

Spondees are two-syllable words spoken with equal stress on each syllable.

The **speech discrimination score**, a term that is not used very often anymore, refers to the percentage of monosyllabic words presented at a comfortable listening level that can be correctly repeated.

Most comfortable loudness level (MCL) is the level at which sound is most comfortable for a listener.

The **uncomfortable loudness level (UCL)** is the level at which sound becomes uncomfortably loud for a listener.

A **dynamic range** is the difference in decibels between a person's threshold for just being able to detect speech and the person's threshold for uncomfortable listening.

Sound Field Testing

Often, tests of speech recognition are presented in sound field as opposed to under headphones. If the patient typically wears a hearing aid, he or she often wears the aid for testing. When recording the results of sound field testing on the audiogram, the audiologist will usually indicate the **loudspeaker azimuth**. This is the direction of the **loudspeaker** in relationship to the patient, measured in angular degrees in the horizontal place. If the loudspeaker is located directly in front of the patient, then the azimuth is 0 degrees. If it is located directly behind the patient, the azimuth is 180 degrees. Sound field measures are typically indicated with the letter *S* on the audiogram. Newby and Popelka (1992) discussed the reasons for sound field testing:

"Testing with a loudspeaker is referred to as **sound field testing** because the sound is not confined, as it is in an earphone, but is circulated in a field about the patient's head. Unless we are talking over the telephone, or for some reason listening through earphones, all our listening throughout the day is of the sound field type. To judge how the patient hears in a typical sound field listening situation is the main reason that we give speech tests through a loudspeaker" (pp. 182–183).

Loudspeaker azimuth is the position of the loudspeaker relative to the listener, measured in angular degrees in the horizontal plane.

A **loudspeaker** converts electrical energy into sound.

Sound field testing determines hearing sensitivity or speech recognition ability by presenting signals in a sound field through a loudspeaker.

Test Environment

Ideally, audiological testing occurs in a sound-isolated chamber so as to obtain the patient's best performance. A sound-isolated chamber is acoustically isolated from the rest of the building through the use of mass (e.g., concrete), insulation (e.g., fiberglass), **dead air spaces**, and doors with tight acoustic seals. Sometimes the ideal test environment is unavailable, especially when conducting on-site assessments in the public schools or in industry. On these occasions, testing might occur in the quietest room available, using specially designed earphone enclosures or insert earphones. A description of the less-than-ideal environment should be included on the audiogram comments section so that the test results might be interpreted accordingly. Sometimes the audiologist opts not to test at 250 Hz as ambient room noise (such as ventilation system noise) may mask presentation of this tone. If background noise is a problem, the audiologist may assume that elevated thresholds that do not exceed 30 dB HL may not be indicative of reduced hearing sensitivity, but rather, indicative of the noisy test conditions.

Dead air spaces are unventilated air spaces.

▨ PURPOSE OF SPEECH RECOGNITION TESTING

When designing an aural rehabilitation plan for a particular patient, a speech and hearing professional will almost always want more information about his or her speech recognition skills than that provided by a traditional audiological examination. There are many ways to use the results of an in-depth assessment. These include the following:

- **To determine need for amplification.** If a person demonstrates reduced speech recognition, then amplification might be considered.
- **To compare performance with a listening aid to performance without an aid and to build patient confidence.** This comparison can be accomplished by measuring speech recognition with and without the device. Sharing the results might motivate a patient to wear a hearing aid and might enhance the individual's confidence for everyday listening tasks.
- **To compare different listening devices.** An individual might be tested with one listening device and then another to determine the device that affords the best performance. This testing is feasible when two or three devices are being compared, but becomes problematic when many devices are under consideration. In recent practice, speech recognition testing has been used less frequently for the purpose of selecting listening devices than in former times (Mueller, 2001).
- **To demonstrate to patients that their ability to recognize speech is diminished.** Especially during counseling, information gained from speech testing can illustrate how speech understanding is impaired relative to persons who have normal hearing.
- **To demonstrate the benefits of visual speech information.** By testing in an audition-only condition and then an audition-plus-vision condition, a speech and hearing professional can gain information that helps the patient realize the importance of visual speech information and the importance of speechreading and focusing on the talker's facial movements.
- **To obtain information that might elucidate environment-related listening issues.** By performing speech testing in the presence of background noise, and comparing the results to performance in quiet, an audiologist can gain information that can be used to counsel patients about their particular listening difficulties. For instance, background noise may be more problematic for certain people, such as older persons, than for others.
- **To assess performance longitudinally.** There may be instances when a speech and hearing professional may want to monitor speech recognition over time and answer questions such as,

"Often . . . we are interested not only in the aided [speech recognition] performance, but also in how much aided performance has changed relative to unaided performance. This is generally referred to as a measure of benefit, rather than performance."

Larry Humes, Professor, Indiana University

(Humes, 2004, p. 12)

"Is the patient's hearing deteriorating because of use of a listening device?" or "Has speech recognition changed as a result of auditory training?" Care must be taken that measurements are not affected by the learning of test materials with repeated administration or, in the case of children, by language growth or cognitive maturation.

- **To determine need for auditory or speechreading training.** If an individual experiences difficulty in recognizing speech, even when using appropriate amplification, then the person may be a candidate for training.
- **To determine placement within a training curriculum.** Not every individual begins a speechreading or auditory training program with the same tasks. People will enter training with different skill levels, and training objectives will need to be selected accordingly.
- **To evaluate the appropriateness of an educational placement setting.** Speech recognition testing may provide one index of how well a child might perform in a school setting that requires good listening skills. Test scores might influence a decision as to whether a child is ready to enter a regular classroom and/or whether a sign interpreter will be required.
- **To determine if expected benefit has been achieved.** One goal of providing a listening aid or providing auditory training is to improve speech recognition. A speech and hearing professional may assess whether individuals obtained expected benefit by comparing their performance with that of a group of persons who have a similar hearing loss or who have received similar interventions.

The purpose may dictate the test. For instance, an audiologist may use one test to determine placement in an auditory training curriculum and another test for assessing benefit from a hearing aid.

PATIENT VARIABLES

In selecting appropriate test materials for assessing word recognition, it is important to consider variables such as cognitive/linguistic level and hearing ability, for these will affect how an individual performs on a particular test. A consideration of patient variables will help a speech and hearing professional choose between test stimuli, response format, testing conditions, and whether to use live or recorded stimuli.

The patient must have the maturity and cognitive skills to take the test. For example, it would be inappropriate to expect a 3-year-old child to repeat a seven-word sentence, as it would be to expect an elderly person with dementia to do so (Figure 2-8). If a young child takes a closed-set test, then it might be necessary that the response items be illustrated by

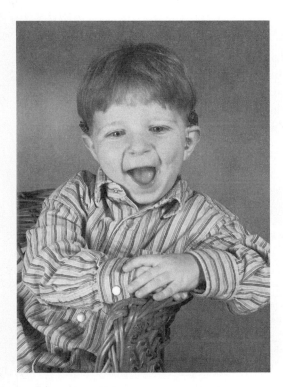

FIGURE 2-8. Selection of stimuli. Stimuli that are selected for speech recognition testing must be appropriate for the maturity and cognitive and linguistic development of the patient. *Photograph courtesy of MED-EL Corp.*

pictures, because the child could not read orthographic choices. Short attention spans and variable levels of compliance may affect performance.

Similarly, the test must present items that are within the linguistic competency of the individual. Otherwise, a clinician may not know whether someone performed poorly on a test because he or she did not know the vocabulary or grammatical structures or because of hearing limitations. For example, a child might be asked to repeat the sentence, *The man ate an artichoke for dinner.* If a child is unfamiliar with the word *artichoke,* it is unlikely the child will be able to repeat it during a speech recognition test, especially if he or she has a significant hearing loss.

The degree of hearing loss and experience with a listening device will affect test selection. For instance, if an adult just received a cochlear implant, it may be inappropriate to administer a monosyllabic word test in an audition-only condition, because the individual likely will exhibit a "floor" performance.

Sometimes there will be a need to consider **communication mode** and other disabilities. For example, if a child uses sign, the test instructions should be presented with sign, and provisions for recording the child's responses must be made (i.e., if the child signs responses, then someone must interpret them). If an individual has decreased speech intelligibility as well as a hearing loss, the responses may have to be written.

Communication mode is the means used by a sender to share information with a receiver and may include speech, sign, writing, hand gestures, or any other system of shared symbols.

STIMULI UNITS

Once the purpose for testing has been identified and patient variables have been considered, test selection can be made. Test stimuli that are used typically to assess speech recognition are summarized in Table 2-2 and shown in Figure 2-9. Examples of tests that correspond with each type are also listed, for both children and adults. Each kind of stimulus presents both advantages and disadvantages.

Table 2-2. Examples of word recognition tests that use phoneme, word, and sentence stimuli for children and adults. These tests typically are administered in an audition-only condition.

TEST	AUTHOR(S)	STIMULUS TYPE	STIMULUS UNITS	RESPONSE FORMAT	TARGET POPULATION
Speech Pattern Contrast Test (SPAC)	Boothroyd, 1994	Phoneme (also includes test of suprasegmental contrasts, such as word stress)	Words and phrases	Closed set	Children over age 10 years
Audiovisual Feature Test	Tyler, Fryauf-Bertschy, & Kelsey, 1991	Phoneme	Rhyming words, including b, c, d, key, me, knee	Closed set (10-choice)	Children
Iowa Consonant Confusion Test	Tyler, Preece, & Tye-Murray, 1986	Phoneme	Nonsense bisyllables, including eemee, eesee, eedee, eebee	Closed-set (13-choice)	Adults
Iowa Vowel Confusion Test	Tyler, Preece, & Tye-Murray, 1986	Phoneme	Monosyllables with an [hVd] format, including heed, who'd, had, head	Closed set (9-choice)	Adults
Nonsense Syllable Test (NST)	Edgerton & Danhauer, 1979	Phoneme	Nonsense bisyllables	Open set	Children and adults
Minimal Pairs Test	Robbins, Renshaw, Miyamoto, Osberger, & Pope, 1988	Phoneme	Monosyllabic word pairs (e.g., pair vs. bear)	Closed set (2-choice)	Children, about age 4 years and older
Auditory Numbers Test (ANT)	Erber, 1980	Word	Numbers	Closed-set (5-choice)	Children
Consonant-Nucleus-Consonant (CNC) Words	Peterson & Lehiste, 1962	Word	Lists of 50 phonemically balanced words, each containing a consonant, vowel or diphthong, consonant	Open set	Adults
Northwestern University Children's Perception of Speech (NU-CHIPS)	Elliott & Katz, 1980	Word	Monosyllables constructed with the most frequently occurring phonemes in the English language, such as fork, dog	Closed set (4-choice)	Children who have the receptive language abilities of age 2.6 years or older
Word Intelligibility by Picture Identification (WIPI)	Ross & Lerman, 1971	Word	Monosyllabic words, such as bear, pear, stair, chair, ear, hair	Closed set (6-choice)	Children ages 5–6 years with moderate hearing loss; ages 7–8 years with severe hearing loss

continues

Table 2-2. *continued*

TEST	AUTHOR(S)	STIMULUS TYPE	STIMULUS UNITS	RESPONSE FORMAT	TARGET POPULATION
Phonetically Balanced Kindergarten (PBK)	Haskins, 1949	Word	Monosyllabic words	Open set	Children, 6 years and older
Northwestern University Auditory Test No. 6 (NU-6)	Tillman & Carhart, 1966	Word	Monosyllabic words	Open set	Adults
Central Institute for the Deaf (CID) Auditory Test W-22	Hirsh et al., 1952	Word	Phonetically balanced monosyllabic word lists	Open set	Adults
Early-Speech Perception Test (ESP)	Moog & Geers, 1990	Word	Words varying in number of syllables	Closed set	Children 6 years and older (there is a version available for children as young as 2 years)
Lexical Neighborhood Test (LNT)	Kirk, Pisoni, & Osberger, 1995	Word	Words, some of which are lexically "easy" and some of which are lexically "hard," with easy words having few other word choices that are phonetically similar (e.g., *thought, live*) and hard words having many words that are similar (e.g., *mole, wed*)	Open set	Children
Bamford-Kowal-Bench Sentences (BKB)	Bench & Bamford, 1979	Sentence	Sentences constructed with vocabulary familiar to 8- to 16-year-old hard-of-hearing children	Open set	Older children and adults
Central Institute for the Deaf (CID) Everyday Speech Sentences	Davis & Silverman, 1978	Sentence	Sentences that vary in length and structure	Open set	Older children and adults
Revised Speech Perception in Noise (SPIN)	Bilger et al., 1984	Sentence	Sentences that have either high context for the last word in the sentence or low context	Open set, presented with a background of speech babble	Adults
CUNY Sentences	Boothroyd, Hanin, & Hnath, 1985	Sentence	Unrelated sentences	Open set	Adults
Hearing in Noise Test (HINT)	Nilsson, Soli, & Sullivan, 1994	Sentence	Unrelated sentences	Open set, presented with a background of noise	13 years and up (there is a version available for children between the ages of 6–12 years)

continues

Table 2-2. *continued*

TEST	AUTHOR(S)	STIMULUS TYPE	STIMULUS UNITS	RESPONSE FORMAT	TARGET POPULATION
The Connected Speech Test (CST)	Cox, Alexander, & Gilmore, 1987	Sentence	Sets of 10 related sentences pertaining to familiar topics	Open set	Adults
The Synthetic Sentence Test (SSI)	Jerger, Speaks, & Trammell, 1968; Speaks & Jerger, 1965	Sentence	Synthetic sentences with minimal contextual cues and minimal redundancy	Closed set	Adults
Quick Speech in Noise Test (QuickSIN)	Etymotic Research, 2001	Sentence	Sets of six unrelated sentences	Open set, presented with a background of noise	Adults
Speech Sound Pattern Discrimination (SSPDT)	Bochner, Garrison, Palmer, MacKenzie, & Braveman, 1997	Sentence	Sets of three sentences, one standard and two comparison (e.g., *Free books are available*, is a standard, *Three books are available* is a comparison)	Closed set, requiring a same or different judgment	Adults
Speech in Noise (SIN)	Killion & Vilchur, 1993	Sentence	Sentences recorded at a variety of signal-to-noise ratios	Open set, presented with varying levels of four-talker babble	Adults, particularly new hearing aid users

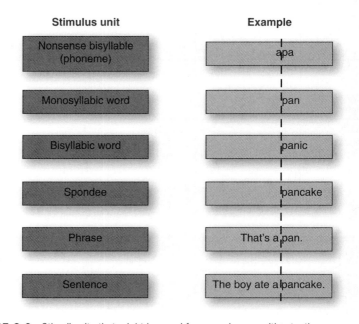

FIGURE 2-9. Stimuli units that might be used for speech recognition testing.

Phonemes and Phoneme Contrasts

Phoneme testing permits phonetic errors to be examined. The items may be designed to assess consonant or vowel recognition. Although often referred to as phoneme testing, technically, these stimuli are **nonsense syllables**.

Test results indicate the kinds of **speech features** utilized during speech recognition. For example, a patient may not have scored high on a test that presents a closed set of items such as *eemee, eenee, eesee, eebee, eepee,* and *eetee*. However, an analysis of errors may reveal that even though overall performance was poor, the individual consistently utilized the voicing feature. For instance, *eepee* may have been heard as *eetee* or *eesee,* both of which contain unvoiced elements, but never as *eebee* or *eenee,* which contain only voiced elements. Thus, in designing auditory training goals, a speech and hearing professional might aim to build on this ability to utilize the voicing feature.

Although a speech and hearing professional can evaluate subjectively an individual's errors and qualitatively assess error confusions, formal statistical and mathematical analyses can be performed on the results. These provide a quantitative indication of the kinds of information an individual utilizes during speech. Such analyses include **information transmission analysis** (Miller & Nicely, 1955), **multidimensional scaling**, and **cluster analysis**.

A feature analysis of consonant phoneme confusion errors indicates which parameters of the speech signal are detected and utilized. Features that typically are considered in this kind of analysis include nasality, voicing, duration, frication, place, and envelope. A commonly used consonant classification system appears in Table 2-3.

For the nasality feature, consonants /m/ and /n/ are classified as nasal consonants. A person who appears to hear the nasality feature is probably responding to the frequencies around and below 300 Hz. Consonants that are aperiodic in nature (/p, t, k, f, s, ʒ/) are grouped together for the voicing feature, whereas the relatively long-duration consonants are grouped together for the duration feature (/z, s, ʒ/). The voicing and duration features probably relate to temporal cues and the voice pitch. Consonants produced with steady turbulence (/v, f, z, s, ʒ/) usually are grouped together for the frication feature. This feature relates to high-frequency turbulence. The place feature, for which consonants are categorized according to whether they are produced in the front, middle, or back of the vocal tract, is cued by spectral or frequency changes over time, particularly in the region of the second vowel formant (see Chapter 4). Finally, the envelope

A **phoneme** is the smallest class of speech sounds in a language.

Nonsense syllables are syllables of speech that have no meaning.

Speech features are categorical properties of phonemes; a phoneme can be described as a bundle of speech features.

An **information transmission analysis** is a statistical procedure that analyzes the transmission of speech features by scoring confusions between test stimuli that are grouped based upon the presence or absence of those features; for example, the phonemes /p/ and /t/ share the feature of being "unvoiced." If a patient confuses *eepee* for *eetee,* the patient will receive credit for having correctly utilized the "voicing" feature but not the "place" feature.

Multidimensional scaling is a statistical procedure whereby data points are represented in a geometric space; for example, two phonemes that sound similar to a patient will be plotted near to each other and two phonemes that sound dissimilar will be plotted far from each other.

Cluster analysis is a statistical approach to information in a database that aims to determine which data points fall into groups or clusters; for example, it is not uncommon for the phonemes /b,d,g/ to cluster together because they often sound similar to people who have significant hearing loss.

Table 2-3. An example of a classification system for consonants that may be used to classify consonant phonemes for a feature analysis. The numbers are arbitrary and serve only to indicate the group to which a sound belongs within a feature.

CONSONANT	VOICING	PLACE	NASALITY	DURATION	FRICATION	ENVELOPE
b	1	0	0	0	0	1
d	1	1	0	0	0	1
g	1	3	0	0	0	1
p	0	0	0	0	0	0
t	0	1	0	0	0	0
k	0	3	0	0	0	0
v	1	0	0	0	1	1
f	0	0	0	0	1	2
z	1	1	0	1	1	1
s	0	1	0	1	1	2
ʓ	0	2	0	1	1	2
m	1	0	1	0	0	3
n	1	1	1	0	0	3

feature reflects time-intensity variations in the audio signal. To recognize words, persons must detect and utilize at least some of these features in the signal. A feature analysis indicates how well a patient can distinguish these cues from one another. The topic of features will be revisited when we consider designing objectives for auditory and speechreading training (Chapters 4 and 6).

An advantage of using phoneme stimuli is that performance is relatively independent of an individual's vocabulary level. It is not important that individuals be familiar with the test stimuli, and indeed, the stimuli are often *nonsense syllables,* such as *eesee* and *eetee.* This same advantage can become a disadvantage when testing young children, who often must be tested with vocabulary they know.

A principal disadvantage of using phoneme stimuli is poor face validity. People do not communicate with these kinds of stimuli typically, and it is not straightforward how recognition relates to conversational speech understanding. For instance, nonsense syllables do not require individuals to organize streams of information into linguistically meaningful chunks, or to process speech information with the same rapidity as ongoing speech.

Advantages of nonsense syllables

- Performance unaffected by a patient's vocabulary level
- A feature analysis can often be performed

Disadvantages of nonsense syllables

- Not appropriate for some children
- Poor face validity

Words

The most commonly used stimuli for assessing speech recognition are monosyllabic words. Many word lists are designed to be **phonetically balanced**, meaning that the words include phonemes in the same proportion in which they occur in spoken English. The *Phonetically Balanced Kindergarten* word lists (PB-K) developed by Haskins (1949) are commonly used to assess spoken word recognition in children. More recently, word lists for testing purposes have been based on principles of **acoustic lexical neighborhoods** (Luce, 1986; Luce & Pisoni, 1998), for example, the *Lexical Neighborhood Test (LNT)* and the *Multisyllabic Lexical Neighborhood Test (MLNT)* (Kirk, 1998; Kirk et al., 1995). Words that have a similar **frequency of occurrence** (i.e., how often the words occur during everyday language use) and that share similar acoustic-phonetic characteristics belong to the same neighborhood. A word that belongs to a **dense neighborhood** (many words that are similar, such as *cat, mat, sat, fat, pat, bat,* etc.) is typically more difficult to recognize than a word that belongs to a **sparse neighborhood** (few words that are similar; the words *thumb, tea,* and *lost* each belong to sparse neighborhoods). Most word lists are comprised of monosyllables that have the phonemic structure of consonant-vowel-consonant (e.g., *cat* or *man*). Word stimuli generally are difficult to recognize, more so than phrases or simple sentences.

One advantage in using real words is that they have somewhat higher face validity than nonsense syllables designed to assess phoneme recognition. People communicate with words in daily conversation. Word tests might be comprised of monosyllabic words, bisyllabic words, and/or spondees. The tests are also easy to score, and allow a wide range of skill levels to be assessed. Responses from a word test can be scored by percentage of words repeated verbatim, or percentage of phonemes correct (e.g., if the word is *bat,* and an individual responds *pat,* two of the word's three phonemes are scored as correct). The reasons that percentage phoneme scores are sometimes computed are to obtain a fine-grained understanding of an individual's performance and to provide a different vehicle for comparing test results. For example, two people might achieve the following scores on the same test:

Person 1: 30% words correct, 40% phonemes correct

Person 2: 30% words correct, 65% phonemes correct

Even though the individuals erred an equal number of times in repeating the words, Person 2's errors better approximate the target than do Person 1's

---

A **phonetically balanced (PB)** word list presents a set of words that contain the speech sounds with the same frequency in which they occur in everyday conversations.

An **acoustic lexical neighborhood** is comprised of a set of words that are acoustically similar and have approximately the same frequency of occurrence.

Frequency of occurrence refers to the frequency in which a word is likely to occur in everyday speech or common usage.

A **dense neighborhood** has many members.

A **sparse neighborhood** has few members.

Simple questions that may reveal presence of hearing loss are:

- Can you hear on the telephone?
- Do people tell you that you set the TV volume too high?
- Do you often ask people to repeat?
- Do you have problems listening in a noisy room?
- Do people seem to mumble?
- Are women and children especially difficult to hear?

Advantages of word stimuli
- Have a somewhat higher face validity than non-sense syllables
- Easy to score
- Permit fine-grained scoring

Disadvantages of word stimuli
- May not index everyday listening performance
- May not be appropriate for some patients who have limited vocabulary

error responses. Thus, the second person may have better listening ability than the first person.

As with phonemes, word stimuli may not reflect adequately how an individual performs in everyday listening situations because people typically listen to connected discourse. For instance, words are presented rapidly during conversation. A person typically does not pause to think about the identity of each word as it is spoken, as one does when taking a test of isolated word recognition. During normal conversation, we might receive speech at between 140 and 180 words per minute (Miller et al., 1984). It is possible for two people to perform similarly on a word test, in which the demands of fast online processing are not great, and yet function differently in everyday conversation. Another problem in using words as test stimuli may arise if the test taker has a language delay because performance on word tests may be influenced by vocabulary. A child who has a limited vocabulary may perform poorly simply because he or she is unfamiliar with the test words. As an example of a word test, lists from the *Lexical Neighborhood Test* (Kirk et al., 1995) are reprinted in the Key Resources.

Phrases and Sentences

A speech recognition test may consist of a series of unrelated phrases or sentences. For instance, the test may commence with the sentence, *The cook cut the apple,* and then continue with, *The boy and girl walked to school,* which is contextually unrelated to the first sentence. Alternatively, the test may present sentences centered on a common theme. For instance, before the test begins, the patient may be informed, "The sentences you will hear concern activities to do at the lake." The first sentence may then be, *We paddled a canoe.* The second sentence may be, *We went for a swim this morning,* and so forth. Performance will be better for topic-related than unrelated sentences.

Sentence stimuli have high face validity because people typically communicate with phrases, sentences, and paragraphs. As such, performance on a sentence test may better reflect how a person performs in the real world than performance on a phoneme or isolated word test. Sentences have the following features, which are characteristic of everyday speech:

- **Prosodic cues:** When people listen to speech, they attend not only to individual sounds, but also to intonation, rate, and duration cues, and these help them identify words and understand meaning. For example, an individual may be presented with a complete sentence, but because of hearing loss, the person may hear only, *mmm mm-mm mmm?* Even though the individual receives a gross approximation of the message, there is still enough information to know that a question is being asked, and that the question contains four syllables, and possibly, enough information to know that it contains three words.

- **Contextual information:** The words in a sentence provide contextual redundancy. Recognition of some words facilitates recognition of other words. If an individual hears, *Mary closed the* _____, it is possible to deduce that the final word is a noun, based on grammatical context, and that the word might be *door,* based on semantic cues.
- **Coarticulation:** When words are spoken in succession as in a sentence, they blend together and vary as a function of what precedes and follows. For example, the schwa sound in the word *the* will sound different if the word *blue* follows than if the word *green* follows. These coarticulation effects provide redundant cues for word recognition.

> **Advantages of sentence stimuli**
> - High face validity
> - Likely to reflect real-word performance
>
> **Disadvantages of sentence stimuli**
> - Performance may be influenced by linguistic knowledge
> - Performance may be influenced by familiarity with the topic

Even though sentences have these features of everyday speech, they also pose some disadvantages for assessment. One disadvantage of using sentence-level stimuli is that performance can be influenced by linguistic knowledge and familiarity with the topic. For example, a young child with limited grammatical knowledge may not perform as well as an older child who has good language skills, even though the two children might have similar perceptual skills. Memory also may affect results. If an audiologist presents a 10-word sentence to a 5-year-old child, the child may forget the beginning of the sentence by the time it ends.

Sentence tests are usually scored by computing a percentage words correct score, although sometimes they are scored for percentage phonemes correct and sometimes only selected key words are assessed. For a word to be scored as correct, it must be repeated verbatim. If the sentence is, *The girls walked to school,* and a person responds, "The girl walked to school," that sentence is scored as four out of five words correct. The omission of /s/ from *girls* makes it an incorrect repetition. As an example of a sentence test, lists from the *CID Everyday Sentence Test* (Silverman & Hirsh, 1955) are reprinted in the Key Resources.

Selection of Test Stimuli

There are no cookbook procedures to follow when deciding which test stimuli to use. However, one guiding principle is that the measures chosen should be informative about how an individual performs in natural situations and should be independent of confounding factors such as vocabulary and grammatical knowledge, cognitive abilities, and memory. Often, clinicians opt to use a test-battery approach, using more than one test so that the aggregate presents different kinds of speech units.

TEST PROCEDURES

Once a test has been selected, decisions must be made about the protocol that will be followed for administering the test. Considerations for assessing speech recognition include the test condition, the type of response set, and whether testing occurs with live voice or recordings.

Test Condition

Tests of speech recognition can be administered in one of three conditions (Figure 2-10):

- Audition-only: Only the auditory signal is presented, usually at a normal or moderately loud conversational level.
- Vision-only: Only the visual signal is presented, usually showing the head and neck of the test talker (this is a lipreading condition).
- Audition-plus-vision: Both the auditory and visual signals are presented (this is a speechreading condition).

Audition-Only

The audition-only condition is most frequently used for speech recognition assessment because it relates most directly to hearing ability. The signal may be presented in quiet or in the presence of noise.

The sound level for presenting the speech stimuli is often at a normal or moderately loud conversational level (60–70 dB SPL). Alternatively, the

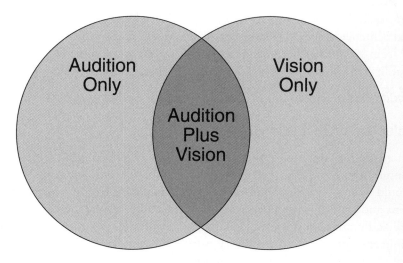

FIGURE 2-10. The test conditions used for speech recognition testing.

level might be set at about 30 to 40 dB above the patient's SRT. When this latter level is chosen, it is said to be 30 to 40 dB **sensational level (SL)**. The intent of using sensation levels is to liken functional listening levels across patients.

Noise may be introduced to increase the difficulty of the listening task or to gain a better understanding of how the person performs in the real world. The noise signal may be talker babble (e.g., six people read text, and their speech signals are overlaid to create a single noise source) or **white noise** (which sounds like a radio off-station). Speech noise and cafeteria noise may also be used. Speech noise has approximately the same energy at each frequency as does running speech, whereas cafeteria noise is noise that was recorded in a cafeteria and then overdubbed several times. Sometimes the competing noise signal is semantically meaningful, say, a single talker reading a passage. A meaningful competing signal might be used to determine how well an elderly individual can tune out distracting competitors.

When a speech recognition test is performed in the presence of noise, the audiologist records the **signal-to-noise ratio (SNR)**, which indicates the difference between the sound level of the signal and the sound level of the noise. Thus, if the signal is presented at 40 dB HL, and the noise is presented at 30 dB HL, the SNR is +10. An example of a sentence test designed to be presented in noise, the *QuickSIN* (Etymotic Research, 2001), appears in the Key Resources.

Vision-Only

Sometimes a test of speech recognition is administered in a vision-only condition. The visual signal typically is comprised of the talker's head and shoulders, with the talker facing the patient head-on. The talker should be well lit, so his or her face is fully visible and not in shadows. The talker usually is placed before a plain, nondistracting background.

Audition-Plus-Vision

Usually, performance for a particular individual will be optimal for an audition-plus-vision condition. This condition is used when best performance is desired or when hearing is so poor that the auditory signal provides only a supplement to lipreading.

Both the vision-only and audition-plus-vision conditions are employed when one is interested in accessing speechreading enhancement or determining goals for speechreading training. **Speechreading enhancement** (sometimes referred to as *auditory enhancement*) is computed by comparing speech recognition scores in a vision-only condition to

---

Sensational level (SL) is the level of a sound in dB above a person's threshold.

"[Sentence tests presented with background noise are] reflective of real-life listening situations. And, because they have good face validity, sentence-length, speech-in-noise tests are excellent tools for establishing realistic expectations, making rehabilitative recommendations, and selecting the best hearing aid technology for each patient."
(Taylor, 2004, p. 24)

White noise is broadband noise that has equal energy at all frequencies.

Signal-to-noise ratio (SNR) is the level of a signal relative to a background of noise.

Speechreading enhancement is the difference or ratio between speech recognition performance in a vision-only condition and an audition-plus-vision condition.

A Brief History of Visual Speech Testing

Visual tests have a history extending almost as far back as the film industry. The first test of vision-only speech recognition was filmed by the lipreading teacher Edward Nitchie (see Chapter 6) in 1913. It included three proverbs: *Love makes the world go around, Spare the rod and spoil the child,* and *Fine feathers make fine birds.* The test had obvious shortcomings. The proverbs were well known to that era's generation, so after recognizing a few words of one, a patient was likely to guess the rest. In addition, performance with just three items probably could not adequately reflect general word recognition ability. Nonetheless, this test represented a beginning. In the 1940s, Utley (1946) developed a test for adults called, *How Well Do You Read Lips?* Well into the early 1980s, it remained a widely used test of vision-only and audition-plus-vision word recognition. It included a word test, a sentence test, and a story test.

The advent of cochlear implants in the 1980s coincided with the development of several new tests (e.g., MacLeod & Summerfield, 1987; Boothroyd et al., 1985; Tyler, Preece, & Tye-Murray, 1987; Walden et al., 1981) whereas advances in computer technology led to more widespread usage. Initially, researchers and clinicians viewed cochlear implants as an aid for lipreading as much as a hearing device per se, so tests were needed to assess how well the electrical speech signal augmented vision-only speech recognition. New computer technologies permitted visual files to be stored digitally and eliminated the need for elaborate test setups comprised of screens and projectors. Computer technology also allowed for faster testing as test items no longer had to be spaced on the recorded film to accommodate slow respondents. Computer-controlled testing allows test item presentation to be paced according to patient performance and allows for online scoring.

scores obtained in an audition-plus-vision condition. It indicates how much better a patient can recognize speech when listening and watching the talker as compared to watching alone, and is often a good indicator of how much benefit a person with significant hearing loss receives by using a listening device during face-to-face communication. Two different computations may yield a speechreading enhancement score. First, a simple difference score may be computed by subtracting the percentage correct score obtained in a vision-only condition (V) from the percentage correct score obtained in an audition-plus-vision condition (AV): AV% correct – V% correct. The greater the difference between the two scores, the greater the amount of enhancement provided by the auditory signal.

Second, a normalized ratio score may be computed. This computation is done by first figuring out how much room for improvement there is in a vision-only condition then referencing the amount of improvement gained with the addition of the auditory signal to that amount available. The formula for computation is: AV% correct – V% correct/100% - V% correct. Table 2-4 presents an example of the two computation methods. In this table, Patient Sam H. recognized 50% of the words correct when a test was presented in a vision-only condition and 75% words correct when the auditory signal was added. Patient Max J. recognized 10% and 55% of the words in the two conditions, respectively. Note that whereas Max J. appears to have achieved greater speechreading enhancement than Sam H. when the simple difference score is used, they appear to have equal gains with the addition of the auditory signal when the normalized difference score is employed.

Tests that are available for assessing speechreading and speechreading enhancement for children include the *Craig Sentences,* the *Craig Words* (Craig, 1964), and the *Children's Audiovisual Enhancement Test (CAVET)* (Tye-Murray & Geers, 2002). Tests for adults include the *Iowa Sentence Test* (Tyler et al., 1986) and the *City University of New York (CUNY) Sentences* (Boothroyd et al., 1985). An example of a speechreading test, the *CAVET*, appears in the Key Resources section. Each test list in the *CAVET* contains words that have been shown to be easy to identify in a vision-only condition and words that have been shown to be difficult to identify in a vision-only condition, so test-takers seldom achieve a floor or ceiling performance level.

Table 2-4. Two different formulas may be used to compute speechreading enhancement. In this example, Sam J. achieved an enhancement score of 25% when it was computed with the difference score formula and an enhancement score of 50% when it was computed with the normalized difference formula. Max H. achieved an enhancement score of 45% when it was computed with the difference score formula and an enhancement score of 50% when it was computed with the normalized difference formula.

PATIENT	V-ONLY SCORE	AV SCORE	DIFFERENCE SCORE: (AV – V)	NORMALIZED DIFFERENCE SCORE: (AV – V) ÷ (100 – V)
Sam J.	50% correct	75% correct	75 – 50 = 25	(75 – 50) ÷ (100 – 50) = 50
Max H.	10% correct	55% correct	55 – 10 = 45	(55 – 10) ÷ (100 – 10) = 50

Hearing Loss Can Be Difficult to Detect in a Good Speechreader

Sometimes mild or moderate and even severe hearing losses go undetected in children because they are proficient speechreaders. Some children may mispronounce some sounds or words, but their parents and teachers do not readily associate their articulation problems with hearing loss. Jeffers and Barley (1971) related the following incident:

> Richard, age five, was [a child whose hearing loss went undetected]. The parents suspected that his younger brother had a hearing loss, but had no idea that Richard might also be similarly involved. His speech was excellent for his age, and his comprehension and recall vocabularies larger than average. His loss was discovered through a whim of the audiometrist who decided that she might as well check Richard's hearing at the same time that she was testing his brother. Richard was found to have a binaural hearing loss of 42 dB [for the pure tone average of 500, 1,000, and 2,000 Hz] . . . and to be severely hard-of-hearing (60 dB or greater) for a good part of the consonant range. A year later his first grade teacher evinced complete disbelief regarding the loss and almost convinced the parents that a misdiagnosis had been made. On a test of speech intelligibility without speechreading given at normal conversational level, he made a score of 48 percent, which would indicate great difficulty in understanding. With speechreading, his score was 84 percent, indicating good comprehension. (p. 10)

Response Format

An **open-set** task or test does not provide choices.

Another important issue to consider when testing speech recognition is what kind of response format will be used to elicit responses. Many standardized tests have an **open-set** format. This format means that no response choices and no contextual cues are provided. The materials are not familiar to the patient, and have never been practiced, say during training.

A **closed-set** is a stimulus or response set that contains a fixed number of items known to the patient.

Closed-set tests often are used with cochlear implant users and with children. These tests provide a limited set of response choices and are easier than open-set tests. Items and foils are presented as written stimuli, pictures, or objects. The members and the size of the response set can be selected to test features of speech recognition and to vary test difficulty. For example, if a teacher is interested in determining whether a new cochlear implant user utilizes suprasegmental cues, the response choices when the test word *ball* is spoken might be *ball, ice cream,* and *tricycle,* words that vary in duration and stress pattern. On the other hand, if the teacher is testing an experienced cochlear implant user, the response set might be *ball, bill, bowl,* and *bell,* which will require the child to attend to more fine-grained segmental cues. The task will be more difficult when there are four response choices as opposed to only three.

Live-Voice Versus Recorded Test Materials

The next issue to consider in regard to selecting speech recognition test materials is whether testing will be performed **live-voice** or whether **recorded stimuli** will be used. As the terms imply, test items can be presented by a live talker or they can be presented via a playback system, such as a computer or compact disc player. The advantages of using live voice are that no playback equipment is required, and the talker can adjust the rate of stimulus presentation to meet performance needs. Many young children are more comfortable with a live-voice test paradigm than a recorded-voice paradigm.

During **live-voice testing**, stimuli are presented by a talker in real time.

Recorded stimuli are presented via a computer, tape recorder, compact disc (CD) player, or a DVD player.

Despite these advantages, there are even more disadvantages associated with using live voice rather than recorded speech. Live talkers can introduce variability from one test session to the next and from one test site to another. Talkers have different speaking styles, and they may vary in their style from one day to another. For instance, test talkers may vary on any of the following variables:

- **Voicing frequency:** Female test talkers usually have high pitches and may be more difficult to understand than male test talkers, who have characteristically low-pitched voices. Most people have better hearing in the lower frequencies than in the mid- and high frequencies.
- **Intonation:** Sentences spoken with appropriate and expressive intonation are generally easier to understand than ones spoken with a monotone or inappropriate intonation. Thus, a test talker who uses more voice inflection while speaking the test sentences will be easier to understand than a test talker who uses less inflection.
- **Speech rate:** Rapidly spoken speech is more difficult to recognize than moderately slow speech. One test talker may speak slowly whereas another may speak more quickly.
- **Clarity of articulation:** Clearly articulated speech is easier to recognize than conversational or mumbled speech. Test talkers may vary in their ability to speak clearly.

- **Physical characteristics:** In an audition-plus-vision or vision-only condition, talkers who have pronounced lip and jaw displacement, no facial hair, and expressive facial movements will be relatively easier to speechread or lipread.

It is important that talker characteristics not confound test results. Otherwise, a clinician will not be able to monitor an individual's performance over time or compare his or her performance to that of other people who have been tested in other clinics. In today's world, most audiology clinics and other hearing-related settings rely exclusively on recorded materials to assess speech recognition. Live-voice testing is rare.

Synthesized and Altered Speech

Most recorded test materials present speech spoken by an adult talker, speaking as clearly as possible. However, there are two other kinds of recorded materials that sometimes are used to assess word recognition: synthesized speech and altered speech.

Synthesized speech is created with a computer or other technological apparatus and not by a human vocal tract. Synthesized speech may be used if the tester wants to determine how a patient utilizes a specific cue for speech recognition. For example, a series of acoustic waveform samples may be created so that there is a systematic variation in the voice-onset time for /b/ in the word *bat*. The tester then might determine at what step in the continuum the patient hears the word *bat* versus *pat*.

Altered speech is human speech that is recorded and then altered in some way, usually by means of computer software. Altered speech may be time-compressed, extended, or filtered. **Time-compressed speech** has been digitized and then processed so that small segments are periodically deleted from the ongoing signal waveform. When it is played back, time-compressed speech sounds like natural speech produced at a fast speaking rate. Conversely, **expanded speech** is created by duplicating small segments of the signal so that the speech sounds as if it were produced with a slow speaking rate. **Filtered speech** is created by passing the speech signal through filter banks. **Low-pass filtered speech** includes the lower but not the higher frequencies, whereas **high-pass filtered speech** includes the higher but not the lower frequencies. Altered speech sometimes is used when the tester is interested in how well the patient can recognize speech when the auditory system is challenged.

In sum, synthesized speech and altered speech often are used to examine the effects of specific acoustic cues on speech recognition or to create a

---

Synthesized speech is created with a computer, not the human vocal tract.

Altered speech is human speech that is recorded and then altered in some way.

Time-compressed speech is speech that has been accelerated by removing segments of the waveform and then compressing the remaining segments together without changing its frequency composition.

Expanded speech is recorded speech that is altered by duplicating small segments of the signal so that it sounds like a slow speaking rate.

Filtered speech is passed through filter banks for the purpose of removing or amplifying frequency bands in the signal.

Low-pass filtered speech has been passed through filter banks that removed the higher, but not the lower, frequencies.

High-pass filtered speech has been passed through filter banks that removed the lower, but not the higher, frequencies.

difficult speech-listening condition. These stimuli might be used to address the following questions:

- Does an individual utilize the plosive burst cue when distinguishing a /t/ from an /s/?
- Even though a young and an aged person have similar hearing thresholds, is the older person less able to understand time-compressed speech, which is a more taxing listening task?

DIFFICULTIES ASSOCIATED WITH SPEECH RECOGNITION ASSESSMENT

There are several problematic issues that should be considered when attempting to evaluate speech recognition and the effects of training on speech recognition performance. Three of the more significant issues are:

- Learning effects
- Test–retest variability
- Clinical significance

Learning Effects

Patients sometimes learn the test items when they are presented more than once, even when several weeks separate the test periods. Thus, because of **learning effects**, performance improves for reasons other than an aural rehabilitation intervention, such as receipt of auditory training. For example, suppose someone was presented with the sentence, *The boy and girl are walking to school* during a speechreading test and recognized the words, *The boy* _____ _____ _____ *walking* _____ _____. If the patient repeated the test 3 months later, he or she might recognize all of the words, because he or she remembered the sentence remnant and used that information as contextual cues for identifying the rest of the sentence. Even recognizing the sentence rhythm and syllabic pattern might trigger recall. It may seem implausible that someone can remember dialogue for that length of time, but one simply need reflect how the words of a song learned in grade school come back after many years of not hearing it, often after just hearing the first couple of words.

Learning effects occur when performance on a test improves as a function of familiarity with the test procedures or items, not as a result of a change in ability.

One way in which the learning problem has been addressed is with the use of **equivalent lists**, that is, sets of sentences that are presumed to be equally difficult to recognize. Equivalency is usually established by playing the separate tests to a large group of participants. If, on average, the participants recognize an equal number of words on each list, then the lists are said to be equivalent.

Equivalent lists contain items that are presumed to be equally difficult to recognize.

The problem with this tactic is that the lists may be equivalent when some listening devices are used but not others. For instance, a group of hearing aid users may perform similarly on two lists of test items, whereas a group of cochlear implant users may not. Similarly, equivalency may vary with the configuration of hearing loss, such that a group of individuals with a sloping mild-to-moderate loss will not perform like a group of individuals who have a flat severe hearing loss. List equivalency also may vary as a function of test condition. For example, two lists may be equivalent when presented in a vision-only but not in an audition-plus-vision test condition.

Some researchers have tried to minimize learning effects by constructing tests that have a large number of items, say 100 or more sentences (Tyler, Preece, & Tye-Murray, 1986). With so many test items, it is thought that patients may be less likely to remember them, even with repeated testing. However, there is little empirical data available to support this assumption. Another tack has been to use a closed-set matrix format (e.g., Gagné et al., 2006; Tye-Murray, Sommers, & Spehar, 2006). A closed set of words is presented in the context of either a constant sentence frame (Gagné et al., 2006) or one of four possible frames (Tye-Murray et al., 2006; Tye-Murray et al., in press). The patient receives several practice items before the test is administered. The closed-set nature of the response set ensures list equivalency, both within and across conditions (e.g., vision-only and audition-only). Learning effects associated with repeated testing are minimized because the patient is familiarized with the matrix of key words prior to each test session by means of the practice session and the same sentence need never be presented twice. Table 2-5 presents the response screen for a matrix test. In this example, every possible sentence has the same syntactic structure (i.e., *The___and the ___watched the ___and the ___*) and contains four key words that may be selected from the response matrix. For instance, one

Table 2-5. Example of a matrix test format. In this example, the matrix includes 32 interchangeable key words for each of the four slots in the sentence frame, where a word can be used only once within a single sentence (adapted from Tye-Murray et al., 2006; Tye-Murray et al., in press). During testing, the matrix appears on a computer touch screen and the patient responds by touching four consecutive choices. The test can be presented in an audition-only, vision-only, or audition-plus-vision condition.

The ___and the ___watched the ___ and the ___.

Please choose from the following words:

Bear	Cat	Deer	Fawn	Men	Saint	Team	Whale
Bird	Cook	Dog	Fish	Mice	Seal	Toad	Wife
Boys	Cop	Dove	Fox	Mole	Snail	Tribe	Wolf
Bug	Cow	Duck	Frog	Moose	Son	Troop	Worm

test sentence might be, *The saint and the wife watched the mice and the mole,* and another might be, *The bird and the boys watched the mole and the cop.* If enough sentences are recorded, than the patient need never hear the same sentence twice, no matter how many times he or she takes the test. For example, the matrix shown in Table 2-5 permits 863,040 different sentences. Although this format ensures list equivalency and minimizes learning effects, it allows for the assessment of only a limited number of words and may be too easy for those patients who have very good listening and/or speechreading abilities.

Test–Retest Variability

Another difficulty related to assessing speechreading performance is that patients, especially children, vary in their performance from day to day. Thus, a patient may achieve a score on one day, then take it on another day and achieve a different score, even though it is the same test. There may be several factors that contribute to **test–retest variability**. One reason for this relates to the individual. For example, on some days a child may be highly motivated to perform well, whereas on others, the child may be restless and uninterested. As such, scores may improve or decrease over time, not as a result of training, but as a result of fatigue, interest, and mood.

Test–retest variability is a measure of the consistency of a test from one presentation to the next.

The nature of the test also may contribute to variability. Most tests are inherently variable, such that simply taking the test two times will yield somewhat different results, even if all testing parameters are held constant. If a test presents a closed set of choices, the patient may perform better on one day than another as a function of chance.

Finally, test conditions can affect variability. Changes in any of the following variables can shift test scores:

- **Mode of presentation:** for example, changing from live-voice stimuli to recorded stimuli may result in a decline in scores.
- **Location:** for example, changing from a sound-treated booth to a clinic office may also lead to decreased performance.
- **Talker:** for example, someone who is familiar versus unfamiliar, and someone who is male rather than female, will typically be easier to understand.
- **The number of times an item is repeated:** for example, presenting a test item twice, or as often as an individual requests, usually leads to better performance than presenting it only once.

Reliability is the degree to which a group of test takers will achieve the same scores with repeated administrations of a test.

Test–Retest Reliability and Validity

An issue closely related to variability is test **reliability**. Reliability of a test relates to the extent that test results are repeatable, and the level of reliability is expressed in terms of a standard error of measurement. Mendel and Danhauer (1997) describe reliability as follows:

> "Reliability concerns the extent to which measurements are repeatable by the same individual using different measures of the attribute, or by different people using the same measure of the attribute without the interference of error (Bilger, 1984). Reliability can be expressed in terms of the standard error of measurement. If a listener is given the same test many times, the score determined from an average of the test scores would approach some value (that is, the true score) more and more closely. The degree to which a single test score approximates the true score determines the reliability of the test" (pp. 10–11).

In addition to being reliable, a test of speech recognition should also have good **validity**, meaning that the corpus of test items representatively sample the domains and indicators of interest and provide a good estimate of the construct of speech recognition ability. Martin and Clark (2006) present three criteria for assessing the validity of a speech recognition test:

1. How well it measures what it is supposed to measure (a person's difficulties in understanding speech).
2. How favorably a test compares with other similar measures.
3. How the test stands up to alterations of the signal (such as distortion or presentation with noise) that are known to affect other speech tests in specific ways. (p. 127)

Validity is the extent to which a test measures what it is assumed to measure.

Clinical Significance

Another difficulty associated with speech recognition assessment relates to clinical significance. It sometimes is difficult to determine whether a small change in performance is clinically significant. For instance, an individual might recognize 30% of the words in a sentence test prior to receiving speechreading training. Afterward, the person might recognize 36% of the words. In this instance, the clinician must determine whether speechreading has improved in a meaningful way.

A within-subject statistical procedure has been used to compare post-training performance to pretraining performance to establish whether a change is statistically significant. The number of words repeated verbatim in each sentence of a pretraining test can be compared to the number of key words repeated verbatim in the same sentence following training. A paired *t* statistic can be computed using all sentences in a list. Although statistical significance does not necessarily equate with clinical significance, it does indicate whether a change is robust.

MULTICULTURAL ISSUES

With the U.S. population becoming increasingly diverse, multilingual testing has gained importance as an issue in aural rehabilitation. When considering multilingual testing, it is important to determine whether the patient is **monolingual** (speaks only one language) or bilingual (speaks two languages). A **bilingual** individual is sometimes described as being a native speaker, such as a native Spanish speaker, to imply proficiency comparable to that of a language speaker who originates from the country where the language is spoken. Performance on a speech recognition test may vary from one patient to another, depending on whether that person is monolingual or bilingual, and on other such language variables as language history (e.g., When did the individual begin to learn English? Which language was learned first?) and competency (e.g., the individual's proficiency in a language). There is evidence that monolingual and bilingual individuals perform differently from each other on speech recognition tests, and Spanish tests of speech recognition yield better performance than English tests for native Spanish bilingual individuals (see Von Hapsburg & Pena, 2002, for a review). Some evidence suggests that Spanish-English bilingual listeners are more adversely affected by background noise than are monolingual English listeners (Von Hapsburg, Champlin, & Shetty, 2004).

There is a demand for speech recognition materials that are appropriate for non-English-speaking patients or patients who use English as a second language. Unfortunately, the demand at present exceeds the supply. The few examples of tests that have been developed for Spanish-speaking patients include the *Spanish Bisyllables* (Weisleder & Hodgson, 1989), 50-word lists of bisyllabic consonant-vowel-consonant-vowel Spanish words presented in an open-set response format, and the **Synthetic Sentence** *Identification (SSI)* test (Benitez & Speaks, 1968).

Monolingual describes a person who speaks only one language.

Bilingual describes a person who speaks two languages.

Synthetic sentences are syntactically correct but meaningless sentences, and usually include a noun, verb, and object.

One difficulty in assessing non-native English speakers for clinicians is that they may not understand the language of their patients, and hence, may have difficulty in scoring responses to test materials. At least one test, *The Spanish Picture-Identification Test* (McCullough, Wilson, Birck, & Anderson, 1995), has been modified to circumvent this problem (McCullough & Wilson, 2001). The test consists of two 50-word lists. The test words (spoken in a carrier phrase context) are common, bisyllabic nouns and verbs that can be easily pictured. The items are presented in a four-choice closed set, with the foils (or alternative responses) rhyming with the target word. The choices are presented in picture form to patients via a computer screen monitor. The advantage of using the picture-based closed-set format is that the clinician administering the test does not need to understand Spanish to test the patient. In addition, the closed-set results compare similarly to results obtained when the test is administered in an open-set format. The word lists appear in the Key Resources as an example of a Spanish-language test.

Bilingualism Defined

"The broadest definition of a bilingual includes anyone who knows two languages (Baker, 1993). Yet, this definition remains too broad to be useful, because the degree to which an individual knows each language depends on many circumstances. Factors such as when the languages were learned, how the languages were learned, what language skills (reading, writing, speaking, listening) were acquired, and how the languages are used on a daily basis affect the state of bilingualism in any individual. Some consider bilinguals only those who are equally fluent in both of their languages, known as *balanced* bilinguals or *ambilinguals.* . . . A functional or holistic view of bilingualism takes into consideration that individuals learn and use each of their languages for different purposes and in different communication contexts. Therefore, a functional view of bilingualism recognizes that a bilingual may become more competent in one language in certain communication contexts and competent in the other language for other contexts. From the functional perspective, then, it becomes important to ask why the languages were acquired, how they were acquired, when they were acquired, and how they are used" (Von Hapsburg & Pena, 2002, p. 203).

CASE STUDY

Reasons to Go with a Test Battery Approach

Lindsey Mooreland, an audiologist, wanted to compare the listening skills of three of her older male patients. At first, she thought she might administer only a word test, the *Children's Audiovisual Enhancement Test (CAVET)*. Because she had extra time, she went ahead and administered a consonant test (*The Iowa Consonant Test*) and a sentence test (*The Iowa Sentence Test*), too. The results for the three real-life patients appear in Table 2-6.

Table 2-6. Percentage correct scores for three patients on three different tests that each present a different stimulus type, presented in an audition-only condition.

TEST AND STIMULUS TYPE	PATIENTS' SCORES IN %		
	Al	Tom	Bob
Iowa Consonant Test (Consonants)	55	61	87
CAVET (Words)	45	45	30
Iowa Sentence Test (Sentences)	58	38	48

If she had administered only the word test, the three men would have appeared similar in their listening skills. Scores ranged from a low of 30% words correct (Bob) to a high of 45% (Al and Tom).

The test battery approach reveals a more complex picture, and the conclusions as to which patient has the best listening skills is not as straightforward as it would have been if she had administered only a word test. In terms of consonant recognition, Bob scored the highest of the three (87% consonant correct), whereas Al scored the lowest (55% correct). For sentence recognition, Al scored the highest (58% words correct) and Tom scored the lowest (38%).

Time available for testing and the purpose for assessment will dictate in large part which and how many tests are administered to a patient. However, if a clinician administers only a single test, it is important to be aware that the test result may not provide a complete picture of the construct of speech recognition for a particular patient.

FINAL REMARKS

In this chapter, we considered in a general way how to assess individuals' ability to recognize speech. We have not focused on particular tests; rather, we have focused on the principles that must be considered when choosing a test for a particular individual. The results of speech recognition testing are invaluable when designing an aural rehabilitation plan.

KEY CHAPTER POINTS

- A typical audiological assessment includes an audiogram, a determination of speech recognition thresholds, and an assessment of speech recognition. The audiogram by itself does not always adequately reflect the magnitude of a patient's communication difficulties.

- The optimal test environment is a sound-treated booth.

- A speech and hearing professional might assess speech recognition abilities for any number of reasons. For instance, an audiologist might be interested in evaluating a patient's need for amplification or assessing the patient's performance over time.

- Patient variables, such as the cognitive/linguistic skill of the test taker, will influence selection of test materials. For example, an audiologist would not select a sentence test for evaluating a 3-year-old child.

- Test stimuli may be phonemes, words, phrases, unrelated sentences, or topically related sentences. Each kind of stimulus offers advantages and disadvantages.

- Once test materials have been selected, decisions can be made about test procedures. For example, an audiologist might opt to present the stimuli in an audition-only condition, using recorded voice and background noise.

- Patients may learn the items in a test with repeated testing.

- A test should have good reliability and validity.

- Test–retest variability sometimes is an important issue. Some people, especially children, may vary in their performance from day to day.

- Although multicultural testing is ever more commonplace, the need for speech recognition tests in languages other than English outstrips the current supply.

- Bilingual individuals perform better on tests administered in their native language than on tests administered in their second language.

TERMS AND CONCEPTS TO REMEMBER

Audiogram

Degree of hearing loss

Effects of hearing loss on word recognition

Test selection

Speech features

Information transmission analysis

Speechreading enhancement

Closed and open sets

Reliability and validity

Bilingual

◢ MULTIPLE-CHOICE QUESTIONS

1. Mrs. Mills complains that she can hear speech with no problem, even if the talker is speaking softly, but that she cannot understand it well. Her configuration of hearing loss is most likely:

    a. Low-frequency
    b. Flat
    c. High-frequency
    d. Saucer-shaped

2. A child who has a severe hearing loss and who is not wearing a hearing aid may:

    a. Recognize speech fairly well in quiet situations, but may recognize only about 50% of the words spoken in the presence of noise
    b. Barely even hear voices, unless the talker is speaking loudly
    c. Perceive speech as vibrations
    d. Get most of the message, unless conversing in group situations

3. The purpose of speech recognition testing:

    a. Will dictate one's choice of test
    b. May vary, but one will always present a phonetically balanced word list
    c. Is often to compare listening devices
    d. Is determined by the native langauge of the patient

4. Stimuli such as *eepee* and *eesee* might be included in a test designed to assess a patient's:

    a. Word recognition
    b. Feature utilization
    c. Nonlinguistic sound recognition
    d. Hearing acuity

5. In speech testing, a neighborhood refers to:

    a. The group of words having similar acoustic-phonetic characteristics
    b. A battery of tests administered for a specific purpose
    c. Test stimuli included on a specific test
    d. A set of phonemes that cluster together in a feature analysis

6. A Spanish bilingual patient:

   a. Will perform the same as an English monolingual patient on *The Iowa Sentence Test*

   b. Must be tested by a clinician who speaks Spanish

   c. Cannot take a word or sentence speech recognition test

   d. Is considered a native bilingual if he or she speaks the language like someone from the country of origin

7. The advantage afforded by adding hearing to vision is known as:

   a. Speechreading enhancement

   b. Speechreading

   c. Audition-plus-vision speech recognition

   d. A normalized ratio

8. Which is seldom true when testing speech recognition?

   a. A closed-set response mode is employed.

   b. The test stimuli are presented live-voice.

   c. Female talkers speak the stimuli.

   d. Stimuli are isolated words.

9. Equivalent lists are sometimes used to bypass the difficulties associated with:

   a. Test–retest variability

   b. Test reliability

   c. Learning effects

   d. Patient variability

10. An audiologist is about to administer a speech recognition test in the presence of background noise. The audiologist has chosen a noise source that best mimics a crowded convention hall. This noise is:

   a. White noise

   b. Pink noise

   c. Competing talker

   d. Speech noise

11. A group of researchers attempted to validate a new test of speech recognition. The test demonstrated poor validity for the following reason:

   a. Persons with severe hearing loss performed about as well as persons with moderate hearing loss.

   b. Test takers performed more poorly on the test when it was administered in white noise than when it was administered in quiet.

c. Persons who recognized many words also recognized many words on the *Lexical Neighborhood Test.*

d. Scores for the test takers improved dramatically when they retook the test on a subsequent day.

KEY RESOURCES

 THE LEXICAL NEIGHBORHOOD TEST

(Kirk, Pisoni, & Osberger, 1995)

List 1

Easy words: juice, good, drive, time, hard, gray, foot, orange, count, brown, home, old watch, need, food, dance, live, stand, six, cold, push, stop, girl, hurt, cow.

Hard words: thumb, pie, wet, fight, toe, cut, pink, hi, song, fun, use, mine, ball, kick, tea, book, bone, work, dad, game, lost, cook, gum, cap, meat.

List 2

Easy words: down, truck, mouth, pig, give, school, boy, put, three, farm, fish, green, catch, break, house, sit, friend, jump, bird, swim, hold, want, snake, more, white.

Hard words: ear, hand, dry, zoo, goat, toy, call, sing, cut, wrong, bed, fat, man, run, hot, read, grow, bag, cake, seat, nine, sun, bath, ten, ride.

 CID EVERYDAY SENTENCES

(Silverman & Hirsh, 1955)

List A

1. Walking's my favorite exercise.
2. Here's a nice quiet place to rest.
3. Our janitor sweeps the floors every night.
4. It would be much easier if everyone would help.
5. Good morning.

6.   Open your window before you go to bed!

7.   Do you think that she should stay out so late?

8.   How do you feel about changing the time when we begin work?

9.   Here we go.

10.   Move out of the way!

List B

1.   The water's too cold for swimming.

2.   Why should I get up so early in the morning?

3.   Here are your shoes.

4.   It's raining.

5.   Where are you going?

6.   Come here when I call you!

7.   Don't try to get out of it this time!

8.   Should we let little children go to the movies by themselves?

9.   There isn't enough paint to finish the room.

10.   Do you want an egg for breakfast?

List C

1.   Everybody should brush his teeth after meals.

2.   Everything's all right.

3.   Don't use up all the paper when you write your letter.

4.   That's right.

5.   People ought to see a doctor once a year.

6.   Those windows are so dirty I can't see anything outside.

7.   Pass the bread and butter please.

8.   Don't forget to pay your bill before the first of the month.

9.   Don't let the dog out of the house.

10.   There's a good ball game this afternoon.

List D

1. It's time to go.

2. If you don't want these old magazines, throw them out.

3. Do you want to wash up?

4. It's a real dark night so watch your driving.

5. I'll carry the package for you.

6. Did you forget to shut off the water?

7. Fishing in a mountain stream is my idea of a good time.

8. Fathers spend more time with their children than they used to.

9. Be careful not to break your glasses.

10. I'm sorry.

List E

1. You can catch the bus across the street.

2. Call her on the phone and tell her the news.

3. I'll catch up with you later.

4. I'll think it over.

5. I don't want to go to the movies tonight.

6. If your tooth hurts that much you ought to see a dentist.

7. Put the cookie back in the box!

8. Stop fooling around!

9. Time's up.

10. How do you spell your name?

List F

1. Music always cheers me up.

2. My brother's in town for a short while on business.

3. We live a few miles from the main road.

4. This suit needs to go to the cleaners.

5. They ate enough green apples to make them sick for a week.

6. Where have you been all this time?

7. Have you been working hard lately?

8. There's not enough room in the kitchen for a new table.

9. Where is he?

10. Look out!

List G

1. I'll see you right after lunch.

2. See you later.

3. White shoes are awful to keep clean.

4. Stand there and don't move until I tell you.

5. There's a big piece of cake left over from dinner.

6. Wait for me at the corner in front of the drugstore.

7. It's no trouble at all.

8. Hurry up!

9. The morning paper didn't say anything about rain this afternoon or tonight.

10. The phone call's for you.

List H

1. Believe me!

2. Let's get a cup of coffee.

3. Let's get out of here before it's too late.

4. I hate driving at night.

5. There was water in the cellar after that heavy rain yesterday.

6. She'll only be a few minutes.

7. How do you know?

8. Children like candy.

9. If we don't get rain soon, we'll have no grass.

10. They're not listed in the new phone book.

List I

1. Where can I find a place to work?

2. I like those big red apples we always get in the fall.

3. You'll get fat eating candy.

4. The show's over.

5. Why don't they paint their walls some other color?

6. What's new?

7. What are you hiding under your coat?

8. How come I should always be the one to go first?

9. I'll take sugar and cream in my coffee.

10. Wait just a minute!

List J

1. Breakfast is ready.

2. I don't know what's wrong with the car, but it won't start.

3. It sure takes a sharp knife to cut this meat.

4. I haven't read a newspaper since we bought a television set.

5. Weeds are spoiling the yard.

6. Call me a little later!

7. Do you have change for a $5 bill?

8. How are you?

9. I'd like some ice cream with my pie.

10. I don't think I'll have any dessert.

THE CHILDREN'S AUDIOVISUAL ENHANCEMENT TEST (CAVET)

(Tye-Murray & Geers, 2002)

List A

Easy to identify, vision-only:	*Difficult to identify, vision-only:*
1. telephone	11. ten
2. elephant	12. hug
3. mouth	13. rock
4. fish	14. talk
5. newspaper	15. sit
6. hamburger	16. cat
7. warm	17. full
8. thumb	18. sing
9. chair	19. birthday cake
10. ship	20. map

List B

Easy to identify, vision-only:	*Difficult to identify, vision-only:*
1. family	11. line
2. remember	12. neck
3. basketball	13. kill
4. bath	14. kiss
5. beautiful	15. dinosaur
6. ice cream cone	16. sock
7. look	17. juice
8. shoe	18. foot
9. light	19. math
10. cheese	20. Mickey Mouse

List C

Easy to identify, vision-only: *Difficult to identify, vision-only:*

1. grandfather
2. fall
3. policeman
4. farm
5. ball
6. butterfly
7. push
8. love
9. hear
10. chocolate

11. down
12. plate
13. six
14. good
15. hill
16. tall
17. sun
18. car
19. pull
20. vegetable

THE QUICK SIN TEST

(Etymotic Research, 2001)

(Note: the sentences are presented in increasing levels of noise. The first sentence is presented with a 25 SNR with the noise level increasing in 5-dB increments such that the sixth sentence is presented at a 0-dB SNR. The test includes 18 lists, consisting of six sentences each.)

A sample list.

1. A white silk jacket goes with any shoes.

2. The child crawled into the dense grass.

3. Footprints showed the path he took up the beach.

5. A vent near the edge brought in fresh air.

6. It is a band of steel three inches wide.

7. The weight of the package was seen on the high scale.

WORDS COMPRISING THE SPANISH PICTURE-IDENTIFICATION TASK

(McCullough & Wilson, 2001)

LIST 1	LIST 1 *(continued)*	LIST 2	LIST 2 *(continued)*
Balón (balloon)	Mono (monkey)	Ala (wing)	Mesa (table)
Barba (beard)	Niña (girl)	Balcón (balcony)	Moto (motorcycle)
Barca (boat)	Ojo (eye)	Barra (bar)	Nota (note)
Besa (kiss)	Oso (bear)	Bastón (cane)	Ocho (eight)
Boca (mouth)	Pala (shovel)	Bata (robe)	Oro (gold)
Bola (ball)	Papa (potato)	Beso (kiss)	Peso (money)
Bota (boot)	Pico (sting)	Bola (ball)	Pino (pine tree)
Caja (box)	Pito (whistle)	Bolsa (purse)	Piña (pineapple)
Canta (sing)	Prisa (hurry)	Cabra (goat)	Piso (floor)
Capa (cape)	Queso (cheese)	Cama (bed)	Plaza (plaza)
Cara (face)	Rama (twig)	Caña (cane)	Riña (fight)
Carne (meat)	Ratón (rat)	Carga (load)	Risa (laugh)
Cárcel (jail)	Reza (pray)	Carta (letter)	Roca (rock)
Coger (catch)	Roja (red)	Casa (house)	Ronca (snore)
Cono (cone)	Ropa (rope)	Coca (Coke)	Rosa (rose)
Corer (run)	Rota (broken f.)	Comer (eat)	Roto (broken m.)
Foto (photo)	Sala (living room)	Coser (sew)	Saco (sack)
Gorro (cap)	Salto (jump)	Dama (lady)	Sapo (frog)
Hueso (bone)	Santo (Saint m.)	Fresa (strawberry)	Santa (Saint m.)
Jota (J)	Talon (heel)	Halcón (hawk)	Tapa (lid)
Ladrón (robber)	Tasa (cup)	Jamón (ham)	Tisa (chalk)
Llama (knock)	Toca (knock)	Llanta (tire)	Tono (note)
Manta (blanket)	Toro (bull)	Lloro (cry)	Trono (throne)
Masa (dough)	Viña (vine)	Mala (sick-f)	Vota (vote)
Misa (mass)	Voto (vote)	Mapa (map)	Zorro (fox)

CHAPTER 3

Listening Devices and Related Technology

OUTLINE

- Hearing aids
- Cochlear implants
- Assistive listening devices (ALDs)
- Case study: Listen to the music
- Final remarks
- Key chapter points
- Terms and concepts to remember
- Multiple-choice questions
- Appendix 3-1

After a patient receives a comprehensive audiological assessment, and before he or she receives auditory or speechreading training, appropriate listening devices are selected and fitted. These systems may include a hearing aid or a cochlear implant, or assistive listening devices (ALDs). The provision of appropriate technical devices is an essential element in the aural rehabilitation plan, whether the patient is an adult or a child. These instruments can minimize conversational difficulties and maximize the use of residual hearing for daily functioning.

The primary objectives for providing an individual with a listening device are twofold:

1. To make speech audible, without introducing distortion or discomfort, and
2. To restore a range of loudness experience

In optimal circumstances, the three kinds of listening devices that are reviewed in this chapter can be selected and fitted to achieve the two objectives just listed.

This chapter presents an introduction for readers who are unacquainted with listening devices and a key-points review for those who are familiar with them. Both related terminology and categories within device types will be considered.

HEARING AIDS

Prior to the 20th century, there were three ways to help a person with hearing loss hear better: (a) speak loudly, (b) talk right into the person's ear, or (c) provide the person with an ear horn, speaking tube, trumpet, or other similar device. The advent of electronic hearing aids revolutionized the methods available to assist patients to hear more. To appreciate the relatively rapid advances that have occurred in hearing aid technology since 1847, it is worthwhile to review Table 3-1. This table highlights some of the landmark events that have occurred in hearing aid design.

Two major trends are evident in modern hearing aid design: miniaturization and enhanced signal processing. Over time, hearing aids have become smaller. Early hearing aids were so large and cumbersome, they were not portable. These tabletop electrical aids often were used only in educational settings where teacher and students might sit around a shared table. The early portable aids were not much of an improvement over the tabletop devices. They were housed in large cases that had to be carried on the body or with the hand and were operated with vacuum tubes. Vacuum tubes were

Table 3-1. Some landmark events in the history of hearing aid technology and marketing. Siemens, Oticon, Telex, Beltone, Maico, Dahlberg, Miracle-Ear, Widex, Starkey, Argosy, Microtronic, Philips, and Danavox are companies that manufacture hearing aids (BTE = behind-the-ear hearing aid; ITE = in-the-ear hearing aid; ITC = in-the-canal hearing aid).

1847:	Siemens is founded in Germany by Werner von Siemens. Makes many improvements in telegraph, telephone, and electric transmission systems.
1890:	National Carbon Company is founded, and later becomes Eveready Battery Co.
1904:	The company that later becomes Oticon is founded by Hans Demant to import American hearing aids to Denmark.
1910:	Siemens makes its first hearing aids for employees, offering them to the public in 1912. Early aids are hand-carried.
1914:	Siemens introduces a small hearing aid receiver fitted close to the auditory canal, with sound carried via an animal membrane.
1919:	Siemens makes the first commercially available audiometer.
1924:	Siemens patents first compact carbon microphone amplifier for use in pocket hearing aids.
1929:	Siemens builds first wearable tube amplifiers with improved response and loudness.
1940:	Maico introduces its first wearable hearing aid (made in three parts) incorporating miniature vacuum tubes.
1944:	Beltone introduces first all-in-one hearing aid, the Mono-Pac.
1953:	Maico markets first completely transistorized hearing aid.
1955:	Dahlberg introduces the Miracle-Ear, the first electronic hearing aid designed to be worn in the ear. That same year, Dahlberg introduces innovative BTE and eyeglass instruments, and begins providing private-level hearing aids to Sears Roebuck. Siemens's first transistor hearing aid introduces the telecoil.
1961:	Siemens introduces Auriculina, the first BTE with frontal sound pickup.
1962:	Miracle-Ear IV is first hearing aid to use integrated circuitry.
1967:	Siemens develops a BTE with push-pull amplifier, and introduces the Fonator speech/auditory training instrument. Widex introduces a sound hook to reduce wind noise.
1971:	Maico patents dephasing microphone that offers directional hearing.
1972:	Starkey establishes right of return policy for its custom full-concha hearing aids.
1976:	Danavox is first hearing aid manufacturer to launch a direct audio input system. Siemens introduces BTE with input compression.
1979:	Oticon introduces E24V, the first hearing aid with a user-operated switch to choose between omni- and directional microphones.
1982:	Argosy Electronics releases the CCA, the industry's first successful in-the-canal instrument.
1986:	Beltone's new Suprimo hearing aid, offering three custom integrated circuits and eight fitting controls, is a long step toward a fully programmable instrument.
1988:	Philips introduces infrared remote-controlled ITEs and ITCs.
1989:	Maico offers the first programmable hearing aid.
1991:	Philips introduces the first very-deep-canal instrument, the XP Peritympanic.
1992:	Danavox introduces DFS Genius, a digital system for suppressing feedback.
1995:	Oticon announces DigiFocus, the first 100% digital ear-level hearing aid. Maico offers the first programmable CIC.
1996:	Telex introduces SoftWear, a completely soft-shelled hearing aid.
1997:	Argosy introduces Quadrasound, a proprietary microchip providing access to four separate signal processors within each hearing instrument. Widex introduces first digital signal–processing instrument in a CIC model. Telex introduces the AcuSound, the first hearing aid to split the incoming signal into two channels based on the signal's amplitude.

continues

Table 3-1. *continued*

2000:	Songbird Medical Inc. offers a disposable hearing aid for about $40, which provides about 40 days of usage.
2001:	Oticon introduces open-ear acoustics, a system designed to use active feedback cancellation to allow for open-ear fittings to eliminate occlusion.
2002:	Active feedback cancellation is introduced into mainline hearing aids, allowing for venting large enough to relieve occlusion for many patients.
2003:	Mini-BTEs with thin tubes enter the market, allowing for significantly improved cosmetics.
2005:	Receiver-in-the-Ear (RITE) hearing aids are released into the market.
2007:	BTEs account for 50% of the hearing aid market only a few years after bottoming out at 20%.

Adapted from "A timeline of the hearing industry" (1991). *The Hearing Journal, 50,* 54–70. Updated with input from Donald Schum, personal communication, [March], 2007.

Signal processing involves manipulation of various parameters of a signal.

Some hearing aids have **multiple memories** that allow the speech signal to be processed in more than one way.

Multiple memory hearing aids allow the user to select the processing strategy according to the listening environment.

Noise reduction is the difference in the sound pressure level (SPL) of a noise measured at two different locations.

Acoustic feedback cancellation is a feature that avoids the annoying squeal produced by hearing aids when the microphone picks up the amplified sound from the hearing aid and reamplifies it.

Programmability in a hearing aid means that several parameters of the instrument, such as gain, are controlled by a computer.

A hearing aid that uses **digital processing** converts the signal from analog to digital form, processes the signal to achieve a target, and then converts the signal back to an analog form.

replaced by transistors, which made it possible for hearing aids to be worn on the head. In the last several decades, there have been advances toward miniaturization so now it is possible to use a hearing aid and have it be completely invisible, unless someone looks directly into the ear. Probably the primary factor spurring this trend toward miniaturization is cosmetic concerns on the part of the users.

Along with miniaturization, there has been another trend evident in hearing aid designs, and that is a growing sophistication in their **signal-processing** capabilities (ability to alter the signal in some way, usually according to a processing algorithm), all in virtual real time. Some of the advances related to developments in signal processing include the following:

- **Multiple memories**, so that a patient might adjust the hearing aid one way when listening in quiet and another way when listening in noise, to maximize sound quality and speech reception. Hearing aids that provide access to different amplification characteristics sometimes are referred to as **multiple memory hearing aids**.
- Sophisticated **noise reduction** circuits, so that the hearing aid amplifies speech and not undesirable background noise (see Yuen, Kam, & Lau, 2006, for a review).
- **Acoustic feedback cancellation**, so that hearing aids will not "whistle" when sound escapes from the receiver.
- **Programmability**, which allows the audiologist to set gain, frequency response, and other electroacoustic properties of the hearing aid. This feature may be especially attractive if the user is experiencing a progressive hearing loss, and the hearing aid must be altered over time to accommodate the changing listening needs.
- **Digital processing**, so that the signal is converted from analog to digital form, processed to achieve a target signal, and then converted back to an analog signal.

- **Multiple channels**, a signal-processing technique wherein the signal is filtered into frequency bands, so that some bands (such as the high-frequency bands or the bands that carry speech information) receive more gain or amplification than other bands (such as the low-frequency bands or bands that contain a high level of noise).

A hearing aid that uses **multiple channels** filters the signal into frequency bands so that some bands (usually the high-frequency bands) can receive more gain than others.

Although these trends are indicative of evolving designs, there are some constants in the components that make up a hearing aid, no matter what the style or special features.

Hearing Aid Components

Figure 3-1 provides a schematic of a generic hearing aid. The **microphone** picks up the acoustic signal from the ambient environment. The microphone component converts the acoustic signal into an electrical signal. The electrical signal then passes to the **amplifier**, where the signal is selectively amplified. For example, only the high frequencies of a signal may be boosted. From the amplifier, the processed electrical signal passes to the receiver. The receiver converts the processed electrical signal back into an acoustic signal and passes it on through any tubing and earmold.

A **microphone** is a transducer that converts an audio signal into an electronic signal.

An **amplifier** increases the intensity of sound.

The hearing aid also carries **batteries**, which provide power for its operation. Batteries come in at least four sizes (denoted by the following codes, from largest capacity or milliamp hours to smallest: 675, 13, 312, and 10). Although battery life is dependent on a number of factors, such as the kind

A **battery** is a cell that provides electrical power.

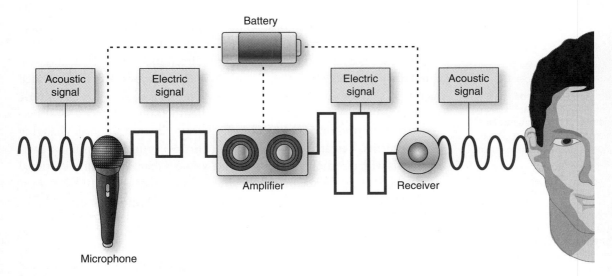

FIGURE 3-1. Schematic of a hearing aid.

of battery it is, the style of hearing aid in which it is used, and the volume control setting, a zinc battery will last about 1 to 4 weeks.

Microphones

Microphones are designed to respond to sound, without distorting it or introducing extraneous noise. The microphone converts the audio signal into an electrical signal. The volume inside of a modern microphone case is divided into two parts by a thin polymer diaphragm. On one side is a thin metal coating that allows the diaphragm to conduct electricity. Parallel to the diaphragm is a metal backplate with an electret coating. This coated backplate can permanently store static electrical charge. The static charge on the electret causes a strong electric field to form between the diaphragm and the backplate. When the diaphragm moves from its resting position, a small voltage develops between the diaphragm and the backplate. So when a microphone is in action, sound waves travel into its front volume, causing the diaphragm to vibrate. These oscillations create an oscillating voltage signal between the diaphragm and the backplate conductor. It is this signal that is passed on to the amplifier.

Directional microphones are more sensitive to sound originating from in front of the user than to sound coming from behind the user.

Omnidirectional microphones are sensitive to sound coming from all directions.

There are two general types of microphones: directional and omnidirectional. **Directional microphones** are designed to respond primarily to sound originating from in front of the user, and not from the back. **Omnidirectional microphones** respond to sound originating from all directions. Directional microphones enhance the signal-to-noise ratio for the user. For instance, a directional microphone will pick up the speech of a talker who stands in front of the user, but not from two individuals who speak about something else in the back of the room. As such, directional microphones are often desirable for listening in noisy situations. Some hearing aids include automatic directional systems, which have a switching algorithm that automatically switches the patient's hearing aid between an omnidirectional microphone mode in quiet situations and a directional mode in noisy situations, according to such factors as signal-to-noise ratio and the level of the sound. Some **automatic directional microphones (ADMs)** even alter their directional response patterns so as to optimize the signal-to-noise ratio in continuously changing environments. Research suggests that patients perform better in noisy environments with directional and ADM microphones than with omnidirectional microphones (e.g., Bentler, 2005; Bentler, Palmer, & Mueller, 2006; Blamey, Fiket, & Steele, 2006; Yuen et al., 2006; Ricketts, Galster, & Tharpe, 2007).

Automatic directional microphones (ADMs) automatically switch between an omnidirectional and directional mode according to environmental conditions.

Amplifiers

The **gain** of a hearing aid is the difference in decibels between the input level of an acoustic signal and the output level.

An amplifier is also a component in all hearing aids. Amplifiers increase the level of the signal. **Gain** describes the amount of amplification provided by an amplifier and is defined as the difference between the hearing aid's input and output. For instance, if an input signal is 30-dB SPL and the output is 60-dB SPL, the gain of the hearing aid is 30 dB.

The signal is selectively processed and amplified. In many hearing aids, the signal passes through three stages of the amplification process. In the **preamplifier stage**, the signal received from the microphone is boosted. During the **signal-processing stage**, the signal is manipulated to enhance the quality of the sound for the patient. Some amplifiers include digital noise reduction (DNR) schemes designed to amplify speech but not background noise. During the **output stage**, the processed signal is amplified and sent to the hearing aid receiver.

> In the **preamplifier stage,** the signal from the microphone is amplified.
>
> In the **signal-processing stage,** the signal is manipulated to enhance or extract component information.
>
> In the **output stage,** the process signal is boosted.

Amplifiers in analog and digital hearing aids process the signal differently. In an analog hearing aid, the signal is amplified as a continuously varying amplitude over time. In contrast, in a digital hearing aid, sound is converted from an analog signal into a digital representation. The processing is performed on this computer language version. The processed signal is then converted back into an analog signal.

Amplifiers may be classified as one of two types: peak-clipping or compression. These terms refer to their mode of limiting the output of the signal so that it is not so loud as to be uncomfortable to the user nor has the potential to cause a noise-induced hearing loss. The goal of peak-clipping or compression is to limit the **maximum power output (MPO)** of the hearing aid, which is the maximum output level a hearing aid will put out in response to a very loud input signal.

> **Maximum power output (MPO)** is the maximum intensity level that a hearing aid can produce.

An amplifier with a **peak-clipping** circuit provides a constant or linear amount of gain (or amplification) across a range of input levels. There is a one-to-one relationship between the input and output, so that the sound is amplified by a consistent amount until it reaches a saturation level. At this **saturation level**, sound coming into the amplifier is so loud that the amplifier begins to "clip" or cut off the peaks of the signal. Although this effectively limits the level of the audio signal, it also introduces distortion; therefore, sound quality decreases. Figure 3-2 presents an example of the relationship between input and output levels of the hearing aid in a peak-clipping system.

> **Peak-clipping** is a method of limiting hearing aid output in which a constant or linear amount of gain is provided across a range of input levels until it reaches a saturation level, at which time the amplifier begins to "clip" off the peaks of the signal.
>
> **Saturation level** is the point at which an amplifier no longer provides an increase in output compared to input.

A nonlinear amplifier system usually functions with a **compression** circuitry. The use of compression has three purposes. One purpose of compression is to limit the maximum output of the hearing aid, so that sound is never so loud as to cause discomfort to the user.

> **Compression** is a nonlinear form of amplifier gain used to determine and limit output gain as a function of input gain.

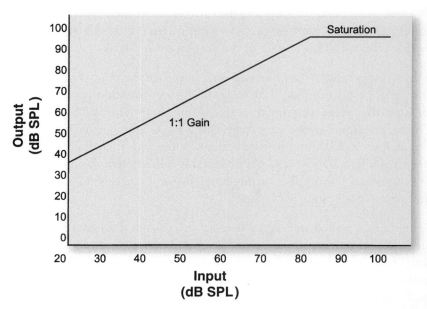

FIGURE 3-2. Input-output loudness function for a hearing aid that uses peak-clipping to limit output.

A second purpose of compression is to provide a range of sounds to the user within the person's dynamic range. As noted in Chapter 2, dynamic range is defined as the difference between a person's threshold for sound and the level at which the sound causes discomfort. In many persons with significant hearing loss, dynamic range is reduced and may be only 40 dB or less.

A third purpose of compression circuitry is to provide a varying amount of gain (amplification) of the speech signal as a function of the input level. Thus, soft sounds are typically amplified more than moderately loud sounds.

Kneepoint is the point on an input–output function where compression is activated.

Compression ratio is the decibel ratio of acoustic input to amplifier output.

In a compression circuitry, sound may be amplified in a linear fashion until it reaches a level of incoming intensity that triggers the compression function. At this point, often referred to as the **kneepoint**, the signal is amplified to a lesser degree, and never amplified beyond a preselected level. This kind of output limiting is used most commonly in today's hearing aids. Figure 3-3 presents the relationship between input and output of a hearing aid that has a compression circuit and indicates the kneepoint. The relation between input and output is referred to as the **compression ratio**, or the ratio of the change in input SPL to the change in the output SPL. For instance, if a sound entering into the amplifier changes by 20 dB but leaves the amplifier changed by 10 dB, that compression ratio is 2:1. The length of time it takes for a compression amplifier to react to a loud sound and

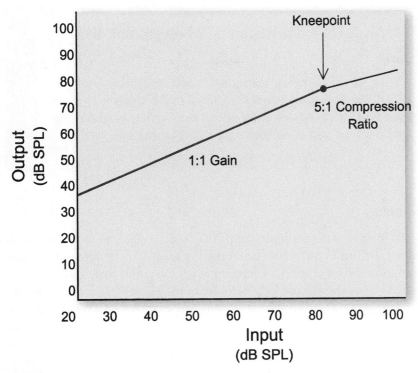

FIGURE 3-3. Input-output loudness function for a hearing aid that uses compression circuitry to limit output.

compress it is referred to as an **attack time**. For example, if it takes 50 ms for a sound of 120 dB SPL to be compressed to a level of 90 dB SPL, than the attack time is 50 ms. Similarly, the **release time** is the length of time for a compression amplifier to increase its gain after a loud sound has ceased. There are different kinds of compression circuits. For example, the K-AMP circuit provides more gain for high frequencies than low frequencies at low-intensity input levels, but not for high-intensity input levels. **Multiband compression** permits different degrees of compression and output limiting for different frequency bands in the incoming signal, so that the growth of loudness in a signal can be controlled, and the signal can be shaped to maximize speech recognition.

Attack time is the time between when a signal begins to the onset of its steady-state amplified value.

Release time is the time it takes for an amplifier to return to its steady state after a loud sound ends.

Multiband compression is a method of shaping the loudness growth of a signal to maximize speech for the listener using different degrees of compression and output limiting for different frequencies.

Receivers

The processed electrical signal enters the other energy transducer of the hearing aid, the receiver, where it is converted back to acoustic energy. In a sense, the receiver is a mini loudspeaker or a microphone in reverse (i.e., whereas the receiver converts the electrical signal into an acoustic signal, the microphone converts the acoustic signal into an electrical signal).

Why Is It Called a Receiver When It's Sending Out Sound?

The tradition of calling the hearing aid's miniature loudspeaker a "receiver" hails back to the telephone industry. The term comes from the speaker in the hand piece of the telephone. The receiver end of the hand piece received an electrical signal from the telephone.

Earmolds

In addition to a microphone, amplifier, and receiver, some hearing aids require the use of earmolds (whereas the casing actually replaces the earmold in many other kinds of hearing aids). Earmolds deliver sound from the receiver to the ear and help hold the hearing aid in place. Earmolds are custom-made to fit into the ear canal of the user. An earmold attaches to plastic tubing, which leads to the hearing aid receiver. It can be constructed in a variety of configurations to suit the needs of the individual user. For instance, some earmolds fill the entire concha of the ear, whereas others consist only of a half-ring that anchors it within the concha. The former style of earmold might be used for a severe or profound hearing loss, and the latter for a mild loss.

Other Features of Hearing Aids

In addition to the components previously shown in Figure 3-1, some hearing aids have additional features. These include an on–off control, a volume control, a telecoil, and a remote control.

On–Off Control

The **on–off control** is a small switch that moves back and forth to turn the hearing aid off when not in use and on when needed; may be incorporated into the volume wheel.

The **on–off control** may be a small switch that moves back and forth to turn the hearing aid off when not in use and on when the hearing aid is needed. The on–off control also may be incorporated into the volume control wheel. When a hearing aid does not have an on–off switch, the hearing aid is activated by inserting the battery.

Audio Input

Many behind-the-ear hearing aids have an audio input that allows an audio signal to be input directly from the signal source. This direct input eliminates distortion from the surrounding environment. For example, a cable may be used to couple the hearing aid directly to a television or radio. The audio input consists of electrical contacts that accommodate a plug or an **audio boot**. It has a separate preamplifier from the microphone.

Telecoil

The **telecoil** (sometimes called a *t-coil* or an *audiocoil*) is an inductive coil within a hearing aid (i.e., a coil of wire wrapped around a magnetized metal rod) that enhances telephone communication. The telephone receiver emits electromagnetic signals, which are picked up by the hearing aid telecoil. The hearing aid microphone thus is bypassed. The signal picked up by the telecoil is amplified and transduced to an audio signal, and then delivered to the ear. If the hearing aid has an on–off switch, it may include a *T* position for *telecoil* and an *M* position for *microphone,* so the user can switch on the telecoil before using the telephone. An *MT* option on the on–off switch allows for simultaneous use of both the telecoil and microphone. Some aids include a "touchless telecoil," where close proximity of a telephone automatically switches the hearing aid's microphone to the telephone mode. Use of a telecoil minimizes acoustic feedback problems and prevents the transmission of ambient room noise. As will be noted later in this chapter, telecoils can be used to pick up signals from assistive listening devices too. Some of the small hearing aid models, such as a completely-in-the-canal style, are too small to incorporate telecoils.

Volume Control

A **volume control** allows the user to adjust the level of amplification. It usually is a rotating wheel.

Remote Control

A **remote control** is a handheld device that can serve two purposes (Figure 3-4). First, it can be used to program the electroacoustic properties of a hearing aid. Second, a remote control can be used to switch the hearing aid from one channel to another, to adjust the volume, and to turn it off and on.

Hearing Aid Styles

Now that we have considered the basic components of a hearing aid, let us review the ways in which the components can be packaged to function as a listening device. There are at least five styles of hearing aids. These are body aids, behind-the-ear (BTE) aids, in-the-ear (ITE) aids, in-the-canal (ITC)

An **audio boot,** also called a *shoe,* is a device that is used with a behind-the-ear hearing aid for coupling to a direct audio input cord.

A **telecoil** is an induction coil that receives electromagnetic signals from a telephone or loop amplification system.

The **volume control** on a hearing aid is used to adjust its output; may be manual or automatic.

A **remote control** is a handheld device that permits adjustments in the volume or changes in the program of a programmable hearing aid.

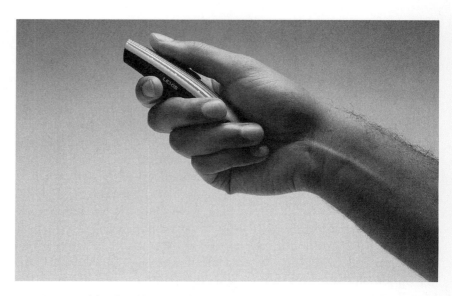

FIGURE 3-4. A hearing aid remote control. *Photograph courtesy of Oticon.*

aids, and completely-in-the-canal (CIC) aids. Most hearing aid manufacturers have a Web site where their products can be viewed and examples of each of these styles are presented. A listing of hearing aid manufacturers and their contact information appears in Appendix 3-1.

Body Aids

The body-aid casement is about the size of a deck of cards and is worn on the torso. The casement leads to a custom-made earmold by means of a long cord. The body-worn casement houses the microphone, amplifier, and receiver. **Body hearing aids** may provide powerful amplification and are useful for severe and profound hearing losses. They also have large controls, so they can be used by individuals who have reduced manual dexterity. Body aids are durable and can be harnessed to a young child so that the likelihood of the hearing aid being lost or damaged may be reduced.

Despite these advantages, body aids are not used often today in either the United States or Europe, although they are more popular in developing countries due to their relative economy. They are somewhat bulky and highly visible. The placement of the microphone on the chest rather than near the ear also may decrease a user's ability to localize sound. They sometimes are used with children who have a pinna that cannot support a BTE hearing aid and with children who have atresia, microtia, or chronic otitis media. For these latter children, the body aid may be attached to a **bone-conductor**, converting it into a **bone-conduction hearing aid**. In this arrangement, sound is delivered to the inner ear via the bone vibrator worn

A **body hearing aid** includes a box worn on the torso and a cord connecting it to an ear-level receiver.

A **bone-conductor** is a vibrator or oscillator used to transmit sound to the bones of the skull by means of vibration.

A **bone-conduction hearing aid** delivers the amplified signal via a bone vibrator placed over the mastoid directly to the cochlea, bypassing the middle ear.

behind the pinna and over the mastoid bone. The vibrations are transmitted through the bones of the skull directly to the cochlea, bypassing the middle ear altogether.

Behind-the-Ear (BTE) Hearing Aids

The **behind-the-ear hearing aid (BTE)** components are built into a small shell that fits behind the pinna (Figure 3-5). The hearing aid case is typically connected to an earmold by a small plastic tube. In BTEs with open-ear fittings, there is no earmold but only a tubing system. This is probably the most flexible style of hearing aid because it can be fitted with many available options, such as a powerful telecoil circuit. In addition, an earmold can be constructed to accommodate the user, which may be desirable for several reasons. For instance, if a child suffers from chronic otitis media, then he or she might not be able to use a device that occludes the ear canal, as does an ITE aid. If a child who uses a BTE is still growing, the earmold can simply be recast when the ear outgrows the existing one. With smaller hearing aid styles, such as ITEs, a new hearing aid must be recast as it becomes too small to accommodate a child's growing skull.

The style of hearing aid known as a **behind-the-ear (BTE)** hearing aid is worn over the pinna and coupled to the ear by means of an earmold.

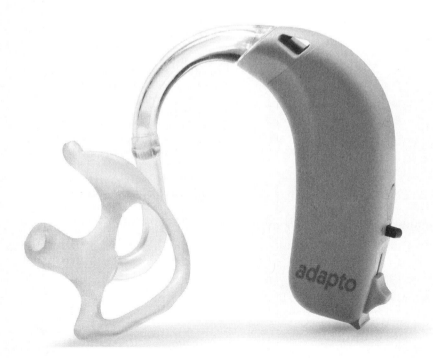

FIGURE 3-5. A behind-the-ear hearing aid and a "skeleton-style" ear mold. *Photograph courtesy of Oticon.*

"Why couldn't hearing technology be as appealing, simple, intuitive and attractive as those mainstream brands [i.e., iPods, MP3s, and cell phones]?" (p. 32)

Suzanne Livingston, co-organizer of a futuristic hearing device exhibit at London's Victoria and Albert Museum

"This exhibit is a step toward [hearing aid stigma] demise. Anything that makes hearing products fashionable or desirable gets my vote. . . . [These designs and concepts] will happen; it's just a matter of time" (p. 34).

Michael Nolan, vice president of European Operations, Starkey Laboratories Inc., commenting on the London exhibit

(Schestok, 2006)

"It was like shopping for sunglasses."

Amy Arra, age 49 years, commenting on the selection of attractive hearing aids available from her audiologist

(Rosenbloom 2007, p. E6)

Other advantages of BTEs include the following:

- When used with a soft earmold, a BTE affords greater safety than ITE hearing aids. This aspect is important especially for children, who may be at high risk for being hit in the ear, say, by a ball in gym class.
- A BTE has the capability of direct audio input, so it can be hardwired to an assistive listening device.
- BTEs have fewer problems with feedback.
- There are fewer repair problems than with other hearing aid styles.
- BTEs are relatively easy to clean, because the earmold can be detached and washed. This aspect is important for individuals who perspire a lot, have wax buildup, or have chronic otitis media.
- A BTE can be used with a nonoccluding earmold, which may be important if the individual has chronic otitis media or is unable to have an occluded ear canal for other reasons.

BTEs may be undesirable if the patient is concerned about cosmetics, as they typically are visible, unless covered by long hair. However, hearing aid designers are increasingly concerned with developing aesthetically pleasing, even trendy, hearing devices (Schestok, 2006) (Figure 3-6). Instead of

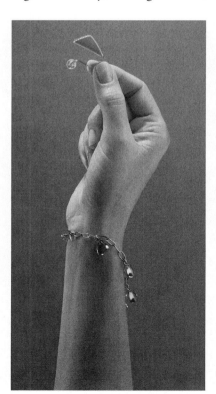

FIGURE 3-6. A hearing aid designed to allay the cosmetic concerns of patients. This stylish triangular design is available in 17 different colors, including *Cabernet Red, Racing Green, Shy Violet,* and *Sunset Orange.* It even comes in an animal print (*Wildlife*) and in checks (*Check*). This is an example of an open-fit hearing aid, a style that is increasingly popular. It has no earmold, and sound is delivered through a thin tubing. This configuration prevents feedback and is cosmetically appealing, although it does not permit a t-coil. *Photograph courtesy of Oticon.*

being stodgy medical devices, the goal is to make them more desirable, like iPods and BlueTooth technology.

In-the-Ear (ITE) and In-the-Canal (ITC) Hearing Aids

In-the-ear (ITE) and **in-the-canal (ITC)** hearing aid styles fit completely in the external ear. A primary difference between the two styles is that the ITC fills less of the concha than does the ITE. The two styles of listening devices must be custom-fitted to the user's ear. The audiologist takes an earmold impression of the ear and then sends the impression to the manufacturer for construction of the aid. The casings of ITEs and ITCs house all of the hearing aid components, and no additional tubing or earmold is necessary. These two styles are the most widely dispensed hearing aids in today's market, probably because of cosmetic reasons. Figure 3-7 presents a photograph of an ITE aid as it is worn in the ear.

The ITC hearing aid offers at least a couple of benefits over BTE aids. The position of the microphone enhances the amplification of high-frequency sounds relative to the BTE aid, and the closeness of the receiver to the tympanic membrane means that less gain is required to provide adequate amplification for a particular level of hearing loss. Although at one time ITC aids did not accommodate telecoils, modern versions include them. Also, earlier versions often did not supply adequate amplification for more severe hearing losses, whereas current versions do. They are not

An **in-the-ear (ITE)** hearing aid fits into the concha of the ear.

An **in-the-canal (ITC)** hearing aid fits in the external ear canal, only partially filling the concha.

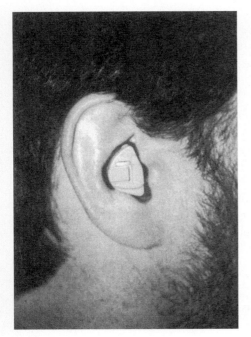

FIGURE 3-7. An in-the-ear hearing aid. *Photograph courtesy of the Central Institute for the Deaf.*

as susceptible to wind noise as are the larger hearing aids. An ITC aid has cosmetic appeal relative to a BTE aid, but does offer some disadvantages comparatively. ITC aids are appropriate for only up to severe hearing losses, and some cannot house telecoils. In the United States, ITE and ITC aids are the most popular styles of hearing aid. They are not quite as popular in Europe, where BTEs lead the market (Vonlanthern, 2000).

Completely-in-the-Canal (CIC) Hearing Aids

A **completely-in-the-canal (CIC)** hearing aid fits entirely within the external ear canal.

Completely-in-the-canal (CIC) aids are worn completely inside the ear canal and do not occupy the concha. They are inserted and removed from the ear canal by means of a short clear cord attached to the hearing aid casement. CIC aids are so small that options often are not available, such as an on–off switch, a volume control, and a telecoil. Some newer devices that use digital technology have remote controls that permit adjustments in gain and program selection. They offer many advantages. They tend to be easy to insert and remove, often more so than trying to insert an earmold, as with a BTE aid. Some people report a better sound quality with CIC aids than with other styles, which is due in part to the absence of an **occlusion effect**. An occlusion effect may occur with most other hearing aid styles. An occlusion effect, caused by plugging the ear canal, may result in speech sounding as if the individual is "listening inside of a barrel." The advantages of CIC aids can be summarized as follows:

In the **occlusion effect,** low-frequency sound in bone-conducted signals is enhanced as a result of closing of the ear canal.

- Easy to handle
- Reduction of an occlusion effect
- Reduction of feedback
- Improved sound localization
- Less electronic gain needed than with other styles, because the volume between the end of the hearing aid and the tympanic membrane (eardrum) is minimal
- Elimination of wind noise
- Enhanced telephone use without the need for additional assistive listening devices
- Virtually invisible to others when inserted into the user's ear canal
- Greater high-frequency gain

Despite the advantages, CIC hearing aids are high-maintenance devices. Cerumen tends to build up, requiring the patient to clean the hearing aid frequently. Current models also do not accommodate directional microphones.

Middle Ear Implants

Unlike conventional hearing aids that pick up sound from the environment, amplify it, and direct it to the tympanic membrane, a middle ear

Binaural Versus Monaural Fitting

Often, the audiologist will recommend that a patient receive two hearing aids instead of one, especially if the hearing loss is moderate or severe (Dillon, 2001). Even though two hearing aids are more expensive than one, and may require more effort to maintain, binaural amplification fitting offers many advantages over a monaural fitting, including the following:

- Elimination of **head shadow:** With one hearing aid, sound coming from the unaided side of the head may be attenuated by as much as 12 to 16 dB, especially high-frequency sounds. Use of two hearing aids allows sound to be received on both sides of the head.
- **Loudness summation:** When sound is received by both ears, a summing of the two signals results. Thresholds for sound may improve by 3 dB or more, as compared to monaural thresholds in either ear.
- **Binaural squelch:** Listening performance will be better in noise when the user wears two hearing aids instead of one. This improvement in signal-to-noise ratio may be 2 or 3 dB.
- **Localization:** A normally hearing person is sensitive to interaural differences in a sound's intensity and phase and this allows him or her, in part, to perceive the direction and the location of a sound source and to segregate one sound source from another. A monaural hearing aid fitting disrupts these cues, whereas binaural hearing aids serve to preserve this localization ability.

Attenuation of sound to one ear because of the presence of the head between the ear and the sound source is called the **head shadow** effect.

Loudness summation is a summing of the signals received by each ear, resulting in a 3-dB advantage for binaural over monaural hearing.

Binaural squelch is an improvement in listening in noise when wearing two hearing aids instead of one, resulting in a 2- to 3-dB improvement in signal-to-noise ratio.

Localization is the ability to locate the source of a sound in space due to the normal ear's sensitivity to interaural differences in phase and intensity.

implant converts the sound signal into a micromechanical vibration and transmits it directly to the ossicular chain. The ossicular chain, comprised of the malleus, incus, and stapes, spans the middle ear volume, stretching from the tympanic membrane to the oval window of the cochlea.

A middle ear implant has outer and inner components. The outer components include the power supply (battery), the microphone, and electronic components that transduce the auditory signal into an electromagnetic signal. The internal components include a receiver, a cable, and a vibrator that deliver the micromechanical vibration to the ossicular chain.

The implantable middle ear device has not been widely used. Most often, it is considered to be appropriate for patients who have moderately severe to severe hearing losses, although some patients who have a mild loss are also candidates (Miller & Fredrickson, 2000). The loss might be sensorineural, conductive, or mixed. The middle ear implant is purported to bypass some of the shortcomings of more traditional hearing aid styles, including problems with feedback, occlusion effects, and buildup of cerumen. They may be particularly successful with patients who suffer recurrent otitis media or chronic suppurative otitis media, both of which preclude wearing a hearing aid in the ear canal. The downside includes high cost and the necessity of undergoing anesthesia for a surgical procedure for the implant.

Selecting a Hearing Aid Style

A consideration of hearing aid styles leads to the question, "How do you determine which style to provide to a particular individual?" There is no pat answer to this question, but the selection of a particular style of hearing aid often is dependent on the degree of hearing loss, the patient's preference, the cost of the device, the person's age and lifestyle, and his or her physical status.

Degree of Hearing Loss

As part of a hearing aid evaluation, an audiologist will obtain an audiogram. The magnitude and configuration of an individual's hearing loss will then help to determine the style of hearing aid selected.

Table 3-2 indicates optimum style options as a function of degree of hearing loss. For example, if an individual has a profound hearing loss, a CIC

Table 3-2. Recommendations for hearing aid style.

STYLE	HEARING LOSS FOR WHICH USE IS OPTIMAL	HEARING LOSS FOR WHICH USE IS APPROPRIATE BUT NOT OPTIMAL	PHYSICAL FACTORS THAT MAY PRECLUDE OR LIMIT USE
Body aid	All degrees, although usually used for severe and profound losses		
BTE	All degrees		Deformed outer ears
ITE	Mild through severe	Severe-to-profound; not recommended for profound	Shallow depression at entry of ear canal
ITC	Mild to moderate-to-severe	Moderate-to-severe; not recommended for profound	Narrow or malformed ear canals; history of cerumen buildup; reduced manual dexterity
CIC	Mild	Moderate; not recommended for severe or profound	Narrow or malformed ear canals; reduced manual dexterity
Middle ear implant	Mild through severe	Profound	

device is not appropriate because it will not provide enough amplification for the person's listening needs.

The recommendations listed in Table 3-2 are generalizations, and audiologists sometimes select these aids even if they are not optimal for the hearing loss because of other considerations, such as user preference.

User Preference

Probably as important as the magnitude and configuration of the hearing loss in selecting a hearing aid style is the preference of the user. The audiologist will talk with the patient, and carefully consider his or her preferences and prejudices concerning hearing aid styles. If user preferences are not considered, the hearing aid may not be used. For example, if an audiologist provided someone with a BTE, and the individual turned out to be too self-conscious to wear it, then the BTE probably was an inappropriate selection on the audiologist's part.

Costs

A closely related issue to preference is cost. CIC and digital hearing aids are the most expensive hearing aids. It is important to explore an individual's financial resources to purchase certain hearing aid styles early in the selection process. Those styles that are deemed too expensive then cannot be considered further.

Lifestyle

Lifestyle is also an important factor to consider during the selection process. For instance, a physician or nurse who often uses a stethoscope, and does not want to use one with a built-in amplifier, may best be served by a CIC aid, because this style can be used with a stethoscope. A person who uses the telephone for a good part of the working day may opt for a BTE hearing aid that has a powerful telecoil circuitry.

Physical Status

Physical status is an important consideration when selecting a hearing aid style. Physical status includes an individual's manual dexterity and the condition of the ear. It is important to assess a person's gross and fine motor skills and to evaluate how well the individual can move his or her hands, fingers, and arms. Both fine and gross motor skills are necessary for putting on and taking off a hearing aid. In addition, fine motor control is necessary for manipulating the controls, changing batteries, and inserting and removing the hearing aid from the ear. If a person has poor skills, it might

Electroacoustic Properties

In addition to selecting a hearing aid style, certain decisions must be made concerning the electroacoustic properties of the hearing aid. These properties affect how the hearing aid processes the audio signal. These properties include saturation sound pressure level and gain/frequency response:

- **Output sound pressure level (OSPL):** Once called the *saturation sound-pressure level (SSPL)*, this term refers to the maximum sound pressure level that can be delivered to the ear, when the volume control is turned full on and the input signal is 90 dB SPL. This value is determined to ensure that the hearing aid's maximum power does not exceed the user's **loudness discomfort level (LDL),** also called uncomfortable loudness level (UCL). The LDL is the threshold at which sound becomes so loud that the hearing aid user cannot tolerate it, even for a brief exposure. An **OSPL90 curve** is obtained by measuring the hearing aid's output in a hearing aid test chamber called a **hearing aid test box.** The hearing aid is connected to a 2-cc coupler that simulates the human external ear canal volume. An input signal then is presented that sweeps across frequencies, at 90 dB SPL. The output of the hearing aid is measured.

- **Gain/frequency response:** The difference between the amplitude of the input signal and the amplitude of the output signal across frequencies is referred to as the gain/frequency response of a hearing aid. Typically, a hearing aid for an individual is adjusted to deliver the greatest amount of gain for those frequencies for which the individual has the poorest thresholds.

- **Total harmonic distortion (THD):** The amplitude distortions in the form of additional harmonic components of an input sine wave. These unwanted signals, created by the hearing aid, typically are reported for the frequencies of 500, 800, and 1600 Hz.

The **output sound pressure level** is an electroacoustic assessment of a hearing aid's maximum level of output signal, expressed as a frequency response curve to a 90-dB SPL signal, with the hearing aid volume control set to full on.

Loudness discomfort level (LDL) is the level at which sound is perceived to be uncomfortably loud.

An **OSPL90 curve** is an electroacoustic assessment of a hearing aid's maximum level of output signal, expressed as a frequency response curve to a 90-dB SPL signal, with the hearing aid volume control set to full on.

Gain/frequency response is the difference between the amplitude of the input signal and the amplitude of the output signal across frequencies.

A **hearing aid test box** is a chamber that provides an electroacoustic analysis of hearing aids and probe-microphone measurements. It provides an off-the-ear determination of OSPL-90 in which the hearing aid is connected to a 2-cc coupler to simulate the human ear canal; an input signal that sweeps across the frequencies at 90 dB SPL is input, and the aid's output is measured.

---

be best to consider a BTE aid, a body aid, or an assistive listening device such as a handheld amplifier. We will revisit this issue of manual dexterity in Chapter 13, when we consider older adults.

An examination of the ear will indicate whether an individual has chronic ear infections or a deformity in the ear canal. Children often have chronic otitis media. If an ITE aid is prescribed, secretions might damage the device. Hence, this is one reason a BTE aid may be more appropriate. A deformed or nonexistent ear canal also may limit (or preclude) the use of certain styles of hearing aids.

In addition to the health of the ear and physical malformations, the curve of the ear canal may influence the selection of hearing aid style. If the individual has a straight ear canal, without a bend, then he or she probably is not a good candidate for a CIC aid. The device will not stay in place. Similarly, if the individual has a shallow concha, an ITC aid may be difficult to keep in the ear.

Selecting the Hearing Aid and Assessing Benefits

Selection of hearing aids typically is based on the audiogram, which indicates the degree of hearing loss and the configuration. Sometimes, a formula for gain is applied, which is a formula used to compute the desired amount of amplification at each frequency This strategy is referred to as **prescription procedures**.

> **Prescription procedures** are strategies for fitting hearing aids by using a formula to calculate the desired gain and frequency response.

Prescription procedures are often used when a hearing aid is to be ordered from a specific manufacturer. A set of optimum electroacoustic characteristics is integrated into the production of a patient's hearing aid. For example, in one procedure, the goal is to restore hearing thresholds to normal. The amount of gain prescribed at each frequency corresponds to the degree of hearing loss. In another prescriptive procedure, high frequencies are amplified more than low frequencies to maximize speech audibility. Incorporated in most prescriptive formulas is the patient's LDL, so sound is not presented at an uncomfortably loud level (see Mueller & Bentler, 2005, and Mueller, 2005, for evidence-based reviews of the effectiveness of prescriptive methods).

Implicit in the use of prescriptive methods of hearing aid selection is the need to verify and validate that the prescriptive targets have been met and that the fitting is appropriate for the particular patient. This **verification** can be done either with behavioral techniques or with probe-tube microphone measurements.

> **Verification** means to determine that the hearing aid meets a set of standards, including standards of basic electroacoustics, real-ear electroacoustic performance, and comfortable fit.

Behavioral techniques may include obtaining an aided audiogram and administering speech recognition tests (Chapter 2). Patients take a speech recognition test with and without their hearing aid, and amount of improvement in percentage words correct on their performance is computed.

The second procedure for evaluating a patient's hearing aid involves **probe microphone** technology. A small flexible tube is inserted into the ear canal

> A **probe microphone** is a microphone transducer that is inserted in the external ear canal for the purpose of measuring sound near the tympanic membrane.

Real-ear measures entail the use of a probe microphone to measure hearing aid gain and frequency response delivered by a hearing aid at the tympanic membrane.

Target gain is the gain prescribed for each frequency of a hearing aid, against which the actual hearing aid output is compared.

and positioned near the eardrum. The tube connects to a microphone, which records the decibels of power delivered at the end of the ear canal. First, sound is measured near the eardrum, so the measure is influenced by the natural resonance of the ear canal. Measurements are then repeated, but this time with the hearing aid worn by the patient. These measures are called **real-ear measures**. Although these measures do not indicate how well an individual can hear when wearing the hearing aid, results indicate whether the prescribed gain at each frequency, also called the **target gain**, is being delivered by the hearing aid.

A subjective procedure to assess hearing aid benefit is the use of a questionnaire or an inventory. The patient may complete a checklist about what he or she can or cannot hear with the hearing aid, and may indicate satisfaction with the device. Cox (2003) identifies seven categories of self-report outcome data. Choice of a particular self-assessment scale might be based on which of these seven categories a clinician is interested in assessing:

1. **Benefit,** or the change in hearing-related disability that has resulted from the use of amplification.

2. **Satisfaction,** or an overview of the physical, social, psychological, and financial changes that have resulted from the use of amplification.

3. **Use time,** which is often related to the severity of the hearing loss and contextual factors.

4. **Residual activity limitations,** or the hearing-related difficulties that the patient continues to experience despite the use of amplification.

5. **Residual participation restrictions,** or limitations that prevent an individual from fulfilling a role in life.

6. **Impact on others,** usually determined by a frequent communication partner (not many instruments are available for this purpose).

7. **Quality of life,** including improvements in social life and mental health.

We shall revisit the topics of benefit, use time, and satisfaction in Chapter 12, when we consider aural rehabilitation plans for adults, as well as the topics of activity limitations and participation restrictions.

Table 3-3 summarizes several self-assessment scales that may be used to assess the goodness of a hearing aid. The scales are designed to measure and validate outcomes following receipt of a hearing aid. Some instruments are geared more to gauging benefit (e.g., *Profile of Aided Loudness [PAL]*; Mueller & Palmer, 1998), whereas others are geared more to assessing satisfaction with the device (e.g., *Satisfaction With Amplification in Daily Life [SADL]*; Cox & Alexander, 1999).

Table 3-3. Examples of self-report measures that have been developed to assess a patient's perceived benefit from a hearing aid.

MEASURE	PURPOSE	REFERENCE
Glascow Hearing Aid Benefit Profile (GHABP) *The prespecified element of the instrument presents four listening situations with six questions about each	To asses individual client concerns and expectations in a variety of difficult listening situations Example: *In this situation [having a conversation with several people in a group] what proportion of the time do you wear your hearing aid? (5-point scale: 1 = never/not at all; 5 = all the time)*	Gatehouse (1999)
Hearing Aid Performance Inventory (HAPI) *64 items, based on 12 bipolar features (e.g., visual signal present/absent)	To assess the benefits of amplification in varying listening situations Example: *You are alone at home talking with a friend on the telephone. (5-point scale: 1 = very helpful; 5 = hinders performance)*	Walden, Demorest, & Helper (1984)
Hearing Aid Users Questionnaire *11-item questionnaire that assesses hearing aid use, benefit, and related problems and satisfactions	To detect problems that affect a patient's ability to use hearing aids and receive benefit Example: *How would you describe your satisfaction with your hearing aid? (4-point scale: 1 = very satisfied;4 = very dissatisfied)*	Dillon, Birtles, & Lovegrove (1999)
Hearing Problem Inventory *50 items about emotional reaction to hearing loss; effect of hearing loss on everyday activities; signal and environmental influences; use of visual cues; use, fit, and care of hearing aid	To assess benefit of using a hearing aid and to identify some of the influences on a patient's perception of his or her problems and hearing aid use Example: *The telephone pickup on my hearing aid is good. (5-point scale: 1 = almost always; 5 = almost never)*	Hutton (1980)
Profile of Aided Loudness (PAL) *12 items across categories of soft, average, and loud sounds	To determine whether amplification has restored loudness Example: *You are chewing soft food: Loudness rating (scale from 0 to 7: 0 = do not hear; 7 = uncomfortably loud); Satisfaction rating (scale from 5 to 1: 5 = just right; 1 = not good at all)*	Mueller & Palmer (1998); Palmer, Mueller, & Moriarty (1999)
Profile of Hearing Aid Benefit (PHAB) *66 items in seven subscales designed to assess the following: familiar talkers, ease of communication, reverberation, reduced cues, background noise, aversiveness of sounds, and distortion of sounds	To generate a measure of hearing aid benefit computed from the difference between aided and unaided conditions Example: *(Answered with and without hearing aid) Women's voices sound shrill (7-point scale: A = always; G = never)*	Cox, Gilmore, & Alexander (1991); Cox & Rivera (1992)

continues

Table 3-3. *continued*

MEASURE	PURPOSE	REFERENCE
Abbreviated Profile of Hearing Aid Benefit (APHAB) *Uses a subset of 24 of the 66 items from the PHAB	To generate a measure of hearing aid benefit in a clinically feasible amount of time Example (see above)	Cox & Alexander (1995)
Profile of Hearing Aid Performance (PHAP) *66 items designed to measure two aspects of performance with a hearing aid, speech communication in a variety of typical workday situations and reactions to loudness or quality of environmental sounds	To generate a measure of performance rather than benefit Example: *When I am in a quiet restaurant, I can understand conversation (7-point scale: A = always; G = never)*	Cox & Gilmore (1990)
Satisfaction with Amplification in Daily Life (SADL) *15 items in four subscales: positive effects, service and costs, negative features, and personal image	To quantify hearing aid satisfaction Example: *Are you convinced that obtaining your hearing aid was in your best interest? (7-point scale: A = not at all; G = tremendously)*	Cox & Alexander (1999)
The Speech, Spatial and Qualities of Hearing Scale (SSQ) *14 items about speech hearing, 17 items about spatial hearing, 18 items about other functions; when applied to aided listening, additional items are included	To assess the recognition of speech in a variety of competing contexts, with particular attention to interventions that involve binaural hearing Example: *Do you have the impression of sounds being exactly where you would expect them to be? (10-point scale: 0 = not at all; 10 = perfectly)*	Gatehouse & Noble (2004)

Hearing Aid Orientation

Once the audiologist receives the prescribed hearing aid from the manufacturer, the patient returns to the clinic to be fitted with the device. At this time, benefit also is assessed, and the patient receives a **hearing aid orientation**. The hearing aid orientation includes the following services:

Hearing aid orientation (HAO) is the process of instructing a patient (and a family member) to handle, use, and maintain a new hearing aid.

- The audiologist describes the function of each part of the hearing aid and ensures that the patient can adjust any controls.
- The patient practices inserting and removing the hearing aid (sometimes with the aid of a mirror) and practices inserting and removing batteries from the hearing aid battery compartment.
- The audiologist reviews basic hearing aid maintenance and ways to clean the device, protect it from moisture, and store it at night, and also discusses battery life, storage, and disposal and how to order new batteries.
- The patient practices using the telephone, using the telecoil switch if the hearing aid has one.

- The audiologist reviews realistic expectations and the limitations of amplification, and why the particular hearing aid was selected.
- The patient and audiologist determine an appropriate use pattern for the first few weeks of using the new hearing aid.
- The patient learns how to **troubleshoot** the device for common problems such as weak or no sound (e.g., one possible solution is to check the battery and replace) and feedback (e.g., one possible solution is to clean the wax guard).
- The patient receives printed information about the hearing aid and warranty.
- The patient and audiologist agree on a follow-up time table and talk about how to monitor performance with the hearing aid.

COCHLEAR IMPLANTS

Not all individuals who have hearing loss have the potential to benefit from using a hearing aid. For instance, someone who has little, if any, residual hearing will probably never recognize the auditory speech signal, no matter how it is processed or how much it is amplified. Another intervention available besides a hearing aid is the cochlear implant. Cochlear implants, virtually unheard of 35 years ago, are now fairly commonplace. Well over 100,000 people worldwide use a cochlear implant (Summerfield et al., 2006).

Most sensorineural hearing loss results from a dearth or absence of hair cells (the sensory receptors of hearing) in the cochlea and not because of a damaged auditory nerve or central dysfunction. A cochlear implant is effective because it replaces the hair-cell transducer system by stimulating the auditory nerve directly, bypassing the damaged or missing hair cells. The nerve impulses are then delivered to the brain, following the route of the neural auditory pathway, as if the cochlea were stimulated in a natural way. Implants are designed to interface with the **tonotopic organization** of the cochlea. The implant divides sound into a series of frequency bands, and it then delivers each band to that region of the cochlea for which it is best suited. For example, high-frequency bands are delivered to the basilar end of the cochlea, whereas low-frequency bands are delivered to the apical end. The level of stimulation serves to code sound intensity.

A Brief History

Although cochlear implants are a relatively new development, scientists have long been tantalized by the idea of providing sound sensation by means of electrical stimulation. One of the first recorded attempts in history to stimulate the ear electrically occurred in 1790, when Volta inserted

Troubleshoot refers to a series of steps to follow when the hearing aid will not turn on, if the sound is faint or distorted, or feedback occurs, the objective being to locate and correct the source of malfunction.

"Most traditional inquiries into hearing disability, in common with all laboratory assessments, tend to regard the world as a static place. In reality, the auditory world is highly dynamic, both in time and in space, and the SSQ [*Speech, Spatial and Qualities of Hearing Scale*] attempts to address these dynamic aspects of hearing function, as well as the static features."

Stuart Gatehouse, co-developer of the SSQ and assistant director of the Medical Research Counsel Institute of Hearing Research in the United Kingdom

(*Gatehouse, 2003, p. 2S80*)

Structures within the peripheral and central auditory nervous system are arranged topographically according to tonal frequency; that is, they have a **tonotopic organization**.

metal rods into each of his ears. The rods were connected to 30 or 40 of his newly invented electrolytic cells. With one deft move, Volta delivered approximately 50 volts to himself. The results were staggering. He perceived a sensation similar to "a blow to the head," followed by "a sound like the boiling of a viscous liquid" (Luxford & Brackmann, 1985, p. 1). The experiment was not repeated.

The more recent history of cochlear implants hails back to France in the 1950s. The electrophysiologist Andre Djourno developed an electrical auditory prosthesis in the mid-1950s for stimulation of motor nerves. He was able to trigger jumping action in both frogs and rabbits. On February 25, 1957, the otolaryngologist Charles Eyries implanted a human with profound hearing loss with an identical device to stimulate the auditory nerve (Seitz, 2002). The patient reported hearing a sound like "crickets chirping" or "a roulette wheel spinning" (Luxford & Brackmann, 1985). Reports of this early implant work filtered to the medical communities in the United States and Australia. Shortly thereafter, in the 1960s and 1970s, much activity was aimed toward the development of wearable devices. Names often associated with this work are Dr. William House of Los Angeles, California, and Dr. Graham Clarke of Melbourne, Australia.

By the 1980s there was widespread use of cochlear implants among adults, and they were in exploratory use with children. The Food and Drug Administration (FDA) approved multichannel cochlear implants in 1990 for children, and now cochlear implants are considered a treatment option for both adults and children who have profound hearing loss. Increasingly, individuals who have severe hearing loss also are considered as candidates for implantation.

Overview

The cochlear implant of the future may be a **completely implantable cochlear implant (CICI),** which will be comprised of only internal components.

In cochlear implants, the **internal components** are implanted within the skull.

Cochlear implants are comprised of internal and external components (Figure 3-8), although soon manufacturers will also be offering a fully implantable cochlear implant, called **completely implantable cochlear implants (CICI)**, with no visible external components. The **internal components** are implanted in the skull, in close proximity to the inner ear. The internal components typically include an internal receiver, which is placed on the mastoid bone, and an electrode array, which is inserted into the cochlea. These components are not visible after implantation, but are covered by skin and hair. The user may have a small incision scar and a slight convex protrusion behind the pinna.

The **external components** are worn on the outside of the body.

The **external components** include a microphone, connecting cables, a speech processor, and a transmitter. The microphone and transmitter typically are worn behind the ear. In older models, the speech processor

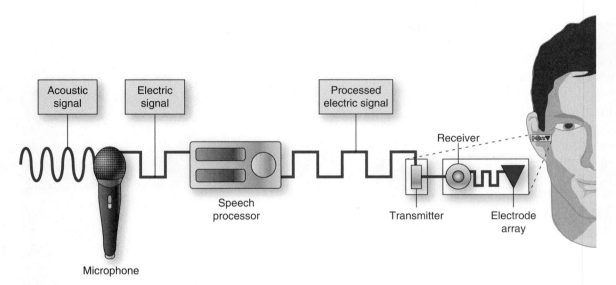

FIGURE 3-8. Schematic of a cochlear implant.

is worn on the chest, similar to a body hearing aid. In newer cochlear implants, the speech processor can be worn behind the ear, like a BTE hearing aid. Figure 3-9 presents a picture of a young student who recently received a cochlear implant. Figure 3-10 presents a photograph of a cochlear implant. As can be seen, the speech processor is about the size of a BTE hearing aid.

The microphone of a cochlear implant picks up sound from the environment, converts it to an electrical signal, and then delivers it via connecting cables to the speech processor. The **speech processor**, as the name implies, processes the signal. Each cochlear implant design utilizes a speech-processing strategy, or algorithm, for determining how the signal is processed. The signal may be digitized, filtered, and then segmented so that different components of the signal are presented to different electrodes in the electrode array.

The processed electrical signal leaves the speech processor and is delivered to the electrode array, via a transmitter and an internal receiver. The transmitter often is worn outside of the head and delivers the signal to an internal receiver. The transmitter may be held in place by a magnet. The electrical signal typically is transmitted across the skin by either electromagnetic induction or radio frequency transmission. From the internal receiver, the electrical signal passes on to the electrode array.

The **electrode array** is a small wire, inserted into the cochlea, usually through the **round window**. The electrode array carries electrode pairs.

A **speech processor** is the component of a cochlear implant where the input signal is modified for presentation to the electrodes in the electrode array.

The **electrode array** is inserted into the cochlea, and is a wire that carries the implant's electrode pairs.

The **round window** is a membrane-covered opening between the middle ear space and the scala tympani section of the cochlea in the inner ear.

"Even after nine years, not a day passes that I don't marvel at the gift of sound and thank all those involved in providing this wondrous technology."

Donna Sorkin, Former Executive Director for Self-Help for Hard-of-Hearing (SHHH) and a cochlear-implant recipient

(*Sorkin, Hearing Loss,* July/August 2002, p. 17)

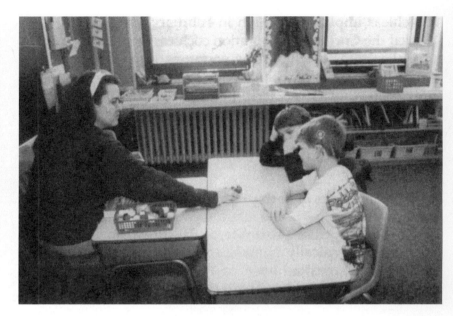

FIGURE 3-9. A young boy wearing a cochlear implant. The microphone is worn behind his ear like a behind-the-ear hearing aid. The external transmitter is held against his head by magnetic induction. This child has only been using the device for a short time, and his scar from surgery is still visible near the base of his skull. *Photograph by Kim Readmond, courtesy of the Central Institute for the Deaf.*

The electrode pairs, which are tiny exposed balls or rings on the wire, are comprised of positive and negative polarity contacts, between which passes current. The current stimulates the fibers of the auditory nerve.

If a device is **multichannel,** it has more than one channel. The term is often used to describe cochlear implants that present different channels of information to different parts of the cochlea.

Most cochlear implants in use in the United States today are **multichannel** devices. This means that the electrode pairs in the electrode array present different information to different regions of the cochlea. In the normal ear, different frequencies of the auditory signal excite different neurons along the cochlea. The goal of a multichannel system is to simulate the normal cochlea and present high-frequency components of the signal to the basal end of the cochlea and low-frequency components of the signal to the apical end.

Interleaved pulsatile stimulation is a cochlear implant processing strategy in which trains of pulses are delivered across electrodes in the electrode array in a nonsimultaneous fashion.

Although there are some variations in the processing strategies used by different models of cochlear implants, many current cochlear implants utilize an **interleaved pulsatile stimulation** algorithm. In this design, each electrode pair in the electrode array is designated to represent different frequency bands. The audio signal is processed and delivered to the electrode array by spreading pulses, in a nonsimultaneous manner (hence, they are interleaved) across the electrode pairs, from high to low or from low to high frequencies.

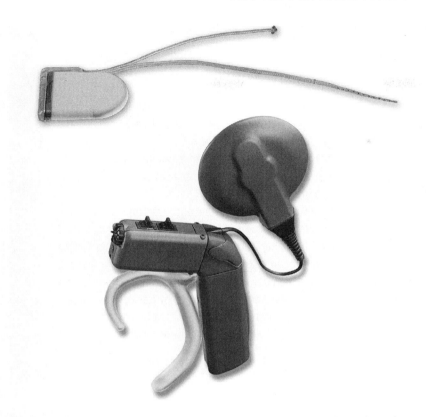

FIGURE 3-10. A cochlear implant. The top image in the figure shows the internal components, which include the receiver and the electrode array. The bottom image shows the external components, which include the microphone and the speech processor. *Photograph courtesy of Med-El Corp.*

The cochlear implant is powered by either a disposable battery or a rechargeable battery. In some cochlear implants, battery life is about 3 to 5 days for disposable batteries and 9 to 17+ hours for rechargeable batteries.

Most cochlear implants can be used in conjunction with an assistive listening device. Direct audio input cables can couple the cochlear implant to CD players, auxiliary microphones, and other portable players. Some devices have an integrated telecoil and some can be plugged into an external telecoil.

In the United States, three manufacturers, Cochlear Corporation, Med-El, and Advanced Bionics, provide most of the devices. Their processing strategies are continually under development. Three processing strategy designs that have been implemented at one time or another are "feature extraction," "continuous interleaved sampling," and analog strategies. The Cochlear Corporation developed the first multichannel cochlear implant, the Nucleus, to receive FDA approval. Early models of the Nucleus cochlear implant were feature extraction devices because they coded first and second formant features (as we will review in Chapter 4, formants refer to vowel resonances).

Hybrid devices are listening aids that combine a cochlear implant system with hearing aid technology.

What's on the Horizon for Cochlear Implant Designs?

Experiments are currently being conducted to evaluate a **hybrid** cochlear implant. This device has a shorter electrode array than traditional cochlear implants (so does not insert as far into the cochlear capsule) and patients hear sounds through a combination of electrical stimulation and traditional acoustic amplification. The goal is to preserve existing hearing sensitivity, which for many people who have hearing loss exists to some extent for low and even mid-frequencies. The device delivers amplified sound for the lower frequencies and electrical stimulation for the higher frequencies. A study of 12 patients who have used the device for at least a year suggests that they achieve very good word recognition as compared to performance presurgery with only a hearing aid, even in the presence of background noise. They experience relatively good music perception, a benefit that eludes many users of traditional cochlear implants (Turner, Gantz, Lowder, & Gfeller, 2005).

Newer models allowed for more sophisticated speech-processing strategies. For instance, the SPEAK strategy, also made available through Cochlear Corporation, divided the incoming auditory signal into 20 frequency bands and cycled through the electrodes on the electrode array, stimulating an average of six electrodes on each cycle (those that corresponded to the frequencies that had the most energy present in the incoming signal). The SPEAK is an example of a continuous interleaved sampling (CIS) strategy. CIS strategies provide interleaved pulsatile stimulation. The company's advanced combination encoder (ACE) strategy stimulates similarly, but uses higher rates of stimulation than the SPEAK. The Advanced Bionics Corporation Clarion device allows a simultaneous analog stimulation (SAS) strategy, which filters the incoming auditory signal and presents it simultaneously to the corresponding bipolar electrodes. A listing of cochlear implant manufacturers and their contact information appears in Appendix 3-1.

Candidacy

The primary candidacy requirements for implantation are the presence of irreversible severe or profound hearing loss and good general health. There is no upper age of implantation, and adults 85 years and older have received implanted devices. The lower age of implantation for certain device types is about 12 months, although children as young as 6 months have received cochlear implants in the United States and in countries such as Australia and Austria (see Watltzman, 2005, for a review). The cochlea is adult size at the time of birth, so implantation for babies is feasible on an anatomical basis.

Table 3-4 presents candidacy requirements for children and adults. For children, it must be demonstrated that they receive little or no benefit from

Table 3-4. Candidacy requirements for cochlear implantation.

CHILDREN (12–18 MONTHS)	CHILDREN (19 MONTHS TO 17 YEARS, 11 MONTHS)	ADULTS
Bilateral profound sensorineural hearing sensorineural loss	Bilateral severe or profound sensorineural hearing loss	Bilateral severe or profound sensorineural hearing loss
Lack of auditory skills development and minimal benefit from using a hearing aid (documented by audiological testing and parent questionnaire)	Lack of auditory skills development and minimal hearing aid benefit (word recognition scores less than 30% words correct or lack of auditory skill development)	Minimal benefit from wearing a hearing aid (word recognition scores less than 50% words correct)
No medical contraindications	No medical contraindications	No medical contraindications
Enrollment in an aural rehabilitation intervention that emphasizes the development of listening skills	Enrollment in an aural rehabilitation intervention that emphasizes the development of listening	

a hearing aid. This typically requires them to undergo a 3- to 6-month trial period with a hearing aid and to receive appropriate aural rehabilitation intervention that encourages listening behaviors. Currently, children who receive a cochlear implant under the age of 18 months must have a profound hearing loss whereas children over the age of 18 months and who have a severe loss may be considered as candidates.

Candidacy requirements for adults have altered since the mid-1980s, when cochlear implantation began to be performed with increased regularity. Early on, adults had to have a profound, postlingual hearing loss and could receive no measurable benefit from hearing aids. For example, if someone recognized more than about 10 or 20% of the words on a monosyllabic word test while wearing a hearing aid, that person was not a candidate. Today, criteria have loosened, in part because advances in speech-processing

Two Versus One

Approximately 4,600 individuals have received bilateral implant surgery and wear a cochlear implant in each ear. There is some evidence that use of two cochlear implants affords a modest increase in speech recognition compared to using only one device, especially when listening in the presence of background noise. Use of two cochlear implants may also enhance sound localization (Litovsky, Parkinson, Arcaroli, & Sammeth, 2006; Wackym, Runge-Samuelson, Firszt, Alkar, & Burg, 2007).

Many other cochlear implant users continue to use a hearing aid in the unimplanted ear (Kirk, Firszt, Hood, & Holt, 2006). When a patient wears binaural hearing aids and then receives a cochlear implant in one ear, the patient typically will experiment with using both the cochlear implant and the hearing aid. In some cases, a patient will find that simultaneously listening to both the electrical and the amplified signals is confusing, and will opt to use only the cochlear implant. In other cases, the patient will find that the simultaneous signals enhance his or her ability to listen in noise and to localize sound, so will opt to use both devices.

strategy design permit greater gains to be realized for persons with profound hearing loss and afford more speech recognition than do most hearing aids. Criteria have also loosened because more clinical research data are available about patient performance on which to make candidacy recommendations. If a patient has a severe or profound hearing loss, and modest word recognition (say, the patient is unable to recognize more than 40% of the words on an open-set sentence test or 30% on a monosyllabic word test), that individual is likely a candidate. Although most adult cochlear implant recipients have postlingual hearing losses, prelingual deafness no longer precludes candidacy (see Dowell, 2005; UK Cochlear Implant Study Group, 2004).

Process

Acquiring a cochlear implant is a multistage process. It often begins with a comprehensive audiological evaluation and, if the patient has never used appropriate amplification (typically a very young child), a trial period with amplification. Once an individual has been deemed a candidate, he or she undergoes surgery at which time the internal components are implanted under the skin behind the pinna. Four to 6 weeks later, the patient returns and the external components of the device are fitted. The audiologist adjusts the stimulus parameters of the speech processor to optimize speech recognition in a process called **mapping**. Ideally, the patient then engages in a comprehensive aural rehabilitation program to develop his or her new listening skills and maintains contact with the cochlear implant center through regularly scheduled follow-up visits.

Mapping is a term used to describe the process of programming the speech processor of a cochlear implant.

How to Establish a Map

Most cochlear implants are established by programming the following parameters:

- Dynamic range: In adjusting the speech processor, each electrode in the electrode array is programmed according to the threshold of stimulation and maximum acceptable loudness level. The difference between these two current levels defines a dynamic range. An **electrical threshold (T-level)** is the amount of current that must be passed through an electrode so the patient is just aware of a sound sensation. **Maximum comfort level (C-level or M-level)** is the maximum current level that can be introduced before the individual experiences discomfort. The thresholds and maximum comfort levels will vary among electrodes and between patients as a function of neuronal survival in the auditory nerve.

- Loudness balancing. Through **loudness balancing,** the speech processor is programmed so stimulation across electrodes preserves the loudness contour of the speech signal. Patients must judge the relative loudness of signals presented to different electrodes in the cochlear implant electrode array. If the electrodes are not balanced, the patient might experience occasional popping sounds and may not hear some speech information.

- Pitch and pitch ranking. Electrodes situated near the basal end of the cochlear are programmed to represent the high-frequency range and those near the apical end represent the low-frequency range. This representation matches the tonotopic organization of the cochlear. **Pitch ranking** determines the ability to discriminate pitch from the basal to the apical electrodes. During pitch ranking, two electrodes are stimulated, one right after the other. The patient's task is to indicate which stimulus pulse has a higher or lower pitch.

The electrical threshold (T-level) is the amount of current that must be passed through an electrode so that the patient is just aware of a sound sensation.

The **maximum comfort level (C-level)** is the maximum current level that can be listened to comfortably for a prolonged duration of time.

Loudness balancing is programming the speech processor so that stimulation follows the loudness contour of the incoming speech signal.

Pitch ranking determines the ability to discriminate pitch from stimulation of the basal to apical electrodes.

〰 ASSISTIVE LISTENING DEVICES (ALDS)

Hearing aids and cochlear implants are listening devices that may be worn during almost all working hours and in almost all communication settings. Assistive listening devices (ALDs) usually are used in specific situations, such as when listening in a public hall or conversing in a restaurant when other kinds of listening devices either are inadequate to permit good communication or are not desirable to the patient. In selecting ALDs for a particular individual, an audiologist will want to consider the person's communication demands in the home, work, community, recreational, or school environments. Table 3-5 presents a list of situations in each of these settings in which use of an ALD may be appropriate. Appendix 3-1 lists sources for obtaining ALDs.

ALDs are especially useful when the audio signal is presented at a distance or when the listening conditions are less than ideal. In such conditions, a hearing aid or cochlear implant may not be adequate to maximize an individual's listening potential. Because the microphone of a hearing aid or cochlear implant is at the level of the individual's ear, it may not pick up sound emanating from a distant source or may deliver not only the desired audio signal, but also any competing background noise to the listener.

Conditions that might compromise a listening environment, and where an ALD may be especially helpful, include the following:

- **Ambient noise:** noise that is present in a room when it is unoccupied. This noise may emanate from open windows, air-handling systems, computers, fluorescent lighting systems, or piped-in music.

Table 3-5. Situations in which use of an assistive device might be appropriate.

HOME	COMMUNITY	WORKPLACE	TRAVEL AND RECREATION	SCHOOL
One-on-one conversation	Medical treatment (visiting a physician, dentist, hospital)	Office conversation	One-on-one conversation, e.g., in the car	Communication with the teacher
Group conversation	Volunteer activities	Lectures	Television reception	Communication with classmates
Television reception	Religious services	Telephone communication	Public spaces	Speech-language therapy
Radio reception	Post office and other community service centers	Conferences and group meetings	Restaurants	
Reception of environmental signals such as the doorbell		One-on-one meetings	Hotel rooms	

- **Reverberation:** Echoes caused by sound rebounding off surfaces such as walls, floors, and ceilings. Rooms that have high ceilings, hardwood floors, and plaster walls tend to be highly reverberant, whereas those that have carpet and heavy draperies tend to have less reverberation.
- **Background noise:** Undesirable noise that masks the auditory signal of interest. For instance, in a classroom, the teacher's voice may be the target signal, and the rustling of paper and the shuffling of feet might be undesirable background noise.

In principle, ALDs work by collecting sound from the sound source (e.g., the talker's mouth) and delivering it to the user's ear. In this way, the audio signal is presented at an audible level, with a favorable signal-to-noise ratio, with minimal ambient noise, without the effects of reverberation, and with little background noise. ALDs can be categorized as one of two kinds: wireless and hardwired (Figure 3-11).

Wireless Systems

As the name implies, a wireless system does not use wire between the microphone and the unit that delivers the signal to the user's ear. Sound is transmitted from the sound source to the individual by means of radio waves or infrared signals. These kinds of systems may be used when the individual is far from the sound source, for example, in a religious service or when attending a theater play or when several people must attend to a talker, as students do when listening to their teacher. A wireless system picks up the audio signal, either through a microphone placed near the sound source or by means of a direct electrical plug-in. The sound is then converted into an electrical signal by a transmitter and delivered through the air to a receiver worn by the user, often by means of radio waves or infrared (invisible light). The signal may be delivered to the ear either via earphones or through the individual's hearing aid. Wireless systems can be further classified as frequency modulation (FM), infrared, induction loop, or simple amplification.

FM Systems

FM (frequency modulation) systems utilize radio waves to transmit sound from the source to the user. The Federal Communications Commission (FCC), which regulates FM systems, has allocated a range of bandwidths for exclusive use by persons with hearing loss (frequencies near 72 MHz and 216 MHz). FM systems are commonly used in classroom settings, and may be described as either a personal FM trainer or a sound-field FM system (Figure 3-12). When using a **personal FM trainer**, the teacher or

Frequency modulation (FM) is the process of creating a complex signal by means of sinusoidally varying a carrier wave frequency.

A **personal FM trainer** is a listening device in which the speaker wears a wireless microphone and the speech is frequency modulated on radio waves transmitted through the room to the listener who wears a receiver.

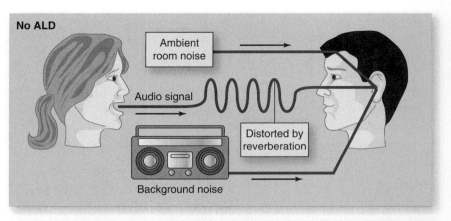

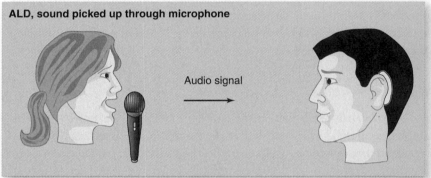

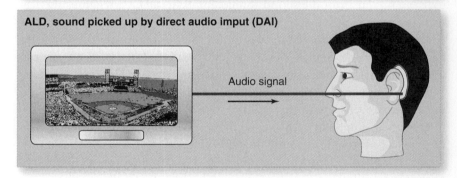

FIGURE 3-11. Schematic of an assistive listening device. In the top third of the figure, no assistive listening device is used, and the signal is distorted by reverberation and masked by background noise. In the center and bottom of the figure, sound is relayed from the source to the listener by means of an assistive listening device. In the center of the figure, sound is picked up through a microphone and transmitted without the use of hardwire to the listener, whereas in the bottom of the figure, sound is picked up by direct audio input.

speech and hearing professional wears a microphone (Figure 3-13), usually on a cord around the neck or clipped onto the shirt. The speech signal is conveyed into a transmitter, where it is frequency modulated on radio frequency carrier waves and transmitted through the classroom to the child,

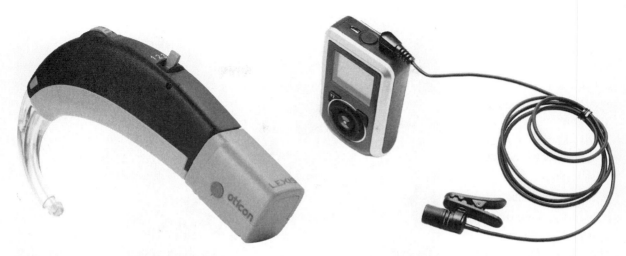

FIGURE 3-12.   A personal FM system. The left side of the figure shows a behind-the-ear hearing aid with an audio boot attached to the base. The right side of the figure shows the lapel microphone and the transmitter. *Photographs courtesy of Oticon.*

who wears a receiver. The receiver may connect to the child's hearing aid by a **direct auditory interface (DAI)** and an audio boot connection, or the child may wear an **FM boot** at the bottom of the hearing aid. Some FM systems utilize a **neckloop** that transmits to the hearing aid via the hearing aid's telecoil. Ear-level FM receiver units and hearing aids with built-in FM receivers are also available. If there is more than one child who has hearing loss in the classroom, then each child wears a receiver and may receive the teacher's signal.

A sound-field FM system operates similarly to a personal FM trainer. A **sound-field FM system** differs from the personal system because the sound is transmitted to loudspeakers that are positioned throughout the room, usually two in the back of the room and one near the front. There, the signal is converted to an audio signal and played into the environment, as with a standard public address system. A child's personal hearing aid microphone picks up the signal. Whereas a personal FM trainer offers better signal-to-noise ratios, the sound-field system is advantageous because it can be beneficial for an entire class, even for those children who do not have a hearing loss, who may have a fluctuating conductive hearing loss, who use a cochlear implant, or who have a unilateral hearing loss. FM sound-field systems also do not require a student to wear a special FM receiver. Hence, the child wears less hardware.

Other situations and settings in which FM systems may be used besides the classroom setting include group lectures, religious services, theaters, and one-on-one communication. Large-area listening environments, such

Direct audio input (DAI) is a hardwired connection that leads directly from the sound source to the hearing aid or other listening device.

An **FM boot** is a bootlike device that houses an FM receiver. It attaches to the base of a behind-the-ear hearing aid.

A **neckloop** is a transducer worn around the neck, often as part of an FM assistive device system. It consists of a cord from a receiver and transmits signals via magnetic induction to the telecoil of the user's hearing aid.

A **sound-field FM system** is a listening system, similar to the FM trainer, in which sound from a microphone is transmitted to loudspeakers that are positioned throughout the room.

"Convince school decision-makers that with sound-field amplification in place, schools can:

- achieve improved test scores
- mainstream students with hearing impairment
- save money
- reduce vocal fatigue
- leverage audiovisual teaching tools"

(Jorgensen, 2005, p. 28)

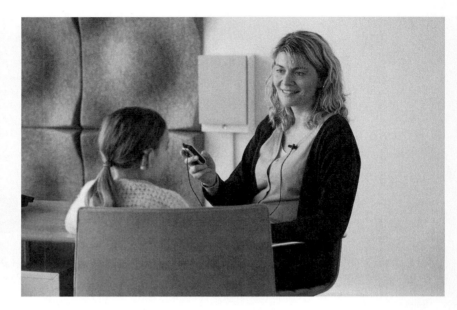

FIGURE 3-13. A personal FM system in use. An audiologist wearing a personal FM trainer microphone clipped to her sweater. She holds the transmitter. The young girl wears an audio boot attached to her behind-the-ear hearing aid. *Photograph courtesy of Oticon.*

as churches and theaters, sometimes incorporate an FM transmitter into their public or large-area broadcasting systems. Listeners then may check out a receiver unit for a particular event or presentation. In one-on-one communication, the person with hearing loss might connect his or her hearing aid to an FM receiver and hold a small FM transmitter toward the talker. The talker then speaks into a small handheld or table-mounted FM transmitter microphone.

Infrared Systems

An **infrared system** is an assistive listening device that broadcasts from the sound source to a receiver/amplifier by means of infrared light waves.

Infrared systems operate similarly to FM units, but use infrared signals to transmit sound. A transmitter/emitter sends the signal encoded in infrared light waves to a wireless receiver, which contains a photo detector diode. A photo detector diode picks up the infrared signal and converts it back to the audio signal. An individual either may wear an infrared receiver that inputs directly into the ears or may receive the signal through a neckloop, DAI, or headphones. Common situations in which infrared systems are used include television watching and movie theaters. Infrared systems are not appropriate for outdoors, as sunlight interferes with transmission. The infrared signals also cannot travel through walls. A "line of sight" is required for the signal to be received.

Question-and-Answer Time

Carol Flexer, a researcher who has studied sound-field FM amplification for more than 10 years, fielded a series of questions about sound-field amplification. Here are a few of the questions and her responses (Flexer, C. [1997]. Sound-field FM systems: Questions most often asked about classroom amplification. *Hearsay*, 11, 5–13).

Question: What exactly is sound-field FM amplification?

Answer: "Sound-field FM technology is an exciting educational tool that allows control of the acoustic environment in a classroom, thereby facilitating acoustic accessibility of teacher instruction for all children in the room. Specifically, frequency-modulated (FM) sound-field amplification systems are similar to small, high-fidelity, wireless, public address systems that are self-contained in a classroom. The teacher wears a small, unobtrusive wireless microphone; thus, teacher mobility is not restricted. His or her speech is frequency modulated onto a carrier wave that is sent from the transmitter to the receiver where it is demodulated and delivered to the students through one to five wall-or-ceiling-mounted loudspeakers."

Question: What's its purpose?

Answer: "The purpose of sound-field FM amplification is to amplify the teacher's voice throughout the classroom, thereby providing a clear and consistent signal to all pupils in the room no matter where they or the teacher are located. The positioning of the remote microphone close to the mouth of the teacher or other desired sound source creates a favorable speech-to-noise ratio (S/N ratio)."

Question: Which populations of children would benefit from learning in a classroom that is amplified?

Answer: "Children with fluctuating conductive hearing impairments, primarily caused by ear infections or ear wax. . . . Children with unilateral hearing impairments. . . . Children with slight permanent hearing impairments (15–25 dB HL). . . . Children who have normal peripheral hearing sensitivity but who are in special education classrooms due to language, learning, attending, or behavioral problems. . . . Children with mild to moderate hearing impairments who wear hearing aids. . . . Children who have normal peripheral hearing sensitivity but who have difficulty processing, understanding or attending to classroom instruction. . . . Children with cochlear implants."

Induction Loop Systems

An **induction loop system** is a system that works by running a wire around the circumference of a room or table that conducts electrical energy from an amplifier and thus creates a magnetic field, which induces the telecoil in a hearing aid to provide amplified sound to the user.

The third kind of wireless system is the induction loop system. For an **induction loop system** to operate, a loop of wire must be placed around the circumference of a room. Sound is picked up by means of a microphone or a direct input (e.g., a television direct connection). Sound is converted into electrical signals and fed through the loop. Electromagnetic energy is broadcast throughout the room and can be picked up by a hearing aid (and some cochlear implants) when the telecoil circuit is activated. The listener must sit either inside of the loop of wire or beside it. Some religious settings, classrooms, and theaters have permanent loop systems

Watching the Tube and Other Pleasures

At one time, persons with significant hearing loss either had to forego watching television and movies altogether or had to struggle to understand the dialogue and other important auditory signals. Thanks to closed captioning, this is no longer true for individuals who can read.

A **closed caption (CC) decoder** in a television set or electronic appliance extracts previously encoded closed caption data from a received video signal and displays it on a screen.

Since 1993, the Americans with Disabilities Act (ADA) has stipulated that all television sets sold in the United States with screens of 13 inches or larger must contain a **closed caption (CC) decoder.** A CC decoder projects dialogue orthographically on the screen and in relative synchrony with the spoken messages as well as a description of relevant sounds, such as a telephone ringing or an alarm. Often, the coding can be activated by means of the television set's remote control.

Some movie theaters also offer closed captioning, using either an open or closed system. In open captioning, subtitles are projected onto the screen, just as in foreign films, and can be seen by the entire audience. In closed captioning (sometimes called rear-window captioning), the captions are available only to individuals who attach a clear acrylic reflector panel to their seats. A rear-window captioner, which displays reversed captions via a light-emitting display (LED) system, is mounted at the back of the theater. It projects the captions onto the reflectors. The result is that the viewer sees captions superimposed on or beneath the movie screen.

"Ever since the first 'talking' motion picture *The Jazz Singer* was released in 1927, individuals with hearing loss have been excluded from the social, cultural and emotional experience of movies."

(Stanton, 2005, p. 14)

Web-based video also permits closed captioning for video. Web-based captioning can be accessed with such technologies as QuickTime (*http://www.apple.com/quicktime/*), RealOne Player (*http://www.rea.com/*), and Media Player (*http://www.microsoft.com/downloads*).

in place. There are portable induction loop systems so that any room can be optimized for communication. A variation of the large-area loop system is the **neckloop**, which is an induction loop wire system that can be worn around the neck. Induction systems are becoming increasingly popular, in large part because they are convenient for the user, who needs only to activate the t-coil on a personal hearing aid. Especially throughout the United Kingdom, Scandinavia, and elsewhere in Europe, it is not unusual to find induction loop systems in banks, post offices, senior citizen centers, train station counters, and tourist information centers.

Simple Amplification

Simple amplification systems merely amplify the audio signal so that it may be more audible to the person with hearing loss. The most common implementation of simple amplification systems is in telephones. **Telephone amplifiers** either replace the telephone handset or clip onto existing handsets. Replacement handsets have built-in amplifiers, so that the signal is amplified before it is delivered to the user's ear. Often, these kinds of handsets have volume controls; therefore, they may also be used by persons who have normal hearing.

Simple amplification systems amplify the audio signal so that it is more audible to a person with hearing loss.

Telephone amplifiers amplify sound from a telephone receiver.

Hardwired Systems

The other kind of assistive listening device can be described as hardwired. **Hardwired assistive listening devices** connect the sound source to the listener by actual wire. A microphone may pick up the audio signal (Figure 3-14) and deliver it to the patient's hearing aid by means of a DAI, or there may be a DAI jack that plugs into a piece of equipment, such as a television. The audio signal is converted into an electrical signal. It travels through the connecting wire, terminating at the user's hearing aid, headphones, or a neckloop. This system provides a favorable signal-to-noise ratio to the user and, usually, an adjustable amount of signal amplification. These kinds of systems are used most often for listening to television, radio, or music. However, such systems are not widely used because they require the user to be tethered to the sound source.

Hardwired assistive listening devices are devices that are directly connected by wires.

Other Kinds of Hearing Assistance Technology (HAT)

Other assistive devices are available that cannot be classified as wireless or hardwired assistive listening devices per se. The term **hearing assistance technology (HAT)** includes the kinds of ALDs we have just considered as

Hearing assistive technology (HAT) is technology that facilitates access to auditory information.

FIGURE 3-14. Hard-wired assistive listening devices. A woman and her daughter are learning to use a hard-wired assistive listening device, while a clinician (standing) provides encouragement. The daughter speaks into a microphone, while the woman listens through headphones. This kind of assistive listening device might be used in restaurants. *Photograph courtesy of the Central Institute for the Deaf.*

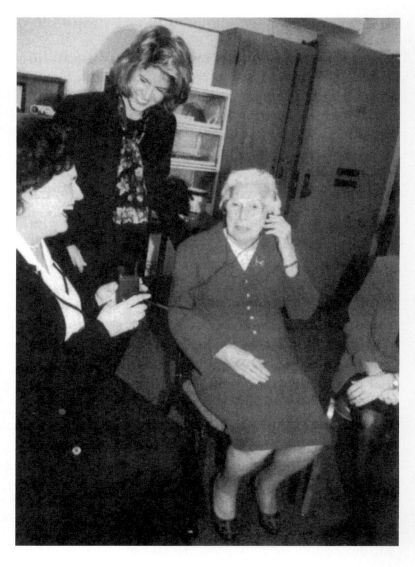

well as devices that facilitate reception of auditory information that is not speech, and auditory information by means other than amplification, such as by vibrotactile stimulation or visual display. One example of a HAT is a vibratory pager, which allows individuals to receive pages. Instead of emitting auditory beeps, a **vibratory pager** vibrates against the user to signal a call. Other examples include:

Vibratory pagers, instead of emitting audible beeps, vibrate against the user's body to signal a call.

- Vibrating alarm clocks, where a vibrator might be placed under the user's pillow
- Flashing alarm clocks, where a flashing lamp or strobe light might signal the alarm

- A doorbell signal coupled to a lamp, which flashes when the doorbell is rung
- A smoke detector, where light flashes signal the presence of smoke
- A baby cry alert system, where a parent can be signaled if a baby begins to cry in another room
- A telephone ring signaler that causes a lamp to flash
- Text messaging with a cell phone and other text message display systems

I Need to Make a Call

Although many persons with significant hearing loss often rely on the Internet for communication at a distance, most persons still have a need to use a telephone. In addition to using a telephone amplifier, these individuals have at least two other options available for using the telephone. These options are:

Text telephones (TTs): A telephone terminal comprised of a telephone, a keyboard, and a message display screen. The telephone handset fits into the terminal cradle. Both parties must have a terminal set. They communicate by typing their messages to one another. The messages are displayed on the message display screen. TTs are sometimes referred to as telecommunication devices for the Deaf (TDDs). Modern systems include features such as automatic dialing, storage of frequently used words and phrases, and personal directories.

Relay systems: All states provide relay systems as a service for their hard-of-hearing residents. A trained operator serves as an intermediary in a telephone conversation. The person with hearing loss communicates with the operator via a TT (and possibly voice), whereas the normally hearing person communicates with the operator via voice. To place a call, the initiator contacts a relay operator, who in turn contacts the recipient of the call.

A **relay system** is a system used by persons with significant hearing loss for telephone access; an individual contacts a relay operator who serves to transmit messages between the caller and the person called by means of teletype or voice.

CASE STUDY

Listen to the Music

Newsweek Magazine (June 14, 2002) featured an article about cochlear implants and included a case study about a woman who longed to listen to music, opera in particular. The case study presented here is much like this woman's story. Added here are references to the literature that support the statements about music perception and music training.

Sally Anderson, a former music teacher from Des Moines, Iowa, went to the opera with her husband, David, and imagined the lyrics and the music. If they went to parties, David would serve as translator and repeat everything that was said in a group conversation. Similarly, on a trip to England, he repeated the tour guides' commentaries during museum and cathedral visits.

Like her aunt, Sally began to lose her hearing in her late 20s and lost much more of it after her second pregnancy. For the next 15 years, Sally graduated to a series of increasingly powerful hearing aids. The realization of deafness occurred when she was sitting next to the telephone one evening while reading the newspaper. "Answer the phone," her teenage daughter said, poking her in the shoulder. Sally had not heard it ringing.

A year ago, her husband convinced her to contact a cochlear implant center after he read an article about cochlear implants in the newspaper. An audiological examination revealed a bilateral profound hearing loss. After a comprehensive medical examination to ensure good health and no cochlear anomalies, Sally signed up for surgery. "It was an opportunity I couldn't pass up. They said I was a prime candidate. I'd had hearing until adulthood, I hadn't been totally deaf for a very long time, and I was highly motivated to hear." She told her audiologist that she could not wait to hear the birds sing or the radio play. The price was off-putting—$50,000 for the surgery alone, and that fee did not include follow-up aural rehabilitation—but the clinical coordinator at the implant center helped Sally determine that her insurance company would provide coverage.

Immediately upon hook-up of the instrument, Sally recognized the sound of chairs scraping against the floor, a door banging, and a telephone ringing. The audiologist administered a sentence test in an audition-only condition, and she recognized about 20% of the words. During her first 6 months of use, her score on the sentence test rose to almost 60% words correct. Her audiologist encouraged her to continue wearing the hearing aid she had long used in her unimplanted ear, as some researchers have shown that a hearing aid provides additional benefit, especially when listening in noisy backgrounds (e.g., Ching, Incerti, & Hill, 2004). Sally eventually discontinued wearing the hearing aid, saying that the little sound she received from it just made listening with the cochlear implant "more confusing" (see also Mak, Grayden, Dowell, & Lawrence, 2006). Over the course of a year she became a telephone user, and was even able to hear the dial tone (e.g., Anderson, Baumgartner, Boheim, Nahler, Arnolder, & D'Haese, 2006; Cray, Allen, Stuart, Hudson, Layman, & Givens, 2004). She occasionally used an FM system (e.g., Schafer & Thibodeau, 2004).

CASE STUDY, *continued*

Listen to the Music, *continued*

Her disappointment with the device pertained to music. It just did not sound like she remembered it (e.g., see Gfeller, Knutson, Witt, & Mehr, 2003; Gfeller et al., 2005). During the second week of implant use, she talked her husband into taking her to a symphony concert. The experience was so disturbing she had to turn her device off midway through the concert.

Sally enrolled in a music-based aural rehabilitation program (e.g., Gfellar, Mehr, & Witt, 2001). A music therapist with experience working with cochlear implant users started Sally on a simple program where she listened to recorded tunes of familiar songs, such as "Twinkle, Twinkle" and "Happy Birthday to You." The renditions of the songs consisted of simple orchestrations and a male solo singer. Sally easily identified the melodies, and this success motivated her to continue with the training. During the past few months, she has graduated from familiar songs (her favorites are Beatles' tunes from the 1960s), to country and western music (which, for many implant users, is pleasurable because of its rhythmicity and repetitiveness), to familiar symphonic pieces.

Last week, David Anderson took his wife to a presentation of the play, *South Pacific.* Following the advice of her aural rehabilitation music therapist, Sally took a score of the music with her. The couple sat in the balcony, where Sally could discreetly set up the music sheets and follow along. This time, she left the auditorium with tears of joy in her eyes. Sally said she recognized some of the tunes and every lyric.

FINAL REMARKS

In this chapter, we have reviewed some of the fundamental aspects of the most widely used technology in aural rehabilitation. We concentrated on hearing aids, cochlear implants, and assistive listening devices. There is one other kind of listening device available for individuals who for some reason cannot use a hearing aid or cochlear implant, and who are not well served by assistive listening devices. This device is a tactile aid.

Tactile aids permit sound awareness by delivering vibrotactile sensation to the user's skin. Most devices look like a body aid, but instead of having a long cord leading to an earmold, they have a cord leading to a vibrotactile or electrotactile array.

These arrays may be placed against the chest or strapped to the wrist. When sound occurs in the environment, the device microphone picks it up. The signal is transduced into an electrical signal and then delivered to the vibrotactile or electrotactile array, where the skin is stimulated. Some of the more sophisticated devices present a spectral display to the skin, and

Tactile aids are aids that transduce sound to vibration and deliver it to the skin for the purpose of gross sound awareness and gross sound identification.

thus may provide some information about the spectral characteristics of the signal. These devices serve primarily as a supplement to lipreading and rarely permit the user to recognize speech without the visual signal. With the advent of cochlear implants, they are not used by many people today.

KEY CHAPTER POINTS

- The objectives for providing an individual with a listening device are to make speech audible, without introducing distortion or discomfort, and to restore a range of loudness experience.

- Hearing aids, cochlear implants, and assistive listening devices are the primary listening devices available to persons who have hearing loss. Tactile aids are used by a small number of people, primarily those who cannot benefit from the more commonly used devices.

- Two major trends in modern hearing aid design are miniaturization and enhanced signal processing.

- Hearing aids have three fundamental components: a microphone, an amplifier, and a receiver. They also have a power source. Microphones may be directional or omnidirectional. Amplifiers may use peak-clipping for output limiting or compression.

- There are five general styles of hearing aids. Selection of style is dependent on the degree of hearing loss, user preference, costs, patient lifestyle, and the patient's physical status.

- Hearing aid benefit may be assessed with behavioral measures, probe microphone technology, and self-assessment scales.

- Cochlear implants provide sound sensation by means of directly stimulating the auditory nerve. Candidacy requirements for implantation include the presence of irreversible sensorineural hearing loss and good general health.

- Most cochlear implants in use are multichannel devices and many of them utilize an interleaved pulsatile stimulation algorithm.

- Assistive listening devices are used to address communication needs related to face-to-face communication, broadcast and other electronic media, and telephone use. General categories of devices are wireless and hardwired.

- Hearing assistance technology includes ALDs as well as devices that facilitate the reception of auditory information that is not speech and that provide auditory information by means other than amplification.

TERMS AND CONCEPTS TO REMEMBER

Miniaturization
Signal processing
Noise reduction

Hearing aid components
Omnidirectional microphone
Gain
Telecoil
Hearing aid styles
Binaural fitting
Prescription procedures
Validation
Tonotopic organization
Cochlear implant components
Cochlear implant candidacy
Compromised listening environments
Wireless systems
FM sound-field system
Induction loop

MULTIPLE-CHOICE QUESTIONS

1. A hearing aid that permits the patient to adjust the way sound is processed, depending on the listening conditions and the sound stimuli, is said to have:

    a. A sophisticated noise reduction circuit

    b. Multiple memories

    c. Digital processing

    d. Multiple channels

2. Mrs. Cantor is a loan officer at a bank. She works at one of several desks that line the bank's main hall. She wants to be able to talk to her clients one-on-one, even though the hall is noisy. Her audiologist most likely would equip her hearing aid with:

    a. An omnidirectional microphone

    b. Peak-clipping circuitry

    c. A volume control wheel

    d. A directional microphone

3. The input SPL compared to the output SPL in a compression circuitry is know as:

    a. Attack time

    b. Compression ratio

    c. Kneepoint

    d. Peak-clipping ratio

4. The receiver of a hearing aid:

    a. Acts as a miniature loudspeaker and delivers sound to the tympanic membrane

    b. Receives signals from the environment

    c. Includes a preamplifier stage

    d. Is also known as a microphone

5. The least popular style of hearing aid sold in the United States is:

    a. ITE

    b. BTE

    c. Body aid

    d. CIC

6. Which statement is true?

    a. The most appropriate style of hearing aid for a young child is an ITE.

    b. If a person has chronic otitis media, then a BTE aid with a nonoccluding earmold may be the most appropriate style of hearing aid.

    c. Most CIC aids have a volume control wheel.

    d. CIC aids create an occlusion effect.

7. An advantage of binaural amplification is:

    a. The enhancement of low-frequency sound reception

    b. Reduction of background noise

    c. Binaural squeal

    d. Elimination of head shadow

8. A middle ear implant:

    a. Directly stimulates the auditory nerve

    b. Is invisible because all of the components are worn internally

    c. Delivers micromechanical vibration

    d. Is relatively inexpensive

9. Mr. Howard has been deemed an appropriate candidate to receive a hearing aid. When considering what kind of hearing aid to prescribe, his audiologist first:

    a. Asks him about his preference

    b. Performs probe-tube measurements

   c. Presents recommendations and reasons for making them

   d. Determines his loudness discomfort level (LDL)

10. Jennifer Martin is an 8-month-old baby. She had her hearing tested
    2 weeks ago. Her audiologist determined she has a bilateral profound
    sensorineural hearing loss. The audiologist would recommend that:

   a. Jennifer be scheduled for cochlear implant surgery

   b. Jennifer be fitted with an ITE aid

   c. Jennifer undergo a trial period with a hearing aid for 3 months and
       then be considered for cochlear implant candidacy

   d. Jennifer be fitted with amplification and then evaluated at age
       2 years for cochlear implantation

11. The component of a cochlear implant that modifies the acoustic signal
    and separates it into frequency bands is called:

   a. The speech processor

   b. The electrode array

   c. The receiver

   d. The transmitter

12. Which of the following is an older development in the realm of cochlear
    implants:

   a. Interleaved pulsatile stimulation

   b. CICI

   c. Feature extraction processing

   d. Hybrid devices

13. Noise that is present in a room, even when it is empty, is referred to as:

   a. Background noise

   b. Reverberation

   c. Static

   d. Ambient noise

14. An example of an ALD wireless system is:

   a. DAIs

   b. Neckloops

   c. Induction loops

   d. Headphones

15. A person with profound hearing loss who wishes to make a telephone call to his or her insurance agent may take advantage of (choose the best option):

    a. A relay system

    b. A text telephone

    c. A telephone amplifier

    d. A telecoil

16. A patient tells her audiologist that she will soon leave her home in Pasadena, California, for a vacation in London. The audiologist likely discusses which of the following topics with her:

    a. The flu virus and its relationship to hearing loss

    b. Her hearing aid telecoil and induction loop technology

    c. European-based cochlear-implant manufacturers

    d. Battery differences between the United States and the United Kingdom

APPENDIX 3-1

Sources for Information About Listening Devices and Related Technology

Hearing aid manufacturers and their contact information. Most of the Web sites include a consumer hotline and a presentation of the company's product line (adapted from Home of the Stars [2005], *Hearing Health, 21*, p. 18).

COMPANY	TELEPHONE NUMBER	WEB SITE
Bernafon	888–941–4203	http://bernafon.com
GNResound	800–248–4327	www.gnresound.com
Interton	800–243–4741	www.interton-usa.com
Micro-Tech	800–745–4327	www.hearing aid.com
Oticon	800–526–3921	www.oticonus.com
Phonak	800–679–4871	www.phonak-us.com
Unitron	800–888–8882	www.unitronhearing-us.com
Rexton	800–876–1141	www.rexton.com
Siemens	800–766–4500	www.usa.siemens.com/hearing
Sonic Innovations	888–678–4327	http://sonici.com
Starkey	800–328–8602	www.starkey.com
Widex	718–392–6020	http://widexusa.com

Cochlear implant manufacturers and their contact information. Most of the Web sites include a consumer hotline and a presentation of the company's product line.

COMPANY	WEB SITE
Advanced Bionics (manufacturer of the Clarion device and the HiResolution Bionic Ear System)	www.bionicear.com
Cochlear Americas (manufacturer of the Nucleus device and the Freedom Cochlear Implant System with SmartSound)	www.cochlear.com
Med-El (manufacturer of the Combi 40+ device and the PULSAR)	www.medel.com

Companies that offer ALD products and their contact information (adapted from Campbell-Angah, 2005, p. 34).

COMPANY	WEB SITE
Adco Hearing Products, Inc.	www.adcohearing.com
Assisted Access Inc./NFSS Communications	http://nfss.com
AssistiveAudio	www.assistiveaudio.com
Associated Dispensing Service	www.aaiaudiology.com/ads.html
Audex	www.audex.com
Audiologydepot	www.audiologydepot.com
Auditory Instrument Distributors	www.auditoryinstruments.com
Center for the Deaf and Hard of Hearing	www.cdhh.org
Centrum Sound Systems	http:www//centrumsound.com
Comtek Communications Technology Inc.	www.comtek.com
Devilbliss Development Co., Ltd.	www.deafmall.net/devilbliss
Duartek Inc.	http://synergy-em,usic.com/duartek.html
Effective Communication Solutions Inc.	www.beyondhearingaids.com
Etymotic Research	www.etymotic.com
Gerferal Technologies	www.devices4less.com
Global Assistive Devices	www.globalassistive.com
HAC of America/HARC Mercantile Ltd.	www.hacofamerican.com
Hal-Hen Co., Inc.	www.hallen.com
Hear More Inc.	www.hearmore.com
Hearing and Communication Technology	www.audiologyshop.com
The Hearing Loss Help Co.	www.hearing-loss-help-co.com
Hearing Products International, Ltd.	www.hear4you.com

continues

continued

COMPANY	WEB SITE
HITEC Group International	www.hitec.com
Lifeline Amplification Systems	www.lifelineamp.com
Listen Technologies Corp.	www/listentech.com
Nady Systems Inc.	www.nady.com
Oval Window Audio	www.ovalwindowaudio.com
Phone-TTY Inc.	www.phone-tty.com
Phonic Ear	www.phonicear.com
Potomac Technology	www.potomactech.com
Premovation Audio	www.premotivation.com
PureDirect Sound	www.purdirectsound.com
Radio Shack	www.radioshack.com
Sennheiser	www.sennheiserusa.com
Silent Call Corp.	www.silencall.com
Sonic Alert Inc.	www.sonicalert.com
Sound Associates Inc.	www.soundassociates.com
TV Ears Inc.	www.tvears.com
Weststone Laboratories	www.westone.com
Williams Sound	www.williamssound.com

CHAPTER 4

Auditory Training

OUTLINE

- Historical notes
- Candidacy for auditory training
- Four design principles
- Developing analytic training objectives
- Developing synthetic training objectives
- Formal and informal auditory training
- Interweaving auditory training with other components of aural rehabilitation
- Auditory training programs
- Benefits of auditory training
- Case studies: Listening with a new cochlear implant
- Final remarks
- Key chapter points
- Terms and concepts to remember
- Multiple-choice questions
- Appendix 4-1
- Appendix 4-2

The goal of auditory training for persons with hearing loss is to develop their ability to recognize speech using the auditory signal and to interpret auditory experiences. Training helps them use their residual hearing to their maximum capability. During formal auditory training, clinicians probably will not encourage individuals to watch the clinicians' mouth movements as they speak. In fact, the clinicians may obscure their mouth, either by covering it or by sitting out of view (Figure 4-1).

Persons should be fitted with appropriate amplification before starting an auditory training program. A hearing aid (or cochlear implant) makes some speech sounds more audible. Auditory training will not change hearing sensitivity, but will enhance a person's ability to utilize whatever sound is available. By ensuring that individuals have the best amplification system possible, an audiologist will increase the raw material they have to work with and enhance their potential to benefit from training.

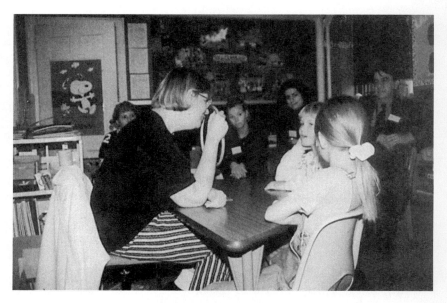

FIGURE 4-1. Formal auditory training. During a typical auditory training exercise, a teacher may cover her mouth movements with a mesh screen held within an embroidery hoop. *Photograph by Kim Readmond, courtesy of the Central Institute for the Deaf.*

HISTORICAL NOTES

The procedures and techniques that speech and hearing professionals use to provide auditory training have evolved gradually over time. Pollack (1970) notes that the value of using residual hearing has long been realized. Archigenes in the first century and Alexander in the sixth century both were known to hold ear trumpets to their ear to intensify the speech signal. Reports of analytic training exercises date back to as early as 1791, when Emaud designed analytic exercises for his deaf pupils. In 1805, Jean Marc Gaspard Itard, at the Paris Institute for the Deaf, provided drill training to children, asking them to discriminate one spoken utterance from another using only their residual hearing. Toynbee noted in 1860 that deaf individuals could learn to attend to their muted voices for the purposes of modulating speech production.

Two of the first schools in the United States to promote auditory training in North America were Currier in New York and Gillespie in Nebraska (Urbantschitsch, 1895). A seminal event in the history of auditory training in the United States occurred when Dr. Max Goldstein left his native St. Louis in 1893 to study with Dr. Adam Politzer, an otologist, and Professor Victor Urbantschitsch, head of the Vienna Otolaryngological Clinic, for 2 years in Vienna. Dr. Goldstein returned to St. Louis, convinced that children with significant hearing losses could learn to talk and to listen. He founded the Central Institute for the Deaf and promoted auditory and speech training for deaf children both nationally and internationally.

Rapid advances in technology during the 20th century increased the potential importance of residual hearing. After World War II, personal hearing aids became more effective and smaller in size so that they could actually be worn throughout the day. At this time, auditory training became a meaningful component of aural rehabilitation for a large segment of the hard-of-hearing and deaf populations. Clarence Hudgins worked with children at Clarke School for the Deaf in Northampton and conducted research that ultimately demonstrated that children who received amplification could increase their speech recognition through listening training (Erber, 1982). Raymond Carhart, a professor at Northwestern University and a man who was often referred to as "the father of audiology," developed auditory training procedures for veterans returning from World War II, many of whom had incurred noise-induced hearing losses from weapons exposure (Kricos & McCarthy, 2007).

The advent of cochlear implants in the latter part of the 20th century led to an explosion in the development of auditory training materials and methods. Computers and training packages founded on sound theoretical underpinnings have changed the complexion of auditory training.

> "In spite of the outstanding technology of modern hearing instruments there is a fundamental problem which no one seems to talk about. Whereas most people who get a new pair of glasses will immediately experience perfect compensation of their poor eyesight—most hearing impaired people have to relearn how to hear in order to fully benefit from their hearing aid."
>
> Harald Seidler, MD, former president of the German Association of the Hearing Impaired and a person with severe hearing loss
>
> (Siemens Audiology Group, 2000, p. 2)

CANDIDACY FOR AUDITORY TRAINING

Auditory training typically is provided to children who either incurred a hearing loss before acquiring speech and language (i.e., children who are prelingually deafened) or incurred their hearing loss afterward (i.e., children who are postlingually deafened). Children who have prelingual and profound losses may have no memory of how speech sounds and may have limited language skills and world knowledge. Thus, they cannot draw on memories of how speech should sound nor utilize acquired knowledge about their world for interpreting the degraded auditory signal. During auditory training, these children first must learn to attend to the auditory speech signal, and eventually they must learn to relate the auditory signal to their vocabulary.

Children who have more hearing, or children who lost their hearing after acquiring some speech and language, often have a larger vocabulary and greater familiarity with grammar and may be better able to deduce meaning from the auditory speech signal, at least initially. The presence of more residual hearing, especially for the mid and high frequencies, portends good progress in auditory skill development. These children will probably begin with more difficult tasks than children who have prelingual, profound hearing losses.

Adults who receive auditory training typically are those who have experienced a recent change in hearing status. For example, someone who has just received a cochlear implant may receive auditory training to accelerate the learning process that often occurs during the first months following implantation (Figure 4-2). Someone who has incurred hearing loss following trauma or use of ototoxic drugs may receive training to adjust to his or her radically altered listening state. Speech through a listening device may sound different from how they remember it, and they must learn to interpret what they hear.

FOUR DESIGN PRINCIPLES

Many auditory training curricula are organized according to four design principles (Table 4-1).

Auditory Skill Level

The first consideration in designing an auditory training curriculum pertains to the person's hearing abilities. Results from an audiological

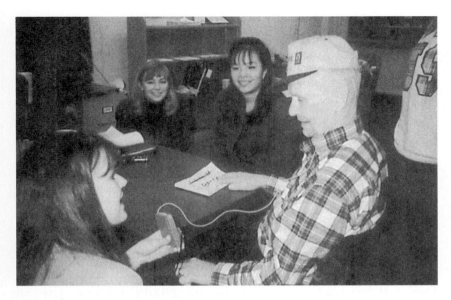

FIGURE 4-2. Auditory training for adults. Adults who may benefit from auditory training are those who have recently received a cochlear implant. *Photograph by Kim Readmond, courtesy of the Central Institute for the Deaf.*

Table 4-1. Four design principles by which activities in an auditory training curriculum may be developed and organized.

A. *Auditory Skill*	**D. *Difficulty Level***
Sound Awareness	Response Set
Sound Discrimination	closed
Identification	limited
Comprehension	open
	Stimulus Unit
	words
B. *Stimuli*	phrases
Phonetic-level	sentences
Sentence-level	Stimulus Similarity
	Contextual Support
	Task Structure
C. *Activity Type*	highly structured
Formal	spontaneous
Informal	Listening Conditions

assessment often are used to assign a student to one of four auditory skill levels (Erber, 1982):

- Sound awareness
- Sound discrimination
- Identification
- Comprehension

As Figure 4-3 indicates, these levels are not discrete benchmarks in auditory development but, rather, represent a continuum of skills. A person may be able to perform some activities associated with a sound discrimination level and some activities associated with identification at about the same time. In this section, the four stages are considered by means of a case study. Table 4-2 presents auditory training activities that may be appropriate for each stage.

Elizabeth Jenkins was diagnosed with a profound, bilateral hearing loss at the age of 13 months. She received bilateral hearing aids within a month following diagnosis. After 5 months of use, her audiologist determined that she was not receiving benefit. Shortly before her second birthday, she received a cochlear implant. Her parents took her to a speech and hearing clinic three times a week, where a speech-language pathologist provided her with auditory training.

During the first few weeks of device use, Elizabeth did not respond spontaneously to sound. For instance, one night her father dropped a stack of plastic dinner plates near the room where Elizabeth was playing. Elizabeth did not turn around to see what had happened. When a telephone rang a few minutes later, she continued playing without a glance toward the sound source.

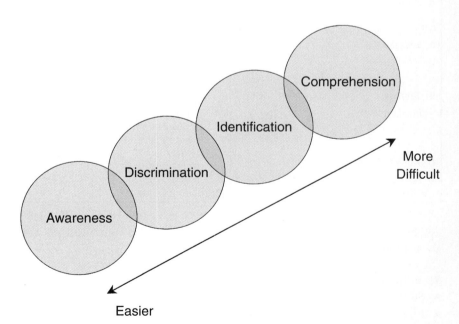

FIGURE 4-3. Four levels of auditory skill development. Auditory skill levels do not represent discrete benchmarks.

Table 4-2. Auditory training activities appropriate for each stage of auditory skill development (for children).

Sound Awareness
Play Peek-a-boo.
Play musical chairs.
March to the beat of a drum.
Push the toy car whenever the clinician says "Vrrrrm."
Sound Discrimination
Play a game with toy animals ("The cow says 'moo'; the sheep says 'baaa'").
Respond to the command ("Give me a crayon"; "Draw").
Play a *Same or Different* game ("boy boy"; "toy boy").
Repeat what you hear ("ma ma ma"; "pa pa pa").
Identification
Play the game *Candyland* and listen for the names of the colors.
Play with sets of postcards or stickers ("Show me the cat").
Play *Go Fish* with cards ("Give me your sevens"; "Give me your twos").
Comprehension
Listen to a read-aloud story.
Play *I Spy*.
Play *20 Questions*.

Several weeks elapsed before Elizabeth consistently demonstrated **sound awareness**, wherein she was aware when sound was present and when it was absent. She searched for sound with eye and head movements or she stopped her activity in response to sound. Sometimes she quieted or startled. She also increased her own vocalizing behaviors. The spontaneous response to sound began to occur once Elizabeth realized that sound has meaning, and that action often produces sound.

Sound awareness is the most basic auditory skill level, and is an awareness of when a sound is present and when it is not.

Elizabeth entered the next auditory skill level, **sound discrimination**, during the latter part of her first year of cochlear implant use. Elizabeth now could recognize when two sounds were the same and when two sounds differed, although sometimes she did not associate meaning with the two sounds or name them. For instance, she could indicate that an "Eeeeeeeeeeeeeee" spoken by her teacher was different from an "Eh." She could distinguish the two-syllable reference to her mother, "Mama," from the single-syllable reference to her father, "Dad." This latter ability is known as **pattern perception**.

Sound discrimination is a basic auditory skill level in which the listener is able to tell whether two sounds are different or the same.

Pattern perception is a kind of discrimination that requires a listener to distinguish between words or phrases that differ in the number of syllables.

After about 10 months of cochlear implant use, Elizabeth entered into the **identification** level of auditory skills development and began to label

Identification is a basic auditory skill level in which the listener is able to label some auditory stimuli.

some auditory stimuli. If her mother asked for a blue crayon, she could pick the blue crayon from a box of four other crayons. This skill relates to an awareness that objects have names, and names have auditory representations. She became aware of suprasegmental nuances in speech, such as changes in her mother's speaking rate, intensity, pitch, and stress. For instance, she could recognize the difference between her mother saying "Elizabeth?" and "Elizabeth!" She could recognize one or two key words in context.

Almost a year and a half elapsed before Elizabeth began to demonstrate some of the listening behaviors associated with the **comprehension** level of auditory skill development, in which she understood the meaning of spoken messages. This stage requires not only advanced auditory skills but some knowledge of vocabulary and grammar as well. At this time, Elizabeth's mother could ask a question with her face not visible and expect that Elizabeth might answer it appropriately, especially if the question was supported by linguistic and environmental context. Elizabeth could follow simple directions such as, "Clap your hands," and recognize familiar expressions such as, "It's all gone." Later, her skills would develop to such an extent that she could understand a series of directions and understand connected narratives.

> **Comprehension** is a higher auditory skill level in which the listener is able to understand the meaning of spoken messages.

Children with significant residual hearing and adults who have had normal hearing before incurring a hearing loss may not progress through these four stages of auditory skill development in the same way as Elizabeth did. For instance, an adult cochlear implant user will be aware of the presence or absence of sound the first time the device is turned on and likely will have some speech discrimination skills. A child who has some residual hearing, or who has incurred a hearing loss gradually over time, also will demonstrate more advanced listening skills.

During the awareness phase of auditory learning, an adult might make a point of showing a child the source and meaning of a sound, and reinforce the child when he or she responds to it. For example, a mother might say:

- "I hear a loud noise. (Point upward.) Look, it's a helicopter."
- "I'm turning on the water. (Turn the handle on a water faucet.) Listen. Now you try it."
- "I hear Janie. She must be coming. Listen."

Activities for sound awareness might include asking a child to drop blocks into a container at the onset of a sound stimulus. With each block drop, the teacher or speech and hearing professional provides animated feedback. It is important that a child be able to recognize when sound is *not* present,

> **Activities for Sound Awareness:**
>
> - The teacher beats a drum; the child indicates onset of sound.
> - The teacher speaks, "ba," with mouth covered; the child indicates when the syllable is spoken.
> - The teacher familiarizes the child with several noisemakers; the child indicates when a noisemaker is sounded and when the noise stops.
>
> *(Stout & Windle, 1992)*

or the absence of sound, as this is an essential skill for participating in a hearing test or the programming of a listening device such as a cochlear implant. This might mean that the child can shake his or her head and know that this is an acceptable response.

Activities for the second level of auditory training task, discrimination, might require a child to first make gross sound discriminations and later, finer discriminations. For instance, early on, the child might be asked to discriminate between syllables that are short and long (e.g., "The car goes *beep* and the cow says *mooooooooo*"), soft and loud (e.g., "The drum beat is *loud* and the drum tap is *soft*"), or continuous and interrupted (e.g., "The whistle goes *eeeeee* and the drum goes *boom-de-boom-de-boom*"). Then the child might discriminate between stimuli that vary in syllable length (e.g., "The dog says *woof* and the cat says *mee-ooow*"). Finally, the child might attend to words that vary in phonetic composition (e.g., "That's a cup and this is a spoon").

In an identification task, older children might play *Bingo,* card games like *Go Fish,* and board games like *Candyland.* In a comprehension task, a teacher might read a story to a child and then ask questions.

Stimulus Units

The second design principle, after a consideration of auditory skills level, pertains to the training stimuli. Although a particular program might emphasize one more than the other, most auditory training curricula include both analytic and synthetic kinds of training activities (Figure 4-4).

During an **analytic training** activity, students' attention is focused on segments of the speech signal, such as syllables or phonemes. As much emphasis is placed on utilizing acoustic cues, such as the presence or absence of voicing in the words *coat* and *goat,* as on gaining meaning from the speech signal. Presumably, one's ability to recognize these segments in isolation enhances real-world communication tasks, allowing students to recognize connected discourse better.

> **Analytic training** emphasizes the recognition of individual speech sounds or syllables.

During **synthetic training**, students learn to recognize the meaning of an utterance, even if they do not recognize every sound or word. They do not perform an analysis of the signal on a sound-by-sound or syllable-by-syllable basis.

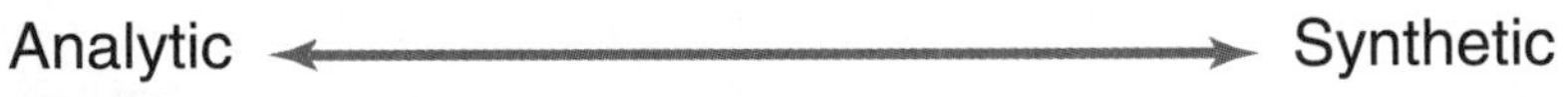

> **Synthetic training** emphasizes the understanding of meaning and not necessarily the identification and comprehension of every word spoken in an utterance.

Analytic ⟵⟶ Synthetic

FIGURE 4-4. Analytic and synthetic training. The distinction between analytic and synthetic activities is a continuum.

There is no clear dichotomy between analytic and synthetic training; rather, this is a continuum, and listening activities will gravitate from focusing attention on acoustic-cue recognition to focusing attention on understanding the gist of a message. In the same lesson, a student might perform analytic training activities and then switch to synthetic activities.

Activity Kind

A third design principle relates to the nature of the training activity (Table 4-1), whether it is more formal or informal. **Formal training** activities occur during designated times of the day, usually with a one-on-one lesson between clinician and student, or in a small group of students. Activities often are highly structured and may involve drill. Students may receive reinforcements for performing a task. For instance, a clinician may speak a series of words without letting the student watch. The student then repeats each word. After every successful repetition, the student drops a coin into a bank. In this example, the speaking of a series of words represents a drill activity. The collecting of coins represents a reinforcement activity.

An **informal training** activity occurs as part of the daily routine and often is incorporated into other activities, such as conversation or academic learning. For instance, a wife may alert her husband when a horn honks or a bird sings after he receives a cochlear implant. She is using informal instruction to draw his attention toward sound and to place names on particular sound patterns.

Except when students are very young, most auditory training programs include both formal and informal training activities. Children who are very young receive primarily informal training. Programs for adults tend to include more formal than informal activities.

Difficulty Level

The final design principle of the four listed in Table 4-1 in which training programs are organized relates to the level of difficulty inherent in the training activity. There are at least six ways to vary training difficulty and to advance students from one skill level to the next (Figure 4-5).

The first way is to vary the size of the stimuli set used for listening tasks. The size of the response set can be varied from a closed set, to a limited set, to an open set. A child might be asked to recognize numbers from a closed set consisting of the numerical digits *one, two, three,* and *four.* A **limited set** is one defined by situational or contextual cues. The set may include words

---

Formal training presents highly structured activities that may involve drill; it usually is scheduled to occur during designated times of the day, either in a one-on-one lesson format or in a small group.

Informal training activities occur during the daily routine and are often incorporated into other activities, such as conversation or academic learning.

A **limited set** of stimuli is defined by situational or contextual cues.

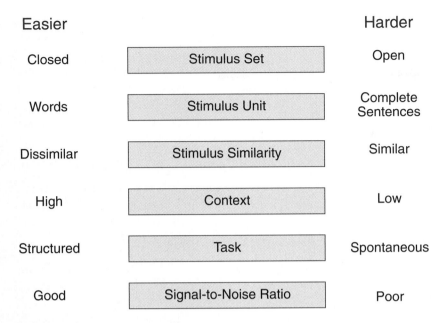

Easier		Harder
Closed	Stimulus Set	Open
Words	Stimulus Unit	Complete Sentences
Dissimilar	Stimulus Similarity	Similar
High	Context	Low
Structured	Task	Spontaneous
Good	Signal-to-Noise Ratio	Poor

FIGURE 4-5. Ways to vary the difficulty of the training task.

pertaining to Halloween, but the student is not briefed about the specific words that might occur during a training exercise. An open set has few inherent constraints; a wide assortment of words are possible as response choices. As a student progresses from closed to limited to open response sets, the listening task becomes more difficult.

A second way to modulate difficulty is to vary the stimulus unit. A clinician might present sentences rather than words and phrases. Students typically perform training activities with words or phrases more easily than with sentences. For instance, a student more likely will identify the word *cat*, from the response set of *cat-mouse-dog* than to identify the sentence, *That's a cat over there,* from the response set of, *That's a cat over there, That's a mouse over there,* and *That's a dog over there.*

A third way relates to stimulus similarity. Most auditory training programs begin with stimuli that differ acoustically and, later, present stimuli that are similar. For instance, initially, when the two items in a training stimulus pair differ, they will be quite dissimilar. A clinician may say the three-syllable phrase, "How are you?" and then the single syllable, "Hi." As a student progresses through auditory training and acquires more listening experience, the items in a stimulus pair will become more similar. The pair might represent a voicing contrast (e.g., *bee* vs. *pea*), a vowel contrast (e.g., *team* vs. *Tim*), or a stress contrast (e.g., *MY dog went home* vs. *My dog went HOME*).

A fourth way to influence difficulty level involves context. Speech stimuli that are supported by either linguistic or environmental context are relatively easy to recognize. For instance, *I had Wheaties for breakfast* is easier to recognize if the talker is standing in the kitchen holding a box of cereal than if the talker is speaking in the office lounge.

A fifth way is to move from structured listening tasks to spontaneous tasks. A student may acquire the skill to recognize a word during a structured activity, but may still not recognize it when it occurs in spontaneous conversation. For instance, a child who is primed to listen for his or her name will be more likely to respond to it than a child who is engaged in quiet play.

Finally, training difficulty can be adjusted by altering the listening environment or the presentation of the stimuli. Background noise, such as the playing of music or talker babble, may be introduced to decrease the signal-to-noise ratio and increase difficulty. The level of the speech may be varied, with a lower level creating greater difficulty.

The level of training difficulty can be varied so that students are challenged but not frustrated. As a general rule of thumb, when providing formal auditory training, the level of difficulty can be increased if someone responds correctly to training stimuli 80% of the time or more. The difficulty level can be decreased if the person responds correctly to less than 50% of the training items.

DEVELOPING ANALYTIC TRAINING OBJECTIVES

At the onset of an auditory training program, a general curriculum is developed or adopted, specifying a hierarchy of training **goals** and **objectives**. If a student has few auditory skills, training typically begins with developing an awareness of sound. Nonspeech stimuli are sometimes used, such as those listed in Table 4-3.

An auditory training **goal** is the result toward which training is directed; it is the desired aim or outcome.

An auditory training **objective** leads to a measurable result, expected within a particular time period and/or after a particular lesson, the accomplishment of which represents a milestone toward achieving the corresponding goal.

Table 4-3. Objects that may promote sound awareness and teach children about the relationship between action and sound.

• Hammer and peg toy	• Computerized game
• Toy drum	• Water faucet
• Piano	• Hair dryer
• Vacuum cleaner	• Whistle

Once sound awareness has been established, early auditory training activities may involve gross discrimination of loudness, pitch, and rate, as in the following examples performed with a xylophone:

- Loudness: Strike a xylophone softly, and ask the student whether the sound is "soft" or "loud."
- Pitch: Play a rising octave, and ask whether the sound is going "up" or going "down."
- Rate: Strike a rapid series of notes, and ask whether the pattern is "slow" or "fast."

Once these kinds of tasks are mastered, then analytic and synthetic training activities might be introduced.

Two kinds of training objectives often are targeted with analytic training: vowels and consonants. Vowels usually are more intense than consonants and have more energy in the low frequencies, so are perceived more readily. For this reason, training for vowel recognition usually begins before training for consonant recognition.

Vowel Auditory Training Objectives

Vowel auditory training objectives typically are designed to contrast vowels that have different formants. **Vowel formants** are the result of resonances in the vocal tract that cause some frequencies to have more energy than other frequencies. The first two formants distinguish one vowel from another. A vowel produced with a wider mouth opening will have a higher first formant than a vowel produced with a narrower mouth opening. A vowel produced with an anterior vocal tract constriction will have a higher second-formant frequency than a vowel that is produced with a posterior constriction. Approximate first- and second-formant values for the vowels of English appear in Table 4-4 (Peterson & Barney, 1952).

Vowel formants are resonances in the vocal tract that cause some frequencies to have more energy than other frequencies.

Training may begin with developing vowel awareness, especially if the student is a young child, and has little experience with the auditory signal. Toys such as farm animals may be used. The child listens as the cow makes a *moooo* sound, the lamb makes a *baaah* sound, and the chick says *cheeeep*.

Once the student demonstrates vowel awareness, vowel training objectives might require students to discriminate between vowel stimuli and then to identify them. Initially, contrasts will concern vowels that differ in first-formant information. For instance, a student might determine whether the words *meet* and *mat* are the same or different. If this proves too difficult,

Table 4-4. Typical first- and second-formant frequency values for the vowels of English, spoken by an adult male talker.

VOWEL	EXAMPLE	FIRST FORMANT (HZ)	SECOND FORMANT (HZ)
/i/	heat	270	2290
/ɪ/	hit	390	1990
/ɛ/	head	530	1840
/æ/	hat	660	1720
/a/	hot	730	1090
/ɔ/	hall	570	840
/ʊ/	hook	440	1020
/u/	who	300	870
/ʌ/	hut	640	1190
/ɚ/	hurt	490	1350

then the contrasts might include words that differ in both initial consonant and vowel—for example, *beat* versus *mat*—and then progress to words that differ only in the first formant of the vowel.

Most persons with hearing loss are more likely to have residual hearing in the low frequencies than the high frequencies; therefore, first-formant contrasts may be more perceptually salient than contrasts that include vowels differing in their second formants. As training progresses, students can discriminate and identify vowel stimuli that differ on the basis of second-formant information, such as *bee* and *boo*. Table 4-5 presents a sample hierarchy of vowel auditory training objectives. These objectives were developed for a child who uses a cochlear implant and who has demonstrated consistent sound awareness.

Table 4-5. A sample hierarchy of vowel training objectives.

The student:

1. Will discriminate vowels that differ in first formant information, using a two-item response set; for example, *meat* from *mat*.
2. Will discriminate vowels that differ in second formant information, using a two-item response set; for example, *bee* from *boo*.
3. Will discriminate words that have vowels with similar first- and second-formant information, using a two-item response set; for example, *met* from *mit*.
4. Will identify words with different vowels, using a four-item response set; for example, *beet* from the response set of *beet, boot, bat,* and *bet*.
5. Will identify words with different vowels, from an open set of vocabulary.

Table 4-6 presents examples of word pairs that might be used for achieving the first three objectives. In typical discrimination exercises, like those required for the first three objectives, a student may sit before two pictures, for example, one of a bat and one of a boot. The clinician might say one of the words, and the student is to point to the correct word. If the student is younger, he or she may place a coin or a piece of cereal on the picture. This provides visible reinforcement, and student and clinician can count the number of markers placed, once the task is completed.

If the student has difficulty in discriminating a stimuli pair, he or she can first practice speechreading (i.e., watching and listening both) the items using a *same/different* task. Figure 4-6 presents a sample response illustration. It has a picture indicating *same* and one indicating *different*. The clinician can speak two words or phrases, such as *That's a pop/That's a peep*, or *That's a pop/That's a pop*. The student then indicates whether the stimuli are the same or different by touching the appropriate picture or by placing a coin on it.

Table 4-6. Vowel and word pairs that can be used for achieving the first three analytic auditory training objectives for vowels.

Objective 1: The student will discriminate vowels that differ in first-formant information, using a two-response set.		
Example vowel pairs:		
/u, i/ versus /a, æ, ʌ, ɔ/		
Word pairs:		
shoe/shop	tube/tub	bean/bun
bee/bat	tooth/tap	moon/mop
boot/bat	shoe/shut	knee/nob
cup/key	three/thumb	bead/ball

Objective 2: The student will discriminate vowels that differ in second-formant information.		
Example vowel pairs:		
/i/ versus /u, ʊ, ʌ, ɔ, a/	/u/ versus /ɪ, ɛ, æ/	
Word pairs:		
bee/boo	seal/soup	feet/foot
soup/sad	key/cup	boot/bit
me/moo	sheep/shop	suit/sat
knee/knot	beet/boot	pot/bean

Objective 3: The student will discriminate vowels with similar first- and second-formant information.		
Example vowel pairs:		
/o/ versus /ɔ/	/ɛ/ versus /e/	
/aɪ/ versus /ɪ/	/a/ versus /ʌ/	
/e/ versus /ɪ/	/i/ versus /ɪ/	
Word pairs:		
pen/pain	hot/hut	ship/sheep
get/gate	beat/bit	fit/feet
ship/sheep	show/shawl	chip/cheap
tin/teen	wet/wait	cake/kit

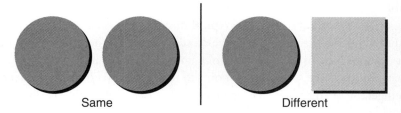

Same | Different

FIGURE 4-6. A response picture for a "same or different" auditory training exercise.

Ideally the words used in a discrimination task should be alike except for the contrasting sounds; for example, the student might discriminate *beet* from *bat,* where the two vowels are contrasting. Such word pairs are relatively easy to construct when the student can read and has an extensive vocabulary. However, when the student cannot read, pictures or objects must be available so that he or she can respond by touching a representation of the word. A list of common one-syllable words that can be illustrated and used for vowel auditory training appears in Appendix 4-1 at the end of this chapter.

For the fourth objective listed in Table 4-5 (i.e., *The student will identify words with different vowels, using a four-item response set*), the response sets increase from two to four choices; for example, the instructor might say the word *beet.* The student's task is to touch one of four pictures: a beet, a boot, a bat, or a bed. For young children, toys or objects may be used in place of pictures.

For the fifth objective, the student must identify words using an open-set format, that is, without a set of response choices. In one exercise, the student might identify words whose vowels have a high-frequency second formant. For example, the instructor might say, "That's a bat," and ask the student to repeat the word without providing a group of words or pictures from which to choose.

Designing Consonant Auditory Training Objectives

Consonant auditory training objectives often are designed to contrast three features of articulation: place, voicing, and manner. Table 4-7 presents a list of consonants grouped together according to these features.

We reviewed the place and voicing features in Chapter 2. For the purposes of auditory training, traditional place classifications include:

- Bilabial, such as /m/ in *man,* wherein the two lips meet to produce the sound
- Labiodental, such as /v/ in *van,* wherein the lower lip and upper teeth contact

Table 4-7. A listing of consonants grouped together according to the features of place of articulation, voicing, and manner of articulation.

A. Consonants classified by manner of articulation
Stops: /p, t, k, b, d, g/
Fricatives and affricates: /f, v, σ, h, s, ʃ, z, dʒ, tʃ, θ/
Nasals: /n, m/
Glides and liquids: /w, j, r, l/
B. Consonants classified by voicing
Voiced: /b, d, g, v, z, m, n, l, w, j, r, θ, dʒ/
Unvoiced: /p, t, k, t ʃ, f, θ, h, s, ʃ/
C. Consonants classified by place of articulation
Bilabial: /m, p, b, w/
Labiodental: /f, v/
Linguadental: /θ/
Alveolar: /t, d, s, z, n, l/
Velar and palatal: /k, g, ʃ, j, tʃ, h, dʒ/

- Linguadental, such as /θ/ in *thumb*, wherein the tongue tip contacts the upper teeth
- Alveolar, such as /d/ in *dot*, wherein the tongue tip approximates or contacts the roof of the mouth just behind the front teeth
- Palatal, such as /ʃ/ in *ship*, wherein the midsection of the tongue body approximates or touches the roof of the mouth
- Velar, such as /g/ in *glove*, wherein the back of the tongue approximates or touches the roof of the mouth

For training purposes, consonants that traditionally are considered palatal are often grouped together with velar consonants.

Manner of articulation is used to classify consonants by the kind of articulatory movements required to produce the particular sound. Consonants can belong to one of five manner groups:

- Stops, such as /p/ and /d/. Stops are produced by completely closing the vocal tract at some point, and allowing pressure to build up behind the constriction. The constriction is released quickly, resulting in a burst of air. Stops are soft sounds and can be produced with or without voicing.
- Nasals, such as /m, n/. They are produced by lowering the velum and allowing air to flow through the nasal cavities. The nasal consonants tend to have high energy in the low frequencies, and they are louder than stops or fricatives.

Manner of articulation is a classification of a speech sound as a function of how it is produced in the oral cavity (e.g., glide).

- Fricatives, such as /f, s/. These sounds are produced by forcing the breath stream through a small constriction in the mouth, which results in a turbulent airflow. Fricatives tend to have a hissing sound. They are louder than stop consonants and longer in duration. They may be produced with or without voicing.
- Affricates, such as /tʃ/. They are produced by combining a fricative with a stop, as in *chop*. For training purposes, fricatives and affricates are sometimes grouped together.
- Glides, such as /w, j, l/. Glides are produced with slow, opening articulatory gestures. For instance, for the word *lot*, the mouth opens more slowly than for the word *tot*. The first word begins with a glide whereas the second word begins with a stop consonant. Glides also are louder than either stops and fricatives and are always produced with voicing.

The easiest features to distinguish for most persons who have hearing loss, even those with significant hearing loss, are voicing cues, and manner cues that signal whether a consonant is a nasal. These distinctions are easiest to hear because voiced sounds and nasals are comparatively loud, and they have energy in the low frequencies. The most difficult cues to hear are those that relate to the place feature. This difficulty occurs because these cues are conveyed by mid- and high-frequency information, and many individuals with hearing loss have their greatest hearing loss for these frequencies.

Knowledge of articulatory features, and how easily they can be heard, can guide the ordering of auditory training objectives. Early auditory training exercises might include consonant stimuli that differ in manner and voice and/or place of production, such as *ta*p and *map*. The sounds /t/ and /m/ differ in terms of manner of articulation, place of articulation, and voicing. Later exercises might require students to identify consonants that differ in place of production but share voice and manner. For instance, they might distinguish between words such as *bag, tag,* and *gag*. These words are similar in their acoustic properties. Table 4-8 presents a sample hierarchy of consonant auditory training objectives for young cochlear implant users.

Table 4-9 presents consonant and word pairs that exemplify the kinds of contrasts and words that might be utilized in achieving the first four objectives. Appendix 4-2 presents a list of common one-syllable words that can be illustrated, which can be used in auditory training activities for very young children who cannot read.

Table 4-8. A sample hierarchy of consonant auditory training objectives.

The Student:
1. Will discriminate nasal versus non-nasal unvoiced consonants that differ in place of production; for example, *mean* from *teen*.
2. Will discriminate nasal versus non-nasal voiced consonants that differ in place of production; for example, *map* from *gap*.
3. Will discriminate unvoiced fricatives versus voiced stops that differ in place of production; for example, *son* from *gun*.
4. Will discriminate unvoiced fricatives versus unvoiced stops that differ in place of production; for example, *sea* from *key*.
5. Will identify words in which the consonants share manner of production from a four-item and then six-item response set; for example, sat from the response set of *sat, fat, shot,* and *van*.
6. Will identify words in which the consonants are all either voiced or unvoiced from a four-item and then six-item response set; for example, *cat* from the response set of *cat, pat, tap,* and *sack*.
7. Will identify words in which the consonants share place of production from a four-item and then six-item response set; for example, *pat* from the response set of *pat, mat, bat,* and *wet*.
8. Will identify words in an open-set format, where the words are familiar vocabulary words.

Table 4-9. Consonant and word pairs that can be used for achieving the first four analytic auditory training objectives.

Objective 1: The student will discriminate nasal versus non-nasal unvoiced consonants that differ in place of production.
Example consonant pairs: /m/ versus /ʃ, s, t, k, tʃ, h, f/ /n/ versus /p, k, f, h, ʃ/
Word pairs:

meat/seat	milk/silk	near/fear
net/pet	news/shoes	no/hose
man/fan	neat/feet	might/fight
may/say	knock/sock	nap/sack

Objective 2: The student will discriminate nasal versus non-nasal voiced consonants that differ in place of production.
Example consonant pairs: /m/ versus /d, g, l, r, θ/ /n/ versus /b, g, w, θ, r/
Word pairs:

nail/rail	nine/wine	note/goat
mail/gate	mice/dice	kneel/wheel
make/rake	knot/rock	make/lake
nail/bail	mow/dough	nap/bat

continues

Table 4-9. *continued*

Objective 3: The student will discriminate unvoiced fricatives versus voiced stops that differ in place of production.		
Example consonant pairs: /f/ versus /d, g/ /s/ versus /b, g/ /h/ versus /b, d/ /ʃ/ versus /b, d/		
Word pairs:		
fun/gun	sell/bell	same/game
shoe/do	heart/dart	shed/bed
she/bee	hay/day	hat/bat
sack/back	song/gone	fall/doll
Objective 4: The student will discriminate unvoiced fricatives versus unvoiced stops that differ in place of production.		
Example consonant pairs: /f/ versus /t, k/ /s/ versus /k, p/ /h/ versus /p, t/ /ʃ/ versus /p, t/		
Word pairs:		
fall/tall	shell/tell	sing/king
fan/tan	sand/can	fat/cat
some/come	show/toe	shine/pine
fin/tin	phone/cone	soil/coil

After the objectives have been achieved with consonants in the initial position, exercises can include them in the final position of words. A carrier phrase such as, *That's a* _____, can be used for presenting noun stimuli.

Alternative Strategies for Designing Training Objectives

The ordering of analytic auditory training objectives described in this chapter is based on comparing sounds based on their similarity and/or dissimilarity from one another. Other strategies for designing auditory training objectives have been proposed. For instance, Miller, Watson, Dalby, and Burleson (2005; also, Miller, 2007) are field testing a computerized program called *Speech Perception Assessment and Training*

DEVELOPING SYNTHETIC TRAINING OBJECTIVES

Depending on the student's skill level, synthetic training objectives might begin with simple discrimination activities that involve suprasegmental aspects of speech. **Suprasegmental** aspects, sometimes referred to as prosodic features, include intonation, stress, duration, and loudness. During training, a teacher might ask a child to move a toy car at a fast or slow pace, depending on whether she or he quickly says, "Go-go-go-go," or slowly says, "Gooo—Gooo—Gooo."

Suprasegmentals are prosodic aspects of speech, including variations in pitch, rate, intensity, and duration, that are superimposed on phonemes and words.

Once these kinds of tasks are mastered, the program can address objectives like those listed in Table 4-10. Students can discriminate and later identify multiword utterances such as *I'm going home* from single-word utterances, such as *home.* This will require them to attend to information about the number of syllables in the phrase. Table 4-11 presents long and short training pairs that can be used for achieving the first objective listed in Table 4-10, and Table 4-12 presents two-syllable spondees that can be used for achieving the second objective listed in Table 4-10.

The next step may be for students to identify simple words from a closed set of choices; for instance, the word *Tom* from the response set of *Tim,*

Table 4-10. A sample hierarchy of synthetic auditory training.

The Student:
1. Will discriminate multiword utterances from single-word utterances, using a closed response set; for example, "How are you today?" from "Hi!" Later, he or she can be asked to discriminate long words from short words; for example, *Halloween* from *cat.*
2. Will discriminate a spondee from a one-syllable word; for example, ice cream from shoe. Later, he or she can be asked to discriminate a spondee from a two-syllable word; for example, "There's a toothbrush" from "There's a pony."
3. Will discriminate between words having the same number of syllables; for example, "That's my cat" from "That's my dog."
4. Will identify simple words from a four-item and then a six-item response set; for example, *cat* from the response set of *cat, dog, elephant,* and *camel.*
5. Will identify picture illustrations from a closed set, after hearing one-sentence descriptions.
6. Will follow simple directions and answer simple questions, using a closed response set.
7. Will listen to two related sentences, and then draw a picture about them; for example, he or she might draw a picture after hearing, "The boy is playing. He has a ball."

Table 4-11. Long and short training pairs that can be used for achieving the first synthetic auditory training objective listed in Table 4-10.

The student will discriminate multiword utterances from single-word utterances:	
How are you/Hi	Beat the drum/clap
See you later/Bye	The cat in the hat/dog
Santa Claus/tree	Give me the crayon/draw
Motorcycle/car	A box of cookies/milk

Table 4-12. Examples of word pairs that can be used for the second objective listed in Table 4-10 for synthetic auditory training.

The student will discriminate a two-syllable from a one-syllable word:	
Airplane/pop	Snowball/ice
Milkshake/cup	Toothbrush/teeth
Flashlight/cake	Popcorn/bowl
Hotdog/bun	Sandwich/gum
Pancake/plate	

John, Don, and *Tom.* As skills progress, the size of the response set can be increased from four to six choices.

Comprehension activities can begin with a closed-set format and move to a more open-set format. Young students might be asked to, *Show me your nose, Show me your ears, Show me your mouth,* and *Show me your hair.* Later, they may be asked to draw a picture, step-by-step, without knowing what the directions might be; for example, *Pick up a blue crayon* (the student demonstrates comprehension by picking it up), *Draw a circle* (the student demonstrates comprehension by drawing the circle), *Put a fish in the circle* (the student draws a fish), and so forth.

If students are adults, a comprehension task might be to listen to a recorded passage and then to answer written questions. Afterward, they listen to the passage a second time, reading a transcript of the passage while listening. The second presentation provides additional listening practice and allows them to check the accuracy of their answers to the questions.

FORMAL AND INFORMAL AUDITORY TRAINING

Once training objectives have been formulated, formal and informal instruction can begin.

Formal Auditory Training

General guidelines for conducting formal auditory training are presented in Table 4-13. Training activities and materials should be appropriate

Table 4-13. Guidelines for conducting formal auditory training.

A. Training stimuli should become more challenging to discriminate over time. Many individuals with hearing loss can determine whether a sound is nasalized or voiced and, less often, whether the sound has frication. They have difficulty in distinguishing place of articulation. In initial training, students may be asked to discriminate between sounds that differ in manner and voice. In late training, they can discriminate between sounds that differ only in place.
B. If feasible, a variety of talkers should speak training items. Students learn that the same sounds or words can be acoustically different when repeated or when spoken by different talkers. This realization allows them to generalize what they learn in training to a variety of talkers. Tape recorders, iPODs, CD-ROMs, and digitized speech samples can be used to present stimuli.
C. A great many training items should be presented during a relatively short period of time. Concentrated training focuses students' attention on listening and maintains their interest, leading to fast learning. Adherence to this guideline means that training reinforcements are provided sparingly, since they may be time consuming and distracting.
D. Nonspeech training stimuli should be used only with young students who are prelingually deaf, and only for a short period. Nonspeech stimuli develop two important concepts: First, sound conveys meaning and second, action often produces sound. The child might turn on and off a water faucet or clap hands. The exception to this guideline is the student who is interested in developing his or her ability to appreciate music.
E. An auditory training exercise can include both analytic- and synthetic-level stimuli. Occasionally the student's attention is focused on recognizing speech sounds and single words or phrases, and occasionally on recognizing words in a meaningful context.
F. Training progresses from closed-set to open-set response modes. Early in training a young student might be asked to color a shape red and therefore need to choose between a red or blue crayon (closed set). Later, the student might be asked to select the red crayon, when crayons from an entire box are available as options (open set).
G. Ten to 15 minutes a day should be devoted to formal auditory training, preferably at the same time every day. Training thus becomes a part of the daily routine.
H. Formal training objectives should be pursued informally throughout the day. When opportunity arises during conversation or academic instruction, the student can be presented with listening tasks that reinforce the formal auditory training objectives.
I. Training activities must be engaging and interesting. Otherwise, the adult may simply pass through the motions of training without receiving benefit; the child may not cooperate.

Table 4-14. An example lesson plan for a formal auditory training session.

Title:

Snake and Ice Cream Game

Goal:

Discrimination

Objective:

The student will discriminate a nasal consonant versus non-nasal unvoiced consonant that differs in place of production.

Materials:

1. a picture of a snake to represent the /s/ sound

2. a picture of a boy about to eat an ice cream sundae to represent the /m/ sound

3. a stack of 26 pennies for reinforcements

Procedures:

1. Introduce the picture of the snake by pointing to it and saying "sssssssss . . ." Ask the child to imitate your production. Similarly, introduce the picture of the sundae, and say "mmmmmm . . ." Ask the child to imitate your production.

2. Say each sound with your face visible. After each utterance, ask the child to point to the corresponding picture.

3. Place 13 pennies on each picture. Cover your mouth. Randomly say one sound after another. After each production, the child may pick up a penny from one of the two pictures. If the child removes a penny from the correct picture, he or she can keep it. If incorrect, the penny must be placed back on the picture.

4. Continue until all pennies are spent.

---

for students' age, gender, language skills, and everyday experiences. For instance, a young boy might respond to materials that concern soccer. An adult might enjoy materials about current news events. If possible, auditory training should occur with no more than one to three students at a time, in a quiet room that offers minimal distractions. The optimal distance between the teacher and student is about 12 inches. A sample lesson plan for a formal auditory training session is presented in Table 4-14.

To make formal auditory training stimulating for children, **reinforcements** are often essential. After students complete a set number of items or perform so many activities, they receive something desirable, such as a sticker or special privilege. The following are general principles to follow when choosing and providing reinforcements:

A. The child should be able to perform a reinforcement activity quickly; he or she should not spend more time with the reinforcement activity than with the training activity.

B. Reinforcement activities should not be too challenging or too absorbing; otherwise the child will not attend closely to the training task.

A **reinforcement** is something desirable provided to a student after he or she performs a training activity or performs in a desired manner.

C. Activities must be varied; drawing lines on a paper may hold a child's interest for a few minutes, but the activity quickly wears thin.

D. Activities should interest the child; for example, if the child enjoys playing with money, he or she might drop coins into a bank.

E. The child should perform the reinforcement activity immediately after responding to a training item correctly.

F. Activities should be appropriate for the child's age and gender.

Informal Auditory Training

Informal auditory training is an effective means of fostering listening skills because listening practice occurs in the context of meaningful communication and is not removed from situational context (Figure 4-7). Informal auditory training can enhance students' confidence in their abilities to engage in conversation and also increase their motivation to rely on hearing for communication.

Reinforcements

Reinforcements are often utilized during formal training activities. Reinforcements must be appropriate for the age and interests of the students. The following two lists present reinforcements that might be appropriate for young children and adolescents:

List 1: Young children
• Collecting stickers in a sticker book
• Putting features onto a Mr. Potato Head
• Placing puzzle pieces one at a time into a puzzle board
• Blowing soap bubbles
• Playing a card game or board game
• Stringing beads onto a bead necklace

List 2: Adolescents
• Earning tokens that can be used to purchase desirable privileges, such as time with a computer game
• Earning tokens that can be used to buy school supplies, such as pencils and notepads
• Earning tokens that can be used to buy extracurricular rewards, such as a gift certificate to a fast-food restaurant

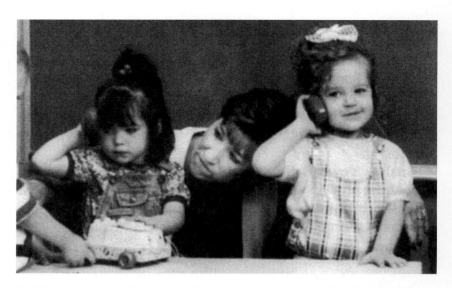

FIGURE 4-7. Auditory training for children. Two children practice their listening skills while playing a telephone game in their preschool class. In this instance, the two girls are listening for their teacher to say the word *phone*. *Photograph by Marcus Kosa, courtesy of the Central Institute for the Deaf.*

Informal auditory training is especially appropriate for babies and young children. By listening to language spoken in meaningful contexts, they will develop speech and language as well as listening skills. Listening and attending to speech will become a part of their self-identity and modus operandi. Parents and caretakers can play an important role in providing listening practice. They may be encouraged to minimize background noise in the home, to speak close to the child's listening device and to speak sometimes with their mouth out of view, and to use language and speech that is repetitive, melodic, expressive, and/or rhythmic. They might draw attention to environmental sounds (e.g., "I hear the telephone ringing.") and engage the child in singing and light conversations (e.g., "I see you!" or "That's a sock. Shall we put on your sock?"). When students are children, classroom teachers can incorporate informal listening practice into the academic curriculum by selecting words, phrases, and sentences that provide listening practice and that also correspond to themes, units, and classroom activities. Theme-based learning is effective because it mimics how children with normal hearing naturally learn to listen. For example, a child might be expected to distinguish between the words *seed, leaf, stem,* and *bud* during a botany unit. The classroom teacher might expect students to comprehend familiar phrases associated with the calendar. The teacher might query, with mouth hidden, "Tell me what today is," "Tell me what day it was yesterday," and "Tell me what will tomorrow be." The teacher may instruct, with face clearly visible, "Go to the chalkboard. I will say a number between one and ten." These instructions establish a context for recognizing her next instruction, which will be spoken while the student faces the chalkboard: "Write the number seven."

INTERWEAVING AUDITORY TRAINING WITH OTHER COMPONENTS OF AURAL REHABILITATION

Auditory training is sometimes provided in conjunction with speechreading training and, if the student is a child, speech therapy. By interweaving auditory and speechreading training, a speech and hearing professional will build a student's associations between corresponding auditory and audiovisual representations of speech. It is common for training stimuli to be presented in the audiovisual condition before being presented in an audition-only condition. Students will recognize considerably more stimuli when they can both see and hear the talker rather than only hear the talker.

There are at least two reasons to incorporate speech production practice into auditory training. First, a child's awareness of oral representations of words may relate closely to the child's ability to identify the words auditorily. For instance, there appears to be an underlying linguistic structure that links speech perception and speech production. This structure reflects a child's knowledge of phonology, as well as grammar (Lachs, Pisoni, & Kirk, 2001). Thus, the gains that children make in their abilities to perceive the sounds of speech develop and fine-tune their phonological representations of words cognitively. In turn, these phonological representations affect the child's ability to produce them. This process likely is a two-way street. As a child's ability to produce sounds improves, the phonological representations of words become more developed and refined, which, in turn, may affect speech perception.

The second reason to link speaking and listening practice together is that by doing so, the child may realize that one purpose of learning to listen is to learn how to utilize auditory information to enhance speech production. Children will develop the habit of monitoring their own speech as they talk. Through auditory training and speech therapy, they can learn to attend to the suprasegmental qualities of their speech outputs (e.g., *Am I talking too loudly? Too softly? Is my voice conveying the nuances of meaning that I intend?*) and attend to the clarity and accuracy of their sound production.

AUDITORY TRAINING PROGRAMS

Although it is important that speech and hearing professionals who provide auditory training understand the general design principles that we have considered in this chapter, they need not "start from scratch" with every student. A number of auditory training programs are available for general use that incorporate some or all of these design principles. These programs can either supplement an auditory training program or comprise its central core. Table 4-15 provides information about a sampling of auditory training resources.

Table 4-15. A sampling of auditory training resources. Additional resources for auditory training are available through several hearing aid and cochlear implant manufacturers (see Chapter 3 Key Resources for their contact information).

RESOURCE	TARGET AUDIENCE	DESCRIPTION
Analytika. Available from Med-EI, http://www.medel.com.	Children and adults	Lists of words contrasting pairs of consonants, vowels, or diphthongs. The lists can be used to provide practice in perceiving specific contrasts. Can be used in developing one's own auditory training program or exercise.
Contrasts for Auditory and Speech Training (CAST). Available from Linguisystems, 3100 4th Avenue, East Moline, IL 61244-9700.	Children ages 3–12	An analytic training program that provides practice in discriminating suprasegmental contrasts (e.g., words differing in number of syllables), dissimilar words, and minimal pair words (e.g., words varying in initial consonant place of production only). Includes a manual and picture cards. Can be used during individualized therapy sessions.
CHATS: The Miami Cochlear Implant, Auditory and Tactile Skills Curriculum. Available from Intelligent Hearing Systems, 6860 SW 81st Street, Miami, FL 33143.	Children who use cochlear implants, hearing aids, and tactile vocoders	A curriculum organized around a flow chart that includes such stages as evaluation, selection of goals and objectives, and selection of activities. A model activity is provided for each objective. Speech perception and speech production goals are interwoven, and a team approach is encouraged, involving audiologist, speech-language pathologist, classroom teacher, and parent or guardian. Can be meshed with the context of classroom instruction.
The Cochlear Implant Auditory Training Guide with CDs (2nd ed.). Available from A. G. Bell Association for the Deaf and Hard of Hearing, 3417 Volta Place, Washington, DC, 20007-2778.	Children aged 5 years and older who use cochlear implants and who may vary widely in their listening abilities	A curriculum that includes hierarchical listening goals, reproducible materials, and game pegs and boards. The CDs include a placement test, lesson plan forms, discrimination cards for words, phrases, and higher language, and listening tasks and activities. Can be used in a therapy setting.
The Developmental Approach to Successful Listening II (DASL). Available from Cochlear Corporation, 400 Inverness Drive South, Suite 400, Englewood, CO 80112.	Children and adults who have hearing loss of every degree	A curriculum that organizes training into sections of sound awareness, phonetic listening, and auditory comprehension. Each of these sections includes a hierarchical list of auditory subskills so progress occurs in each of the three sections simultaneously. Can be used in a therapy or classroom setting.

continues

Table 4-15. *continued*

RESOURCE	TARGET AUDIENCE	DESCRIPTION
Listening and Communication Enhancement (LACE). Available from Neurotone, 2317 Broadway, Suite 250, Redwood City, CA 94063.	Adults	A Web service that provides practice in listening to a variety of speech stimuli, including speech in babble, time-compressed speech, and sentences with missing words. Training is home-based, self-paced, and occurs in half-hour sessions.
The *Speech Perception Instructional Curriculum and Evaluation (SPICE).* Available from Central Institute for the Deaf, 825 South Taylor Avenue, St. Louis, MO 63110.	Children 3–12 years	A curriculum that provides training for four levels of auditory skill level: detection, suprasegmental perception, vowel and consonant perception, and connected speech. The program includes goals, objectives, and activities as well as toys and illustrated word and phrase cards. Initially, training occurs in formal training sessions that focus on a single skill and then training becomes more informal and emphasizes more natural language. Can be used in a therapy or small classroom setting.
SKI-HI. Resource manual is available from The SKI-HI Institute, 6500 Old Main Hill, Logan, UT 84322-6500.	Children birth to 5 years	A comprehensive developmental program that provides audiological services and complete home intervention programming. It includes an auditory stimulation training program. This program is organized around four stages of development and targets 11 skills, including attending, recognizing, locating, and speech sound discrimination and comprehension. The overall program is meant to provide services to large areas, such as districts and states, and includes a home intervention resource manual.

For many auditory training curricula (e.g., Erber, 1982; Moog, Biedenstein, & Davidson, 1995; Vergara & Miskiel, 1994), the first step is to determine the placement of the student within the program. For instance, in the *Developmental Approach to Successful Listening (DASL) II* (Stout & Windle, 1992), the student might be tested to determine if he or she can indicate when a continuous environmental sound stops. If yes, the student is then tested to determine if he or she can indicate when a sustained speech syllable or word stops (the next objective in the hierarchy of objectives). If no, the student begins auditory training with an exercise focused on developing environmental sound awareness.

After placement is determined, goals are identified. In most programs, the goals represent global speech perception skills and are ordered hierarchically in terms of difficulty. They often correspond to the four levels of auditory skill that we considered earlier. For instance, the *Speech Instructional Curriculum and Evaluation (SPICE)* (Moog, Biedenstein, & Davidson, 1995) has four general goals: detection, suprasegmental perception, vowels and consonants, and connected speech. Similarly, the *DASL II* organizes exercises according to the three goals of sound awareness, phonetic listening (which includes discrimination and identification), and auditory comprehension.

Objectives (and some curricula refer to these as *goals within goals* or *subgoals*) and corresponding activities are serially ordered to achieve the auditory training goals. Objectives in most curricula are a measurable means for achieving a goal, and for many programs, they are ordered in a similar manner as the objectives that we considered earlier for vowel and consonant analytic training and synthetic training. The first four objectives for *phonetic listening* in the *DASL II* program, for instance, include (a) discriminate a short staccato sound from a long continuous sound, (b) discriminate between a continuous sound and repeated syllables, (c) discriminate between one short syllable and two short syllables, and (d) discriminate between two long, continuous syllables and two short, staccato syllables. The criterion for achieving each of these objectives is 50 consecutive correct responses with a variety of stimuli. Notice how these goals progress students from one level to the next in small, incremental steps. Table 4-16 presents an example of a lesson plan designed to be taught in the context of a classroom lesson about the seasons. In this example, auditory training is interlaced with speech production practice. The lesson includes a goal, an objective, and activities.

Table 4-16. Example of an auditory training lesson that includes a goal, objective, and activities and is meant for a class setting (adapted from Vergara & Miskiel, 1994, p. 241).

Goal:

Perception of Sentences

Title:

The seasons

Objectives:

Recognizes phrases in a six-choice task.

Materials:

Season story (select a story about the seasons); sentence strips (written with phrases chosen from season story).

Content:

(1) Review seasons with students (summer, fall, winter, spring); (2) Read and discuss story about the seasons; (3) Review selected phrases written on sentence strips (e.g., hot sun; snow is cold; beautiful flowers; bright yellow leaves; fun swimming; trick or treat); (4) Ask students to initiate and imitate each phrase; (5) Repeat phrases, ask students to name the season associated with each phrase; (6) Repeat above without lipreading; (7) Give each child an opportunity to be the teacher; (8) Observe and note each child's response.

Tips:

Remind students to listen to the salient features of each phrase. Emphasize the syllable number of the words to help with discrimination.

A student does not necessarily have to meet one training objective before progressing to the next one. The *CHATS* (Vergara & Miskiel, 1994) utilizes cycling:

> "**Cycling** involves presenting a skill within a specified time period and then moving on to another objective. . . . For example, after targeting one objective for two weeks, the teacher may choose to move on to another objective returning to the original objective at a later date. . . . Cycling provides the opportunity for students to process new concepts. For example, after an initial introduction, children are provided with opportunities to experiment with a particular task so that at the time of the second presentation, they may experience a higher level of success." (p. 58)

Cycling entails the coming back to a training objective that has been achieved with some success in order to provide reinforcement and additional learning.

Cycling is a means to build listening skills and is effective in helping students overcome a plateau in their listening performance.

A number of newer auditory training curricula utilize computerized training (e.g., Fu & Galvin, 2007; Sensimetrics, 2006; Tye-Murray, 2002). For example, the *Listening and Communication Enhancement* program (LACE, Sweetow, 2006) is a packaged computerized auditory training curriculum geared for adults. Training presents words and sentences in the presence of speech babble, and requires patients to identify missing words in sentences, to recognize time-compressed speech, to perform a short-term memory task, and to attend to competing talkers. The program also includes communication strategies training in the form of "tips."

BENEFITS OF AUDITORY TRAINING

Efficacy of auditory training is difficult to assess. Many of the extant studies have methodological flaws, such as the failure to monitor outcomes for extended periods of time, use of inadequate sample sizes, failure to establish whether treatment effects generalize beyond the training parameters, inadequate description of the training program, or some combination of these (see Sweetow & Palmer, 2005, for a review). Blamey and Alcantara (1994), commenting on the apparent contradictory results of some investigations, suggest that whether or not auditory training is found to be effective relates to the varying types and amount of practice provided, the skill of the clinician who provides training, the different kinds of listening skills that are evaluated, and the varying level of performance of the students at the time of their entry into a training program. Despite these daunting experimental design hurdles, there are several studies that support the efficacy of training.

> "Even if later, more thorough studies of auditory training may correct some judgments rendered in this paper or even if they are completely repudiated, it is of no consequence to the cause itself. I ask only that the subject be thoroughly examined from a great many sides. . . . It is my heartfelt conviction that general application of auditory training will lead to its general acceptance."
>
> Victor Urbantschitsch (1847–1921), first head of the Department of Otology of the Vienna Otolaryngological Clinic and mentor to Dr. Max A. Goldstein, the St. Louis physician who introduced Dr. Urbantschitsch's auditory training methods to the United States
>
> *(from Auditory Training for Deaf Mutism and Acquired Deafness by Victor Urbantschitsch, 1895, preface)*

Adults

Sweetow and Palmer (2005) surveyed the literature to address the following question: "Is there evidence of improvement in communication skills through individual auditory training in an adult hearing-impaired population?" (p. 494). Only 6 articles out of a possible 213 met their criteria of providing sufficient detail and methodological rigor to obtain evidence-based assessments of the benefits of auditory training. The training methods were similar across the programs, providing analytic and/ or synthetic training. Of the six investigations reviewed, four provided evidence that auditory training enhances the listening performance of adults who have hearing impairment (Bode & Oyer, 1970; Montgomery, Walden, Schwartz, & Prosek, 1984; Rubinstein & Boothroyd, 1987; Walden et al., 1981), one did not (Kricos, Holmes, & Doyler, 1992), and one reported mixed results (Kricos & Holmes, 1996).

Since publication of this review, additional studies have suggested that auditory training is beneficial (e.g., Sweetow & Sabes, 2007; Woods & Yund, 2007). For instance, Burk, Humes, Amos, and Stauser (2006; and in a similar study, Burk & Humes, 2007b) demonstrated that the word recognition performance of seven older adults (ages 65–75 years) with mild-to-moderate hearing loss improved following auditory training. Improvements occurred for the testing of words, both when they were spoken by the female talker who spoke during training and when they were spoken by novel female and male talkers. Six months after completing this experiment, five of the seven students returned for additional testing. The participants had retained about half of their level of improvement. However, at this later test date, it was revealed that the students had not transferred benefits to sentences that contained the target training words or sentences that were spoken by novel talkers. In another study, Tobey et al. (2005) examined whether cochlear implant users who received auditory training while under the influence of d-amphetamine received greater benefit than a comparable cohort with no drug enhancement. Participants engaged in 16 one-hour training sessions. Both groups showed a significant improvement in their posttraining test measures as compared to the pretraining test measures, and the test group showed more improvement than the control group. Finally, in perhaps the most comprehensive study, Sweetow and Sabes (2006) provided computerized training to 65 experienced adult hearing aid users. Training was conducted with a home-based computer for 30 minutes per day, 5 days each week, for a total of 4 weeks. Half of the participants received training immediately after the pretest session whereas the other half received training 1 month later. Testing included two sentence tests and questionnaires that were administered immediately after the 4-week training program and then again 4 weeks later. Data were reported for 42 of the participants. Results indicated improvement for the trained participants based on all but one of the outcome measures 4 weeks posttraining.

In addition to the studies cited previously, additional support for the potential effectiveness of auditory training comes from the neuroscience and cochlear implant literature. It appears that adults retain neural **plasticity** in relationship to auditory learning (Palmer, Nelson, & Lindley, 1998; Tremblay, Piskosz, & Souza, 2003). For instance, brain activity has been shown to change as a result of auditory training (e.g., Kraus et al., 1995; Russo, Nicol, Zecker, Hayes, & Kraus, 2005; Tremblay & Kraus, 2002; Tremblay, Kraus, Carrell, & McGee, 1997). Some adults who receive cochlear implants continue to improve their listening performance for periods of 9 months or even longer following device hookup (Tye-Murray, Tyler, Woodworth, & Gantz, 1992).

Plasticity is a term used to refer to the physiological changes in the central nervous system that occur as a result of sensory experiences.

Children

Little research has been performed on the benefits of auditory training per se for children. As with adults, the research is difficult to conduct because many variables may influence the effectiveness of training. For instance, the kind of listening aid that the student uses may affect outcome. Current cochlear implants allow many users to hear mid- and high-frequency components of the speech signal. These users may hear more information about place and frication, as well as other parameters of speech, than individuals who have similar hearing loss and use hearing aids. Progress also may be influenced by the student's age, motivation to receive training, age at which the hearing loss was incurred, duration of hearing loss, family situation, and the student's personality. For example, a teenager who has had a hearing loss since birth probably will receive less benefit from auditory training than a small child who recently incurred a hearing loss. An outgoing, extroverted child who frequently interacts with children who have normal hearing might have a greater intrinsic desire to develop listening skills than an introverted child who prefers solitary activities.

Some evidence suggests that auditory training is beneficial for the pediatric population. Children who use aural/oral communication and rely on listening and speechreading for recognizing messages tend to perform better on tests of speech recognition than children who use total communication and rely on speech and sign language (Geers & Moog, 1992). Children in an aural/oral educational program often receive more auditory training than children in a total communication program, so one interpretation is that

"We're seeing a resurgence of training programs designed to improve the speech perception of people with hearing loss. One reason for this resurgence, I believe, is all the information we have acquired recently about brain plasticity. . . . The ability to alter neural response patterns, through training, is provocative and the translation of this basic science to auditory rehabilitation is obvious for those of us interested in the rehabilitation of hearing-impaired patients."

Kelly Tremblay, PhD, associate professor at the University of Washington in Seattle and internationally known researcher in the area of electrophysiological measurement

(Tremblay, 2006, p. 14)

aural/oral children perform better on speech recognition tests because of the increased amount of auditory training they receive. Hnath-Chisolm (1997) provided auditory training to 17 children, who ranged in age from 4 to 8 years. They listened to isolated word stimuli in a Phase 1 and then words in sentence contexts in a Phase 2, for a total of 4 weeks of training. Significant improvements occurred in recognition of minimally contrasted word pairs and sentences. Results suggested that greater improvements occurred as a result of training with sentence-level stimuli than isolated word stimuli.

CASE STUDY

Listening with a New Cochlear Implant

This section focuses on two children who were described by Ertmer, Leonard, and Pachuilo (2002). At the onset of the description, both children had received cochlear implants. These two examples demonstrate how an auditory training program might be implemented and adjusted to meet the specific needs of the individual. The first child, Drew, had experience with normal hearing and then usable residual hearing for many years before incurring a profound hearing loss. His preimplant experiences with hearing allowed him to quickly associate the electrical signal with his memories of how speech used to sound. In contrast, the second child, Bobby, suffered a hearing loss much earlier in life, and his auditory skills emerged more slowly.

Case Study 1: A Child with Prelingual Onset of Deafness

Drew had normal hearing until shortly after his third birthday, when he contracted meningitis. He suffered a moderate sensorineural hearing loss in his right ear and a severe loss in his left ear. He received binaural hearing aids and joined a preschool for children who have hearing impairments. His family and teachers used total communication with him (i.e., communicated using both spoken language and sign language that has English syntax), although he expressed himself only with speech.

At the age of 7 years, Drew lost his hearing completely and thereafter received a cochlear implant. He began individualized intervention sessions with a speech and hearing professional, twice weekly for 1-hour periods. This intervention lasted 20 months.

Speech sounded qualitatively different to Drew through a cochlear implant than through the hearing aids he had used prior to his complete loss of hearing. Thus, the primary goals of intervention were to "help Drew make sense of the new signal" (p. 206) and to increase his hearing performance so as to improve speech and language skills. His intervention integrated activities in auditory training and speech and language therapy.

For auditory training, Drew participated in both analytic and synthetic listening activities. The analytic auditory training focused on the parts of speech so as to enhance Drew's ability to distinguish between vowel and consonant features. The program objectives were similar to those presented in this chapter, in Tables 4-5 and 4-8. Speech sound contrasts progressed from requiring Drew to make gross distinctions to fine

CASE STUDY, *continued*

Listening with a New Cochlear Implant, *continued*

distinctions, and the number of choices in a response set increased as Drew became more proficient in his listening skills. He had to meet a criterion of 80% accuracy for two consecutive intervention sessions initially for a contrast (e.g., distinguishing pair /t/ words from /d/ words). As his skills developed, this criterion level was raised to 90% accuracy for a single session. This upgrade was done to allow Drew to spend the majority of his time working on difficult contrasts and less time on those that were perceptually salient for him already.

Drew's progress for analytic listening tasks concerning consonants is plotted in Figure 4-8. Similar progress was noted for vowel discriminations. The light bars indicate his average score for a specific consonant contrast prior to training, and the darker bars indicate his performance following training. The number of sessions devoted to establishing the contrasts is denoted in parentheses above the bars.

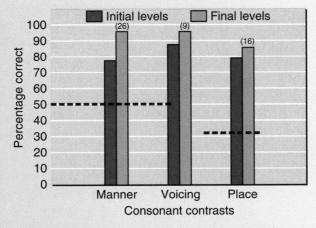

FIGURE 4-8. Drew's scores for percentage correct consonant features at the onset and the termination of auditory training intervention for each contrast (dashed lines = chance-level performance; numbers in parentheses = number of sessions devoted to the contrast). Modeled after Ertmer, Leonard, and Pachulio (2002, p. 207).

Drew's initial scores ranged from 70% to almost 90% correct after just one training session. He received training only for those items that did not meet the 80% criterion level. Some of the contrasts that needed three or more sessions to establish included the following contrasts: /e/ versus /æ/ and stops versus fricatives.

For synthetic auditory training, an emphasis was placed on comprehension of meaningful speech. Training tasks included repeating and completing sentences and answering questions about spoken material, which allowed Drew to utilize contextual and syntactic cues.

continues

CASE STUDY, *continued*

Listening with a New Cochlear Implant, *continued*

Case Study 2: A Child with Prelingual Onset of Deafness

Bobby lost his hearing when he was 5 months of age, after a bout of spinal meningitis. He received a cochlear implant at the age of 3 years, and in the interim received approximately a year of family-centered speech and language intervention. Those around him used manual sign language to communicate with him, and he mainly expressed himself through gesturing and pointing. He wore a hearing aid for only a few weeks following his illness. He was described as shy and reluctant to try new tasks.

At the onset of intervention (which did not start until about a year following implantation), Bobby demonstrated some sound awareness. For example, he alerted to the ring of the telephone and the sound of water running. However, he did not respond to sound in a meaningful way and he did not respond to his spoken name.

The initial auditory training goals were designed to teach Bobby to identify nonspeech sounds, such as a drumbeat or a bell ring. Training with speech stimuli began with asking Bobby to identify words that differed in syllable number and to recognize frequently occurring words, including his name, the clinician's name, and the names of familiar toys. He worked on recognizing familiar phrases, such as *Sit down*.

During the analytic segments of training, Bobby initially could not perform a two-choice listening task. The clinician used praise, encouragement, and reinforcers (e.g., puzzle pieces) to maintain Bobby's attention and to motivate him. When he misidentified items, the clinician presented the items audiovisually and then presented an auditory-only model again to reinforce contrasts between phonemes.

Word pairs that differed in number of syllables (e.g., *orange* vs. *strawberry*) were first presented and practiced for about 10 to 15 of the 22 intervention sessions. By the end of the intervention, he identified syllables differing by number of syllables with about a 75–81% accuracy. Once this milestone was achieved, Bobby began to focus on discriminating between phonemically dissimilar words that have the same number of syllables (e.g., *car* vs. *sheep*).

His auditory training program also focused on enhancing auditory comprehension in meaningful contexts. His synthetic training activities included practice in recognizing names, phrases, and statements and questions. He listened to simple books, where the clinician and his mother took turns reading pages. The readings were recorded, and Bobby took home the audiocassette for home practice.

CASE STUDY, *continued*

Listening with a New Cochlear Implant, *continued*

After 2 years of experience with his cochlear implant, Bobby was just beginning to discriminate between gross acoustic patterns consistently. He demonstrated improved awareness of speech and environmental sounds, but he still had only emerging abilities in associating speech with meaning.

Comments About the Case Studies

Drew and Bobby present different challenges for auditory training intervention. Whereas with a child like Drew, a clinician will be hard-pressed to keep up with his rapidly emerging listening skills, a child like Bobby will progress slowly and may require the clinician to develop novel ways of motivating and keeping him interested in intervention.

Synthetic Auditory Training Procedures

In an auditory training program for Drew, one of their students, Ertmer, Leonard, and Pachuilo (2002) implemented these four procedures:

Picture [vocabulary] books . . . were particularly useful during the first months after implantation because they contained abundant vocabulary words for everyday situations and allowed auditory training to be game-like. For example, after reviewing the vocabulary words on a given page, . . . Drew and the clinician took turns making up sentences such as, "I see a red hat on the table." The listener would then find the corresponding picture. At first, a short, simple sentence format was used repeatedly (e.g., "I see X." or "Can you find X?"). As Drew's auditory, syntactic, and semantic skills improved, more complex and varied sentences were introduced.

Conversations about selected topics (e.g., basketball, vacation plans, school) also provided practice in auditory comprehension. . . . A topic was selected and then discussed for a few minutes. Drew was encouraged to guess if he did not understand what was said.

continues

Tips for Cochlear Implant Users About Listening to Music

- "Practice listening to music that was familiar prior to hearing loss.
- Begin with music played by fewer instruments, such as solos or small ensembles, rather than music by large bands or orchestras.
- Try songs that have many repetitions of musical patterns or words [e.g., children's songs] . . .
- Use visual cues, such as watching a singer's lips and the rhythm of the piano player's fingers, to help make sense of the music.
- Read along with the lyrics . . .
- Don't give up! Many people report that music sounds better the more they listen to it."

Gfeller, 2005, p. 2

Synthetic Auditory Training Procedures, *continued*

A [continuous discourse] tracking procedure . . . was used with high-interest stories to improve sentence comprehension and syntax skills. During this activity, Drew was asked to repeat sentences exactly as they were read to him. He was also encouraged to ask for repetitions and clarifications. This task was often difficult when Drew was unfamiliar with the story. He was most successful when the page had been read with the clinician before the sentence repetition task.

Riddles and jokes provided challenging material for synthetic auditory training during the second year of intervention. The clinician would read a riddle or joke and then Drew would repeat what he heard before guessing the answer. (p. 208)

FINAL REMARKS

When individuals have hearing loss, listening skills often do not emerge spontaneously. Deliberate and systematic auditory training is required to foster listening potential.

Auditory training need not be confined to speech and environmental stimuli. Some individuals with hearing loss may desire instruction that will enhance their recognition and appreciation of music. For instance, adult cochlear implant users who enjoyed music before losing their hearing often wish to begin listening again once they have received their implants. Work is currently under way in some cochlear implant programs to develop music training programs and to evaluate the efficacy of this kind of program for enhancing music enjoyment (Gfeller & Witt, 1999; Gfeller, Mehr, & Witt, 2001; Gfeller et al., 2002).

KEY CHAPTER POINTS

- Usually, children with significant hearing losses receive auditory training. Adults are less likely to receive training.
- Most auditory training curricula are designed to progress a student from one auditory skill level to the next. The four skill levels underlying most programs are sound awareness, sound discrimination, identification, and comprehension.

- Many auditory training curricula include both analytic and synthetic kinds of training activities, and formal and informal activities.

- Difficulty of training can be adjusted by varying the size of the stimuli set used for listening tasks, the stimulus unit, stimulus similarity, context, structure, and the listening environment. As a general rule of thumb, a clinician will want to alter the level of difficulty if a student responds correctly to training stimuli 80% of the time or more, or responds correctly to less than 50%.

- A hierarchy of specific training objectives typically is developed at the onset of a student's auditory training program. The objectives are targeted with both analytic and synthetic training.

- Analytic vowel auditory training objectives are often designed to contrast vowels with different vowel formants. Consonant auditory training objectives are often designed to contrast features of articulation, such as place, voice, and manner. Alternative strategies for designing analytic training objectives focus on the frequency of occurrence of particular sounds and on word frequency.

- A variety of auditory training programs are available. These include the SPICE, the DASL II, LACE, and CHATS.

- Several published reports suggest that auditory training is beneficial. In addition, brain activity appears to change as a result of auditory learning.

- Students may vary widely in how quickly they progress, in part as a function of their hearing history, their personalities, and their listening environments.

TERMS AND CONCEPTS TO REMEMBER

Sound awareness
Sound discrimination
Identification
Comprehension
Analytic training
Synthetic training
Difficulty level
Formants and features
Goals
Objectives
Guidelines for formal auditory training
Theme-based learning
Interweaving
Brain plasticity

MULTIPLE-CHOICE QUESTIONS

1. Which modification would make an auditory training activity more difficult?

   a. Switching from an open response set to a limited response set

   b. Switching from a spontaneous activity to a highly structured activity

   c. Contrasting words beginning with /m/ and /n/ rather than words beginning with /d/ and /ʃ/

   d. Asking a child to determine whether two phrases are the same or different rather than asking the child to answer questions presented auditorily

2. Which statement best captures what research tells us about the efficacy of auditory training:

   a. The preponderance of the evidence suggests that it is beneficial for both children and adults, but there are some data to the contrary.

   b. Auditory training is beneficial for children but not for adults.

   c. Auditory training is beneficial for adults but not for most children.

   d. No evidence-based research exists.

3. Saundra dropped the lid to a pan onto the tile kitchen floor. Her daughter, playing in the room next to the kitchen, turned her head. The daughter's response is best described as:

   a. Sound awareness

   b. Sound identification

   c. Sound discrimination

   d. Analytic listening

4. An activity where a student is asked to discriminate word pairs is best described as:

   a. Introductory

   b. Analytic training

   c. Synthetic training

   d. Phonemic training

5. A clinician can decrease the level of training difficulty in an auditory training intervention session:

   a. By decreasing the signal-to-noise ratio

   b. By decreasing the task structure

    c. By increasing stimulus similarity

    d. By changing the number of items in the stimulus set

6. Which of the following tasks is likely to be included later rather than earlier in an auditory training intervention?

    a. Discriminating vowels that differ in first-formant information

    b. Discriminating vowels that differ in second-formant information

    c. Discriminating monosyllables from bisyllables

    d. Discriminating vowels with similar first- and second-formant information

7. The consonant feature that is typically most difficult for persons with hearing loss to hear is:

    a. Manner of articulation

    b. Place of articulation

    c. Voicing

    d. Nasality

8. The activity that a beginning student most likely will perform early on in auditory training is the following:

    a. Discriminate nasal from non-nasal unvoiced consonants.

    b. Discriminate unvoiced fricatives from unvoiced stops that differ in place.

    c. Identify words in which the consonants are all either voiced or unvoiced, from a four-item response set.

    d. Discriminate words varying in place of production.

9. Ms. Hoffman has prepared a reinforcement for her 5-year-old student. Every time the child recognizes a word correctly, she will get to make an animal out of clay. This activity is:

    a. Not an optimal reinforcement activity because it is not age-appropriate

    b. Not an optimal reinforcement activity because it is too time consuming

    c. An optimal reinforcement activity because it is challenging

    d. An optimal reinforcement activity because it takes no advanced preparation on Ms. Hoffman's part

10. Which of the following statements about informal auditory training is false?

    a. Parents can be encouraged to speak in an expressive, melodic, and rhythmic voice.

    b. The general classroom is an ideal site for providing informal auditory training because listening practice can be incorporated into meaningful themes and units.

    c. Children may be distracted by the content of the speech and, thus, may not attend to its acoustic qualities, thereby diluting benefit.

    d. Adults are more likely to receive formal auditory training than informal auditory training in a clinic setting.

11. Which curriculum was designed to be used for children ranging in age from birth to 5 years?

    a. SKI-HI

    b. LACE

    c. CHATS

    d. DASL II

12. "The student will discriminate minimal pair words differing in nasality" is an example of a(n):

    a. Goal

    b. Activity

    c. Objective

    d. Criterion

APPENDIX 4-1

Words That Can Be Illustrated and Used for Vowel Auditory Training Exercises

/u/		/ʊ/		/i/	
soup	goose	book	hood	beak	geese
boot	tool	hook	wood	wheat	feet
food	moon	foot	pull	sleep	peel
suit	pool	full	shook	seat	sheet
shoe	fool	bull	cook	bean	peas

/ɪ/		/ɛ/		/æ/	
bit	six	net	ten	bat	patch
sit	mitt	bell	men	bag	gas
lid	pill	belt	nest	man	hat
pin	fish	bed	egg	cans	pan

/ʌ/		/a/		/ɚ/	
gun	brush	jar	doll	bird	worm
gum	one	top	sock	shirt	girl
duck	bun	rock	knot	burn	church
bus	gun	pots	mop	pearls	purse

/e/		/o/		/ɔ/	
rake	cake	bow	coat	shawl	lawn
eight	rain	soap	bone	long	fawn
lake	grapes	pole	boat	cross	ball
tape	chain	hose	goat	walk	chalk

APPENDIX 4-2

Words That Can Be Illustrated and Used for Consonant Auditory Training
Exercises

/p/		/b/		/t/	
pan	pea	bee	boot	tea	tool
peach	patch	ball	bell	top	toes
pool	pill	bat	boat	tooth	two
pen	pin	beet	bed	tack	toad

/d/		/k/		/g/	
dog	doors	K	clouds	gas	gum
ducks	deer	crown	corn	goose	loves
dots	dice	cake	keys	green	girls
doll	D	cat	clown	gun	goats

/tʃ/		/d/		/f/	
church	cheese	jar	J	frame	farm
chair	chips	jump	jug	foot	feet
chick	chain	jeep	jeans	fan	fox
chin	cheek	jet	juice	fish	face

/v/

vase	vault
van	vane
veil	vest
vine	valve

/h/

hose	horse
hit	house
ham	hip
heel	hand

/m/

mouse	moon
mitt	mat
man	mice
mail	match

/r/

red	rope
rain	rose
rake	rice
rat	rock

/θ/

thumb	three
thigh	thick
thin	thorn
thread	thief

/s/

seal	sail
stars	socks
stairs	school
seeds	sled

/n/

nail	net
knot	nuts
knees	nine
knife	nose

/l/

leg	lamp
lake	leaf
lamb	light
lock	lime

/ʃ/

sheep	shorts
shoes	shirt
sheet	shack
shell	ship

/w/

wheat	web
wig	witch
wave	wire
wine	wood

CHAPTER 5

Speechreading

OUTLINE

- Speechreading for communication

- Characteristics of a good lipreader

- What happens when someone lipreads?

- The difficulty of the lipreading task

- What happens when someone speechreads?

- Importance of residual hearing

- Factors that affect the speechreading process

- Oral interpreters

- Case study: An exceptional lipreader

- Final remarks

- Key chapter points

- Terms and concepts to remember

- Multiple-choice questions

Lipreading is the process of recognizing speech using only the visual speech signal and other visual cues, such as facial expression.

Speechreading is speech recognition using both auditory and visual cues.

The terms lipreading and speechreading often are used interchangeably. In our discussion, we will follow the conventions of Thorn and Thorn (1989), Walden, Prosek, Montgomery, Scherr, and Jones (1977), and Lansing and Helgeson (1995). When **lipreading**, a person relies only on the visual signal provided by the talker's face for recognizing speech (Thorn & Thorn, 1989). When **speechreading**, the person attends to both the talker's auditory and visual signals, as well as the talker's facial expressions and gestures, and any other available cues. These clues include the setting in which the conversation is occurring or what has been discussed beforehand (Walden et al., 1977).

SPEECHREADING FOR COMMUNICATION

Persons with normal hearing routinely rely on speechreading. Consider these examples: When we are at a noisy restaurant, we understand more if we watch the talker's face while we listen (MacLeod & Summerfield, 1987; Sumby & Pollack, 1954). We may feel unsettled when we view dubbed foreign films because the words we hear do not match those we see. A raised eyebrow imparts additional meaning to the question, "You're not working today?" A number of experimental paradigms have been developed that demonstrate that even if an individual has normal hearing, that person relies on visual speech information to recognize and comprehend a message. If someone reads aloud Kant's *Critique of Pure Reason,* which is difficult-to-grasp philosophy, the audience will better understand the content if the members see and hear the reader than if they only hear the person's voice (Arnold & Hill, 2001; Reisberg, McLean, & Goldfield, 1987). If a talker "shadows" someone who is reading a passage, that is, attempts to repeat each word the reader speaks as quickly as possible, the individual will do so at a faster rate if he or she sees and hears the reader than by listening alone (Reisberg et al., 1987). Evidence that visual information is used routinely for speech recognition also comes from studies employing **functional magnetic resonance imaging (fMRI)**, a noninvasive means of mapping brain activity. When someone tries to recognize speech using the visual signal only, the **auditory cortex** becomes activated. Activation will not occur if the research participant simply watches a face make rhythmic movements of the jaw and mouth without opening the lips (see Campbell, 1998, for a review). Even infants engage in speechreading. If a 5-month-old baby hears someone phonate "eeeeeee," and simultaneously views a side-by-side projection of the same talker, on one side saying "eeeeeee" and the other side saying "aaahhhh," the baby most likely will fixate on the visual signal that corresponds to the acoustic signal (Kuhl & Meltzoff, 1982).

Functional magnetic resonance imaging (fMRI) is an imaging technology used to study the activity of the brain; the computerized images show which brain structures are active during a particular mental activity.

The **auditory cortex** is the region of the brain that is responsible for processing auditory information and is located in the temporal lobe of the cerebral hemisphere, just forward of the occipital lobe.

A person with hearing loss will depend more on the visual signal for speech recognition than will individuals who have normal hearing. Whereas most persons can converse on the telephone with ease, or follow a news broadcast on the radio, a person with hearing loss will experience decreased speech recognition when only the auditory signal is presented. The greater the hearing impairment, the more an individual will rely on visual information for communication.

CHARACTERISTICS OF A GOOD LIPREADER

A plethora of research has revealed that it is difficult to predict lipreading performance. Performance cannot be predicted by an individual's intelligence, educational achievement, presence of and duration of acquired hearing loss (and hence, practice with the lipreading and speechreading tasks), age at hearing loss onset, gender, or socioeconomic status (Hygge, Rönnberg, Larsby, & Arlinger, 1992; Jeffers & Barley, 1971; Lyxell & Rönnberg, 1990; Rönnberg 1995; Rönnberg, Öhngren, & Nilsson, 1982, 1983; Tye-Murray, Sommers, & Spehar, 2007a; 2007b). Even with additional information about verbal abilities, cognitive skills such as visual memory, and personality, it is not possible to make an infallible prediction (see Summerfield, 1989, for a review).

Some research suggests that particular cognitive skills might correlate with lipreading. These skills include visual word decoding, **working memory**, lexical identification speed (e.g., how quickly a person can determine whether a string of letters constitutes a word), phonological processing (e.g., how quickly a person can decide whether two words rhyme), and verbal inference making (e.g., how well a person can complete sentences that have missing words) (Andersson, Lyxell, Rönnberg, & Spens, 2001).

Working memory refers to one's ability to store simultaneously and manipulate items in memory.

A handful of other variables may be somewhat predictive. Young adults lipread better than elderly adults (Farrimond, 1959; Honnell, Dancer, & Gentry, 1991; Sommers, Tye-Murray, & Spehar, 2005). Figure 5-1 shows the difference between how well young and old adults lipread consonants, words, and sentences. These individuals have normal hearing and no visual impairment. As the figure suggests, the younger adults can lipread all three types of speech stimuli better than the older adults. There is some evidence that age yields an influence on lipreading performance on the other end of the life span as well. Younger children do not recognize some phonological contrasts or words in a carrier phrase context as well as older children do (Hnath-Chisolm, Laipply, & Boothroyd, 1998; Kishon-Rabin & Henkin, 2000; Mauzé, Tye-Murray, & Jerger, 2007). For instance, children between

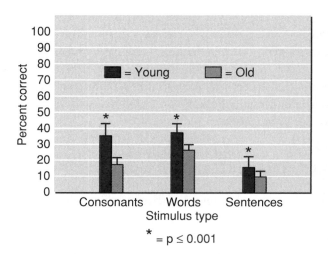

FIGURE 5-1. Percentage correct scores for a group of 45 young lipreaders (ages 18–24 years) and a group of 45 older lipreaders (ages 65 years and older). The asterisk indicate a significant difference in performance between the two groups.

the ages of 5 and 7 years appear not to recognize the place of production of final consonants as well as children between the ages of 9 and 11 years do. Finally, even though individuals who have acquired hearing loss do not appear to develop superior lipreading skills to those individuals who have normal hearing (e.g., Tye-Murray et al., 2008), some evidence suggests that individuals who have congenital hearing loss lipread better than do individuals who are born with normal hearing (Bernstein, Demorest, & Tucker, 2000; Mohammed et al., 2005). Bernstein, Auer, and Tucker (2001; see also Auer & Bernstein, 2007) compared the lipreading performance of eight individuals with prelingual profound hearing loss to that of eight individuals with normal hearing using a sentence test. The groups did not differ in their percentage word correct scores, but when the responses were scored in terms of phonemes correct, the group with hearing loss performed better.

There is also some evidence, albeit conflicting, that neurophysiological measures relate to performance. The latencies of recorded electrical potentials made at the cortex following stimulation of the eye by a flash of light may correlate with lipreading performance (Rönnberg, Arlinger, Lyxell, & Kinnefors, 1989; Shepherd, 1982; Shepherd, DeLavergne, Frueh, & Colbridge, 1977; but see Samar & Sims, 1983; Summerfield, 1992), with shorter latencies being characteristic of good lipreaders. Shorter latencies indicate more rapid transmission of neural impulses from the eye to the brain and are unlikely to be affected by an individual's experiences, personality, or circumstances.

Possible predictors of lipreading skill:

- Age
- Prelingual hearing loss
- Certain cognitive skills
- Willingness to guess

Some speech and hearing professionals have cited more nebulous characteristics that may relate to lipreading performance, including individuals' ability to capitalize on contextual cues, their willingness to guess, their mental agility, and their willingness to revise interpretations of a partially recognized message (e.g., Jeffers & Barley, 1971; Lyxell & Rönnberg, 1987). Especially in children, linguistic and world knowledge can constrain proficiency. Someone who has a limited vocabulary, limited knowledge of grammar, and limited world knowledge will likely experience lipreading difficulties. For instance, if a child has a limited knowledge of geography, the child will not readily recover the word missed when lipreading the sentence, "_____ *is the capital of the United States.*"

Predicting Lipreading Performance

People vary widely in their lipreading performance. Some individuals can score 80% words correct or better on a vision-only test condition, as measured by verbatim repetition of test words, whereas others score 5% or worse on the same stimuli (Bernstein, Demorest, Coulter, & O'Connell, 1991). The amount of practice in lipreading does not account for variability. Some college students who have normal hearing and who have never received lipreading training perform better on a sentence recognition test presented in a vision-only condition than adults who have an acquired hearing loss, and who have been deaf (and hence, speechreading for communicative purposes) for many years (Hanin, 1988).

WHAT HAPPENS WHEN SOMEONE LIPREADS?

A talker's face presents salient cues for recognizing the sounds of speech and the prosodic patterns of sentences. For instance, when a talker speaks the sound /m/, the lips press together. When the talker makes the /u/ sound, the lips pucker slightly. The eyebrows rise when a talker incredulously asks a question (e.g., *You did what?*). When someone lipreads, the person's eyes scan the talker's face, seeking both phonetic and prosodic cues as to what is being said. Eyes may stabilize, for an eye fixation, or rotate in quick, high-velocity shifts.

Researchers have studied eye movement behavior during lipreading using equipment that tracks the center of the pupil. In one study, it was found that lipreaders monitor different regions of the face, according to the kind of information they seek (Lansing & McConkie, 1999). Research participants were asked to discriminate either phonetic contrasts (e.g., *Ron ran* vs. *We won*) or to discriminate between questions and statements (e.g., *Ron ran?* vs. *Ron ran*). In general, subjects tended to direct their eye gaze toward the talker's eyes, nose, and mouth, with occasional shifts to the regions of the forehead, cheeks, and chin. When seeking prosodic information about questions versus statements, they focused more on the upper face (most likely monitoring events such as forehead wrinkling, eyebrows raising, and eye widening), and when making phonetic judgments, they focused more on the lower face, monitoring lip and jaw movement. Eye gaze tended to shift to the talker's eyes at the end of an utterance, regardless of what the subjects' lipreading task happened to be.

Speechreading as an Art Form

Evelyn Glennie is a classical percussionist who has a profound hearing loss. In a radio interview (KMOX, St. Louis), she was asked why she lipreads so well. Ms. Glennie replied that she approaches lipreading in the same way many people with normal hearing listen to music. At a symphony, audience members do not necessarily attend to every note, but rather, attend to the structure of the music and the interplay of the various instruments. Similarly, Ms. Glennie explained, she does not try to lipread every word. She follows the message as it is conveyed by the words she recognizes; by what has been said beforehand; and by the talker's facial expressions, head nods, body posture; and hand gestures.

THE DIFFICULTY OF THE LIPREADING TASK

When lipreading, most people recognize less than 20% of the words they see. (Look back at Figure 5-1 and examine the percentage correct scores for words in a sentence context.) Why is lipreading so difficult? The answer to this question relates to the variables listed in Table 5-1. In this section we consider five variables that compound the difficulty of the lipreading task: visibility of sounds, rapidity of speech, coarticulation and stress effects, visemes and homophenes, and talker effects.

Table 5-1. Factors that influence the difficulty of the lipreading task.

FACTOR	EFFECT
Visibility of sounds	Many sounds are not associated with visible mouth movement.
Rapidity of speech	Often, sounds occur in sequence faster than the eye can resolve them.
Coarticulation and stress effects	The appearance of words vary as a function of how they are spoken.
Visemes and homophenes	Many sounds and words appear alike on the face.
Talker effects	Talkers speak sounds and words with different mouth movements.

Visibility of Sounds

Many sounds entail minimal visible mouth movement. Woodward and Barber (1960) estimated that 60% of speech sounds are not visible on the mouth or cannot be seen readily.

Words that are more visible on the face tend to begin with consonants that are made with bilabial closure (/p, b, m, w/), the lower teeth pressing the upper lip (/f, v/), or the tongue tip contacting the upper teeth (/θ, ð/). Consonants with limited visibility include sounds that are produced within the mouth, such as /k, g, t, n/. Some features of phonemes are simply not visible at all. For instance, there is no visible evidence indicating that a phoneme is either voiced (e.g., /b, d, g/) or unvoiced (e.g., /p, t, k/). Figure 5-2 presents

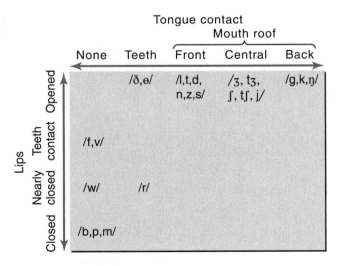

FIGURE 5-2. Consonant production as a function of tongue and lip activity.

the consonants (excluding /h/) according to the activity of the lips and tongue. Those consonants that have lips closing during production tend to be more distinctive than those that do not; the consonants that are produced with tongue activity toward the front of the mouth tend to be more distinctive than those produced at the back of the mouth.

Vowels are considered not to be highly visible. They may or may not be distinguished by lip spreading (e.g., *beak* vs. *book,* where /i/ involves more lip spreading than /ʊ/), tongue and jaw height (e.g., *bit* vs. *bought,* where /I/ is associated with greater tongue and jaw height than /ɔ/), and lip rounding (*boot* vs. *bet,* where /u/ is associated with more lip rounding than /ɛ/) (see Figure 5-2). Fortunately, even though vowels are not associated with distinctive mouth movements, they tend to be acoustically salient to individuals who have hearing loss. Vowels are relatively intense, change slowly over time in their frequency composition, and are relatively long in duration (see Figure 5-3).

Rapidity of Speech

When speaking conversationally, a talker may speak anywhere from 150 to 250 words per minute, or roughly four to seven syllables per second, excluding time spent pausing. Greenberg (1999) analyzed a large corpus of spontaneous speech and found that although the average syllable duration was about 200 milliseconds (or 5 Hz), speaking rate varied as a function of emotion, social formality, fatigue, and style of articulation. Whereas a typical talker may produce an average of 15 phonemes per

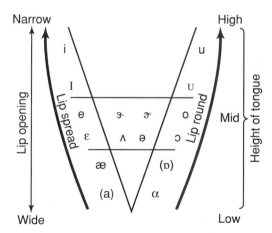

FIGURE 5-3. Vowel production as a function of lip opening, lip spreading, and tongue height. Modeled after Berger (1972, p. 78).

second, the human eye may be capable of registering only about 9 or 10 discrete mouth movements in this time interval. Thus, the lipreader (speechreader) has little time to ponder the identity of a particular word and even may not realize the occurrence of every word. The individual may have difficulty determining when one word ends and the next word begins as word boundaries may not be clearly demarcated visually.

Coarticulation and Stress Effects

Coarticulation and stress effects may result in the same sound looking different depending on its phonetic and linguistic context. For example, the sound /b/ looks different in the word *boot* versus *beet.* The lips begin to round in anticipation of the following /u/ in the first case; the lips begin to spread in anticipation of the following /i/ in the second case. If an alveolar consonant follows a rounded vowel such as /u/ in the word *hoot,* the lip rounding may hide the tongue and the teeth.

Stress can also affect the appearance of a word. The word *you* looks different in the following question, depending on the talker's stress pattern:

What did ya do yesterday?

What did YOU do yesterday?

Visemes and Homophenes

The fact that sounds belong to viseme groups and many words are homophenous increases lipreading and speechreading difficulty. **Visemes** are groups of speech sounds that look alike on the face (Fisher, 1968). The sounds /b, m, p/ comprise a viseme. When these sounds are spoken without voice, as in *bat, mat,* and *pat,* they are indistinguishable on the mouth. There is some disagreement among researchers as to which sounds constitute a viseme, although all agree that there are fewer visemes than phonemes (e.g., Binnie, Montgomery, & Jackson, 1974; Erber, 1974; Lesner, Sandridge, & Kricos, 1987). Two listings of consonants grouped as visemes as compiled by two different sources appear in Table 5-2.

> **Visemes** are groups of speech sounds that appear identical on the lips (e.g., /p, m, b/).

Homophenes are words that look the same on the mouth. It is not always intuitively clear which words are homophenous and which words are not. For example, as different as the words *grade* and *yes* sound, they are nonetheless homophenous. When only the visual signal of the talker is presented, an individual will likely not discriminate one word from the other. On the other hand, even though the words *boon* and *doom* sound similar, and might be confused with one another if the listening environment is

> **Homophenes** are words that look identical on the mouth.

Table 5-2. Consonants grouped as sets of visemes. Reports from two different research groups.

ERBER (1974)	LESNER, SANDRIDGE, AND KRICOS (1987)
/p, b, m/	/p, b, m/
/f, v/	/f, v/
/θ, ð/	/θ, ð/
/ʃ, ʒ/	/ʃ, ʒ, dʒ, tʃ/
/w, r/	/w, r/
/l/	/l/
/n, d, t, s, z/	/t, d, s, z, n, k, g, j/
/k, g/	
/h/	

Source: Adapted from Lesner, K., Sandridge, S., and Kricos, P. (1987). Training influences on visual consonant and sentence recognition. *Ear and Hearing, 8,* 283–287; and Erber, N. P. (1974). Visual perception of speech by deaf children: Recent developments and continuing needs. *Journal of Speech and Hearing Disorders, 39,* 178–185.

noisy, an individual will have no problem in distinguishing one from the other if the talker's face is visible.

Table 5-3 presents a list of other homophenous word pairs. If a speech and hearing professional wanted to sensitize a patient to the existence of homophenous words, the professional might use these word pairs to perform an exercise like this (Kaplan et al., 1985, p. 100):

- I say, *rise.* The word that is a homophenous to this word is (circle one on your answer sheet):
  - a. pies
  - b. mine
  - c. rice (*correct answer*)
  - d. lice

Table 5-3. Examples of homophenous word pairs.

HOMOPHENOUS WORD PAIRS (WORDS THAT LOOK ALIKE ON THE FACE)	
Rise	Rice
Perch	Merge
Marry	Bury
Mat	Man
Bind	Mite
Aunt	Hand
Van	Fat
Pass	Ban
Down	Stout

- I say, *merge*. The word that is homophenous to this word is (circle one on your answer sheet):
  a. lunch
  b. perch (*correct answer*)
  c. worst
  d. burn

Somewhere between 47% and 56% of words in the English language are homophenous (Auer & Bernstein, 1997). Grammatical sentence cues and other linguistic and situational cues can decrease the confusion about word identity, and some talkers will better distinguish words on the basis of the visual signal than will other talkers. Nonetheless, the existence of homophenous words often makes lipreading difficult. Often, the word choices that a lipreader must consider are numerous, as illustrated in the example, "Pat sat on a log." Table 5-4 is a matrix of possible confusions that could be made for each word.

The lipreader might come away with any number of meanings after lipreading this simple sentence, including:

- Matt sat by ad.
- Bess stacked hot dogs.
- Brad tanned on a dock.
- Paul set its lock.

Talker Effects

Talker effects may confound lipreading efforts because the same sound may look different when spoken by two different people (e.g., Lesner & Kricos, 1981; Montgomery, Walden, & Prosek, 1987). For instance, two talkers may differ in the degree of mouth opening used for speaking the vowels in the sentence, *"That is Pat's."* A person who has a pronounced accent may appear different when talking than a person who has the same regional accent as the lipreader. For instance, a native of Minnesota may not recognize visually the word *rice* when it is spoken by a Texan.

Table 5-4. Confusions Matrix.

PAT	SAT	ON	A	LOG.
Matt	set	in		dog(s)
Brad	tanned	hot		sock
Bess	stacked	his		dock
Paul	tracked	its		lock

"They're losing sensitivity to this as they grow older. There's really no reason for them to hang onto this ability if they are only going to be learning one language."

Whitney Weikum, lead scientist on a study demonstrating that monolingual babies can visually discriminate one language from another at the ages of 4 and 6 months but not at the age of 8 months

(Fountain, 2007)

Even Babies Lipread

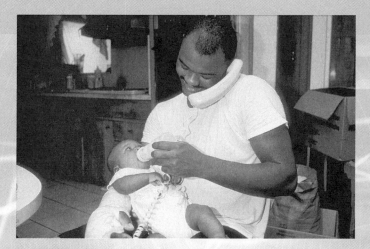

FIGURE 5-4. Infants and speechreading. Infants attend to the visual speech signal as they learn their native language.

Have you ever held an infant and noticed how the baby gazes intently at your mouth while you speak (Figure 5-4)? A recent study suggests that one reason babies attend to faces is that visual speech may play a critical role in helping them to narrow down their perceptual sensitivities to match the phonetic and linguistic distinctions of their native language. In a study performed in British Columbia, researchers presented videotaped sentences to babies in a vision-only condition (Weibum et al., 2007). The sentences were spoken in English (or French) until the baby became bored or looked away. That was followed by the same talker speaking the same sentences but in the other language in order to determine whether the change in languages caught the infant's attention. The results showed that babies who were being raised in a monolingual household were sensitive to the change in language at the ages of 4 and 6 months, but were no longer so at the age of 8 months. Conversely, babies who were being raised in a bilingual household remained sensitive to the change even at 8 months. The authors concluded that bilingual infants "advantageously maintain the discrimination abilities needed for separating and learning multiple languages" (p. 1159).

WHAT HAPPENS WHEN SOMEONE SPEECHREADS?

When someone speechreads, the person must integrate what is heard with what is seen. For instance, if someone were to hear a burst of air followed by an audible low-pitched sound and simultaneously see the lips press together and then release, the individual would most likely experience the percept of a /b/ sound. The person's brain would have combined the sounds that were heard with the facial movements that were seen.

Models of Audiovisual Integration

How does audiovisual integration happen? We don't know, although many research teams have devoted a good deal of effort trying to sort out this issue. One widely explored puzzle is, at what point do we integrate auditory and visual information? Do we process the two signals independently and then combine them, or do we process them interactively? For instance, it may be that visual and auditory information are mapped onto some kind of "phonetic prototype" at the same time, or it may be that vision biases phonetic decisions about the auditory signal before a decision is made about what is being heard (see Bernstein, Auer, & Moore, 2004, for a review).

What we do know unequivocally is that what we hear influences what we see, and what we see influences what we hear. Sometimes, the whole is difficult to predict from the parts. One of the most influential experimental paradigms that illustrates this assertion is the "McGurk Effect," so called because it was discovered in an experiment reported by McGurk and MacDonald (1976). McGurk and MacDonald presented discrepant auditory and visual speech stimuli to a group of research participants who had normal hearing. The stimuli were consonant-vowel monosyllables. For example, a participant may have heard the syllable *ba* while simultaneously seeing someone speak *da*. For some combinations of consonants, participants perceived a third consonant that differed from the two syllables. When they heard *ba* and saw *ga,* they typically perceived the syllable *da.* These results suggest that, when we recognize speech, we integrate auditory and visual speech information as we decode the signal and that this integration is obligatory (i.e., we cannot help but do it).

A number of investigators have proposed that **audiovisual integration** occurs at a distinct stage of the speech recognition process (e.g., Grant, Walden, & Seitz, 1998; Massaro, 1998; Ouni, Cohen, Ishak, & Massaro, 2007). For instance, Figure 5-5 illustrates three stages, including an initial stage of perceiving the auditory and visual signals, a second stage where integration occurs, and a third stage where discrete phonetic and

> "I can hear you and I can watch your mouth move, and then I put together the sounds and the visual image, and I can understand the words as I integrate the two signals."
>
> Marlee Matlin, Academy Award–winning actress and person with significant hearing loss
>
> (Accessed August 1, 2007, http://www.brainyquote.com/ quotes/authors/m/marlee_matlin.html)

Audiovisual integration occurs when information from the auditory and the visual signal combine to form a unified percept.

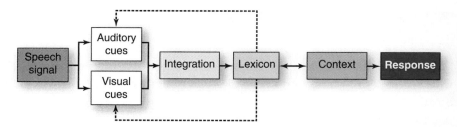

FIGURE 5-5. A model of audiovisual speech recognition, similar to that proposed by Grant et al. (1998). The model includes distinct stages for perceiving the auditory and visual speech cues, for integrating the two kinds of cues, and for accessing the mental lexicon. The dotted lines indicate that the words in the lexicon, in some instances, might affect the perception of auditory and visual cues.

lexical decisions are reached. The possible existence of a distinct stage of integration has motivated some investigators to evaluate whether an integration ability is a quantifiable skill and whether it might be amenable to intervention. For instance, if someone has poor integration, then perhaps aural rehabilitation and speechreading training might be directed toward enhancing this skill. Although means have been developed for quantifying integration (e.g., Braida, 1991; Tye-Murray, Sommers, & Spehar, 2007a), questions have arisen as to whether a distinct stage, as shown in Figure 5-5, is the most accurate way to conceptualize how individuals combine the auditory and visual speech signals. In particular, age has been shown to impact negatively upon one's ability to lipread but it has either minimal or modest impact upon one's ability to integrate (Cienkowski & Carney, 2002; Sommers, Spehar, & Tye-Murray, 2005), at least in optimal viewing and listening conditions, and older individuals with age-appropriate hearing loss have integration abilities similar to those of older individuals who have normal hearing (Tye-Murray et al., 2007). Perhaps there are minimal or modest differences between older and younger persons' abilities to integrate and no difference between individuals with normal hearing and hearing loss because there is no distinct stage of integration. An alternative view of audiovisual speech recognition appears in Figure 5-6.

The model of audiovisual speech recognition presented in Figure 5-6 is based on the Neighborhood Activation Model (NAM; Luce & Pisoni, 1998). In this model, presentation of a spoken word activates a set of lexical candidates, or a lexical neighborhood, the members of which "compete" as a match for the incoming stimulus. As noted in Chapter 2, an acoustic lexical neighborhood of words is comprised of words that sound alike with the exception of a single phoneme (e.g., *kit, can, cab,* and *scat* are all neighbors of the auditory word, *cat*). In an auditory-only condition, members of the neighborhood are activated with the onset of the spoken word and candidates are eliminated as the word unfolds until only one word remains.

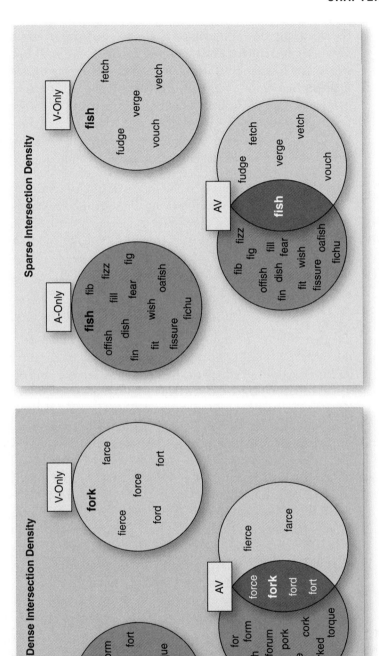

FIGURE 5-6. An alternate model of audiovisual speech recognition. The left half of the figure illustrates the auditory and visual lexical neighborhoods for the word *fork* whereas the right side of the figure illustrates the auditory and visual lexical neighborhoods for the word *fish*. The upper half of the figure indicates that both words have similar densities for their auditory and visual neighborhoods. However, the lower half of the figure illustrates that the two words have different intersection densities. In less than ideal viewing and listening conditions, a patient would likely recognize the word *fish* more readily than the word *fork*. Adapted from Tye-Murray, Sommers, and Spehar (2008, p. 236).

Words with a **high frequency of usage** are words that occur frequently in everyday conversation.

Words with a **low frequency of usage** are words that occur infrequently in everyday conversation.

Visual lexical neighborhoods are groups of words that look alike on the face and have approximately the same frequency of occurrence.

So-called "top-down" information affects recognition. For instance, a word with a **high frequency of usage** will receive more activation than a word with a **low frequency of usage**. A neighborhood may be dense or sparse. A member of a dense neighborhood (such as the word *cat*) has many words that sound like it whereas a member of a sparse neighborhood (such as the word *telephone*) has few words that sound like it. A listener who has hearing loss is more likely to recognize *telephone* than *cat* because the former word has fewer lexical neighbors that serve as competition.

Evidence suggests that words belong not only to auditory lexical neighborhoods, but also to **visual lexical neighborhoods** (Mattys, Bernstein, & Auer, 2002; Tye-Murray, Sommers, & Spehar, 2007b). For instance, a word like *elephant* has few words that resemble it visually and so it is much more likely to be recognized by a lipreader than a word such as *cheese,* which has many words that resemble it visually (Tye-Murray & Geers, 2002; Tye-Murray et al., 2008).

Figure 5-6 shows how the NAM might apply to audiovisual integration. The left side of the figure shows a lexical neighborhood schematic for the word *fish*. The first sphere in the top half of the diagram represents the auditory lexical neighborhood whereas the second sphere represents the visual lexical neighborhood. The bottom half of the figure demonstrates what happens when someone speechreads. The candidate choices are fewer than for either the auditory-only or visual-only conditions but ambiguity still exists. As such, if the individual has a hearing loss, the individual might well misperceive the word. The right side of the figure shows a lexical neighborhood schematic for the word *fish*. Again, the first sphere represents the auditory lexical neighborhood whereas the second sphere represents the visual lexical neighborhood. The bottom half of the figure demonstrates what happens when the word is presented audiovisually. Only one choice is available at the intersection. As such, the word *fish* is much more likely to be recognized by someone who has hearing loss than the word *fork*. Consistent with this portrayal and interpretation, Tye-Murray et al. (2008) showed that words having few items in the overlapping regions of their intersections are more likely to be recognized correctly than words having many items in an auditory-plus-vision condition. This finding suggest that during speechreading, there occurs a simultaneous activation of acoustic and visual lexical neighborhoods, leading to a winnowing of members in the intersection of the auditory and visual neighborhoods as the speech signal unfolds.

Audiovisual speech recognition is not quite as simple as depicted in either Figure 5-5 or Figure 5-6. As we shall see in the following sections, both residual hearing and a number of other factors can influence the process.

Quantifying Audiovisual Integration

A number of researchers have attempted to develop ways to quantify a person's ability to integrate the auditory and visual speech signals (e.g., Blamey, Cowan, Alcantara, Whitford, & Clark, 1989; Braida, 1991; Massaro & Cohen, 2000). The general approach has been to derive a measure of predicted audiovisual performance by assessing speech recognition performance in an auditory-only and a vision-only condition and then comparing how actual performance in an auditory-plus-vision condition differs from that predicted by the two unimodal performance scores. If an obtained audiovisual score is poorer than a predicted score, than an individual is said to have displayed less than optimal integration skills (Braida, 1991). A limitation of these approaches is that they can be used only with tests that utilize consonant stimuli (e.g., *eepee, eemee*) because they require consonant confusion matrices to predict audiovisual performance. Moreover, they require extensive testing to obtain stable estimates of performance. For example, if the consonant has 13 consonant samples, as in the *Iowa Consonant Test* (Tyler et al., 1986), patients must receive about 170 items in each of the three test conditions, auditory-only, vision-only, and auditory-plus-vision.

An alternative measure of integration, termed integration enhancement (IE), was developed so that a patient's integration ability could be assessed using a variety of test stimuli, including consonants, words, and sentences (Tye-Murray et al., 2007a). IE is based on predicting audiovisual performance using a simple probability (p) formula. Patients are tested in three conditions, auditory-only (A), vision-only (V), and auditory-plus-vision (AV Observed). Predicted audiovisual performance (AV Predicted) is computed with the percentage correct scores from the auditory-only and vision-only test conditions, using the following formula:

$$(p)AV\ Predicted = 1 - ((1 - (p)A)(1 - (p)V)).$$

In this calculation, it is assumed that auditory and visual speech recognition are independent events and a patient makes an error only when he or she fails to get accurate phonetic information in both auditory and visual modalities. IE is calculated according to this equation:

$$IE = (p)AV\ Observed - (p)AV\ Predicted/(1 - (p)AV\ Predicted).$$

The AV Predicted is typically less than the AV Observed. As such, IE can be described as the benefit or boost in audiovisual speech recognition beyond what is already accounted for by auditory-only and vision-only performance. The utility of an integration enhancement formula is that it can be used to quantify a patient's IE ability and may be helpful in understanding performance on an audiovisual speech recognition task. For instance, a patient may experience difficulty because of unimodal performance (e.g., the person may be a poor lipreader) or because of problems in integration, or both.

IMPORTANCE OF RESIDUAL HEARING

Persons who are most dependent on the visual signal for speech communication are those who have only a minimum of residual hearing. Even a little hearing can be helpful.

Rosen, Fourcin, and Moore (1981) asked a test talker to produce a series of nonsense syllables with varying medial consonants, such as /apa/, /ama/, /ada/, and /asa/. A laryngograph was placed on his throat, which reflected vocal fold vibration, and the output was used to develop an auditory signal that reflected the changes over time in the talker's fundamental frequency (voice pitch). As such, the speech signal sounded as if someone were speaking with his or her hand clamped over the mouth. When the test subjects (who had normal hearing) saw but did not hear the talker, they identified 44% of the consonants correctly. When they saw the talker speak and heard the concomitant changes in fundamental frequency, their performance improved to 72% consonants correct. Similar results have been found for conversational sentence of known topic (Boothroyd, Hnath-Chisolm, Hanin, & Kishon-Rabin, 1988).

The results of these two experiments help to explain why so many people with profound hearing losses are dependent on their hearing aids for successful communication. Even though they receive minimal auditory information, their ability to speechread is enhanced by the amplified signal. In listening to connected speech, such as sentences, residual hearing can help to extract suprasegmental patterns, which can convey information about syllabic structure and word boundaries as well as information about syntax (e.g., a question vs. statement) and semantics (e.g., a word spoken with emphasis may have a different meaning than the same word spoken without emphasis). The degraded auditory signal may provide segmental information as well, such as whether a sound is voiced or unvoiced.

FACTORS THAT AFFECT THE SPEECHREADING PROCESS

How well someone speechreads in a particular situation is influenced by at least four factors. As Table 5-5 indicates, these factors are the talker, the message, the speechreading environment and communication situation, and the speechreader.

Table 5-5. Factors that influence the speechreading task.

TALKER	MESSAGE	ENVIRONMENT	SPEECHREADER
Facial expressions	Length	Viewing angle	Lipreading skill
Diction	Syntactic complexity	Distance	Residual hearing
Body language	Frequency of word usage	Background noise	Use of appropriate amplification
Speech rate	Shared homophenes	Room acoustics	Stress profile
Familiarity to the speechreader	Context	Distractions	Attentiveness
Accent			Fatigue
Facial characteristics			Motivation to understand
Speech prosody (intonation, stress, and rhythm)			Language skills
Objects in or over the mouth			

Table 5-6. Speaking behaviors that impede the speechreading task. This list was generated during a group discussion with adults who are hard of hearing.

I have a difficult time speechreading when the talker:

- mumbles
- doesn't look at me when talking
- chews gum
- has an unusual accent
- has a speech impediment
- smiles too much
- moves around while talking
- uses no facial expressions
- shouts
- has a high-pitched voice
- talks too fast
- uses long, complicated sentences and obscure vocabulary words
- has a beard and/or mustache
- wears dark glasses

The Talker

The talker can increase or decrease the difficulty of the speechreading task (Table 5-6). For instance, many audiologists and speech-language pathologists have learned to speak with clearly articulated speech and ample, albeit not exaggerated, mouth movements. Patients sometimes complain to their clinician,

"I can speechread you just fine. It's when I get out in the real world, talking to people that I don't know, and who don't move their lips, that I get into trouble with my speech understanding." Often, the aural rehabilitation plan might include training for frequent communication partners about how to speak with clear speech and appropriate speaking behaviors (Schum, 1997).

Talker Behaviors

A talker who uses appropriate but not exaggerated facial expressions, who speaks with clear and not mumbled speech, and who uses body language is relatively easy to speechread. The following behaviors make a talker difficult to speechread:

- Shouting
- Mumbling
- Turning away
- Speaking rapidly
- Covering the mouth with a hand
- Smiling simultaneously while talking

Clear speech is a way of speaking to enhance one's intelligibility; it entails speaking with a slowed rate and good but not exaggerated enunciation of words.

"Communication partners should be instructed to both speak clearly and allow access to visual speech information."
Karen S. Helfer, research at the University of Massachusetts, Amherst
(Helfer, 1997, p. 442)

People who speak with clear speech include:
- An elementary school teacher
- A newscaster
- An airport employee who announces airline arrivals and departures
- A public radio broadcaster
- A politician
- Queen Elizabeth

Auditorily, **clear speech** has been shown to be more intelligible than speech that is spoken conversationally (e.g., Picheny et al., 1985; Uchanski et al., 1996). Clear speech is characterized by a somewhat slowed speaking rate and good (although not exaggerated) enunciation. Some sounds might be slightly longer than normal and more fully differentiated. Key words are emphasized and pauses are inserted at clause boundaries. Overall, the duration of utterances are longer (Picheny et al., 1986, 1989; Uchanski et al., 1996). An utterance that is spoken with clear speech is also more likely to be recognized in a vision-only condition (Gagné & Boutin, 1997) and in an audition-plus-vision condition (Helfer, 1997) than when it is spoken conversationally. For instance, on a sentence recognition test, a group of participants recognized 34% more of the words when the sentences were spoken with clear speech in an audition-plus-vision condition than when they were spoken conversationally in an audition-only condition. The biggest effects in both the auditory-only and audition-plus-vision conditions occurred for words in the middle of sentences, suggesting that clear speech helps to demarcate word boundaries (Helfer, 1997). The following represents examples of conversational speech and the more intelligible clear-speech counterpart:

D'yeet yet? For *Did you eat yet?*

Go-in fishin' 'morrow af'ernoon. For *I'm going fishing tomorrow afternoon.*

D'yever see 'em? For *Did you ever see them?*

Gestures and facial expression can influence speechreading performance. For instance, a talker who speaks a happy script with a happy facial expression will be more intelligible than one who speaks it with a sad facial expression. Similarly, a talker who speaks a somber script with a sad facial expression will be more intelligible than one who speaks it with a happy facial expression (Rönnberg, 1996). Facial expression can also serve to convey prosodic cues, such as a question versus a statement intonation (Srinivasan & Massaro, 2003).

Familiarity

Persons who have hearing loss will have an easier time recognizing the speech of someone who is familiar, such as a family member, than someone who is unfamiliar, because they are accustomed to the talker's mouth movements and speech patterns. There is some evidence that thin lips are easier to speechread than thick or immobile lips and that a foreign accent increases difficulty (Berger, 1972).

Gender

Talker gender influences the difficulty of the task. Females tend to be easier to lipread than males (Bench, Daly, Doyle, & Lind, 1995; Daly, Bench, & Chappell, 1996). However, even though females' speech may be more recognizable when it is presented in a vision-only condition, it may not necessarily be easier to recognize in an audition-plus-vision condition, as the higher fundamental frequency of the female voice is harder for most persons with hearing loss to hear than the lower fundamental frequencies associated with male voices. The average fundamental frequency of males is about 117 Hz whereas the average fundamental frequency for females is 217 Hz (Fitch & Holbrook, 1970). For male talkers, the presence of facial hair, as with a mustache or beard, can impede speechreading by obscuring lip and jaw movement (Kitano, Siegenthaler, & Stoker, 1985).

How Something Is Said Will Affect How One Speechreads It

Try this experiment. Say to a friend, without using your voice, "Oh my aching back." As you speak, use minimal facial expression and body movements. Ask your friend to guess what you have said. Chances are, the guess will be incorrect. Now mouth the phrase again, but this time, assume a pained expression and rub your back with your hand. The odds are high that the friend will quickly recognize your utterance this second time around. This experiment reveals an important principle in speechreading: *Context cues can dramatically affect an individual's ability to speechread.*

The Message

The second factor that can influence speechreading performance is the message that a talker presents. The structure and the component words affect recognition. For example, if a talker were to say, "The elephant is big," a person with hearing loss would likely recognize what was said, especially if the talker were standing in a zoo next to an elephant cage when he or she said it. The word *elephant* is highly visible on the face, and has few words that look similar to it. The sentence is short and syntactically simple, and the adjective, *big,* begins with the highly visible phoneme, /b/. The setting of the zoo provides situational clues for understanding the sentence. On the other hand, if out of the blue someone were to say, "The hen sat on the cart," most persons with hearing loss would be at a loss. The component words do not entail many highly visible mouth movements. Production of the /h/ in *hen* is invisible, and the tongue humping associated with production of /k/ in *cart* cannot be seen. The words are also one-syllabic, and most have other words that look similar on the face and are acoustically similar. Words that look like and sound like the word *cart* include, among others, *kit, heart, cot,* and *hot.* The message's structure, frequency of use of the component words, the number of similar-looking words, and the supporting context all affect speechreading performance.

Structure

Some messages are easier to speechread than others, depending on their length, syntactic complexity, frequency of use, similarity to other words, and linguistic context. As a general rule, the longer the sentence and the greater its syntactic complexity, the more difficult it will be to speechread. Words that have two syllables tend to be easier to recognize than monosyllables spoken in isolation.

Frequency of Usage

Commonplace words, such as the word *sweater,* have a higher probability of being recognized than words that are used less frequently, such as the word *cardigan.* We say that the word *sweater* has a greater frequency of usage than *cardigan,* because it is more likely to be spoken in everyday conversation.

Neighborhoods

Words that have fewer response possibilities are also easier to recognize. For example, the word *bat* may be difficult to recognize, even though it begins with a highly visible mouth movement, because many other words are similar both visually (e.g., *bad, bet, mat, met, pat*) and acoustically (e.g., *cap, cat, scat, bad*). On the other hand, the word *telephone* is easier to recognize, even though it is less commonplace than the word *bat,* because not many words look or sound similar to *telephone* (e.g., Kaiser, Kirk, Lachs, & Pisoni, 2003). As noted earlier, lexically easy-to-recognize words have few lexical neighbors, or few words that are acoustically (or visually) similar, whereas lexically difficult-to-recognize words have many neighbors (Greenburg & Jenkins, 1964; Kirk, Pisoni, & Osberger,1995).

Linguistic Context

Words that are specified by linguistic context typically are easiest to recognize (e.g., Garstecki & O'Neill, 1980; Grant & Seitz, 2000; Lansing & Helgeson, 1995; Marslen-Wilson, Moss, & Van Halen, 1996; Züst & Tschopp, 1993). For example, the word *table* is harder to identify when embedded in the sentence *Candace will buy the _____,* than in the sentence, *Candace will set the _____ and chairs in the kitchen.* Context cues provide cues for a word missed. Although *table* and *sable* are homophenes, and are acoustically similar, an individual probably would not mistake one word for the other because *table* makes more sense in this second sentence context. Grammatical structure also provides contextual cues. For instance, in the sentence, *The _____ read the book,* grammatical sentence structure specifies that the missing word is a common noun.

Topical Cues Can Help

Simply knowing the topic of conversation can enhance a speechreader's performance. For example, if an audiologist allows someone to read the word *homes* before asking the person to speechread the sentence, *She just moved into a three-bedroom apartment,* the person will speechread more words correctly than if no topical word is presented beforehand (Hanin, 1988). The sentence, *I cut my finger with a knife,* will be easier to speechread if it is preceded with a related sentence such as, *I was careless with a sharp blade,* than if it is preceded by an unrelated sentence such as, *You need special watering tools* (Gagné, Tugby, & Michaud, 1991).

The Speechreading Environment and Communication Situation

The third factor that can affect speechreading performance is the environment. Patients often avoid social situations because they cannot hear in certain environments. "I hate parties," a patient may complain. "The lighting is always dim and the music is too loud."

Another may say, "I bought a round dining table. With our old rectangular one, I could never read anyone's lips."

The viewing angle, the distance from the talker, room conditions, and the presence or absence of background noise may all affect how well patients speechread in any given environment or communication situation.

Viewing Angle

Viewing angle may affect how well the speechreader can recognize the speech signal (Figure 5-7). A number of investigators have suggested that the best angle for speechreading is a frontal viewing angle (0 degrees azimuth) and that an intermediate angle (30–45 degrees) is better than a lateral angle (90 degrees) (e.g., Erber, 1974; Neely, 1956). In contrast, Ijsseldjik (1992) found that children were equally as adapt at lipreading words, phrases, and simple sentences presented at a 0-degree viewing angle as at a 60-degree angle. Bauman and Hambrecht (1995) reported similar data from a single adult (as did Jordan & Beven, 1997, who assessed the performance of adults using nonsense stimuli).

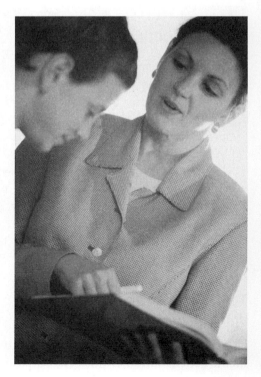

FIGURE 5-7. Viewing angle. Here, the talker is standing above the speechreader and at a 90° angle, so performance might be less than optimal.

If a conversation is occurring in a group setting, as in a conference held around a rectangular table, the speechreader may miss the beginnings of many utterances, as one person and then another interjects comments in the discussion, because the speechreader must locate the talker first. The individual often may not have an advantageous viewing angle of the talker, particularly if the talkers turn their heads toward various participants as they speak.

Distance from the Talker

Distance from the talker may affect performance, particularly if the speechreader is too far away to view the talker's mouth movements (Figure 5-8). Common wisdom suggests that a child speechreading from the back row of a classroom will not recognize as much of the teacher's spoken message as one who sits in the front row, and who has **favorable seating**.

Viewing distance may affect lipreading and speechreading in different ways. In one study, Erber (1971) presented vision-only speech signals over a range of distances using two live (not videotaped) talkers. Children who had profound hearing loss could recognize about 75% of common nouns spoken at a distance of 5 feet but only about 11% of the words at a distance of 100 feet. A more recent study (Gagné, Charest, Monday, & Desbiens, 2006)

Favorable seating for speechreading includes being close enough to see the talker's lip movements, being able to see the talker full-face rather than in profile, and having the talker's face well lit.

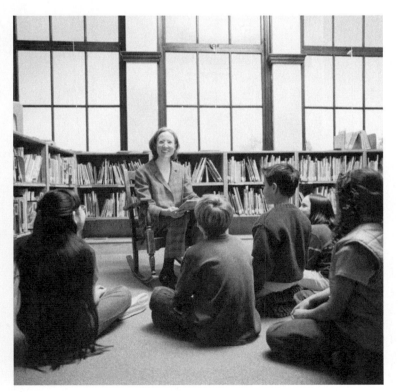

FIGURE 5-8. Distance. A child should have favorable seating in a classroom in order to optimize speechreading performance.

revealed a similar finding. A group of 16 young adults scored about 16% better when they were separated from the recorded talker by a distance of 1.8 meters than when they were separated by a distance of 7.3 meters. In contrast, a study that assessed audiovisual speech recognition (Jordan & Sergeant, 2000) presented nonsense syllable stimuli such as /bi/ to individuals who had normal hearing. No decrement in performance occurred as the distance of the recorded talker varied from 1 meter to 10 meters. Likewise, Small and Infante (1988) found that a distance up to 18 feet did not affect speechreading performance. These latter two studies suggest an important role for "coarse" visual cues during speechreading, when the auditory speech signal is also available.

Room Conditions

A poorly lit talker, who speaks in front of a light source so that shadows appear on the face, will be relatively difficult to speechread (Figure 5-9) and so will one who stands before a bright window in a room with no

FIGURE 5-9. Illumination. Poorly lit talkers are difficult to speechread.

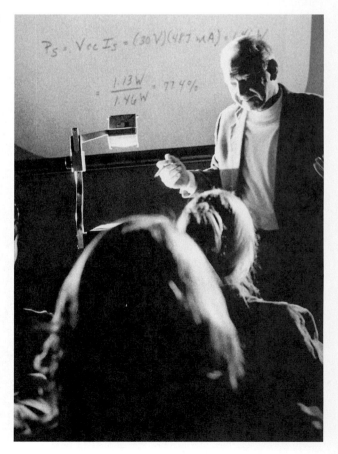

Talking with a Guy Named Baldy

Domnic Massaro, PhD, a psychologist at the University of California, Santa Cruz, has spearheaded the development of a computerized talking head. He calls his creation "Baldy," most likely because his creation looks like a flat-cheeked Yul Brynner. The three-dimensional head floats on the computer screen. When he talks, his lips move and pucker, his eyebrows raise, and his chin and facial features vary, depending on what he is saying. Baldy can be made to look like he's made of a scaffolding of triangles or a flesh-covered face that looks like its been covered in shrink-wrap. The latter result looks fairly human, almost like an animated storefront mannequin, and it is possible to lipread the head's words. The program user can change Baldy's mood (he can smile, he can frown, he can looked surprised, he can look angry), his skin coloring, and his ethnic identity and even species (it's possible to convert Baldy into a talking monkey). The user can type in a word or sentence, and Baldy will speak it.

There are several possible uses for animated synthetic speech such as Baldy. The most obvious is for speechreading practice using a computer. The Baldy system has also been used to study the basic process of audiovisual speech perception and audiovisual integration. For instance, it is possible to make Baldy's lips appear to say one thing and the accompanying sound to say another (as when performing a McGurk Effect experiment). It has also been used to teach speech production and speechreading to children at an oral school for children who are deaf and hard of hearing, Tucker Maxon Oral School in Portland, Oregon. The version of Baldy used at the school allows the user to remove the skin off the head and thereby view the activity of the tongue body, either head-on or in a half-sagittal view. By watching the movement of the lips, lower jaw, and tongue, children learn to place their articulators during speech production.

overhead lights. Light shining in the eyes of the speechreader can impair performance. Erber (1974) found that speechreading performance varies as a function of the contrast between the light reflected from the face of the talker and the light reflecting from the wall surface behind the talker. High background brightness, with a corresponding reduction in facial **luminance,** leads to a significant reduction in speechreading accuracy. Gagné, Doucet, and Potvin (2006) showed that low levels of illumination

Luminance is the intensity of light per unit area of the source.

decrease speechreading performance, and that the effect is more pronounced if the talker has dark skin rather than light.

Just as with listening performance, the presence of background noise can impair someone's speechreading performance. Table 5-7 lists common sources of room noise that can interfere with the speechreading task. A noisy environment can mask speech and decrease the speechreading enhancement effect afforded by residual hearing, as well as distract the speechreader from the speech recognition task (Figure 5-10).

Other factors that exert an effect include excessive room reverberation, the availability of assistive devices, and interfering objects such as a support beam extending from a room's floor to ceiling. The presence of visible movement, such as movement by others in the room or activity seen from a window, also can be distracting.

The Speechreader

Finally, variables related to the individual can affect the person's speechreading performance.

Innate Skill and Hearing Acuity

Speechreading performance relates to lipreading skill, as well as to an individual's hearing acuity. Generally, the better the lipreading skill and the greater the amount of residual hearing, the better the speechreading

Table 5-7. Examples of noise sources common to various communication settings.

HOME	RESTAURANTS	WORKPLACE	CLASSROOM
Kitchen sink/running water	Dishes/silverware	Computers	Children talking
Washer/dryer	Music	Printers	Paper rustling
Air conditioner	Guests talking	Machinery	Shoes scuffling
Furnace			Chairs moving
Vacuum cleaner			Projectors
Television			Fans, ventilator, furnace, air conditioner
Radio			Hall noise
Family members talking			
Open window/door (lawn mower, leaf blower, traffic)			
Refrigerator			

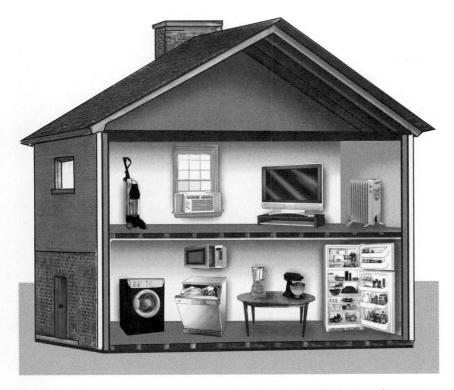

FIGURE 5-10. A sample of noise sources that may be present in the home environment.

performance (e.g., Sommers et al., 2005). However, the nature of the hearing loss also affects performance. For example, two persons may have severe hearing losses. If one has a conductive loss and the other has a sensorineural loss, the latter individual may have poorer speech discrimination and therefore may perform more poorly on a speechreading task.

Speechreading performance also is influenced by individuals' use of appropriate amplification and use of eyeglasses when needed. Poor visual acuity, such as that stemming from cataracts, will of course hinder performance.

Emotional and Physical State

An individual's level of stress, fatigue, and attentiveness can affect performance. For example, if the speechreader is engaged in a job interview, anxiety may impair his or her speechreading performance. A businessman may not speechread family members well at home because he is fatigued from a long day of concentrating on coworkers' auditory and visual signals.

> ## Miss America: It's Not Always Glamorous
>
> Heather Whitestone was crowned Miss America in 1994, and became the first woman with significant hearing loss to win the honor. Her talent was ballet dancing, which she learned as a child, becoming attuned to the vibrations of the music. Here is what she had to say about speechreading:
>
> I find lipreading very stressful and frustrating because I am often confused. For example, if you look at person's lips saying *dog* and *saw*, they look the same. With my hearing aid alone, I do not hear "s" or "d" sounds. So usually I have to use my common sense. For example, if someone said, "The dog is running across the street," then I know it was not the saw who ran across the street—it was the dog. Most hearing people do not understand that people in my position have to think incredibly fast in order to keep up with conversations. . . . Lip reading is a grueling and exhausting mental exercise and lip readers are constantly thinking and trying to discern what is actually being said. I get real mad at those who think that I am stupid simply because I cannot hear. The truth is I get exhausted after a while and simply cannot keep up. At that point, I begin to guess at what is being said and eventually give up and choose to be quiet.
>
> (Accessed August 1, 2007 *http://www.heatherwhitestone.com/site/content/faqs.shtml*)

Situations where an oral interpreter might be required:

- A classroom
- A convention hall
- A conference room
- A conversation where one of the talkers is not present, as in a conference call
- A conversation with someone whose speech is difficult to speechread, as with someone who has an unfamiliar accent

ORAL INTERPRETERS

An **oral interpreter** sits in clear view of a person who has hearing loss and silently repeats a talker's message as it is spoken.

Oral transliteration is the act of lagging a talker by a few words, mouthing or speaking the words with a normal speaking rate and good enunciation. Although oral transliteration usually does not entail the use of sign language, natural body language, expressions, and gestures are typically presented that support the content of the words.

The final topic to be considered in this chapter concerning speechreading is the oral interpreter. Because many persons who have hearing loss rely on the visual speech signal, situations may arise when an oral interpreter is helpful or even essential. Speech and hearing professionals may be asked on occasion to help locate an oral interpreter. An **oral interpreter** (also called an oral transliterator) is someone who sits in clear view of the individual with hearing loss and silently (or softly) repeats a talker's message as it is spoken, often lagging behind by only one or two words. Through this process of **oral transliteration**, an oral interpreter attempts to convey a talker's mood and intent. National certification is available through the Registry of Interpreters for the Deaf (RID), and includes the Certificate of Transliterating (CT) and the Oral Interpreter Certificate

(OIC). Certified interpreters must adhere to a Code of Ethics (1984), which dictates their professional code of behavior. This code includes the following guidelines:

- They cannot share with other individuals information they learn during an interpreting assignment.
- They cannot change the meaning of a message as they interpret it for the person who has hearing loss.
- They cannot add their opinions or personal commentary to a message.

CASE STUDY

An Exceptional Lipreader

A few studies have focused on exceptionally good lipreaders (e.g., Andersson & Lidestam, 2005; Lyxell, 1994; Rönnberg et al., 1999) in an effort to understand what makes some people particularly facile at deciphering the visual speech signal. For example, Lyxell (1994) studied a 56-year-old woman, SJ, who lost her hearing at the age of 16, following a bout with meningitis. On a sentence test administered in a vision-only condition, SJ scored 57% words correct. By comparison, the average performance of a control group of 119 participants (49 who had hearing loss and 70 who had normal hearing) was 24% words correct. They identified roughly half as many words as SJ. Interestingly, her ability to discriminate words, which means her ability to indicate whether two words spoken in a pair are the same or different (Chapter 4), was no better than the average control subject. Thus, even though she is skilled at lipreading sentences, this skill does not transfer to word discrimination.

SJ has developed a specific strategy for lipreading. She reported that when she lipreads, she tries to repeat each spoken word as soon as she can after it is spoken. When possible, she tries to summarize the words into meaningful units, for instance, during pauses in the talker's speech. She purposefully fills in missing pieces of information and updates misperceived words.

A cognitive test battery revealed that SJ has a better than average ability to comprehend read sentences and to recall the last words of a series of sentences presented in text format. This performance suggests that she has a good short-term working memory for complex tasks. For more simple tasks, such as repeating back strings of digits presented sequentially on a computer screen, her performance was unremarkable. She was also found to have an excellent ability to fill in missing words in printed sentences, although she did not exhibit extraordinary skill in filling in letters in words.

The results from the cognitive tests mesh well with her reported strategy for lipreading. She has a large working memory that allows her to buffer information as she lipreads. She can use this stored information

continues

CASE STUDY, *continued*

An Exceptional Lipreader, *continued*

to catch up on what she missed and to correct what later turns out to be a misperception. The author notes that she deviates from the general case, where working memory tends not to be predictive of lipreading performance. We will return to the topic of working memory in Chapter 13, when we consider older adults who have hearing loss.

FINAL REMARKS

Intuitively we associate speech recognition with the sense of hearing. However, as we have learned in this chapter, the sense of sight also can be an important component in our everyday communication. In fact, persons with hearing loss may be reliant on their vision for recognizing spoken messages. A topic that currently is receiving much attention in the research literature pertains to audiovisual integration; that is, how we combine the disparate auditory and visual signals of a talker into a unified percept. The answer to this question may have important theoretical implications for models of speech perception. For our present purposes, this is an interesting question because exploring the answer may help us design more effective speech reading training protocols.

KEY CHAPTER POINTS

- Even persons with normal hearing rely on speechreading to some degree.
- Some people are better speechreaders than others. The reasons for this are unclear. Performance cannot be predicted by such factors as intelligence or practice with the speechreading task.
- When we lipread, our eyes both fixate and perform quick shifts. They often focus on talker's eyes, nose, and mouth.
- Infants appear to rely on the visual speech signal for learning their native language.
- Lipreading is difficult. Some of the factors that may compound the lipreading task include the partial visibility or nonvisibility of many speech sounds on the face, the rapidity of speech, coarticulation, the visual similarity of many sound groups, and talker eccentricities. For instance, the words *Bob* and *Mom* are indistinguishable on the lips. The word *hick* requires minimal visible mouth movement.

- Some models of audiovisual integration suggest that the ability to integrate is distinct from the abilities to recognize speech auditorily or to recognize speech visually. An alternative model, based on the concept of lexical neighborhoods, posits that a distinct stage of integration may not be a part of the speech recognition process.

- A little residual hearing can increase markedly one's ability to recognize speech when looking and listening simultaneously.

- The talker, message, environment, and state of the person affect how well the individual will recognize a spoken message. For instance, a talker who mumbles will be difficult to understand.

- A talker's use of clear speech can effect a dramatic improvement in a patient's ability to lipread and speechread.

TERMS AND CONCEPTS TO REMEMBER

Speechreading
Lipreading
Variability in individual skill levels
Sound visibility
Coarticulation and stress effects
Visemes
Homophenes
Models of audiovisual integration
Neighborhood Activation Model (NAM)
Intersection density
Variables affecting performance
Clear speech
Frequency of usage
Oral interpreter
Code of Ethics

MULTIPLE-CHOICE QUESTIONS

1. Which statement below is false?

   a. Older adults tend to be poorer lipreaders than younger adults.

   b. If you have normal hearing, you will probably comprehend more if you hear and see a talker who is reading aloud than if you only hear the reader.

   c. Intelligence quotient correlates positively with lipreading ability.

   d. Infants have been shown to engage in speechreading.

2. When someone lipreads, the person's eyes:

   a. Fixate on the talker's mouth.

   b. Scan the entire face in rhythmic saccades.

   c. Focus primarily on the mouth, nose, and eye regions.

   d. Focus on the eyes for phonetic content and the mouth for prosodic nuances.

3. Mr. Simmons is taking a lipreading test. Which word is he most likely to identify incorrectly?

   a. Hornet

   b. Elephant

   c. Bathtub

   d. Thumb

4. One reason lipreading is so difficult is because:

   a. People rarely pause between sentences.

   b. Sounds look different on the mouth depending on the phonetic context of a word.

   c. Residual hearing does not supplement the visual signal.

   d. The visual signal doesn't convey place of articulation information.

5. Which two sounds are examples of a viseme?

   a. /l, w/

   b. /f, t/

   c. /m, n/

   d. /p, b/

6. The McGurk Effect is an example of:

   a. Audiovisual integration

   b. Lipreading

   c. Viseme confusion

   d. The benefits of residual hearing for lipreading

7. Who would be the most difficult person to speechread?

   a. A woman

   b. A spouse

   c. A store clerk with a foreign accent

   d. A speech-language pathologist

8. Typically, a word that has a high frequency of usage is easier to identify on the face than a word that has low frequency of usage. An exception to this rule of thumb is:

   a. The word with a high frequency of usage has more than one syllable.

   b. The word with low frequency of usage has far fewer lexical neighbors than the word with a high frequency of usage.

   c. The word with a high frequency of usage begins with a visible sound.

   d. The word with a low frequency of usage is spoken in a sentence context.

9. A man who speaks with clear speech:

   a. Speaks with a slow speaking rate, with good enunciation and appropriate pausing.

   b. Expresses himself with short statements and concise language.

   c. Speaks so that his face is clearly visible to the person who has hearing loss and so that his mouth is not obscured by a hand or other objects.

   d. Speaks at a loud level so that the patient can better understand his words.

10. The research is ambiguous on which of the following issues?

    a. Optimal angle for speechreading the talker

    b. Clear speech and its effect on the intelligibility of an utterance

    c. Lexical neighborhood density and its effect on the likelihood of a word being recognized correctly

    d. The existence of a McGurk effect

11. An oral interpreter:

   a. Signs and speaks the message.

   b. Mouths the message of a talker, or quietly repeats it, so that the patient can lipread it.

   c. Is typically a frequent communication partner of the patient who desires to facilitate the communication interaction.

   d. Acts as an intermediary between a persons who has a congenital hearing loss and uses sign language and a person who has an adventitious hearing loss and communicates with speech.

CHAPTER 6

Speechreading Training

OUTLINE

- Candidacy
- Traditional methods of speechreading training
- Developing speechreading skills
- Analytic speechreading training objectives
- Synthetic speechreading training objectives
- Computerized instruction
- Efficacy of speechreading training
- Case study: Targeting training
- Final remarks
- Key chapter points
- Terms and concepts to remember
- Multiple-choice questions

At the beginning of the 20th century, speechreading training was a principal component of most aural rehabilitation programs, in large part because there were few alternative means for alleviating communication problems experienced by persons with hearing loss. Professionals simply did not have the technology to reduce hearing difficulties. In those times, persons would attend speechreading classes and perform drill activities at home.

With the advent of hearing aids, cochlear implants, and assistive listening devices, individuals are better able to use their residual hearing. Concomitantly, the popularity of speechreading training has waned, so that now it rarely is found as the sole element of an aural rehabilitation program.

CANDIDACY

Who is a candidate for speechreading training? The answer to this question depends in part on whom is asked. In this text, it is suggested that children may benefit from training, especially if they use total communication (Chapter 14) and do not rely solely on speechreading for everyday communication (e.g., children who use both speech and manually coded English to communicate). Adults who have recently lost their hearing also may be candidates for training. In addition to improving their speechreading skills, they may receive psychological benefits from participating in a program, feeling they have taken constructive action to deal with their hearing losses.

TRADITIONAL METHODS OF SPEECHREADING TRAINING

In the last century, four speechreading training methods were popular in the United States (Berger, 1972; Jeffers & Barley, 1971). These methods were advocated originally by Bruhn, the Nitchies, the Kinzes, and Bunger.

In 1902, Martha Emma Bruhn introduced the Mueller-Walle method to North America, a method that originated in Germany. She published three textbooks, the last of which was the *Mueller-Walle Method of Lip Reading for the Hard of Hearing* (Boston: Leavis, 1947). The hallmark feature of this program was an emphasis on rapid syllable drill, such as *she-ma-flea* and *she-may-free*. Students also practiced recognizing homophenous words, using sentence context cues to distinguish between possible meanings.

Edward B. Nitchie, who published his first book, *Lip-reading Principles and Practices,* in 1912, rarely employed syllable drill. Instead, he emphasized

Meuller-Walle Method

- Speech sounds categorized according to their visible characteristics
- Lessons based on a sound movement or group of movements
- Rapid, rhythmic syllable drills
- Simple sentences

the importance of psychological processes of speechreading. Practice usually centered on sentence materials and the identification of homophenous words through contextual cues. Students sometimes practiced speechreading themselves by talking before a mirror. Training materials were presented without voice. He placed emphasis on focusing on speech movements as opposed to static articulatory postures. Nitchie's text was updated by his wife Elizabeth in 1940, and it was one of the most widely read texts on the subject in the 20th century.

Cora Kinze studied with both Bruhn and Nitchie before establishing her own school for speechreading training with her sister Rose in 1917. Not surprisingly, the sisters developed an eclectic method, combining the analytic syllable drill of Bruhn with the more synthetic exercises of Nitchie. The Kinze sisters also developed materials specifically for preschool and elementary school children.

The Jena Method was developed by Karl Brauckmann who lived in the city of Jena, Germany, and published two brief textbooks in 1925. The Jena method was introduced to the United States by Anna Bunger in 1927. A hallmark of Brauckmann's approach was its emphasis on **mimetic** and **kinesthetic** forms and sensations, and the recognition that our ability

Nitchie Method

- Mirror practice
- A synthetic approach in later years
- Speech movements as opposed to static postures
- Importance of grasping the whole
- Use of stories, humorous anecdotes, and sentences to effect "mind training"

The Jena Method

- Sounds described according to whether movement involves lips, tongue, or tongue-soft palate
- Syllable drill
- Student speaks in unison with the clinician
- Student concentrates on his or her kinesthetic and tactile sensations

Mimetic means imitating or copying movements.

Kinesthetic relates to the perception of movement, position, and tension of body parts.

A Look Back to 1942

In discussing basic principles of learning how to lipread and speechread, a U.S. government handbook offered this advice:

> Under all systems of [lipreading/speechreading] instruction the student spends much time in observing and interpreting syllables or monosyllabic words containing the sounds being studied. Although systems vary in the degree of emphasis placed on various factors in the training, the leading teachers agree that, in order to become a proficient lipreader, one must not only train the eye for accuracy, quickness, and visual memory, but also must train the mind to understand, by the context, those words which cannot be recognized by the movements of the mouth. Finally, the student must be fortified by courage, patience, and a determination to learn. He must practice his new art interminably, with his friends in conversation, in the church or lecture hall, and watching strangers on the street.

(U.S. Government Printing Office, 1942, p. 47)

to produce speech relates to our ability to perceive it. In this method, students focus on the mouth movements of the instructor, while simultaneously speaking the training materials. Training materials include repeated syllables and then words derived from the syllables.

Some of the fundamental principles underlying these seminal training programs are evident in more modern training curricula. Students' attention typically is focused on sound identification (as in the Mueller-Walle method), as well as on recognizing the gist of a sentence (following Nitchie). Most contemporary programs recommend that training items be presented with both auditory and visual signals. The notions of kinesthetic awareness of one's own speech production and of lipreading one's own speech via either a mirror or videotape has enjoyed some attention (as with the Jena method), as investigators have attempted to show that production practice enhances perception performance, with modest success (De Filippo, Sims, & Gottermeier, 1995).

⬛ DEVELOPING SPEECHREADING SKILLS

The first class of a communication strategies training program often is informational in nature and includes a consideration of the speechreading process. A handout like the one reprinted in Table 6-1 might be used to guide discussion among adult clients. This handout reviews factors that affect the speechreading process and the importance of using speechreading cues maximally.

In addition to considering the principles outlined in Table 6-1, class participants also might be asked to reflect on their speechreading habits and listening difficulties. They often review rules to follow when speechreading, such as those listed in Table 6-2. For instance, although *Watch the talker's lips,* the first rule presented in Table 6-2, seems like an obvious recommendation, some people become distracted by watching the talker's hand gestures or they have a habit of listening with lowered eye gaze instead of concentrating on the talker's mouth movements. As a result, their speechreading performance is not as good as it could be.

Finally, during an introduction to speechreading, class participants might review charts like the one presented in Figure 6-1 to identify difficult listening situations and to formulate solutions for rectifying the difficulties. They might be asked to identify which seats in Figure 6-1 present the most favorable circumstances for lipreading and speechreading, and which seats present the least favorable. This kind of activity sensitizes students to the concept of favorable speechreading conditions.

Table 6-1. A handout that might be distributed at an adult rehabilitation class to stimulate discussion about the speechreading process.

Speechreading is a process of attending to auditory and visual information to recognize a spoken message. Speechreading is not just watching others' lips to identify the words they are saying. It also consists of making the most of your hearing, and using your mind to collect all the information available to make a "best guess." Speechreading includes the following:

1. Lipreading: Watch the mouth movements of the talker, including the lips, jaw, and tongue tip. It is impossible to identify every word, but you can identify some words and sounds that will help you ascertain what is being said.

2. Facial expression: It is possible to identify people's moods or how they feel by the expression on their faces. You can also glean subtle nuances of meaning in their messages by attending to facial expressions.

3. Gesture, posture, and movement: What people are doing, how they are sitting, and the gestures they make give clues to what they are thinking about and what they might say.

4. Situational cues: You can anticipate what a person is going to talk about by the situation or place they are in and the relationships of the people present.

5. Knowing the topic: It is easier to follow conversation when you know what the talker is talking about. The easiest way to find out is to ask someone else who is listening. You might say, "What are we discussing?"

6. Knowledge of language: You might be able to make educated guesses about a particular word missed on the basis of sentence structure.

7. Keeping informed: Knowing what news items or subjects are of current interest to people may help you to anticipate what will be talked about. Read newspapers and magazines and watch the news on television.

8. Emotional factors: Keep motivated and develop self-confidence even though there will be times that you make errors.

9. Use your hearing: Although you have a hearing loss, you may be able to hear sounds and words that help you to identify the message or idea.

Until now, you have been taking advantage of these clues to some extent. One goal of this class is to make you more conscious of them so you use them maximally. Using these clues, much of the message can be predicted. Some parts of the message are less predictable (e.g., hearing a new name), making them more difficult. Therefore, you must use two kinds of information: (a) the part of the message you did understand and (b) any additional knowledge that can help you to fill in the gaps in order to figure out the whole message.

Source: Adapted from "Speechreading instruction for adults: Issues and practices," by R. Cherry & A. Rubinstein, 1988, p. 302. *Volta Review,* 289–306.

How to Practice Speechreading:

- Work with a partner.
- Talk about real-life things.
- Practice viewing the speaker from various angles and distances.
- Know the subject at hand.
- Speechread for overall content rather than individual words.
- If you cannot fill in the missing pieces, ask the speaker to reword the entire sentence [rather than] single words.
- If you are unable to understand, do not [automatically] interrupt . . . because you may be able to comprehend the meaning once the sentence is complete.
- After you have gained a level of competency, practice with background noise.

(Alexander Graham Bell Association for the Deaf and Hard of Hearing, 1988, p. 1)

Following this kind of introduction, the class may (or may not) receive formal speechreading training. In today's world, rarely if ever do participants in an aural rehabilitation class practice lipreading (vision-only speech recognition). Rather, they practice recognizing speech using both auditory and visual signals. As noted, children are more likely to receive formal speechreading training than are adults. This is especially true for those who have received a cochlear implant. As with formal auditory training, formal speechreading training objectives can be divided into two categories: analytic and synthetic.

Table 6-2. Rules to follow when speechreading. A handout like this might be discussed during a group class.

---

1. **Watch the talker's lips.**
   This seems obvious, but often, a speechreader can be distracted by other events in the room, or the talker's hand gestures. Also, there may be a tendency to watch the talker's eyes instead of the mouth.

2. **Provide information to the talker about how to communicate with you.**
   This may include asking the talker to speak clearly and at a slightly louder than normal conversational level. The talker should not shout or exaggerate lip movements. The talker should face you when speaking, and should not chew or cover the mouth, such as with a hand.

3. **Try to ensure that the room is well-lit and that your position in the room allows for optimal speechreading performance.**
   You will want to find a seat where light does not shine in your eyes and adjust light sources so they do not cast shadows on the talker's face. Position yourself near enough to the talker so you can clearly see the talker's mouth and facial expressions.

4. **Try to minimize background noise.**
   Background noise might be minimized by ensuring that radios and televisions are turned down or off. Favorable seating, say at a table away from the kitchen in a restaurant, may also minimize background noise.

5. **Know the topic of conversation.**
   During a conversation, ask someone the topic of conversation. It is much easier to recognize a message if you know what is being discussed. If you know in advance that a specific topic will be discussed, try to learn something about it beforehand.

6. **Pay attention to context cues.**
   The situation in which the conversation occurs may provide information about what is being said. The talker's facial expressions and what has been discussed beforehand may also be informative.

7. **Keep a positive attitude.**
   Speechreading can be tiring. Stay motivated, and do not be distracted by your own anxiety and self-doubts.

ANALYTIC SPEECHREADING TRAINING OBJECTIVES

Analytic speechreading training objectives are directed toward developing vowel recognition and consonant recognition skills. The logic underlying many speechreading curricula is gradually to increase patients' reliance on the auditory signal for discriminating phonemic contrasts while they speechread (Figure 6-2).

Vowel Speechreading Training Objectives

If a person has only rudimentary speech recognition skills, initial speechreading training objectives might focus his or her attention on distinguishing /i/, /u/, and /a/. These sounds differ both in their formant structure and in how they appear on the mouth. The /i/ is produced with a narrow mouth opening, with some spreading of the mouth corners. It has a first formant of low frequency, and a second formant of high frequency.

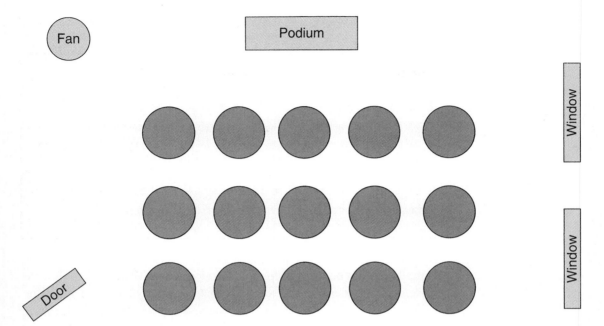

FIGURE 6-1. A chart for discussing listening environments and ways to minimize speechreading difficulties. Students might be asked to identify where they might sit to optimize speechreading performance.

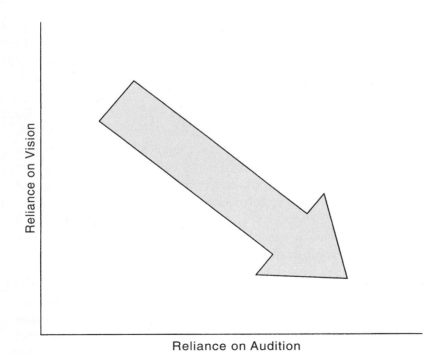

FIGURE 6-2. Increased reliance on the auditory signal for speech recognition.

Table 6-3. Vowel analytic training objectives that were designed for young cochlear implant users. These objectives are also appropriate for adults who have significant hearing loss.

The student:

1. Will discriminate words with /i/ and /u/; for example, *me* from *moo.*

2. Will discriminate words with /i/ and /a/; for example, *keep* from *cop.*

3. Will discriminate words with /u/ and /a/; for example, *coop* from *cop.*

4. Will identify words with /i/, /u/, and /a/, using a four-item and then six-item response set; for example, *bean* from the response set of: *bean, pot, pit,* and *pool.* The vowels in the response set may include vowels other than /i, u, a/.

5. Will identify words with /u/, /i/, and /a/ from an open set of familiar vocabulary.

Subsequent training that contrasts other vowels can be incorporated into consonant training activities.

Typically, the lips pucker and form a narrow opening when a talker phonates /u/, and both first and second formants have a relatively low frequency value. For /a/, the lips form a moderate opening and appear relaxed; the formants have midrange values. Table 6-3 presents one possible hierarchy of analytic speechreading training objectives based on these three distinctive vowel types.

Consonant Speechreading Training Objectives

In Chapters 2 and 4, we considered three different types of speech features: manner, voice, and place of articulation, and noted that consonants can be characterized in terms of these three features. It is fortuitous that the visual signal associated with consonant production ideally complements the auditory signal. Cues that signal manner and voice often are easier for persons with hearing loss to hear than are cues that signal place of articulation. For instance, someone with a severe hearing loss who uses amplification is likely to hear the difference between the words *bat* and *pat.* However, if presented with only the visual signal, these two words will be indistinguishable. In contrast, cues about place of articulation tend to be somewhat visible, but place of articulation is difficult to determine through listening alone for persons who have significant hearing loss. A person with hearing loss might discriminate the words *pat* and *sat* if he or she can see the talker, but may not be able to discriminate them if the individual only hears the talker.

A list of consonant speechreading training objectives appears in Table 6-4. The first speechreading consonant training objectives may involve discriminating consonants that differ in place of production, and that share either voice or manner (Table 6-4). For example, a student may be asked to discriminate between the /p/ in *pay* and the /s/ in *say.* The clinician speaks the two items and the student then indicates whether they are the

Table 6-4. Consonant analytic speechreading training designed for young cochlear implant users. These objectives also are appropriate for adults who have significant hearing loss.

The student:

1. Will discriminate consonant pairs that differ in place of production and share either voice or manner, for example, *tag* from *bag*.

2. Will discriminate consonant pairs that share similar place of production but differ in manner and voice, for example, *pan* from *man*.

3. Will discriminate consonant pairs that share place and manner or voice, for example, *park* from *bark*.

4. Will identify consonants that share manner of production, using a four-item and then a six-item response set; for example, *tag* from the response set of: *tag, bag, back,* and *gas*.

5. Will identify consonants from a four-item and then a six-item response set of voiced or voiceless consonants; for example, *pop* from the response set of: *pop, cop, cap,* and *top*.

6. Will identify consonants that share place of production, using a four-item and then a six-item response set: for example, *pan* from the response set of: *pan, man, bat,* and *mat*.

7. Will identify words from an open set of familiar vocabulary.

---

same or *different.* The clinician attempts to speak with constant loudness and intonation. The next two objectives require students to discriminate between consonants that share place, but that differ on other signal parameters (Objectives 2 and 3 in Table 6-4).

After a student achieves the first three consonant speechreading training objectives, intermediate objectives in a speechreading curriculum (Objectives 4 and 5 in Table 6-4) might focus attention on identifying consonants that share manner or voice. The student will progress from performing a discrimination task, as in the first three speechreading training objectives, to performing a closed-set identification task. For example, individuals might identify the word *cat* from the response set of *cat, pat, pet,* and *kit,* words that all begin with voiceless consonants. Following a discrimination activity, they then may perform an identification activity, using a closed-set response format. For this kind of training activity, the clinician might set before the individual a set of five or six picture cards, such as the set shown in Figure 6-3. The clinician then speaks one of the items, and the student indicates which item was spoken. This kind of task is a precursor to open-set word recognition.

Advanced objectives for consonant speechreading training (Objectives 6 and 7 in Table 6-4) often focus attention on identifying consonants that share place and manner, place and voice, or place, manner, and voice in a closed-set and then an open-set format. For example, students may be asked to identify /p/ as in *pole* when one of the foils is *bowl*. The /p/ and /b/ sounds are visually and acoustically similar.

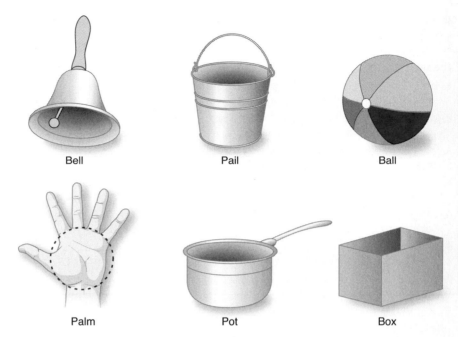

Bell   Pail   Ball

Palm   Pot   Box

FIGURE 6-3. Illustrations (*bell, pail, ball, palm, pot, box*) for a closed-set identification task when the target phonemes are /p/ and /b/. A clinician might present each item five or more times during the training session. When the student can read and has fairly good listening skills, the response set can be expanded and the response choices can be presented orthographically.

SYNTHETIC SPEECHREADING TRAINING OBJECTIVES

In comparison with sentence-level auditory training objectives, sentence-level speechreading training objectives will begin with more challenging tasks (Figure 6-4). This is because most people can recognize more speech when they can both see and hear rather than only hear a talker. For example, if the student is a child, the first task in a speechreading training curriculum may be to practice recognizing simple directions. Such a task would occur much later in an auditory training curriculum.

Table 6-5 presents a sample hierarchy of synthetic speechreading training objectives. The first objective requires students to follow simple directions, in a closed-set format. Initially, the set might be small. For example, two crayons, blue and orange, might be placed before a young child. The clinician asks the child to draw a blue beach ball. As the student advances, the set is enlarged, and the directions become more complex. In more advanced exercises, the clinician might present the following directions:

1. Color the ball orange.
2. Color the sand yellow.

3. Color the shovel purple.

4. Color the sky blue.

5. Color the water blue.

The second and third objectives listed in Table 6-5 require the individual to identify sentence illustrations from a set of pictures. The clinician might lay a set of pictures on a table (Figure 6-5) that might be used in a sentence recognition exercise. These are placed in front of the individual, and

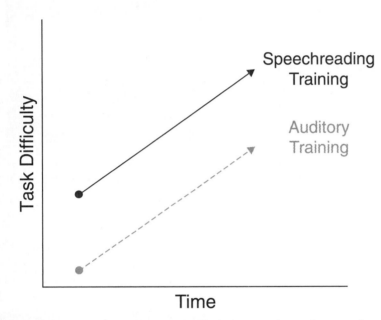

FIGURE 6-4. Task difficulty. Greater task difficulty is appropriate at the onset of speechreading training than at the onset of auditory training.

Table 6-5. Synthetic speechreading training objectives designed for young cochlear implant users. These objectives can be modified to meet the maturity and cognitive levels of adults who have significant hearing loss.

The student:

1. Will follow simple directions using a closed response set.

2. Will identify a sentence illustration from a set of four dissimilar pictures.

3. Will identify a sentence illustration from a set of four similar pictures.

4. Will listen to topic-related sentences, and repeat or paraphrase them.

5. Will listen to two related sentences, and then draw a picture about them or paraphrase them.

6. Will speechread a paragraph-long narrative and then answer questions about it.

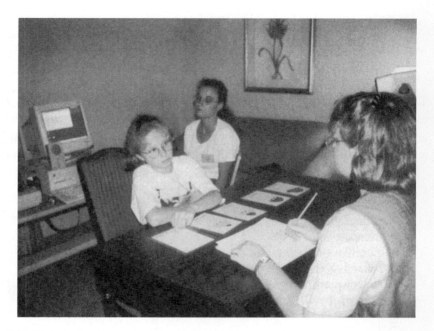

FIGURE 6-5. Synthetic speechreading training. A clinician and child perform a sentence recognition task using picture cards. *Photograph by Kim Readmond, courtesy of the Central Institute for the Deaf.*

then the clinician speaks sentences that correspond to each picture. The student's task is to speechread the clinician and then touch the picture that illustrates the sentence. Postcards, snapshots, or magazine pictures can be used to construct picture sets. Several sentences can be developed for each picture so that a single set can provide practice for speechreading a large number of sentences.

The fourth objective for synthetic level training requires the student to recognize topic-related sentences. These are sentences that concern a common theme. A set of topic-related sentences appears in Table 6-6 as an example.

The final objectives for formal synthetic speechreading training require students to speechread paragraphs. The clinician might present a picture that provides contextual cues for recognizing the passage. As in a continuous discourse tracking task, the student must repeat (or in this task, paraphrasing is also permitted) each sentence after speechreading the clinician speak sentences one at a time from a paragraph. Quite often, speechreading training includes extensive use of continuous discourse tracking (e.g., Alcantara, Cowan, Blamey, & Clark, 1990; Pichora-Fuller & Bengueral, 1991; Pichora-Fuller & Cicchelli, 1986; Plant, 1998), a training procedure that we will consider more fully in Chapter 9.

Table 6-6. Example of a set of topic-related sentences that can be utilized in achieving the fourth objective for synthetic speechreading training: The student will listen to topic-related sentences, and repeat or paraphrase them.

Sentences Concerning Cooking

1. I added a cup of flour.
2. The bread is in the oven.
3. Will you hand me the measuring cup?
4. I need the box of sugar.
5. The mixer is in the cabinet.
6. The oven is set to 300 degrees.
7. Put the bowl in the sink, please.
8. The pan is filled with batter.
9. I will beat the eggs.
10. Please pour a cup of milk.

A Holistic Approach to Speechreading Training for Children

Yoshinaga-Itano (1988) describes a **holistic approach** that can be used to teach children speechreading. The training goals of this approach can be summarized as follows (Yoshinaga-Itano, 1988):

- Increase the child's knowledge of the speechreading process.
- Increase the child's ability to generate strategies to facilitate more successful communication.
- Increase the child's tolerance for communicative situations that have a higher degree of frustration.
- Increase the child's ability to generate personal goals for improving speechreading.
- Increase the child's motivation to improve speechreading abilities. (p. 244)

In implementing a holistic approach, Yoshinaga-Itano suggests that children should participate in setting goals and should make a commitment to accomplish them. The holistic program should allow for both self-evaluation and clinician evaluation, and speechreading practice should be provided in real-life versus drill situations.

A **holistic approach** to speechreading incorporates several methods and includes the child in setting goals.

COMPUTERIZED INSTRUCTION

The ubiquity of home-based and laptop computers, as well as the capability of today's computer technology to accommodate massive amounts of audiovisual speech materials, has rendered computerized instruction possible. The clinician may work with the patient, or a small group of patients, in the clinical setting (see Figure 6-6). Alternatively, the patient may take the program home (Figure 6-7) or may use it in a school or work setting.

Two examples of computerized programs are the *Dynamic Audio Vision Interactive Device (DAVID)* developed at the National Technical Institute for the Deaf at the Rochester Institute of Technology (Sims, Dorn, Clark, Bryant, & Mumford, 2002; Sims & Gottermeier, 2000) and *Conversation Made Easy,* developed in part at University of Iowa Hospitals and available through the Central Institute for the Deaf in St. Louis (Tye-Murray, 2002b). *DAVID* presents sentences centered around everyday topics, such as going shopping or going to the bank. The student watches a sentence and then types a response into a keyboard. Depending on the level of difficulty, the student either selects a response from a closed set of choices (easy level of difficulty), types in content words (intermediate level of difficulty), or types in the complete sentence (challenging level of difficulty). The program provides "help" alternatives, such as the option to have a sentence repeated, to have a word spoken in isolation in clear speech, or spoken

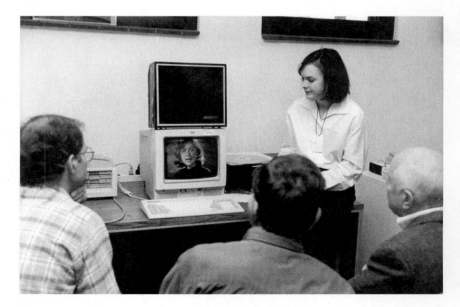

FIGURE 6-6. Computer-based instruction. A clinician uses a computer-based program to provide speechreading instruction to a small group of adult patients. *Photograph by Kim Readmond, courtesy of the Central Institute for the Deaf.*

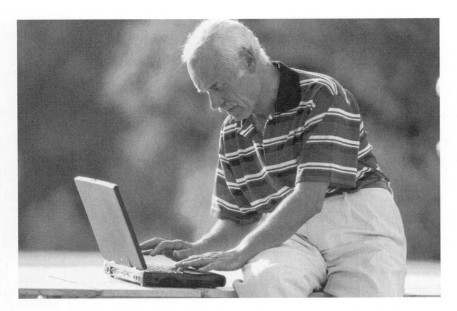

FIGURE 6-7. Speechreading training exercises in the home setting, conducted with a laptop computer.

with the talker seen at a 45° azimuth view. A student's performance on the program may be documented in terms of how long it takes in seconds (i.e., response time) to get the item 100% correct.

Three versions of *Conversation Made Easy* are available: one for adults and teenagers, one for children who have low-level language skills, and one for children who have high-level language skills. In this program, students need not know how to type or spell, which makes use by children and aging adults who have dexterity problems possible. Students can enter their responses either by clicking on a picture response with the mouse or by typing a single key on the keyboard. Three kinds of exercises are provided in each version. First, students receive analytic practice, where they learn to discriminate and identify sounds, words, and simple phrases. In one analytic activity, a man appears on the computer monitor and says the word *cat,* and then a woman appears and says the same word. The student's task is to indicate whether the two words are the *same* or *different.* Even though words spoken by a man and woman are acoustically different, they are phonetically the same. This is an important concept to realize, especially if training is to generalize to real-world contexts. In the second kind of exercise, students recognize unrelated sentences. A talker appears on the computer monitor and speaks a sentence. Afterward, four pictures appear, one of which illustrates the sentence. The student clicks on an alternative. If the response is correct, the text of the sentence appears on the screen, and the talker reappears and speaks the sentence.

If the response is incorrect, five repair strategies are offered: Repeat the original sentence, rephrase it, simplify it, elaborate on it, or provide a key word (topic word). Whichever option the student selects, it happens right away. The talker reappears on the monitor and performs the selected option. This continues for a particular sentence until the student selects the correct alternative or until no picture alternatives remain. The third program provides synthetic speechreading practice for sentences that are related by context (e.g., for children, one exercise concerns math class; for adults, one exercise concerns a visit to the physician). The materials provide a simulation of real-world listening environments. In addition to using the repair strategies, the student may also use facilitative strategies. For example, if the teacher is filmed from the back of the classroom, the student can request to "move to the front of the classroom." If this option is selected, the "teacher" reappears on the computer monitor and repeats the sentence, this time filmed at a closer range.

There are several advantages to using computerized instruction to supplement other aural rehabilitation efforts. These include the following:

- Many items can be presented in a short period of time. For example, we found that in 3 days, adult patients working on Program 1 of *Conversation Made Easy* completed an average of 1,800 training items. Concentrated training may lead to faster learning and maintains a student's interest.
- For most available programs, the computer keeps a record of the student's responses during training. Thus, even though the student may perform the training exercises at home, the clinician can still monitor training progress.
- The student can practice speechreading many people without leaving the clinic or home. For example, in the program for children in *Conversation Made Easy,* 16 different people in the second program alone speak training sentences. In the third program, many of the talkers are children, because children need practice in speechreading other children.
- For most programs, training is interactive, which is not always possible with standard audiovisual recorded materials. This interaction means that a student's response to one training item determines what will happen next. Response contingency is an important element in any instructional design.
- Instruction is self-paced. Students can proceed through an exercise as slowly or as quickly as they choose.
- Training can occur at the student's convenience. For many people, such as those who work during the day or those who do not have

transportation, coming to a speech and hearing clinic for speechreading training poses logistical problems. By using a computerized program, students can choose where and when to receive practice.

The speech and hearing professional need not be present in the room while the student performs the training activities. Because aural rehabilitation is often labor-intensive and expensive, the use of computerized instruction may be one means of establishing better cost–benefit ratios. The speech and hearing professional might be available to discuss the training goals and training results with the student and might role-play and practice some of the training activities with the student.

EFFICACY OF SPEECHREADING TRAINING

Many researchers have considered whether lipreading and speechreading skills can be developed through training and practice. Investigations aimed at assessing efficacy are difficult to design because the outcome can be influenced by a number of variables, including the heterogeneity of the research participants (including such factors as age, degree of hearing loss, level of motivation to participate in training), variations in training stimuli and methods, variations in the duration of intervention, and the talent of the instructor. For instance, a participant who has engaged in 6 weeks of speechreading training may be more motivated to perform well on a post-training test of audiovisual speech recognition than a control participant who has received no training. Table 6-7 summarizes several of the investigations that have been reported during the last three decades, and reflects how experiments might differ in their designs and outcomes.

A relatively large number of investigators report that training improves performance (e.g., Bernstein, Auer, & Tucker, 2001; Sims et al., 2002; Walden et al., 1977, 1981), whereas others report that speechreading training provides little or only marginal benefit (e.g., Lesner et al., 1987). When improvements do occur, they are often, although not always, modest. For instance, some investigators have demonstrated that adults with hearing impairment show only small improvement following training, typically improving by 10–15% in their ability to recognize speech stimuli (e.g., Alcantara et al., 1990; Gagné, Dinon, & Parsons, 1991; Walden et al., 1981). It appears that tutored self-instruction that occurs in the home with videotaped stimuli is effective in teaching skills (Lonka, 1995; see also Dodd, Plant, & Gregory, 1989), which bodes well for the feasibility of computerized instruction.

Some investigators have shown that training programs that include a kinesthetic component might be effective (De Filippo, Sims, & Gottermeier, 1995; Novelli-Olmstead & Ling, 1984; Small & Infante, 1988). These kinds of

Table 6-7. An overview of several investigations that have focused on the effectiveness of lipreading and speechreading training, arranged here in chronological order (V = vision-only; AV = audiovisual; CV = consonant-vowel; VC = vowel-consonant; AR = aural rehabilitation).

AUTHORS	PARTICIPANTS	GENERAL PROCEDURES	FINDINGS
Binnie (1977)	12 adults with hearing loss (mean age = 63 years)	a) Participants attended 1½ hour-long speechreading classes weekly for 12 weeks.	Performance did not change on V tests of monosyllables and sentences. A posttraining questionnaire revealed that participants had a more assertive approach to their communication difficulties and a more positive opinion of their communication skills.
Walden, Prosek, Montgomery, Scherr, & Jones (1977)	31 adults with hearing loss	a) All participants received the same training. b) Participants received 14 sessions of individualized instruction, which included 38 exercises geared to train V recognition of CV and VC syllables.	Performance was assessed by looking at within-cluster responses for nine viseme groups. On average, the percentage score changed from 91% to 99%.
Walden, Erdman, Montgomery, Schwartz, & Prosek, 1981	35 male new hearing aid users (age from 19 to 68 years), assigned to one of three groups: standard AR; AR plus (AR+) auditory consonant recognition training; or AR plus lipreading training	a) Participants in the AR(+) groups received 7 hours of either auditory or visual consonant recognition training over 10 days. b) Participants were trained individually and viewed the clinician via closed-circuit television. c) The training tasks included discrimination and identification.	Both AR(+) groups improved their scores on an AV sentence test (about 23–28% words correct on average) and did so significantly more than the AR group. Consonant viseme recognition, which was assessed only in the group that received lipreading training, improved from 83% to 93%.
Danz & Binnie, 1983	Eight young adults with normal hearing, four received speechreading training and four served as controls	a) The participants who received training completed 18 individual sessions during a 14-day period. b) Training consisted of continuous discourse tracking, where participants viewed the talker in an AV condition in noise via closed-circuit television. The control participants received no training.	The training group demonstrated improved performance in an AV condition with noise on the continuous discourse tracking procedure and significant improvement on a consonant recognition test. They showed no improvement on a sentence recognition test. The control group did not change on any measure.
Montgomery, Walden, Schwartz, & Prosek, 1984	24 adults (age from 24 to 60 years) with hearing loss and 10 adults with normal hearing (the control group); 12 of the adults with hearing loss received AR and 12 received AR(+)	a) Training was similar to that provided by Walden et al. (1977) but also included speechreading training for sentence-length and conversational materials. b) Nonsense syllables were presented with the vowel portion audible and the consonant portions inaudible.	The two AR groups demonstrated significant improvement on a sentence test in an AV condition following training whereas the control group of participants with normal hearing did not.

continues

Table 6-7. *continued*

AUTHORS	PARTICIPANTS	GENERAL PROCEDURES	FINDINGS
Lesner, Sandridge, & Kricos, 1987	30 young adults; 10 received videotaped analytic training for consonants in a V condition with feedback; 10 received the same training without feedback; 10 received no intervention	a) The training group with feedback received 14 hours of videotaped training whereas the training group without feedback received 7 hours. b) Training included same–different discrimination and identification tasks.	All three groups showed significant improvement on a consonant recognition test in a V condition (between about 9% and 15%), and the two training groups improved significantly more than did the control group but did not differ from each other. No group demonstrated improvement on a sentence test.
Small & Infante (1988)	30 university female students; 15 received lipreading training; 15 received no training	a) Participants in the training group were asked to imitate the talker's articulatory movements after each stimulus. b) Group training was provided, divided into four 1½-hour sessions over the course of 2 weeks. c) The distance from the talker and the viewing angle varied during training.	The participants who received training improved their performance on a sentence test, for each of three visual distances assessed. For instance, they recognized an average of 6.5 more words following training at a distance of 3–6 feet. The participants who received no training demonstrated no improvement.
Dodd, Plant, & Gregory, 1989	45 participants; all but 13 (who were in the control group) had postlingual hearing loss; participants were divided into four groups: a control group that received no training (mean age = 36 years); AR class and video training at home (mean age = 50 years); video training at home (mean age = 64 years); and AR class (mean age = 64 years)	a) The "lipreading package" consisted of a videocassette and a manual. The video held nine lipreading lessons, each 20 minutes long. b) Exercises included 52 lipreading tasks spoken by 20 different speakers, including word discrimination, sentence recognition, and sentence comprehension. c) Training occurred over a 5-week period.	One test required participants to respond to questions and a second assessed recognition of words in sentences. The three test groups improved following training (13–14%) whereas the control group did not change significantly on the second test administration. There were no differences between test groups.
Warren, Dancer, Monfils, & Pittenger (1989)	20 young adults with normal hearing	a) Participants saw the same recorded list of sentences in a V condition every day for 5 consecutive days or they saw a different list every day. b) Participants were instructed to "mouth" the sentences as they viewed.	Participants in the same-list group improved their percentage words correct score by 13.6% whereas those in the different-list group improved by 9.2%.
Gagné, Dinon, & Parsons, 1991	Two groups of eight young-adult participants with normal hearing; one group received lipreading and speechreading training	Training was provided with the CAST computerized program (Pichora-Fuller & Cicchelli, 1986). a) Activities included an automated continuous discourse tracking procedure. b) Participants completed eight lessons over a 10-week period.	The two groups did not differ in their mean improvement scores for a consonant test or for two sentence tests presented in a V condition. The training group demonstrated faster tracking rates following training whereas the control group demonstrated no change.

continues

Table 6-7. *continued*

AUTHORS	PARTICIPANTS	GENERAL PROCEDURES	FINDINGS
Gesi, Massaro, & Cohen, 1992	35 college students with normal hearing, divided into three groups; two groups received lipreading training and one served as a control	a) Training stimuli included CV syllables spoken by four different talkers. b) The training groups received 3 days of training. The *discovery* group received only enough information to perform the tasks whereas the *expository* group received explicit lessons about how the sounds were produced and the visual characteristics of the sounds.	Both training groups demonstrated significant improvement in identifying CV syllables and retained the improvements 4 weeks following training. However, they did no better in identifying monosyllabic words than did the control group.
Lonka, 1995	76 Finnish participants with mild-to-moderate hearing loss, divided into four groups of 16–20	a) Groups received either individual speechreading training with a clinician and personal counseling and auditory training; individual speechreading training with a clinician; speechreading training at home with video tapes; or no treatment. b) Training included both analytical and synthetic exercises.	The three groups that received training demonstrated significant improvements on a sentence test (about 6–14% words correct) whereas the control group did not.
De Filippo, Sims, & Gottermeier, 1995	Four groups of 12 males (age from 18 to 34 years old), with profound prelingual or perilingual hearing loss; groups varied as to whether they received self or trainer video feedback and whether they receivedl feedback during or after production	The two *feedback-during-production* groups spoke and lipread either themselves or the trainer via video at the same time. The two *feedback-after-production* groups spoke the items first and then viewed either themselves or the trainer speak the items via video.	Overall, performance improved on the trained items, scored as percentage consonants correct. The group that viewed self-speech following speech production also improved on the untrained test items.
Bernstein, Auer, & Tucker, 2001	Eight adults with normal hearing and eight adults (age from 18 to 40 years old) with prelingual and profound deafness who use spoken English as their primary mode of communication with family members	a) Training items included sentences spoken by a male and a female. b) Participants completed six sessions of lipreading training during a period of up to 5 weeks.	The two groups did not enhance their performance on a sentence test when it was scored in terms of percentage words correct but showed small and comparable improvement when the test items were scored in terms of phonemes correct.

programs request students to shadow the speech of their teacher, attending to the feel of their own speech gestures as they do so, and/or to watch themselves speak in a mirror or via video feedback. These procedures are reminiscent of the methods promoted by Nitchie and Brauckmann, both of whom were considered at the onset of this chapter. For example, Small and Infante asked their participants to imitate the talker's articulatory movements simultaneously with the talker's utterance or immediately afterward. De Filippo, Sims, and Gottermeier asked their participants to speak training items and allowed them to either watch themselves speak the items by means of a video monitor or to watch their instructor speak the items. Small and Infante reported gains as a function of training and De Filippo et al. reported an advantage for individuals who had received the opportunity to practice lipreading their own speech production (see Table 6-7).

Often, results are inconclusive or present contradictory findings. Some people may not show improvement in their performance on a test of audiovisual speech recognition. However, if asked whether they believe they benefited from speechreading training, they may provide an ardent testimonial in support of training or will report benefit via a questionnaire (e.g., Binnie, 1977).

Some individuals may become better test takers, so their speechreading skills only appear to improve, rather than actually improving. Gagné et al. (1991) evaluated the effectiveness of a computerized speechreading training program in which participants received speechreading practice by using a modified continuous discourse tracking procedure. Changes in speechreading performance were determined by comparing scores on standard speech recognition tests obtained prior to the training program to scores obtained after training. The participants did not improve on most of the standard tests. However, they were able to repeat more words verbatim per minute during the continuous discourse tracking task posttraining than pretraining. The researchers cautioned that the improved tracking rates might have resulted from 25 to 30 hours of practice with the tracking procedure during training and familiarity with the talker, rather than from improved visual speech recognition skills. Tye-Murray and Tyler (1988) discuss these and other drawbacks of using continuous discourse tracking as a test procedure.

Only a few investigators have examined the extent to which children improve following training (e.g., Novell-Olmstead & Ling, 1984; Massaro & Light, 2004; Novell-Olmstead & Ling, 1984). For instance, Massaro and Light, using a computer-animated talking head named Baldy (Chapter 5), found that children improved their recognition of phonemes following training. It is possible that children have more potential to benefit from training than do adults, although this possibility has not received much attention. Some of the studies that have been conducted have focused on whether speechreading training, in conjunction with the use of a tactile aid, is beneficial. It appears that the results are positive (e.g., Kishon-Rubin, Heras, & Bergman, 1997; see also Alcantra et al., 1990, who provided training to adult users of tactile aids).

CASE STUDY

Targeting Training

A case study presented by Witt (1997) tells an unusual story about a man (JT) who had used a cochlear implant for 9 years. He was considered by his audiologist to be neither a "star" user nor a "poor" user, but reflective of the average adult who uses a cochlear implant. What makes the case study unusual is that JT had used his implant for 9 years prior to entering an intensive 6-day aural rehabilitation program, where he received approximately 40 hours of aural rehabilitation therapy. It is more common for adult cochlear implant users to engage in aural rehabilitation immediately following implantation.

At the time of the study, JT was 51 years old. Although he was diagnosed with a mild hearing loss at the age of 5 years, his hearing did not worsen until he was 28 years old. He had lost his hearing completely by the time he was 41 years old.

The aural rehabilitation program included auditory training, speechreading training, assertiveness training, and telephone training (i.e., how to converse effectively on the telephone using conversational strategies). For the speechreading component, the audiologist identified those sounds that JT had the most difficulty recognizing auditorily (e.g., /k, g/). Those sounds were targeted during analytic speechreading training. In addition, the synthetic training materials were heavily weighted with these target sounds. JT practiced speechreading both with a clinician and with computerized materials (at the time, available in laser video disc format and now available in CD-ROM format; Tye-Murray, 2002c).

At the beginning of training, JT appeared intent on recognizing every sound in a message. For instance, the following exchange occurred between JT and his clinician (pp. 37–38):

Clinician:	I said, "Is he "ill?" You thought I said, "Is she Gill?"
JT:	I know.
Clinician:	Okay, maybe *Gill* is a female name. I thought it was a male name.
JT:	I knew I had it wrong when I said it, but the /s/ and the /h/ kind of all merge together here and I just said what I heard.
Clinician:	Okay, and now that you think about it and look at it, well, *Gill* is an odd name. If I would have said, "Is he Bob?" you probably would not have said, "Is she Bob?"
JT:	I might have because I'm not thinking of the meaning in this exercise.
Clinician:	Okay.
JT:	I'm just repeating what I heard.
Clinician:	Okay, you're just repeating what you heard.
JT:	Yeah.
Clinician:	Okay, so you're not necessarily comprehending.
JT:	Right.

At the end of training, JT engaged in a synthetic training exercise that required him to answer questions. He responded correctly to all of the questions, demonstrating that he both recognized the speech and comprehended the message. Afterward, he commented, "The hearing part wasn't the effort; the effort was the explaining. As we got into it I kind of relaxed and had fun."

Two measures suggest that his ability to comprehend speech in an audition-plus-vision condition improved as a result of training (a standard test of speechreading was not administered before and after intervention). First, a test assessing how well JT could speechread and simultaneously perform a hand task *(Color Change-Dual Task)* demonstrated that he did not have to devote as much attention to recognizing utterances following training. He showed improvement on this test both immediately after training and 2 months later. Hence, he could devote greater mental energy to comprehending what he was speechreading and formulating an appropriate response. Similarly, his performance increased on a short-term memory test following training, suggesting that he maintained more of what he speechread. Apparently, he was able to allocate more mental energy to storing information and less to recognizing the message on the face and with his residual hearing. At the end of training, JT recorded in his diary, "I try listening to my wife and kids. . . . My confidence is much higher. . . . I have confidence that I will recognize sounds and that recognition provides useful information to me. I think that before rehab I lacked confidence."

This case study demonstrates one of the more subtle benefits of speechreading training. With some patients, the speechreading task seems to become less effortful following training, allowing them to devote more mental energy to comprehending the message and less to identifying sounds and words. In part, this gain may relate to an increase in confidence and, in part, to an increased facility to recognize speech audiovisually. This study also demonstrates how a clinician has the opportunity to tailor the aural rehabilitation program to meet the individual needs of the patient. JT had expressed frustration with using the telephone, so his program included telephone training. He had difficulty recognizing specific speech sounds, so his program included a preponderance of these sounds during speechreading training.

FINAL REMARKS

At one time, many adults received aural rehabilitation that was comprised primarily of speechreading training. With the advent of sophisticated listening devices, and the increase of communication strategies training, few adults receive a great deal of speechreading training, and rarely is it provided in the absence of other aural rehabilitation services. Nonetheless, it is important for persons with hearing impairment to understand why speechreading is so difficult. The emphasis of speechreading training may be on ways to minimize the difficulty of the task, such as ways to manage the environment or ways to encourage appropriate speaking behaviors on the part of their communication partners.

KEY CHAPTER POINTS

- Speechreading training was popular in the first half of the 20th century. The advent of more sophisticated listening devices, and questions about the benefits of training, have led to a reduced emphasis on speechreading training in most aural rehabilitation programs.

- As with auditory training, a speechreading training program typically includes both analytic and synthetic training objectives.

- The logic underlying many speechreading curricula is gradually to increase students' reliance on the auditory signal for recognizing phonemic contrasts.

- Speechreading training often includes continuous discourse tracking tasks.

- Computerized speechreading training offers many benefits, including intensive practice and schedule flexibility.

- A relatively large number of investigators have attempted to evaluate the efficacy of speechreading training, using a variety of training methods and tests and focusing on a number of different participant groups.

- Extraneous variables, such as patient motivation, complicate assessments of speechreading training efficacy.

- Speechreading training appears to provide modest benefits to most patients.

- Several training programs that include kinesthetic components have been shown to be effective.

TERMS AND CONCEPTS TO REMEMBER

20th-century methods

Kinesthetic

Class handouts

Complementary signals

Formal speechreading training objectives

Holistic approach

Computerized instruction

Efficacy

⬙ MULTIPLE-CHOICE QUESTIONS

1. If a person is a candidate for intensive speechreading training, this person is most likely to be:

    a. A new recipient of a cochlear implant

    b. An experienced hearing aid user

    c. A younger adult

    d. A graduate of an oral school

2. Which of the following statements is false?

    a. The visual speech signal complements the auditory signal.

    b. The visual speech signal is redundant with the information provided by residual hearing.

    c. The visual signal presents a good deal of information about place of production.

    d. The visual signal presents information that helps the speechreader distinguish /i/ from /u/ from /a/.

3. Which exercise might appear later during a speechreading training curriculum rather than earlier?

    a. The student will discriminate consonant pairs that differ in place of production.

    b. The student will discriminate consonant pairs that share place of production, but that differ in voice and manner.

    c. The student will identify words that begin with consonants that share place of production, from a six-item response set.

    d. The student will identify words that begin with consonants that do not share place of production, from a six-item response set.

4. Asking a child to color in the states of a map of the United States (e.g., *Color Maine with the color red.*) is an example of what kind of training activity?

    a. Synthetic

    b. Analytic

    c. Synthesis

    d. Discrimination

5. The advantages of computerized instruction include:

    a. Patients can become familiar with a talker's facial movements.

    b. Patients can forgo interactions with a speech and hearing professional.

    c. Training can occur outside of the clinical setting.

    d. Patients can design their own exercises.

6. The best way to describe the data about the efficacy of traditional analytical and synthetic speechreading training is:

    a. Most data are supportive.

    b. Most data are nonsupportive.

    c. Analytic training is superior to synthetic training.

    d. The results are equivocal.

7. A number of studies of speechreading training that included kinesthetic elements:

    a. Have required participants to feel the neck of the talker as the talker speaks.

    b. Have shown it to be more effective than either analytic or synthetic training.

    c. Have been found to be methodologically flawed.

    d. Have shown it to be effective in enhancing speechreading performance.

8. A class handout in a speechreading class would likely not include the following tip:

    a. Wear your hearing aid whenever you are going to be speechreading.

    b. Pay attention to the talker's facial expression.

    c. Ask for a key word because knowing the topic of conversation will likely help you to speechread.

    d. Ask a communication partner to mouth speech silently so that you can practice your lipreading skills.

PART 2

Conversation and Communication Behaviors

CHAPTER 7

Communication Strategies and Conversational Styles

OUTLINE

- Conversation
- Facilitative communication strategies
- Repair strategies
- Research concerning repair strategies and communication breakdowns
- Conversational styles and behaviors
- Case study: A couple conversing
- Final remarks
- Key chapter points
- Terms and concepts to remember
- Multiple-choice questions

Successful everyday communication for individuals with hearing loss is influenced by many variables, including the effectiveness of their listening device, their speechreading skills, and the amount of residual hearing. In addition, success in communication is affected greatly by how well people use communication strategies. A **communication strategy** is a course of action taken to facilitate a conversational interaction or to rectify a problem that arises during conversation. During **communication strategies training**, patients receive instruction about how to manage their conversational interactions effectively. Many speech and hearing professionals recognize that communication strategies training is a powerful way to enhance individuals' abilities to manage everyday listening problems.

In this chapter, the foundation will be laid for the next chapters about conversational fluency and hearing-related disability assessment and conversation strategies training. First we will consider general issues related to conversation and then focus on communication strategies and conversational styles. The included conversations actually occurred. Some have been edited for brevity or clarity for the present purposes.

A **communication strategy** is a course of action taken to enhance communication.

Communication strategies training is instruction provided to a person with a hearing loss to maximize his or her communication potential.

CONVERSATION

Much of the fabric of human relationships is woven by our conversations—by what we say, how we say it, and how we listen. We engage in conversation for several reasons (Figure 7-1):

- To share ideas
- To create meaning
- To relate experiences
- To tell stories
- To express needs
- To effect a result
- To instruct
- To influence
- To establish intimacy
- To build understanding

"In everyday talk, storytelling is ubiquitous: 'You'll never believe what happened today.' 'I'll never forget the time when . . .' 'Did you hear the one about . . . ?' When in doubt—or at loose ends or in the need of attention—we narrate."

O. Scott, film critic for the *New York Times*

(Scott, 2007, p. 11)

The way people talk with others is guided by their knowledge of implicit **rules of conversation**. A metaphysical reflection about the way we converse might indicate that most of us typically adhere to culturally established conventions. For example, when two or more people begin a conversation, they each:

Conversational rules are implicit rules that guide the conduct of participants in a conversation.

- **Tacitly agree to share one another's interests.** They commit their mental resources to attending to their communication partner's

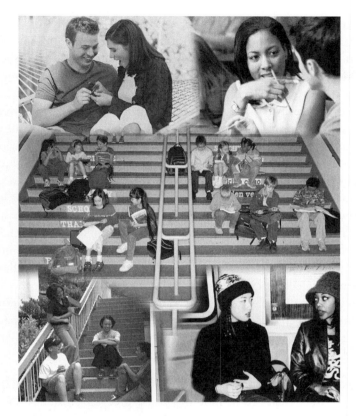

FIGURE 7-1. Reasons to engage in conversation: to share, to inform, or to instruct.

messages, and respond to the messages in a way that furthers the discussion.

- **Ensure that no single person does all of the talking.** Most people do not dominate the conversation with their own talking, and they do not expect their communication partners to bear the onus of continuing the conversation alone. They share speaking turns. A communication partner should not leave a conversation thinking, "I didn't get a word in because that man wouldn't stop talking," or thinking, "He sat like a piece of furniture, as if he didn't care."

- **Participate in choosing what to talk about, and participate in developing the topic.** Typically, there is not a "chief" who leads the conversation, and who alone decides what is talked about and how that subject is developed. Rather, all participants play a role, at some point or another, in deciding what is talked about and in shaping the direction in which the discussion progresses.

- **Take turns in an organized fashion.** Conversation often unfolds in either a turn-taking or an overlapping style. In a turn-taking interaction, one person finishes speaking before the next person begins and

Four Often Quoted Maxims (Rules) of Conversation

- Maxim of Quantity: Avoid wordiness
- Maxim of Quality: Be truthful
- Maxim of Relation: Be relevant
- Maxim of Manner: Be perspicuous (orderly, clear in statement, not obscure or ambiguous)

Paul Grice, English language philosopher

(Grice, 1975)

interruptions are infrequent. In an overlapping interaction, it is acceptable for two or more communication partners to speak simultaneously or for one partner to start speaking before another finishes. This latter style might predominate in conversations that are more intimate, spontaneous, and energetic.

- **Try to be relevant to the topic of conversation (topic coherence).** If a conversation is centered on automobiles and someone abruptly begins to talk about a recipe for cornbread, that individual has violated an implicit rule of conversation by not being relevant to the discussion. A sequential ordering principle is in play throughout most conversations. An utterance is usually made in response or in relation to someone's preceding utterance. Even when topics change, the change is typically accomplished in an orderly way. A communication partner may remark, "Which reminds me, . . ." or in some such way explicitly or implicitly explain why he or she is not adhering to a relatedness expectation.
- **Provide enough information to convey a message without being verbose.** In a conversation, people expect our communication partners to deliver their messages in a fairly succinct way and in a manner that maintains their interest in listening.

If one participant in a conversation has a hearing loss, some of the rules of conversation may have to be modified or adapted. For instance, interruptions may occur more frequently because the individual must frequently ask for clarification of a misperceived message. Other participants may have to exert a greater effort to ensure that the person has an opportunity to contribute to a topic's development. If he or she did not understand or misunderstood something that has been said, the person with hearing loss may sometimes contribute remarks that are not relevant to the ongoing discussion. The individual may also have to use communication strategies, ideally in a way that does not violate the more universally established rules of conversation.

The quality of conversations experienced by persons with significant hearing loss often differs from that experienced by persons who have normal hearing. They may not hear the rhythms created by the ups and downs of a talker's prosody and the alternation of speech and small pauses, those musical elements of spoken language that sweep a listener along during the telling of a narrative or story. Emotional nuances and subtle meaning, say affection or sarcasm, might be lost if the listener cannot register the talker's tone of voice or lexical emphasis. Consider the utterance (spoken with a high pitch), "You're NOT going to give me a birthday present AGAIN?" and the same utterance (spoken with a low volume), "You're not going to

With a Wave of the Hand

Most of us supplement our words with complex hand gestures. We might spread our palms wide apart when we say the word *big,* or shake our finger for emphasis. These gestures can be quite helpful to persons with hearing loss as they try to understand spoken messages. Sometimes, conversations involving someone with hearing loss will incorporate more hand gestures than usual. Researchers have classified hand gestures into at least six categories (e.g., Cassell, 2001):

- **Emblematic:** culturally specified gestures, e.g., the "V" gesture might symbolize *victory* to some citizens living in the United Kingdom but *peace* to some citizens living in the United States.
- **Iconic:** gestures that depict an item, action, or feature of something being described; e.g., a talker might slide a hand through the air as he describes a slide into home base that happened at a baseball game.
- **Metaphoric:** gestures that depict a metaphor; e.g., a talker might make a corkscrew whirling motion with an index finger at her temple while simultaneously saying the word *crazy.*
- **Deictic:** gestures that locate items, places, or people in space; e.g., a talker might hold out his left palm when referring to people living in the western suburbs of a city and his right palm when referring to persons living in the eastern suburbs.
- **Beat:** gestures that provide emphasis and serve an evaluative or orienting function; e.g., a talker might flick her wrist as she stresses the unimportance of completing a particular task.
- **Regulatory:** gestures that help guide the flow of conversation; e.g., a talker may let her hands fall as she nears the end of a speaking turn.

give me a birthday present again." The first version is **keyed** as an introduction to an argument while the second is keyed as a gentle remonstration.

From a broad-brush perspective, the content of a conversation might be limited or its fluency stunted when one of the participants has a hearing loss. Conversations involving someone who has a hearing loss may have any of the following characteristics:

- **Disrupted taking of turns.** When someone comes to an end of a speaking turn, the person often begins to speak slower and his or her intonation contour begins to fall. The person with hearing loss

Keying occurs when a talker's tone of voice, cadence, lexical emphasis, prosody, and other speaking characteristics imbue an emotional stance to an utterance.

may not hear these signals and thus, inappropriate silences may occur because he or she does not initiate a conversational turn on cue. In addition, if the person has not understood the message, he or she may be unable to formulate a response or be slow in doing so, and so again, silence ensues. Inappropriately long pauses may cause the communication partner to conclude, " 'You're withholding,' 'You're hostile,' 'You never tell me what's on your mind,' or even 'You have nothing on your mind!' " (Tannen, 2000, p. 393).

- **Modified speaking and listening styles.** Communication partners may speak slowly with precise articulation in order to facilitate speech recognition for the person with hearing loss. They may rely more on nonverbal behaviors to convey their messages, such as more frequent and elaborate hand gestures, and exaggerated facial expressions. The listener with hearing loss may utilize unusual eye gaze patterns. For instance, the person might stare at the talker's mouth and make infrequent eye contact.

- **Modified conversational style.** Communication partners might refrain from an overlapping style of turn taking because the person with hearing loss is unable to speechread two or more people simultaneously (if more than two people are in the conversation) or the person might miss the beginning of their remarks if they overlap.

- **Less rich imagery.** The communication partner might omit the details that make a story colorful; for example, a talker might describe a motor vehicle as "a junk heap on wheels" to a listener who has normal hearing but as "a car" to the listener who has difficulty in recognizing any but the most common of words. The two descriptions certainly evince different mental images.

- **Inappropriate topic shifts.** The person with hearing loss may not recognize previous remarks and may inadvertently (and inappropriately) change the subject.

- **Superficial content.** Because speech recognition is difficult for the individual who has hearing loss, the participants in a conversation may avoid certain topics for discussion and avoid topics that might evoke unusual vocabulary or complex syntax. A spouse might decide that it is not "worth the effort" to describe the intricacies of a business meeting in response to her husband's question, "How was your day?" Instead, she might simply say, "Fine," and leave it at that.

- **Frequent clarification.** Misunderstandings are commonplace in conversations, even when all participants have normal hearing. When someone has a hearing loss, misunderstandings may become even more frequent. Both the person with hearing loss and the communication partner may need to engage in clarification more often, and diversions from the topic may occur regularly.

- **Violation of implicit social rules.** The person with hearing loss may talk too loudly and may appear as "not paying attention" or as "not caring about what is said."
- **Disrupted grounding.** When people engage in conversation, they often employ a **grounding** process, wherein they incorporate a bit of information into the conversation as "common ground" and then this information is presupposed throughout the remaining interaction. A person with hearing loss might miss out on important information early on in a conversation or inadvertently indicate that he or she has understood shared information because of bluffing behavior. The person may then misunderstand later remarks. In a related sense, if the person has a prelingual or perilingual hearing loss, he or she might lack general world knowledge that most people acquire

"Conversation about the weather is the last refuge of the unimaginative [. . . or the person who has a significant hearing loss]."
Oscar Wilde, 19th-century playwright

Grounding is a conversational occurrence in which communication partners establish a body of information as shared common ground for an ongoing conversational interchange. It usually entails the presentation of information by one communication partner and the confirmation of mutual understanding by another.

Older Persons and Persons with Hearing Loss: Commonalities in Conversation

Takeoka and Shimojima (2002, p. 189) suggest that conversations with older persons are often slow-paced and filled with repetitions, with the unwanted outcome of being "boring." Communication problems may arise not only because of the presence of hearing loss, but also because of older persons' alleged slowness to understand or stubbornness to accept new ideas. The researchers note that younger people, when conversing with older persons, sometimes adopt a "patronizing speech style." The patronizing style may include:

- Talking only about restricted topics
- Using directive speech
- Using childlike expressions
- Speaking very slowly
- Exaggerating their nonverbal signals
- Paraphrasing frequently
- Decreasing their grammatical complexity
- Talking about fewer topics

Compare this list with the list we have just reviewed about how conversations involving a person with hearing loss might differ from the norm. Note the similarities. Speech and hearing professionals may find that some of their younger adult patients are frustrated by how some people react to them during conversation.

through incidental listening. This person may have an even greater danger of not sharing "common ground." A communication partner might come to realize that grounding must be more deliberate and may have to state assumed information explicitly and/or state common ground information more than once.

FACILITATIVE COMMUNICATION STRATEGIES

In Chapter 5, we noted that four factors influence the speechreading task, the talker, the message, the environment, and the listener. In a communication strategies training program, patients learn to use facilitative strategies. **Facilitative strategies** are used to influence these four factors. Table 7-1 summarizes four types of facilitative communication strategies, each designed to influence each of these four factors. Figure 7-2 summarizes the process that persons might engage in when they experience difficulty in recognizing speech during conversation. The individual identifies the source of difficulty, implements a facilitative strategy, and determines whether the difficulty is resolved. If it is, then the conversation can continue. If it is not, the person might implement another strategy.

> **Facilitative strategies** include instructing the talker and structuring the listening environment, to enhance the listener's performance.

Strategies That Influence the Talker

Persons with hearing loss use **instructional strategies** to influence communication partners' speaking behaviors. A person asks the talker to change the delivery of the message, as in these examples:

> When implementing an **instructional strategy**, the listener asks the talker to change the delivery of the message.

Table 7-1. Facilitative and repair strategies.

Facilitative strategies may be used to influence:

- **Patient's speech recognition skills**
  Adaptive strategies: The individual with hearing loss implements relaxation techniques.
  Anticipatory strategies: The individual prepares for conversational interactions in advance by anticipating conversational content and potential listening difficulties.

- **Communication environment**
  Constructive strategies: A person structures the environment to optimize communication by minimizing background noise and ensuring a favorable view of the talker.

- **Communication partner**
  Instructional strategies: A person influences the communication partner's speaking behaviors by asking the partner to speak clearly, facing forward.

- **Message**
  Message-tailoring strategies: Individuals encourage communication partners to use short sentences and they employ closed-ended questions.
  Acknowledgment gesture: A person provides feedback to the communication partner by a nod or shake of the head.

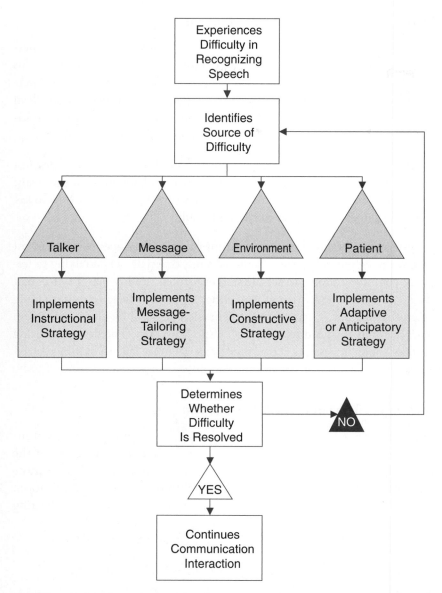

FIGURE 7-2. Process someone may follow when encountering a communication difficulty.

- "When you cover your mouth with your hand, I have a hard time speechreading you."
- "Could you face me please?"
- "Please slow down your talking. I understand more that way."

To use instructional strategies, persons must identify behaviors that impede their speech recognition efforts. Then they may instruct the communication partner about how to change the behavior.

Strategies That Influence the Message

Message-tailoring strategy is a way of phrasing one's remarks to constrain the response of a communication partner.

Message-tailoring strategies influence the way someone constructs a message. A person might ask, "Did you go swimming or biking last night?" This question sets the stage for one of two responses, *swimming* or *biking.* Alternatively the individual may not use a message-tailoring strategy, and instead ask, "What did you do last night?" which opens the floodgate for a multitude of answers and a greater likelihood of communication breakdown.

Metacommunication is communication about communication.

Using a message-tailoring strategy requires a kind of **metacommunication** skill. That is, not only must persons be able to think about what they want to say, but also they have to consider in their own minds how best to say something in order to effect the desired result.

An **acknowledgment gesture** may consist of a head nod or a head shake. It is often made in response to a remark from a frequent communication partner, who is familiar with the signaling system.

Another way to tailor a communication partner's messages is by means of an **acknowledgment gesture.** Some patients, especially when talking to frequent communication partners, learn to nod their heads when they feel that they have understood a remark and either shake their head or quit nodding when they do not. Their partner might then respond by clarifying the remark without the need to relinquish a speaking turn. The danger of using acknowledgment gestures is that they can sometimes lead to bluffing behaviors, a kind of maladaptive communication act that we will consider shortly.

Strategies That Influence the Environment

A **constructive strategy** is a tactic designed to optimize the listening environment for communication.

One uses a **constructive strategy** to enhance the communication environment. The success of constructive strategies hinges on the ability of the person to analyze the communication environment and to identify those elements that can be modified or exploited to optimize communication. Table 7-2 presents a list of constructive strategies that persons with hearing loss may use to optimize communication.

Strategies That Influence the Reception of a Message

Adaptive strategies are methods of counteracting maladaptive behaviors that stem from hearing loss.

Adaptive strategies serve to counteract maladaptive behaviors and include relaxation techniques and other means of dealing with emotions and negative behaviors that stem from hearing loss. For example, some persons with hearing loss feel anxious during a conversation with someone who is unfamiliar to them, and they worry about what they might miss or what their communication partners think of them. In these instances, they might have to take a deep breath, consciously relax, purposefully redirect their thoughts toward the present conversation, and attend to the talker's lip movements. This adaptive behavior not only can decrease anxiety, but also can enhance message recognition.

Table 7-2. Examples of constructive strategies that can be used to optimize the listening and speechreading task. This list might be reviewed with the person who has hearing loss, as well as with the person's frequent communication partners.

- If possible, ensure that the talker is well-lit so that you watch the talker's face.
- If the talker is far away, move closer.
- If background noise is present, try to either reduce the noise or move to a quieter setting. Turn down the television set or turn it off; close a door to eliminate unwanted noise; choose a quiet restaurant rather than a noisy one.
- Try to avoid rooms or auditoriums that have sound reverberation. You might request that a meeting be held in a room with good acoustics—typically, a room that has carpet, draperies, and minimal noise from air conditioners and radiators.
- Arrive early so that you can get favorable seating, near the talker.
- Eliminate visual distracters, such as a curtain flapping in an open window.
- Position yourself in relationship to the talker so as to minimize glare. For example, if the talker is standing before a sunlit window, you might ask that you be able to change places.

Maladaptive Strategies

Sometimes people who have hearing loss adopt **maladaptive strategies** to cope with their communication difficulties. These strategies include bluffing and pretending to understand, social withdrawal to avoid communication difficulties, dominating conversations so as to be aware of what is being talked about, and succumbing to feelings of anger, hostility, or self-pity. Some individuals become unduly anxious and tense, either as they anticipate an upcoming communication interaction (such as a meeting with their boss) or during the interaction itself, as problems in understanding begin to arise. It is well within the purview of a communication strategies training program to encourage alternative behaviors in lieu of maladaptive strategies.

A **maladaptive strategy** is an inappropriate behavioral mechanism for coping with the difficulties caused by hearing loss in a conversation; they sometimes yield short-term benefit but incur long-term costs.

An individual uses an **anticipatory strategy** to prepare for a communication interaction. These strategies include anticipating potential vocabulary and conversational content. For example, before a job interview, a person with hearing loss might study related information about the company, such as employee handbooks or news clippings. The individual might buy books about recruitment procedures and learn what kinds of questions are standard during interviews. Should the interviewer mention names of key employees, the person may thus recognize the names because they are already familiar. When the interviewer asks routine questions, they also may be

Anticipatory strategies are methods of preparing for a communication interaction.

Ready? Set? Go!

People with hearing loss can implement anticipatory strategies prior to a communication interaction and enhance their probability of recognizing spoken messages. Examples of anticipatory strategies that might be reviewed with a patient are listed below:

- Obtain a synopsis of a play before going to see it. Knowing the plot may help you follow the dialogue that occurs between the play's characters.
- Learn the names of key players and products before you go on a job interview. These words will then likely be more recognizable on the talker's face. Also know how job interviews are structured, from beginning, to middle, to end. This information will help you anticipate what may be said during each segment.
- Keep abreast of current events and movies. If these topics arise during group conversations, you will be better able to fill in the blanks when you miss words here and there.
- Read the textbook before a subject is covered in class (good advice for any student). Knowing the subject matter in advance will help you to follow it in class.

Aside from enhancing actual speech recognition, there may be psychological advantages to using anticipatory strategies. A person with hearing loss might feel more comfortable during an interaction if the person has practiced speechreading the vocabulary that might occur and if the person has obtained some background information. Moreover, simply having a definitive course of action may make individuals feel more in charge of their communication interactions.

easier to recognize because the person has the appropriate framework in which to listen. More global preparatory work may include considering what vocabulary is likely to occur (e.g., *popcorn* at a movie theater concession stand) and then practice speechreading that vocabulary with a partner. Someone can anticipate spoken remarks by attending to situational cues (e.g., talking with a ticket seller at a movie theater). Predictions can be made on the basis of "knowledge of a partner's typical conversational style (e.g., use of colloquialisms or gestures); common conversational sequences (e.g., as in greeting rituals); and expected responses to utterances of particular types (e.g., to choice questions)" (Erber, 1996, p. 42).

There are mixed findings about the effectiveness of anticipatory strategies. One study showed that anticipatory strategies are not effective in enhancing speech recognition when a person is about to enter into a familiar communication situation, as when preparing for an appointment with a physician or a visit to a bank or a gas station (Tye-Murray, 1992e). However, when the situation is unfamiliar, use of anticipatory strategies appears to be effective in preparing individuals to recognize speech (Rubinstein, Cherry, Hecht, & Idler, 2000). For instance, if people learn the plot of a theretofore unfamiliar story, they will later recognize sentences about the story better than if they had not reviewed it.

REPAIR STRATEGIES

Communication strategies training also may teach patients to use **repair strategies** to repair **communication breakdowns**. After signaling the occurrence of a communication breakdown, people can request information by using one of many possible **receptive repair strategies** (Table 7-3). The word *receptive* indicates that the repair strategy is used to rectify a communication breakdown when the recipient of a message (in this case, a person with hearing loss) does not recognize the sender's (talker's) message. Examples include: "Could you say that again?" (the *repeat repair strategy*), "Who is going to give you a ride?" (the *request for information repair strategy*), and "I missed that completely; what are you talking about?" (the *key word repair strategy*). An individual also might ask for more information (the *elaborate repair strategy*): "Tell me more; I didn't catch that."

Repair strategies are tactics implemented by a participant in a conversation to rectify a breakdown in communication.

A **communication breakdown** occurs when one communication partner does not recognize another's message.

A **receptive repair strategy** is a tactic used by an individual when he or she has not understood a message.

Table 7-3. Repair strategies that can be used to repair communication breakdowns.

Specific repair strategies request the communication partner to:
- Repeat all or part of message: *Can you say that last part again, please?*
- Rephrase the message: *Please say that in a different way, I didn't catch what you said.*
- Elaborate the message: *Tell me more.*
- Simplify the message: *I didn't hear you properly. Can you try that again with fewer words?*
- Indicate the topic of conversation: *I'm not sure I'm following you. You're talking about . . . ?*
- Confirm the message: *You said we're going on Tuesday, right?*
- Provide feedback: *I got the part about Janice. What will she be doing this afternoon?*
- Write
- Fingerspell (if both parties know the manual alphabet) or spell

Nonspecific repair strategies ask:
- *What?*
- *Huh?*
- *Pardon?*

Depending on how well individuals know their communication partners, they might feel comfortable in asking them to write, to use gestures and hand signals, or to spell important topic words. Selection of a particular repair strategy may hinge on a variety of factors, including how useful a particular strategy has been in the past, how much of the message was understood, and an assessment of how well a communication partner might follow the instructions.

Stages of Communication Breakdown

Figure 7-3 suggests at least three stages are involved in repairing a communication breakdown. First, the breakdown must be detected, then one of the communication partners chooses a course of action, and then the action is implemented. When communication breakdowns occur, persons with hearing loss might detect immediately that they did not recognize the message. In such cases, an individual might alert the partner and seek repair. "Hold on," the person might say, "I missed that." It sometimes happens that an individual does not realize a breakdown has occurred until much later in the conversation, as in the following example:

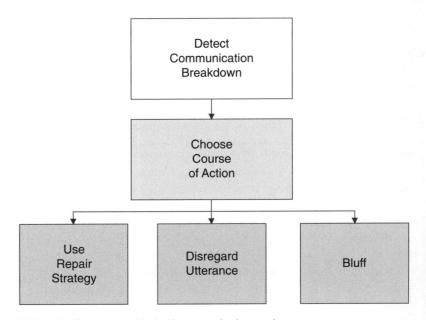

FIGURE 7-3. Stages associated with communication repair.

Professor:	(who has a hearing loss) What was your last assignment?
Film student:	I did a 10-minute educational film on Arctic moss.
Professor:	(thinking the film student said Arctic *moths*) Oh, you must have had to do that over the summer then.
Film student:	Believe it or not, some species live embedded in ice crystals, so we did some shots in early November.
Professor:	What do they do, live in caverns?
Film student:	Huh?
Professor:	(beginning to wonder whether he has missed something) Live in caverns?
Film student:	Well, I guess there's some moss in caverns up there, but I've never seen any caves.
Professor:	*Moss?* [blushing] Oh, I thought we were talking about *moths!*

As the professor sensed an incongruence between the film student's and his own remarks, he gradually realized that he misunderstood an utterance earlier on in the conversation. This is a prime example of not realizing that a breakdown has occurred at its onset.

Often the communication partner is the first to recognize that a communication breakdown has occurred, as in this example:

Classmate:	So the midterm exam is next Friday?
James:	I'm going to be working on my report on Friday.
Classmate:	No, I'm *asking* you if the exam is on Friday.

In this example, the classmate intended her statement to be a yes–no question. Although it is unclear whether James, who has a hearing loss, understood the remark and misconstrued its intention or whether he simply did not understand it, the classmate recognized that a communication breakdown occurred and initiated a repair.

Once a misunderstanding becomes apparent, an individual might alert the communication partner and provide instruction about how to repair it. For instance, he or she may ask about the topic of conversation (e.g., "What are you talking about?"). This is actually a form of metacommunication between two people because it entails discussion of a communication act.

Usually, breakdowns are repaired with the use of one or two repair strategies, as in this interchange when a request for a partial repetition is made:

Coworker: I'll get a copy of the fax to you tomorrow.

**Person with
hearing loss:** A copy of what tomorrow?

Coworker: The fax. The fax sent by Mr. Roberts.

There are occasions when several exchanges are required. In the worst of circumstances, these interchanges can be awkward for all parties involved in the conversation, as in the following example in which a husband and wife (who recently received a cochlear implant) talked while seated in a speech and hearing test room:

Husband: Laura is going to catch the train on Tuesday.

Wife: (uses a *nonspecific repair strategy and the feedback repair strategy*) "What? I didn't catch any of that."

Husband: I said, Laura is going to catch the train on Tuesday.

Wife: (uses the *feedback repair strategy*) No, none of it.

Husband: Laura . . .

Wife: (uses the *feedback repair strategy*) Something about more?

Husband: No, watch me. Laura is going to get the train.

Wife: (uses the *feedback repair strategy*) Oh, yeah. I got 'train.'

Husband: Yes, a train. Laura is . . .

Wife: (uses the *spelling repair strategy*) (shaking her head) Nope, nope, none of it. Spell it.

Husband: (spelling) L-A-U-R-A.

Wife: (uses the *feedback repair strategy*) Oh Laura! What about Laura and the train?

An **extended repair** occurs when many repair strategies are needed to mend a communication breakdown.

At this point, several repair strategies have been implemented and the message is still not conveyed. This is an example of an **extended repair**. It would be easy for both participants in the conversation to abandon repair, and say, "Never mind, it's not that important." Indeed, in situations such as this, that is often exactly what happens.

Sometimes when someone uses a repair strategy, the topic of conversation shifts, as indicated in Figure 7-4. Ideally, people use repair strategies in such a way that they do not cause the conversation to stagnate or veer off into a different direction. For example, a student with a hearing loss, Janet, did not use a repair strategy effectively in the following exchange:

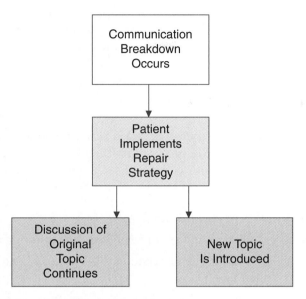

FIGURE 7-4. Possible effects of using a repair strategy.

Cynthia: I got my grades in the mail last Saturday.

Janet: Grapes? Why are you getting grapes in the mail?

Cynthia: No, I said *grades*, not *grapes*.

Janet: Oh, I know you make wine, so I thought you had joined some kind of mail-order program. By the way, when am I going to get my bottle?

The problem with this interchange is that the topic of conversation changed inappropriately (from grades to a promised bottle of wine) as a result of the repair strategy used. A seemingly more cooperative and congenial way to repair this communication breakdown is as follows:

Cynthia: I got my grades in the mail last Saturday.

Janet: Grapes?

Cynthia: No, I said *grades*.

Janet: Oh, you got your grades in the mail. How did you do?

In this latter version, Janet asked for confirmation and then steered the conversation back on track.

Sometimes patients bluff and pretend to understand following a communication breakdown, nodding and smiling in agreement with what they do not know. The consequences of **bluffing** can be negative. The person may

Bluffing is pretending to understand an utterance and behaving in a way that suggests that understanding occurred, even if little or none of the message was recognized.

appear insensitive, uninterested, dull, or inattentive. He or she may begin to feel powerless to manage communication difficulties. When bluffing is used excessively, conversation may leave the person feeling like a failure or angry at him- or herself.

Bluffing

The following conversation, which occurred between two women who had just met, presents an instance in which bluffing led to the appearance of insensitivity. Woman 2 has just said that she is about to take a trip. Woman 1 has a hearing loss:

Woman 1: Where are you going?

Woman 2: To Portland to see my daughter. She is having a baby.

Woman 1: (nodding; she understood the word *baby*, but not much else) I see.

Woman 2: She has been bedridden for several weeks because she has diabetes and high blood pressure, and now the doctor says they are going to have to induce or the baby you know might be in trouble if it goes much longer than it's been going, even though it will be 4 weeks premature which we are pretty worried about especially since it's her first.

Woman 1: (lost by the length and convoluted syntax of her partner's utterance, and still not understanding much) Oh, how nice.

Woman 2: No, not really, this is pretty serious.

Inadvertently, Woman 1 has created an unfavorable impression because she bluffed and pretended to understand instead of repairing the communication breakdown.

One reason that someone may bluff is because use of a repair strategy may require a person to acknowledge a hearing loss. For instance, an individual might say, "Can you say that again please?" and the communication partner might respond, "What's the matter?" For some people, it is difficult to acknowledge, "I have hearing loss, and I can't always catch all that is said to me."

Social stigma is having a condition that is devalued because it deviates from a societal norm and results in a negative status being placed upon a person or group of persons.

Self-stigma occurs when a person stigmatizes one's own condition by feelings of shame and embarrassment, and develops a spoiled self-identity by virtue of having a shortcoming or disability.

Many persons are reluctant to admit a hearing loss, in part because of personal vanity and perceived **social stigma** and/or **self-stigma** (Blood, Blood, & Danhauer, 1978; Danhauer, Johnson, Kasten, & Brimacombe, 1985; Hétu, Riverin, Getty, Lalande, & St-Cyr, 1990). Unfortunately, many people have stereotypical views of persons with hearing loss. Some see them as difficult to communicate with or as deserving pity. For many people, revealing

I'll Never Tell

The following summary was included in a report about the communication problems experienced by inpatients at a hospital. This section dealt with reluctance to admit a hearing loss:

Patients who conceal their hearing loss do so for a variety of reasons, but the most common one is self-consciousness. Some go to great lengths to conceal their disability. Some are very skillful at this concealment, not appreciating how dysfunctional it is. Female patients often adopt hairstyles that cover their hearing aids. One patient admitted that she disliked wearing a hearing aid, because her hair was no longer thick enough to cover it. Many hearing-impaired people pretend to understand what is being said, rather than admit to their difficulties. This can be very misleading and create many problems. One patient said: "My reticence to make my hearing loss known made me the victim of my own vanity." A patient who finally decided to admit to his problem was agreeably surprised that both the doctors and nurses were helpful and understanding. In some cases patients' deceptions were unexpectedly exposed. (Hines, 2000, p. 35)

a hearing loss to someone who does not know them is a daunting challenge and, hence, they may be reluctant to use repair strategies. Hallberg (1996) suggests that the driving force for all coping strategies, including bluffing and pretending to understand, lies in an individual's efforts to maintain a positive and "I am normal" self-image and to avoid being considered as deviant or deficient by others. Acknowledging a hearing loss, and putting a spotlight on the loss by signaling communication breakdowns and using repair strategies, may result in a spoiled self-identity. These behaviors may also lead others to view the person with hearing loss as an undesirable social deviation from a normal state, a situation that most people would like to avoid. In addition, Hallberg suggests that the reluctance to admit a hearing loss might stem from self-deception or a distortion of reality. There may be a discrepancy between a person's desired self-image and actual circumstances, and the self-deception protects the self-image and helps the individual maintain a positive or normal self-image in the face of hearing loss.

Another reason why people may bluff relates to a desire to be cooperative and agreeable. Some people are unwilling to use repair strategies and bluff because they feel guilty and embarrassed about introducing difficulties into a conversation. Typically, when we converse, we engage in a cooperative enterprise as we try to ensure that a conversation is as pleasant and rewarding an experience for our communication partner(s) as it is for ourselves. If someone frequently halts the conversation for clarification, it may become less pleasant and less rewarding (Figure 7-5), as in the following exchange:

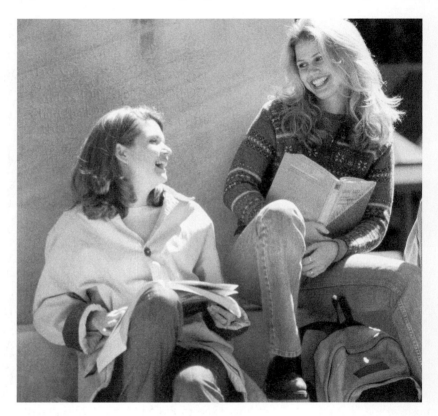

FIGURE 7-5. Spirit of cooperation during conversation. When we engage in a conversation, we usually try to be cooperative and help make the conversation a pleasurable or meaningful experience for all participants.

Patrick:	I am going on spring break next week.
Richard:	Huh?
Patrick:	I said *spring break.*
Richard:	Oh.
Patrick:	We are driving to Florida in Jason's parents' car.
Richard:	Huh?
Patrick:	We are driving to Florida in Jason's parents' car.
Richard:	Oh.
Mary:	I wish I were going somewhere.

Richard:	Huh?
Mary:	I wish I were going somewhere.
Richard:	Yeah, me too.

As the interchange unfolds, the spontaneity of the conversation becomes stifled by the continual requests for clarification. Maintaining continued conversation will prove laborious and effortful for all involved. It is for such reasons that many persons with hearing loss opt to bluff, particularly when talking to people they do not know well.

While bluffing is generally not a good idea, some patients believe that bluffing is sometimes acceptable, as when they are in a group situation or when they are tired of paying attention. Patients may decide to bluff because they think that if they wait a moment, the meaning of an utterance will register with them or subsequent remarks will clarify what was missed. The challenge, of course, is to know when bluffing is appropriate and when it is not (Wyant, 2007).

Expressive Repair Strategies

In addition to using receptive repair strategies, many children who have hearing loss need to use expressive repair strategies. **Expressive repair strategies** are used to rectify a communication breakdown that occurs because the person with hearing loss (the sender) produces an unintelligible utterance, and the communication partner (the receiver) is unable to recognize it.

Many children who have hearing loss have limited language skills or poor articulation. As a result, their communication partners often may not recognize their spoken messages. They can learn how to cope with these kinds of communication breakdowns by using expressive repair strategies. Expressive repair strategies include repeating their original message using their best speech (e.g., they might slow down their speaking rate and emphasize important key words), breaking their longer sentences into shorter sentences, using another communication modality such as writing or mime, and using supplemental hand gestures, such as pointing.

Expressive repair strategies are used when the sender produces an unintelligible utterance and the communication partner cannot understand it.

RESEARCH RELATED TO REPAIR STRATEGY USAGE AND COMMUNICATION BREAKDOWNS

Although communication breakdowns may occur in any conversation for any variety of reasons, certain conditions increase the likelihood of their occurrence. As noted earlier, environmental conditions, message content, and speaking behaviors all influence how well a person with hearing loss recognizes a spoken message. A study by Caissie (2001) suggests that the dynamic nature of the conversation also affects when communication breakdowns are most likely to occur. For instance, if two people are engaged in a conversation, and they limit themselves to talking about a single topic, they are less likely to experience communication breakdowns than if they jump from one topic to the next. As the two individuals exchange remarks on their chosen topic, there is more contextual information available to resolve potential misunderstandings.

Topic Shading

Abruptly shifting from one topic to another is more likely to cause communication difficulties than discussing only one topic. Interestingly, even more disruptive than topic changing is topic shading. **Topic shading** happens when a new topic is introduced, but is a direct offshoot of something that was just being discussed, as in the following example:

> **Topic shading** occurs when a new emphasis is derived from an ongoing topic of conversation such that the topic remains the same but the relevant details shift.

Janice:	(who has hearing loss) I'm going to Chicago tomorrow.
Robert:	Are you driving or flying?
Janice:	Flying.
Robert:	I've got to get my tickets for my New York trip.
Janice:	Huh?

In this example, the two participants are still talking about traveling when the topic shifts, but instead of talking about Janice's trip they are now talking about Robert's need to purchase airline tickets. It may be that when an entirely new topic is introduced, the person with hearing loss can contribute a relevant comment, even if she or he has not understood every word. For example, if instead of mentioning his airline tickets, Robert had said, "What are you doing tonight?" Janice might have caught the general gist of his message and might have responded with an appropriate response (e.g., "Not much."). When topics shift subtlety, individuals may request clarification to ensure they are following the direction the conversation is veering toward (Caissie, 2001).

Frequency of Bluffing

Hétu et al. (1987) studied workers with occupational hearing loss. They found that 67% of the respondents when at a family gathering, a party, or a social meeting were likely to *pretend to be understanding while keeping silent* (see also Stephens, Jaworski, Lewis, & Alsan, 1999); that is, they engaged in bluffing.

Use of Nonspecific Repair Strategies

Research suggests that most individuals are more likely to ask their communication partners to repeat a message following a communication breakdown than to simplify it, restructure it, or elaborate (Caissie & Gibson, 1997; Hétu, Lalande, & Getty, 1987; Tye-Murray et al., 1993; Tye-Murray, Purdy, Woodworth, & Tyler, 1990; Tye-Murray & Witt, 1996). Moreover, their most common repair tactic is to say, "What?," "Huh?," or "Pardon?" This kind of repair strategy (i.e., what-huh-pardon) is called a **nonspecific** as opposed to a **specific repair strategy**. When using a specific repair strategy, the person with hearing loss often provides explicit instruction to the communication partner about how to repair the breakdown.

Consequences of Using Repair Strategies

When a person uses a repair strategy, how is a communication partner likely to respond? One of the most noteworthy findings pertains to the use of the repeat repair strategy and nonspecific repair strategies. When these are used following a communication breakdown, the communication partners typically repeat the original message verbatim (Caissie & Gibson, 1997; Tye-Murray, Witt, Schum, & Sobaski, 1995). Thus, if someone says "Huh?" there is a high probability that the communication partner will repeat exactly what he or she has just said.

Additional research suggests that someone is more likely to understand a message following a communication breakdown if the communication partner restructures it rather than simply repeats it (Gagné & Wyllie, 1989), especially if the talker already has repeated the message one time and the person with hearing loss still has not recognized it. For instance, someone says, "I bought a new car," and a person responds, "Huh?" Then the first communication partner repeats, "I bought a new car." A third verbatim repetition may be less helpful to a person with hearing loss than if the communication partner had rephrased the message as, "I bought a Buick." New words, especially the more visible word *Buick* as opposed to *car,* may be easier for the patient to recognize audiovisually. Caissie and Gibson (1997) found that the most effective repair of communication breakdowns occurred when communication partners either paraphrased or confirmed the message. Repeating the message one time was almost equally effective. The least effective strategies appeared to be elaboration.

There may be an additional drawback to using nonspecific repair strategies, but there may also be some positive aspects of doing so, too. When persons often say "What?" or "Huh?" during a conversation to rectify communication breakdowns, their communication partners are more likely to perceive

Nonspecific repairs simply indicate a lack of understanding.

Specific repairs provide explicit instructions to the communication partner about how to repair the breakdown.

them unfavorably and to enjoy the interaction less (Gagné, Stelmacovich, & Yovetich, 1991; Tye-Murray, Witt, Schum, & Sobaski, 1995). In the experimental paradigm that was used in these experiments, audiovisual recordings were made of spontaneous conversations between two people, one of whom had a real or simulated hearing loss. The recordings were then shown to a team of judges who were asked to rate each person with hearing loss on a personality 6-point rating scale (e.g., *this person is competent-incompetent*). The judges also rated them on a scale of emotional responses, using a second 6-point rating scale (e.g., *this person makes me feel composed-irritated*). When individuals used nonspecific instead of specific repair strategies, they were rated more unfavorably, and they elicited more unfavorable reactions from the judges, perhaps because such use placed the onus of repair on the communication partner.

Despite the drawbacks, there may be some positive outcomes of using nonspecific repair strategies in some contexts. First, communication breakdowns that occur during spontaneous conversation between adults in which one partner has a hearing loss often are resolved after the use of a single repair strategy, even if it is a nonspecific strategy (Lind, 2006; Tye-Murray, Witt, Schum, & Sobaski, 1995). These data suggest that nonspecific repair strategies can be effective. Second, a nonspecific repair strategy is minimally disruptive to the flow of ongoing conversation. When an individual asks, "Huh?" he or she assumes the speaking floor briefly, and the communication partner can easily continue a speaking turn. However, when someone uses other repair strategies such as, "I missed that, can you tell me what you are talking about?" and uses them frequently, a conversation can become stilted and less fluent. By using a nonspecific repair strategy, the individual takes a phantom speaking turn and may appear more cooperative in the conversational interchange. Third, the use of nonspecific repair strategies might facilitate the grounding process, wherein one partner presents a bit of information and the other partner provides an acknowledgment (in such instances, the nonspecific repair strategy assumes the same purpose as an acknowledgment gesture). The nonspecific repair strategy might serve to acknowledge that information was not conveyed successfully and thereby establish a lack of common ground. Finally, a nonspecific repair strategy might indicate the location of a problem. Lind (2006) examined the frequency and effectiveness of repair strategies that occurred during an approximately 20-minute conversation between a cochlear implant user and his wife and found that nonspecific repairs were effective in pinpointing the location of difficulty. The husband sometimes said "Huh?" in the middle of his wife's utterance. Even though he did not identify the source of the breakdown, indicating the time of occurrence led to successful repair.

Mentioning a Hearing Loss

One investigation examined what happened when adults who use cochlear implants talked with someone they did not know, and who did not know about the hearing loss (Tye-Murray & Witt, 1996). In this investigation, one patient was seated at a table with someone who had normal hearing. The normally hearing person was told that he or she was participating in a study about conversation, but did not know that his or her communication partner had a hearing loss. Each dyad tested in the experiment talked for 10 minutes. The conversations were videotaped and later analyzed. Analyses showed that only 44% of the patients revealed their hearing losses, even though most experienced many communication breakdowns during the course of the 10-minute conversation. What is perhaps most interesting is what happened when a patient did reveal a loss. Once the patient did so, the conversation began to center around the topic of hearing loss and difficulties associated with hearing loss, rather than other shared topics of interest. This change may be yet another reason why people are reluctant to reveal a hearing loss—they do not want the loss to become the focus of discussion.

Who Is Likely to Use Repair Strategies

Some individuals are more likely than others to use a repair strategy than to say nothing following a communication breakdown. Individuals who use repair strategies also are less likely to feel frustrated with their speechreading skills and less likely to avoid social interactions than individuals who say nothing. Persons who are least likely to use communication strategies tend to share certain characteristics (Tye-Murray et al., 1993; Tye-Murray, Purdy, & Woodworth, 1992):

- They have attained lower levels of education.
- They have experienced a sudden hearing loss.
- They receive minimal benefit from their listening devices.

You Say, I Say

When persons with hearing loss implement a repair strategy, they invite a response from their communication partners, thereby establishing a linked speaking turn. Schegloff and Sacks (1973) call linked speaking turns **adjacency pairs**. Examples of adjacency pairs include question–answer (e.g., "Who asked?"—"Bob asked."), greeting–reciprocation (e.g., "Hey there."—"Hi."), and summons–acknowledgment

continues

Adjacency pairs are linked speaking turns.

You Say, I Say, *continued*

combinations (e.g., "Can you come over here?"—"Sure."). Particular repair strategy–response adjacency pairs often emerge when a person with hearing loss interacts with a person who has normal hearing. These include (see Tye-Murray & Witt, 1996, p. 467):

1. *Nonspecific repair strategy–message repetition response.* When an individual with hearing loss implements a nonspecific repair strategy following a communication breakdown, the communication partner typically repeats the original message.
2. *Request for information repair strategy–provide information response.* When an individual requests specific information, the communication partner typically provides it.
3. *Confirmation repair strategy–feedback response.* When an individual restates the message content, the communication partner usually either confirms or corrects the statement.

Research with Children

Some research has concerned children's use of specific kinds of repair strategies and communication breakdown management. Some findings suggest that children who are hard of hearing and deaf tend to provide nonlinguistic information to clarify their spoken messages (e.g., Ciocci & Baran, 1998; Givens & Greenfeld, 1982) or to repeat the message (Most, 2002, 2003). For instance, Baylock, Scudder, and Wynne (1995) reported that children were most likely to physically show their communication partner what was needed or wanted after the partner said, "What?" or "I don't understand." When children do not recognize their communication partners' messages, they more often rely on nonlinguistic responses when seeking clarification than do children with normal hearing; for instance, they might signal a misunderstanding by a confused look or a shoulder shrug.

One investigation examined the conversations of 181 children who use cochlear implants and compared their performance to 24 children who have normal hearing, using both objective and subjective measuring procedures (Tye-Murray, 2003). The children engaged in conversations with a clinician, using an aural/oral mode of communication. Audio-videotapes of the conversations were analyzed to yield the following measures: percentage of time the child and clinician spent trying to repair a breakdown in communication, percentage of time the two spent sitting in silence, and the ratio between the amount of time the child spoke and the amount of time the clinician spoke (as we see in the next chapter, these measures are related to a construct called *conversational fluency*). The cochlear implant users spent significantly more time in communication breakdown and in silence than did the children with normal hearing. Speech intelligibility and receptive language were the best predictors of communication breakdown, with children who had better speech and language skills experiencing fewer and shorter breakdowns in communication. These results underscore the importance of providing explicit instruction to manage communication difficulties because even children who have state-of-the-art listening technology still experience more difficulties than children who have normal hearing.

CONVERSATIONAL STYLES AND BEHAVIORS

Many communication strategies training curricula include materials that are aimed at developing desirable conversational styles and conversational behaviors. Although there are no right and wrong ways per se of engaging in conversation, and what is appropriate will vary with the situation, some conversational styles and behaviors are nonetheless more effective when communication is hampered by the presence of hearing loss than are other styles and behaviors.

Conversational Styles

Conversational style refers to the set of behaviors and methods that a person implements to relay and receive information during communication activities. Adults who have significant hearing impairment, and even children and teenagers, may exhibit at least four kinds of conversational styles: (a) passive, (b) aggressive, (c) passive-aggressive, and (d) assertive.

A person with a **passive conversational style** is someone who wants to appear cooperative at all costs and avoid misunderstandings and conflict. This style entails little risk and is very safe in the short term, but it can be counterproductive in the long term. Someone who engages in a passive conversational style often does the following:

A person with a **passive conversational style** tends to withdraw from conversations and social interactions rather than attempt to repair conversations.

- Withdraws from conversation.
- Frequently bluffs and pretends to recognize utterances.
- Speaks with a quiet tone and uses little eye contact; the facial expression may be sheepish or expressionless in response to a message.
- Avoids social interactions and group gatherings in order to avoid communication difficulties.

Someone who sits at the bridge table, smiling and quietly nodding, is probably someone who can be characterized as having a passive conversational style. The person gains little by being in the game. The individual may begin to feel frustration, victimization, resentment, and helplessness. After having been passive for too long, the person might display a burst of anger. This person may have a difficult time recognizing his or her own communication needs and knowing how to get them met more effectively.

Persons with an **aggressive conversational style** represent the opposite extreme of persons with a passive conversational style. They may protect their rights at the expense of others and feel a need to come out "on top" of a conversation at all costs. They may exhibit some of the following characteristics during conversation:

A person with an **aggressive conversational style** may blame others for misunderstandings.

- Hostility, regardless of the message, and belligerence and a bad attitude
- Shouting or "soapbox" speech
- Excessive or expansive body gestures
- An intimidating demeanor, such as directing an intense stare at the talker and/or leaning into the talker or standing stiffly erect

The person may purposely or inadvertently embarrass, hurt, or anger his or her communication partners and blame others for communication difficulties. "Quit mumbling, and try to help me out!" someone may demand, or, "You never told me that!" The first utterance is a tacit insult (i.e., it implies, "You could help me out but you have chosen not to."), whereas the second is an accusation ("It's not that I didn't hear you, it's that you never told me in the first place!"). These kinds of utterances have the potential to alienate communication partners and may result in the person with hearing loss being ineffective and even avoided.

A **passive-aggressive conversational style** is one in which aggression is expressed in indirect ways.

Some individuals with hearing loss adopt a **passive-aggressive conversational style**, which incorporates elements of both a passive and aggressive style. They may forfeit their right to understand a message initially and then manipulate the conversation or take vengeance later. The goal is to avoid communication breakdowns and communication difficulties and then make the communication partner sorry that they occurred and/or that they were not rectified. The person might say, "I can't understand what you're saying but I realize that it's probably not important." Sometimes the person might act passively to a person's face and then aggressively later. "Yes, yes," an older man might say to a doctor. He then may complain bitterly to his adult daughter later that the doctor was insensitive to his hearing loss and that he will not be returning for follow-up visits. The person with an passive-aggressive communication style may:

- Use sarcasm.
- Behave passively to someone's face and then aggressively when they are gone.
- Exhibit sullenness, stubbornness, or procrastination.

During communication strategies training, patients often are encouraged to minimize their use of passive, aggressive, and passive-aggressive conversational styles and instead implement an assertive style. The goals of the assertive conversationalist are to communicate effectively and to find solutions that minimize or prevent communication breakdowns. Persons who adopt an **assertive conversational style** usually follow these guidelines during conversation. They:

A person who adopts an **assertive conversational style** takes responsibility for managing communication difficulties in a way that is considerate of communication partners.

- Respect the rights of their communication partners, while honestly and openly expressing their own needs and emotions.
- Take responsibility for managing communication difficulties, but do so in a way that is considerate of their communication partners.
- Use eye contact when speaking with a person and have facial expressions appropriate to the message.
- Use body language that conveys receptiveness and openness.
- Acknowledge their communication partner's efforts to promote good communication when appropriate.

"Let's get a seat away from the stereo speaker," an assertive person may suggest, "and then you won't have to repeat everything you say." This remark is courteous and provides direct explanation of how to remedy a communication problem.

These four types of conversational styles (passive, aggressive, passive-aggressive, and assertive) may be reviewed in a communication strategies training program. One goal is to make patients aware of their communication styles so that they can learn to communicate more effectively and so that they can recognize ineffective communication behaviors in others. Through practice and hard work, they can develop assertive ways of rectifying their communication problems. They can also learn how to respond effectively to their communication partners when they implement passive or aggressive behaviors.

Sometimes, the aural rehabilitation plan includes **psychosocial therapy** (e.g., Hogan, 2001). One of the primary goals of this type of intervention is to encourage assertive behaviors. Participants explore the psychological and

Psychosocial therapy challenges erroneous assumptions and develops self-image.

social ramifications of hearing loss and some of the underlying reasons why they may not engage in assertive behaviors. For instance, some people who behave passively may do so because they feel they burden other people when they ask for assistance. These underlying assumptions are challenged during psychosocial therapy.

Communication Behaviors

Figure 7-6 presents three constellations of behaviors that complement the model of conversational styles just reviewed. The model consists of three circles that are labeled interactive, noninteractive, and dominating.

Interactive behavior is the use of cooperative conversational tactics, consistent with an assertive conversational style.

Persons who fall within the **interactive behavior** circle use cooperative conversational tactics, which are consistent with an assertive conversational style. These individuals share responsibility with their communication partners for advancing a topic of conversation and selecting topics of conversation. They do not dominate discussion, and they show interest in what their communication partners say and attempt to respond appropriately to their remarks.

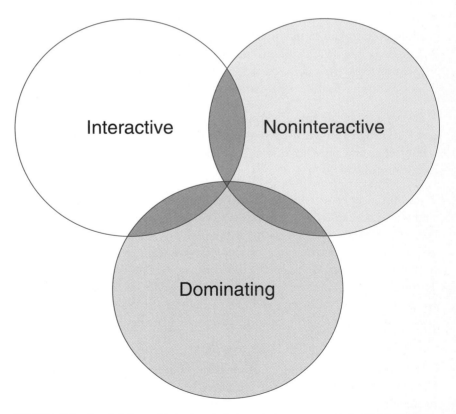

FIGURE 7-6. Constellations of behaviors that characterize some persons with hearing loss.

Persons who fit the **noninteractive behavior** constellation often can be characterized as having a passive conversational style. They may bluff following a communication breakdown. They may not contribute much to the development of a conversation topic, and they may not participate in selecting a topic to talk about. They also may not respond to turn-taking signals. For instance, a communication partner may say, "So . . . you know . . . hmmm," hoping that the person with hearing loss will contribute a remark. The following interchange illustrates a noninteractive conversational style (exhibited by Rose, who has a hearing loss):

Marie:	I saw a great movie last night.
Rose:	Oh.
Marie:	It was on the old-movies channel on cable.
Rose:	Hmmm.
Marie:	It had Fred Astaire and Ginger Rogers, lots of dancing and, you know, that kind of old-movie stuff . . .
Rose:	(nods)
Marie:	I just love that . . .
Rose:	(nods)
Marie:	I guess it takes me back to when I was going to the movies as a kid.

In this interchange, Rose does not express interest in Marie's remarks and does not share in advancing the topic. Marie begins to talk more in order to fill in the silences.

A noninteractive conversational style often yields unfavorable consequences. In a series of interviews with adults who have hearing loss, Cowie and Douglas-Cowie (1992) were told by one participant, "There are many occasions when I would like to ask questions, but in case I don't hear the answer I just don't do it. I think that probably gives the impression that I'm not interested, which isn't the case, it's just to save embarrassment" (p. 269). An individual's withdrawal can elicit negative reactions from communication partners and create an internal source of stress for oneself.

There is some evidence that two characteristically passive behaviors, avoidance and pretending to understand, are commonly used by persons who have hearing loss. Stephens et al. (1999) provided a questionnaire to 100 consecutive patients attending an audiological rehabilitation clinic in Cardiff, Wales. The patients were asked how often they exhibited certain behaviors in 11 different communication interactions. The most commonly cited behavior (in addition to asking people to repeat a

Noninteractive behavior is characteristic of a passive behavioral style and is one in which the individual does little to advance the course of the conversation.

misunderstood message) was *avoidance,* defined as "deliberately avoiding conversations with other people in certain circumstances to avoid the embarrassment of having to ask them to repeat what they say." Another commonly cited behavior was *pretend,* defined as "pretending they are hearing even when they don't, to avoid asking people to repeat themselves."

Dominating conversational behaviors are characteristic of an aggressive conversational style and may include interrupting, taking long speaking turns, and dominating the topic of conversation.

The final constellation in Figure 7-6 denotes a constellation of **dominating conversational behaviors**, which are characteristic of an aggressive conversational style. Persons who fall into this circle may take extended speaking turns, interrupt, and use abrupt topic changes. They may try to dominate the conversation, in order to always be aware of what is being talked about. Sometimes they will avoid asking questions so that they do not have to give up the speaking floor to hear the answers. Here is an excerpt from one conversation in which Deidre, an older woman with hearing loss, was conversing with her friend's daughter, Carrie:

> **Deidre:**   Sharon says you are going on vacation.
>
> **Carrie:**   Yes, I am flying with my brother to . . .
>
> **Deidre:**   (interrupting) Oh, I went on a plane once, to see my brother in South Carolina. He has a house down there, one he built himself on a lake.

With one remark, the two are suddenly talking about Deidre's plane trip and her brother rather than Carrie's upcoming travels.

As is the case with a passive conversational style, a dominating conversational style also may have undesired effects. One participant in the interviews conducted by Cowie and Douglas-Cowie (1992) reported, "I have to dominate the meeting, I make myself the artificial center of attention so that people will just speak to me . . . instead of speaking to the chairman they would be speaking to me" (p. 269). One can surmise that colleagues (or at least the chairman) might react unfavorably to such a dominating conversational style.

In the model illustrated in Figure 7-6, the three circles overlap for two reasons. First, an individual usually demonstrates behaviors that are characteristic of more than one constellation. An individual's use of conversational behaviors may vary during a conversation, as the person becomes more comfortable or the dynamics of the interchange are established. Behavior may vary as a function of the familiarity of the communication partner too, as well as the circumstances in which the conversation is occurring. For instance, someone who typically exhibits dominating communication behaviors may exhibit interactive behaviors when trying to talk his or her way out of a speeding ticket with a policeman. The second reason for the overlap is that some people, such as those who have a passive-aggressive conversational style, might demonstrate communication behaviors that appear on a superficial level to be interactive but at a deeper level are actually noninteractive or dominating.

CASE STUDY

A Couple Conversing

In the case study reported by Lind et al. (2006), a 55-year-old cochlear implant user spoke with his wife of 33 years for 23 minutes in an unstructured conversation. They sat in a quiet, well-lit room and spoke face-to-face about any topic they chose to discuss. Despite the optimal communication conditions and their familiarity with one another, they experienced 47 communication breakdowns. The repair activity or repair sequences occupied all or part of 67.7% of their conversational turns. They initiated their repair sequences with specific repair strategies, roughly 60% of the time. Below are excerpts from three of the repair sequences (punctuation added). For each one, consider the kind of repair strategies used and the type of conversational style exhibited by the husband. Were the strategies specific or nonspecific? Was the conversational style more characteristic of an aggressive, passive-aggressive, assertive, or passive style? Were all of his remarks consistent with the same style? What style of turn taking predominated?

Excerpt 1 *(p. 38)*:

Wife:	Doesn't sound very profitable. I s'pose they make profit on the coffee.
Husband:	Don't mumble, what?
Wife:	I said I guess they make a profit on the coffee even if they don't sell the book.
Husband:	Even if they don't sell the book, yeah.

Excerpt 2 *(p. 43)*:

Wife:	We always used to camp in the winter so camping in the winter in Victoria is, is not different?
Husband:	Sorry I'm not following.
Wife:	I mean if you're going to end up south sooner that's no different to short holidays we used to have, we always used to go away in the winter *time* . . . .
Husband:	(overlapping with *time*) Yeah.

Excerpt 3 *(p. 44)*:

Wife:	Yeah but these are the phone calls that I have to *make* . . .
Husband:	(overlapping with *make*) See you keep dropping, I'm losing you.
Wife:	These are the phone calls that I have to make so you know (etc.)
Husband:	(overlapping with final word in wife's utterance) Yes.

FINAL REMARKS

In this chapter, we have considered communication strategies and conversational styles and behaviors. People have a myriad of means for managing their communication difficulties. Although many of the strategies we considered in this chapter seem like common sense, it is surprising that many people either have not explicitly thought about them or do not use them effectively. Moreover, many people are not aware they may be using a conversational style or conversational behaviors that alienate(s) their communication partners. Although these behaviors may have been adopted as a means of coping with hearing-related difficulties, they may create problems in and of themselves.

KEY CHAPTER POINTS

- Face-to-face conversation usually proceeds in an orderly fashion, with communication partners adhering to implicit rules of conversation.

- Grounding occurs when one communication partner presents information and another partner acknowledges understanding. This information is then presupposed throughout the remaining conversation.

- The accepted rules of conversation often must bend when one of the communication partners has a hearing loss. The overall quality of conversation also may be diminished. For instance, there may only be superficial content and grounding may be disrupted.

- There are two classes of communication strategies, facilitative and repair. Within each of these classes are several kinds of strategies that individuals with hearing loss can use to facilitate conversational interchanges.

- There are at least three stages involved in repairing a communication breakdown: detection, selection of a course of action, and implementation.

- Persons who have hearing loss often bluff and pretend to understand. They may do this because they are reluctant to admit a hearing loss or because they do not want to appear uncooperative.

- Much research has centered on the use of repair strategies. One conclusion that emerges is that the most commonly used repair strategy is the repeat strategy.

- There are both advantages and disadvantages in using nonspecific repair strategies.

- Anticipatory strategies are more effective when used before unfamiliar communication interactions than when used before familiar ones.

- Persons may be assertive, passive, aggressive, or passive-aggressive in their conversational styles.

- Constellations of communication behaviors might be described as interactive, noninteractive, dominating, or some combination of the three.

TERMS AND CONCEPTS TO REMEMBER

Rules of conversation
Hand gestures
Modifications in conversation
Grounding
Message reception
Facilitative strategies
Expressive and receptive repair strategies
Maladaptive strategies
Stages of repair
Nonspecific repair strategies
Social stigmata
Cooperative enterprise
Conversational styles
Communication behavior constellations

MULTIPLE-CHOICE QUESTIONS

1. Marcus Jones has a significant hearing loss. The tacit rules of conversation may be violated when he talks to an unfamiliar communication partner because:

    a. Marcus will probably change the topic of conversation inappropriately.

    b. Marcus will slow his speaking rate.

    c. The communication partner will repeatedly confirm that Marcus has recognized his or her message.

    d. The communication partner will provide too much information and border on verbosity.

2. The two stages of grounding are:

    a. One communication partner presents a bit of information and the other acknowledges receipt.

    b. One communication partner suggests a topic of conversation and the other tacitly agrees to discuss it.

    c. A communication breakdown is detected and a repair strategy is employed.

    d. Following a communication breakdown, a repair strategy is implemented and the conversation resumes.

3. Two classes of communication strategies are:
   a. Anticipatory and facilitative
   b. Environmental and corrective
   c. Specific and nonverbal
   d. Facilitative and repair

4. Which of the following messages might be easiest for a person with hearing loss to recognize?
   a. John gave the baseball to Tom and asked him to take it home last night.
   b. He took it home.
   c. He tossed the baseball to Tom. "Take it home," he said.
   d. John had the baseball. John gave the baseball to Tom.

5. Which question might reflect a message-tailoring strategy?
   a. Who did you see at the game?
   b. Where were you this morning?
   c. Did you find my list?
   d. How do you get to Toledo?

6. Moving to a seat that is close to the podium during a lecture is an example of:
   a. An anticipatory strategy
   b. A constructive strategy
   c. An instructional strategy
   d. An attending strategy

7. Which of the following is a disadvantage of using a nonspecific repair strategy following a communication breakdown?
   a. Your communication partner may react unfavorably to the conversation.
   b. You might elicit a simplified version of what was originally said.
   c. You take a "phantom" speaking turn.
   d. You are viewed as taking away your communication partner's speaking turn.

8. Which of the following is an advantage of using a nonspecific repair strategy during a conversation?
   a. It elicits a rephrasing from the communication partner.
   b. It may indicate to the communication partner the point in time that the breakdown occurred.

    c. You are viewed as assertive.

    d. It gives the communication partner a choice in how to repair a communication breakdown.

9. A person who frequently interrupts may be said to have what kind of conversational style?

    a. Passive

    b. Assertive

    c. Uncooperative

    d. Aggressive

10. A person who has a passive-aggressive conversational style would most likely utter which of the following lines?

    a. "Whatever you decide is fine by me."

    b. "I have a hearing loss so let's move over here where it is more quiet so we can talk."

    c. "I know you two have a lot of catching up to do, so just pretend that I'm not here."

    d. "If you wouldn't talk so fast, I could speechread you better."

CHAPTER 8

Assessment of Conversational Fluency and Communication Difficulties

OUTLINE

- Conversational fluency
- General considerations for evaluating conversational fluency and hearing-related disability
- Interviews
- Questionnaires
- Daily logs
- Group discussion
- Structured communication interactions
- Unstructured communication interactions
- Case study: A school boy opens up
- Final remarks
- Key chapter points
- Terms and concepts to remember
- Multiple-choice questions
- Key resources

Typically, a communication strategies training program begins and ends with an assessment of individuals' conversational fluency and hearing-related disability. The goals of the initial assessment are to:

- Determine the communication demands placed upon individuals in their everyday life.
- Evaluate the impact of hearing loss on daily activities.
- Identify the settings in which communication problems are likely to arise.
- Document the kinds of social activities in which a person is likely to engage.
- Assess how effectively they use communication strategies in a variety of settings.
- Chronicle their employment responsibilities.

The goals of assessment will guide the selection of which measures are administered. For example, if the goal of assessment is to identify communication problems that are especially troublesome, a speech and hearing professional might interview the patient or administer a questionnaire. On the other hand, if the goal is to document conversational fluency, the clinician might determine how well information can be exchanged between two communication partners, while maintaining a give-and-take dialogue. Assessment techniques for this purpose may include structured communication interactions or informal conversations.

The final assessment indicates whether a person's actual or perceived conversational fluency has improved and communication difficulties have diminished as a result of an aural rehabilitation intervention. Some of the original measures might be repeated to determine whether performance has changed. One-time-only measures also might be administered, such as a questionnaire, in which participants can critique the success of an aural rehabilitation plan.

Typically, a speech and hearing professional will want to know what the patient's audiogram looks like, both aided and unaided. In addition, the clinician will assess a patient's ability to recognize words in an audition-only condition and in an audition-plus-vision condition. In Chapter 2, we considered the audiogram and assessment of word recognition. In this chapter, we consider those assessment instruments that pertain to hearing-related communication difficulties in everyday situations and conversational fluency.

CONVERSATIONAL FLUENCY

The following factors help to define conversational fluency (Erber, 1996, pp. 204–205; Erber, 1998):

- *Time spent in repairing communication breakdowns.* If during the course of a conversation, numerous communication breakdowns occur and they require many interchanges between the person with hearing loss and the communication partner before they are resolved, then conversational fluency is low. On the other hand, if need for clarification is minimal, conversational fluency is high. When analyzing communication breakdowns, consider (a) the proportion of time spent in communication breakdowns, (b) the total number of breakdowns, and (c) the average duration of a breakdown.
- *Exchange of information and ideas.* If the participants in a conversation successfully and easily share information and ideas, and the conversation seems to them to be spontaneous and not stilted, then conversational fluency is high.
- *Sharing of speaking time.* When conversation is smooth-flowing, participants have ample opportunity to speak, and no one person dominates with protracted speaking times. Prolonged silences or frequent interruptions are not characteristic of fluent conversations.
- *Time spent in silence.* If the participants sit in awkward silence for an inordinate amount of time, then conversational fluency is poor.

Sociolinguists often index the sharing of speaking time with a measure called **mean length turn ratio (MLT ratio)**. To determine this ratio, **mean length of speaking turn (MLT)** is first computed for each participant in a conversation by determining the average number of words each person speaks (or average duration in seconds of a conversational turn) for some set number of conversational turns (often 50 turns). A **conversational turn** begins when one communication partner starts to speak. The turn ends when the person stops talking, and someone else responds to the remark. The MLT ratio is computed by taking a ratio between the MLTs of the two communication partners. Table 8-1 illustrates how MLT and MLT ratio are determined.

The dialogues in Table 8-1 also illustrate two different levels of conversational fluency. In the first example, conversational fluency is high. The two communication partners exchange information with ease, and they share responsibility in advancing the topic of discussion. They talk about a fairly uncommon conversational topic, period furniture, which entails using unusual vocabulary such as *French regency* and *deco*. The MLT ratio

Sociolinguists are scientists who belong to a branch of linguistics that studies the effects of social and cultural differences within a community on its use of language and conversational patterns.

Mean length turn ratio (MLT ratio) is the ratio of the MLTs of two speakers in a conversation.

Mean length (speaking) turn (MLT) is computed by determining the average number of words spoken during a set number of conversational turns, or the average duration of conversational turns in seconds.

Conversational turn is the period during which a participant delivers a contribution to the conversation.

Table 8-1. Dialogues that illustrate two levels of conversational fluency. Example 1 presents a sample with high conversational fluency, whereas Example 2 presents a sample with low conversational fluency.

EXAMPLE 1
Joan: Has your new furniture arrived yet?
Ann: Yes, and I'm thrilled with it.
Joan: You said that it was going to be French regency.
Ann: No, I didn't go with that. My husband wanted a deco look.
Analysis: Joan's MLT = 8.0 words (16 words divided by 2 utterances)
Ann's MLT = 9.0 words (18 words divided by 2 utterances)
MLT ratio: 0.9, where 1.0 = equal length speaking turns

EXAMPLE 2
Martha: Has your new furniture arrived yet?
Tom: Huh?
Martha: Your furniture?
Tom: (looks around, shakes head)
Martha: How are you doing? How is your wife? . . . Mary?
Tom: Fine.
Analysis: Martha's MLT = 5.6 words (17 words divided by 3 utterances)
Tom's MLT = 0.7 (2 words divided by 3 utterances)
MLT ratio: 6.2, where 1.0 = equal length speaking turns

MLT = mean length turn

Why traditional audiological tests might not reflect conversational fluency:

- Most require patients to repeat exactly what they heard; engagement in a conversation usually does not require that.

- Most assess recognition of unrelated words and sentences; conversation is comprised of utterances related by linguistic and situational context.

- Most do not allow for the use of repair and facilitative strategies; in conversation, a patient may ask communication partners to modify an utterance or modify their speaking behavior.

for this conversation is approximately equal, which is often characteristic of fluent interchanges.

The second conversational excerpt in Table 8-1 presents a sample of low conversational fluency. The topic of discussion quickly becomes superficial, as communication breakdowns occur. In this conversation, Martha bears the onus of responsibility for advancing the conversation. She must fill in the awkward silences and develop the topic. Conversational fluency of this type is not uncommon when one of the communication partners has a significant hearing loss.

GENERAL CONSIDERATIONS FOR EVALUATING CONVERSATIONAL FLUENCY AND HEARING-RELATED DISABILITY

Conversational fluency and the communication difficulties that are associated with hearing-related disability can be challenging for a speech and hearing professional to assess for a number of reasons.

First, conversational fluency and success in managing communication difficulties vary as a function of the conversational setting and situation and as a function of the communication partner. For instance, conversational fluency may be high when an individual talks with a seasoned speech and hearing professional but low when the person converses with an unfamiliar store clerk. The speech and hearing professional is likely to be accustomed to talking to persons with hearing loss and probably speaks slowly and clearly and checks for comprehension. The store clerk may not know how to facilitate speech recognition for the person with hearing loss, may turn away when talking (and hence limit the person's ability to speechread), and may speak quickly. A measure of conversational fluency taken from the same patient probably would be high for the first communication partner but low for the second.

A second reason that assessment of conversational fluency may be problematic is because measures vary with the topic of discussion. For instance, conversational fluency may be high for a superficial topic such as the weather but low for a topic centering on local politics. Thus, depending on what was discussed, a speech and hearing professional might rate conversational fluency with a particular patient as either high or low.

A third reason is because communication difficulties do not always arise during a conversation. A person may experience numerous difficulties in conversing in the workplace, but none while talking to a family member in a speech and hearing clinic test room. If communication breakdowns do not occur during the course of an assessment, a speech and hearing professional may not gain an appreciation of how an individual manages communication difficulties.

Finally, no one measure can capture adequately the **construct** of conversational fluency or hearing-related disability because both are defined by several dimensions. That is, both are abstractions that reflect a multitude of factors (i.e., the occurrence of breakdowns and pauses, the fluidity of conversation, MLT ratio, amount of time spent in silence, and the superficiality of discussion). A number of measures typically must be performed, and the results aggregated and then interpreted.

A **construct** is an abstract or general idea that is inferred or derived from a constellation of measures or from a group of specific instances.

In the next sections, we consider specific assessment procedures that may be used. These procedures are listed in Table 8-2, along with some of their advantages and disadvantages.

Table 8-2. Some general procedures for measuring conversational fluency and communication needs, and one advantage and disadvantage of each.

PROCEDURE	ADVANTAGE	DISADVANTAGE
Interview	Yields patient-specific information	Difficult to quantify information
Questionnaire	Quick and easy to administer	May miss patient-specific information
Daily log	Provides quantitative information about an extended time period	Can be a reactive procedure
Group discussion	Stimulates patients to introspect and reflect	Some patients may be reluctant to participate
Structured communication interaction	Has good face validity because assessment is based on actual conversational interactions	Can be time-consuming to score
Unstructured communication interactions	Good ecological validity because it best mimics real-world interaction	Results may vary as a function of the communication partner

INTERVIEWS

Interviews are a basic assessment procedure used to elicit specific information about an individual's hearing-related communication difficulties.

The most straightforward assessment procedure is the **interview**. Individuals talk about their conversational problems, and they consider possible reasons as to why communication breakdowns happen (Figure 8-1). They comment on their subjective impressions of conversational fluency in a variety of settings (e.g., the workplace, the home). "Are you able to use the telephone?" a clinician might ask, or the clinician might ask a more open-ended question, such as,

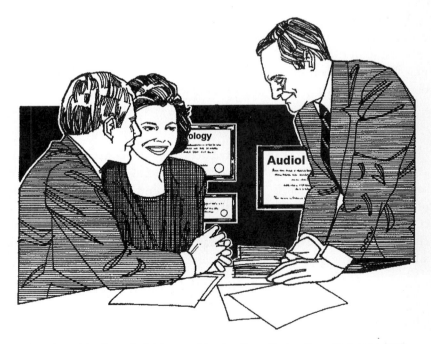

FIGURE 8-1. Interviews. A clinician may interview the patient or the patient and a family member to learn about communication difficulties that are being experienced.

"Tell me about your listening difficulties." People's answers will indicate their particular concerns and their perceptions of their situation and problems. As a speech and hearing professional interacts with the patient, the professional will acquire a sense of how well the patient can converse informally.

Interviews are effective because they elicit information that is specific to an individual. For instance, an individual may report experiencing difficulty communicating during office conferences, whereas another may report experiencing problems while watching television. An open-ended discussion about the workplace may trigger a patient to reflect about particular instances in which communication was difficult in his or her recent past and may provide direction for the aural rehabilitation plan.

The disadvantage of interviews is that remarks cannot be quantified. This is problematic when changes in communication behaviors that result from intervention must be documented. Documentation is essential when a speech and hearing professional seeks reimbursement for providing sevices to patients from third-party health care providers.

> "Functional tests cannot tell the story of disabilities and handicaps, since these are to do with the person's actual experiences in the world. Thus that experience must be tapped, and the only way to do it is by asking people to make accounts of it."
>
> William Noble, Professor of Psychology at the University of Manchester
>
> *(Noble, 1996, p. 9)*

Conducting the Interview

Often, interviews are semistructured and unfold in a conversational format. Broad topics are covered, such as communication difficulties that occur in the home, social settings, school, or the workplace. When interviewing a patient, a speech and hearing professional engages in "generous listening," listening in a way that lets people know they are being heard, without being judged, and provides positive attention, regard, and acknowledgment.

Generous Listening

Here are specific tips to keep in mind as you interview a patient for the first time (Gitles, 1999):

- Do not get involved writing information and do not turn away from the patient. Continue to look at the person, and, most important, listen as if your life depended on it. Listen as if you have never heard any of this before, because you haven't, not from this person.
- If the patient pauses, stifle the impulse to ask the next question, interpret what the person is saying, or change the subject. Instead say something like, "Is there anything else?" or "What else can you tell me about that?" or "Tell me more about that."

continues

Generous Listening, *continued*

- Use how, what, and when questions and avoid why questions. People will reveal more to you if they do not feel the need to justify their actions or defend their behavior.
- Encourage patients to talk until they have nothing left to tell you.
- When people answer questions, the more you listen, the greater the depth of the information they will reveal. That is where connectedness and relatedness occur. The more that patients reveal, the more they feel it is safe to talk to you, the more they get to weave and listen to their own story about their hearing (which they may have never told a soul), and the greater realization they have of the extent of their problem. As a result, the less reluctant they are about receiving help and the more they begin to let you help them.
- Listen to patients without judgment, evaluation, or opinions. Listen for the emotion and feelings in their expression and be aware of what is *not* being said. Acknowledge patients for having the courage to come in for help and let them know you will support them in whatever way you can.
- The more that you, as a professional, reveal your passion and commitment to helping people—perhaps through a personal story about someone you have helped—the greater the intimacy and relatedness with your patient (pp. 54–56).

Excerpts from two sample interviews demonstrate how an interview may be unsuccessful or successful. In the first interview, the clinician asks a preponderance of yes–no questions. It is almost as if she knows the answer before the patient even responds. A following question is not influenced by the patient's response to a previous question. By the end of the interview, the clinician has gained little information about the patient's communication difficulties or conversational fluency, and the patient probably feels like he has been cycled through a pat list of questions that the clinician fires away at everyone who comes in for a hearing test.

Clinician: (Leads Mr. Brown to the testing suite. When he is seated in the testing chair, the clinician begins the interview.) So, you think you have a hearing loss?

Mr. Brown: My wife seems to think I do.

Clinician:	(The clinician makes a tick mark with her pen on the yellow notepad she is holding.) You have trouble hearing at home?
Mr. Brown:	I do okay.
Clinician:	(The clinician makes a tick mark.) What about work?
Mr. Brown:	Yeah, that's okay too.
Clinician:	(The clinician makes a tick mark.) You can use the telephone?
Mr. Brown:	Yeah.
Clinician:	(The clinician makes a tick mark, tucks the pad of paper under her arm.) Fine. Let's test your hearing and see what we find.

In contrast, in the excerpt from the second interview, which appears next, the clinician engages in "generous listening." She asks open-ended questions and encourages the patient to elaborate on his responses. Because there is a genuine dialogue occurring, the clinician has a first-person opportunity to observe the patient experience a communication breakdown, giving her some insight as to how the individual handles breakdowns and the ease with which they can be repaired.

Clinician:	(Greets the patient in the waiting room and asks him to follow her to her office for a conversation.) Good morning, Mr. Andrews. What brings you here today?
Mr. Andrews:	My wife says I have a hearing loss.
Clinician:	(Nods, continues to look Mr. Andrews in the eye.)
Mr. Andrews:	I think she mumbles a lot. But then again, I guess I'm cranking up the volume of the TV too high. That probably means something.
Clinician:	What happens when she tries to talk to you from another room?
Mr. Andrews:	Huh?
Clinician:	Say you are in the living room. Your wife is talking to you from the hallway. What happens?
Mr. Andrews:	I can't hear her. Same as when she's talking in the kitchen with the water running. I can't hear her.
Clinician:	Tell me more about listening at home.
Mr. Andrews:	(Describes his difficulties with hearing the doorbell and listening on the telephone. They then discuss the challenges he encounters when listening in the workplace.)

Simply by listening, and treating the person as a unique individual and not as Mr. or Mrs. Joe/Jane client, a clinician will learn much about a patient's communication difficulties. Moreover, the clinician will establish a bond of human contact that lets the individual know that the professional genuinely cares about his or her hearing health and communication needs. The topic of interviews will be revisted in Chapter 12 when we consider aural rehabilitation plans for adults.

QUESTIONNAIRES

Another assessment instrument that is used to assess conversational fluency and hearing-related disability is the questionnaire (Chapter 3). Questionnaires might query respondents about how often communication breakdowns occur and whether they typically attempt to repair communication breakdowns and how. Questionnaires are a means of gathering general information easily and quickly (Figure 8-2).

One drawback in using questionnaires is that it is possible to miss important information about communication difficulties that are specific to an individual simply because they are not covered by items in the questionnaire. A true–false statement such as, *I always verify what I understood during a meeting with a coworker afterward,* is irrelevant to the respondent who does not work or does not attend meetings. Moreover, responses to questionnaires may not

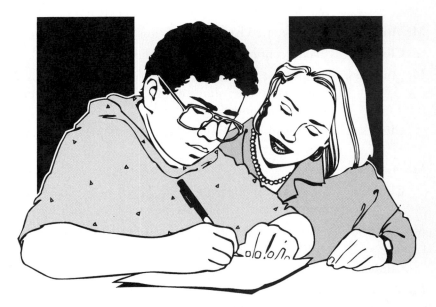

FIGURE 8-2. Questionnaires are an effective means of obtaining information about communication and conversation in an easy and fast way.

reflect the importance of each communication difficulty or communication situation to the individual. An inability to talk on the telephone may be disruptive to the lifestyle of one person but only a minor annoyance to another.

A number of self-assessment questionnaires have been developed. Members of the Academy of Rehabilitative Audiology consider at least four instruments to be valid and useful: the *Hearing Handicap Inventory for the Elderly*, the *Self-Assessment of Communication*, the *Hearing Handicap Inventory for Adults*, and the *Communication Profile for the Hearing Impaired* (Dancer & Gener, 1999). The first three appear in the Key Resources at the end of this chapter, and the fourth is available for purchase (CPHI Services, 1498 Goodbar Avenue, Memphis, TN 38104). Table 8-3 reviews many of the available questionnaires. The last two instruments in the table were specifically developed to be used with children.

Table 8-3. A list of self-report questionnaires.

TEST	PURPOSE	REFERENCES
Abbreviated Profile of Hearing Aid Benefit (APHAB) 24 items, four subscales (ease of communication, reverberation, background noise, aversiveness of sounds)	To measure the disability associated with hearing loss and the amount by which use of hearing aid reduces disability. Example: *(answered with and without hearing aid)* I can communicate with others when we are in a crowd. *(Always, almost always, generally, half the time, occasionally, seldom, never)*	Cox & Alexander (1995) Paul & Cox (1995)
Amsterdam Inventory for Auditory Disability and Handicap 30 items, six factors (detection of sounds, distinction of sounds, auditory localization, intelligibility in noise and in quiet, intolerance of noise)	To identify factors that affect the patient in daily life and to assess hearing handicap. Example: *Can you carry on a conversation with someone in a busy street? (Almost never, occasionally, frequently, almost always)*	Kramer, Kapteyn, Festen, & Tobi (1995) Kramer, Kapteyn, Festen, & Tobi (1996) Kramer, Kapteyn, & Festen (1998)
Client Oriented Scale of Improvement (COSI) 16 standardized listening situations	To identify up to five areas of listening difficulty and the degree of benefit obtained compared to that expected for similar persons in similar situations (see Chapter 12).	Dillon, James, & Ginis (1997) Dillon, Birtles, & Lovegrove (1999)
Communication Profile for the Hearing Impaired (CPHI) 145-item questionnaire dealing with four areas: communication performance, communication environment, communication strategies, and personal adjustment	To assess a broad range of communication problems. Example: *One way I get people to repeat what they said is by ignoring them. (5-point scale ranging from "rarely" to "almost always")*	Demorest & Erdman (1987)
Communication Scale for Older Adults 72 items divided into two scales: communication strategies and communication attitudes	To provide in-depth information about the effects of aural rehabilitation on daily life and to evaluate use of communication strategies and an individual's feelings about hearing loss. Example: *I become angry when people do not speak clearly enough for me to understand. (scale ranging from "always" to "never")*	Kaplan, Bally, Brandt, Busacco, & Pray (1997)

continues

Table 8-3. *continued*

TEST	PURPOSE	REFERENCES
(Revised) Communication Self-Assessment Scale Inventory for Deaf Adults (CSDA) 125 items, four scales (difficult communication situations, importance of each situation, communication strategies, communication attitudes)	To measure the communication abilities of adults who have prelingual deafness. Example: *You have difficulty hearing music when it is loud enough for other people. (Almost always, sometimes, almost never)*	Kaplan, Bally, & Brandt (1995)
Denver Scale of Communication Function-Modified (DSCF-M) 34 items concerning four areas (attitudes towards peers, socialization, communication, difficult listening situations)	To assess communication skills of older patients. Example: *The people I live with are annoyed with my hearing loss. (5-point scale ranging from "definitely agree" to "definitely disagree")*	Kaplan, Feeley, & Brown (1978)
Glasgow Hearing Aid Benefit Profile (GHABP) four prespecified/four subject specified items across six dimensions (disability, handicap, hearing aid use, benefit, satisfaction, residual disability)	To measure disability/handicap and benefit from use of hearing aid(s). Example: *The people I live with are annoyed with my hearing loss. (5-point scale ranging from "not satisfied at all" to "delighted with it")*	Gatehouse (1999)
Gothenburg Profile (GP) 20 items, two scales: Experienced disability (being able to hear speech, being able to localize sounds) and experienced handicap (impact of hearing impairment, how you perform and react)	To measure experienced hearing disability and handicap. Example: *Do you find hearing problems an obstacle to your social life? (11-point scale, ranging from "never" to "always")*	Arlinger, Bellermark, Oberg, Lunner, & Hellgren (1998) Ringdahl, Eriksson-Mangold, & Andersson (1998)
Hearing Aid Needs Assessment (HANA) 11 items, three ratings per item: (1) How often (hardly ever, occasionally, frequently); (2) How much trouble (very little, some, very much); (3) How much help expected (very little, some, very much)	To compare perceived communication needs with actual benefit eventually achieved with hearing aids. Example: *You are at home listening to your stereo system. (Ratings for how often, how much trouble, and how much help expected)*	Schum (1999)
Hearing Attitudes in Rehabilitation Questionnaire (HARQ) 40 items, seven scales measure attitudes toward: hearing impairment (e.g., personal distress, hearing loss stigma, minimization of hearing loss) and hearing aid (e.g., hearing aid stigma, hearing aid not wanted, pressure to be assessed, positive expectation of aid)	To measure older people's attitudes toward hearing loss and use of a hearing aid. Example: *If I wear a hearing aid, people will probably think I'm a bit stupid: (1) not true, (2) partly true, (3) true.*	Hallam and Brooks (1996)
Hearing Coping Assessment (HCA) 21 multiple-choice items covering problem-focused coping and emotion-focused coping	To evaluate how well the patient thinks he or she can cope with hearing impairment. Example: *(1) I never had any problem talking to one person . . . (4) I have much trouble talking to one person.*	Andersson, Melin, Lindberg, & Scott (1995)
Hearing Disabilities and Handicaps Scale (HDHS) 20 items, three factors (speech perception, nonspeech sounds, handicap)	To assess the severity of the most common disabilities and handicaps associated with hearing impairment. Example: *Is it difficult for you to ask people to repeat themselves? (Never, seldom, often, always)*	Hétu, Getty, Philibert, Desilets, Noble, & Stephens (1994) Hallberg (1998)

continues

Table 8-3. *continued*

TEST	PURPOSE	REFERENCES
Hearing Handicap and Disability Inventory (HHDI) 40 items, four scales (performance, emotional response, social withdrawal, perceived reaction of others)	To assess the consequence of hearing impairment in the elderly and to identify aural rehabilitative needs and effect of inter- vention. Example: *My hearing loss discour- ages me from using the telephone. (Almost never, sometimes, often, almost always)*	VanderBrink (1995)
Hearing Handicap Inventory for Adults (HHIA) 25 items with two subscales (emotional consequences, social and situational effects)	To quantify perceived handicap and to assess benefit of hearing aids. Example: *Does a hearing problem cause you to feel embar- rassed when meeting new people? (Yes, sometimes, no)*	Newman, Weinstein, Jacobson, & Hug (1990) Newman, Weinstein, Jacobson, & Hug (1991)
Hearing Handicap for the Elderly (HHIE) 25 items with two subscales (emotional consequences, social and situational effects)	To assess older person's perceptions of hearing loss, used with noninstitutional- ized individuals. Example: *Does a hearing problem cause you to use the phone less often than you would like? (Yes, sometimes, no)*	Ventry and Weinstein (1982) Weinstein, Spitzer, & Ventry (1986)
Hearing Handicap Scale (HHS) 20 items	To measure disadvantage caused by the presence of hearing loss during everyday listening. Example: *When you ask someone for directions, do you understand what he or she says (5-point scale, ranging from "practi- cally always" to "almost never").*	High, Fairbanks, & Glorig (1964) Tannahil (1979)
Hearing Performance Inventory (HPI) 158 items that assess understanding of speech, speech intensity, response to auditory failure, and social, personal, and occupational issues	To evaluate problem areas experienced during everyday living. Example: *You are with a male friend or family member and several people are talking nearby. Can you understand him when his voice is loud enough and you can see his face? (4-point scale ranging from "practically always" to "practically never")*	Giolas, Owens, Lamb, & Schubert (1979)
Open-ended Problems Questionnaire One item is used to assess various groups (e.g., cochlear implant users, frequent communication partners)	To measure what people consider are the main problems as a result of hearing im- pairment. Example: *Please make a list of difficulties you may have as a result of your hearing loss. List them in order of importance starting with the biggest difficulties. Write down as many as you can think of.*	Barcham & Stephens (1980) Stephens, Jaworski, Kerr, & Zhao (1998)
Listening Inventories for Education (LIFE) Three inventories about classroom listening completed by student and/or teacher, includes both rating scales and picture prompts	To provide a behavioral evaluation of the quality of the classroom listening environ- ment and to assess the effectiveness of interventions. Example: *(student views a cartoon of a teacher at the front of a class) The kids are going to take a test. The teacher is giving directions. Tell me how well you can hear the words the teacher is saying.*	Anderson & Smaldino (1998)

continues

Table 8-3. *continued*

TEST	PURPOSE	REFERENCES
The Children's Version of the Abbreviated Profile of Hearing Aid Performance (CA-PHAP) 24 items, four subscales (ease of communication, reverberation, background noise, aversiveness of sounds)	To measure the disability associated with hearing loss and the amount by which use of hearing aid reduces disability. Example: *(answered with and without hearing aid) I miss a lot of what the teacher says in my classroom. (Always, almost always, most of the time, half –the time, once in a while, hardly ever, never)*	Kopun & Stelmachowicz, 1998

Source: Adapted from Bentler, R. A., & Kramer, S. E. (2000). Guidelines for choosing a self-report outcome measure. *Ear and Hearing,* 21, 375–495.

The popularity of these instruments relates in part to the fact that subjective impressions of communication difficulties often do not correspond to patients' audiograms (Brainerd & Frankel, 1985; Demorest & Walden, 1984; Speaks, Jerger, & Trammell, 1970; Weinstein & Ventry, 1983). An audiogram may indicate that a person has a significant hearing loss. However the individual, when completing a questionnaire, may describe the loss as a minor nuisance, but not overly problematic. In considering the discrepancy that sometimes exists between audiological and questionnaire information, Erdman (1994) notes:

> Self-reports simply constitute different measures; the method of measurement differs as does the content of the measurement. Audiometric tests assess maximum potential or best performance of the central or peripheral hearing mechanism. Self-report instruments, on the other hand, assess typical performance in behavioral utilization of hearing ability. (p. 69)

Open-ended questions elicit qualitative information.

Questionnaires may yield either quantitative or qualitative information, depending on the design of the questionnaire items. **Open-ended questions** typically elicit qualitative data. Examples of open-set items include the following:

- Describe the situations wherein you typically have problems communicating.
- What do you usually do when you do not understand someone?

Closed-ended questions are used to gather quantitative or categorical information.

Closed-ended questions may be used to gather quantitative or categorical information. An example of a quantitative questionnaire item appears next. On this item, the respondent's task is to write a number between 1 and 10 on each response blank, where *1* means *never* and *10* means *always:*

I am at a department store. The clerk asks me a question, but I do not understand her. I am most likely to:

_____ *ask the clerk to repeat the question*

_____ *ask the clerk to say the question in a different way*

_____ *shake my head to indicate that I missed what the clerk said*

_____ *say and do nothing*

Both kinds of questionnaire items offer advantages and disadvantages. Open-ended items are less restrictive and might yield information from a patient that could not have been anticipated. However, sometimes answers to open-ended items are rambling or off-topic, and they may be difficult to quantify, which may be important if a clinician desires to compare pre- and postintervention performance. Closed-ended items allow for a quantitative analysis of responses. However, important information may be missed if the questionnaire does not include items that tap information relevant to a patient's communication difficulties.

DAILY LOGS

In completing a **daily log**, respondents perform a self-monitoring procedure regarding behaviors of interest, and provide self-reports. For example,
they may log how many times a day they experience communication difficulties, and in which communication settings (e.g., the home, the workplace). In completing logs, patients may answer a series of questions about
their communication difficulties or behaviors every day for a set number
of days. Example items from a daily log appear in Table 8-4.

Daily logs are self-reports of behavior used by respondents for self-monitoring.

When patients complete a log for several consecutive days, their responses
provide a general index of their daily use of communication strategies, their
conversational fluency, and their communication difficulties. Responses
also may provide information about their aural rehabilitation needs. For
example, if an individual reports that he never spoke on the telephone during 6 consecutive days, it might be inferred that this person may be unable
to use the telephone successfully, and therefore avoids telephone conversations. The aural rehabilitation plan may thus be designed to provide telephone training and a telephone receiver amplifier.

Individuals can perform a daily-log activity before and after participating in
a communication strategies training program, and trends in responses can
be compared before and after training. For example, if after completing a
communication strategies training program and after receiving a telephone
receiver amplifier, the man just discussed reported he used the telephone
an average of two times every day (as compared to never), then it might be
concluded that intervention provided some benefit to this individual.

Table 8-4. Example items from a daily log designed to monitor someone's communication behaviors.

1. **Think about your communication interactions today. For the following situations, circle the term (never, a few times, many times) that best describes how much time you spent a talking today (beyond a greeting). Circle one response for each condition:**

In a quiet place	Never	a few times	many times
In a noisy place	Never	a few times	many times
On the telephone	Never	a few times	many times
From another room	Never	a few times	many times
In a group of people	Never	a few times	many times

2. **For the following two situations, write down a number between 0 and 100 (0 = nothing and 100 = everything) that indicates how much of what was said to you today you believe you understood.**

   _____ while watching the talker and listening

   _____ while listening only

3. **Did you ever indicate that you did not understand a spoken message today (Yes or No)?**

   _____

4. **What did you do when you did not understand a message? (Check all that apply.)**

   _____ I asked the talker to repeat the message.

   _____ I said "Huh" or "Pardon."

   _____ I asked the talker to rephrase the message.

   _____ I asked the talker to indicate what he or she was talking about.

   _____ I decided the message was not important enough to keep trying.

   _____ I asked the talker to spell or write the message.

   _____ Other (describe) _____

5. **Consider the conversations that you had with relatives today. Check all of the statements below that apply.**

   _____ I felt anxious when I tried to talk with my relative today.

   _____ I was able to understand my relative's spoken messages.

   _____ I felt satisfied with the success of our communication interactions.

   _____ I avoided talking about unimportant topics.

Guidelines for Constructing a Daily Log

Although there are a few examples of daily logs for aural rehabilitation applications available in the literature (e.g., Palmer, Bentler, & Mueller, 2006), a speech and hearing professional may have to design them and tailor them to track the pertinent activities and behaviors of each

Guidelines for Constructing a Daily Log, *continued*

patient. Next are five guidelines to consider when developing a daily log:

1. Include detailed instructions at the beginning of the daily log and at the start of each section that initiates a new format. Make the instructions clear and concise.
2. Use active sentences rather than passive sentences when writing daily log items.
3. Log items should have a minimum of prepositional phrases.
4. Avoid professional jargon or terms used often within the speech and hearing communication field but not by the general public.
5. Limit the number of items in a daily log to a maximum of seven. Otherwise, it may be too taxing for a patient to complete or too much of an imposition in the daily routine.

Self-monitoring can be a **reactive** procedure because it may influence a person's communication behaviors and how he or she uses communication strategies. For example, researchers have shown that when individuals complete self-monitoring diaries, they often improve their academic performance, reduce their consumption of alcohol, or decrease the number of cigarettes smoked (e.g., Johnson & Wilhite, 1971; McFall, 1970). Similarly, by monitoring use of communication strategies, patients may actually improve their use of them. As such, the use of daily logs can be used as a training procedure as well as an assessment procedure. However, for this very reason, it can be problematic when one is trying to assess the effects of an intervention program.

Self-monitoring can provide a **reactive** procedure as it may influence how a person uses communication behaviors and strategies.

🌀 GROUP DISCUSSION

In a **group discussion** (Figure 8-3), usually convened on the first meeting of a communication strategies training program, members of the class construct a list of their communication problems and the topics they would like included in the syllabus. The remainder of the program then focuses on these issues. This procedure can be used any time that instruction occurs in a group setting as opposed to one-on-one. Table 8-5 lists some concerns that have emerged during this kind of group session.

Group discussion provides a forum for class members to discuss communication issues.

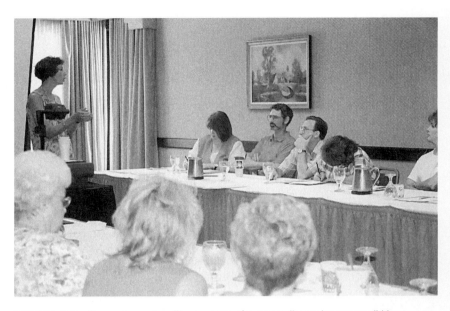

FIGURE 8-3. Group discussion. The success of a group discussion may well hinge on the skill of the group leader. In this session, the clinician is using an overhead projector to record the group participants' comments. *Photograph by Kim Readmond, courtesy of the Central Institute for the Deaf.*

Table 8-5. Common concerns that might be identified during a group discussion.

- Difficulty talking on the telephone
- Impatience on the part of a spouse
- Inability to manage communication breakdowns effectively
- Avoidance by old friends
- People talk to my spouse instead of me
- Feelings of isolation and loneliness
- Feelings of incompetence and anger
- Difficulty conversing in noisy settings
- Difficulty in communicating with my coworkers
- Anxiety about not being able to hear warning signals
- Frustration that family does not understand my hearing loss
- Frustration that most people do not know what it is like to have a hearing loss
- Feelings of being "left out"

Source: Adapted from Trychin, S. (1994). Helping people cope with hearing loss. In J. G. Clark & F. N. Martin (Eds.), *Effective counseling in audiology: Perspectives and practice* (pp. 247–277). Englewood Cliffs, NJ: Simon & Schuster.

Tips on Conducting a Group Discussion

The success (or failure) of a group discussion often hinges on the skill of the speech and hearing professional who conducts the session. Procedures that might be followed when conducting a group discussion include the following:

- Establish the ground rules at the very beginning. Ground rules might include, *Avoid interruptions* or *Raise your hand before you speak so everyone will be looking at you when you start talking.*
- Encourage everyone to participate in the discussion, perhaps by asking group members to take turns one at a time around the table.
- Record remarks on a chalkboard, on an overhead projector slide, or on an oversize hanging notebook, even if they seem off-topic or minor.
- Make sure that no one is made to feel embarrassed or foolish for making a contribution.
- Ask some questions that guide the discussion and engage the students in the discussion. For example, you might say, "Mrs. Smith, you work in a pharmacy. What kinds of listening difficulties do you experience when you are behind the counter?"
- Come to the class prepared to draw specific material from the participants.

〰 STRUCTURED COMMUNICATION INTERACTIONS

Structured communication interactions also can be used during both assessment and training. **Structured communication interactions** are simulated conversations that reflect some of the difficulties that actually occur in a patient's typical day. *TOPICON* (Erber, 1988) is an example of a structured communication interaction activity that may be used for both assessment and training purposes. In this procedure, the patient carries on a conversation with the clinician. The clinician monitors and evaluates conversational difficulties that occur. Afterward, the clinician and student discuss the fluency of the interaction. They talk about the problems that arose and alternative ways of handling them. They consider who spoke more during the interaction and why. They discuss the direction of information flow, and they identify which communication strategies

Structured communication interactions are simulated conversations used to reflect a patient's communication difficulties.

TOPICON is an example of a structured communication interaction activity. The clinician and patient are independently provided with conversational topics. One of them selects a topic and initiates a conversation about it. The two then conduct a brief conversation on the chosen topic, during which the clinician monitors and evaluates the events. The clinician might evaluate "naturalness" and "topic maintenance" and might maintain a count of communication breakdowns.

Example topics for *Topicon*

- Babies
- Types of cheese
- Going shopping
- Tennis
- Books
- Today's news
- Car repair

Erber (1996, p. 92)

During a **referential communication** interaction, one communication partner is expected to convey information to another partner by means of an interactive exchange.

Quest?AR is a structured communication procedure that can be used to assess communication difficulties.

were applied and whether or not they were effective. Conversation fluency can be evaluated with a consideration of the following: (a) number of prolonged pauses, (b) number of restarts, (c) number of topic shifts, (d) interruptions of turn taking, (e) level of abstraction and superficiality, (f) presence of self-consciousness, and (g) the degree of understanding (Erber, 1988, p. 79).

Another kind of structured communication interaction activity is called **referential communication**, and concerns the transmission of information between two communication partners. For example, both patient and clinician might sit before an array of photographs. The clinician describes one of the photographs. The patient's task is to identify the intended referent. When the patient does not understand one of the clinician's descriptions, he or she is expected to use repair strategies.

Question–Answer Sessions (Quest?AR)

Quest?AR is a structured communication procedure that can be used to assess communication difficulties. In the procedure, the clinician asks a series of scripted questions, and the patient responds. Occasionally, listening difficulties are added to induce communication breakdowns. Performance is then evaluated in terms of the frequency of communication breakdowns, and the patient's facility in repairing them. An example of the procedure is presented next (quoted from Erber & Lind, 1994, p. 280).

	Difficulty Added	Difficulty Identified
1. Why did you go there?	_____	_____
2. When did you go?	_____	_____
3. How many people went with you?	_____	_____
4. Who were they (relations/names)?	_____	_____
5. What did you take with you?	_____	_____
6. Where is (the place where you went)?	_____	_____
7. How did you get there?	_____	_____
8. What did you see on the way?	_____	_____
9. What time did you get there?	_____	_____

UNSTRUCTURED COMMUNICATION INTERACTIONS

As the name implies, an unstructured communication interaction is a fairly spontaneous interaction that has few external constraints. Typically, it is a free-flowing conversation between a patient and a communication partner that is most often scored after the fact, although sometimes it is evaluated as it unfolds. In order to ensure that communication breakdowns occur, a clinician might decide to use an **elicitation technique.** To observe a patient's use of a receptive repair strategy, the speech and hearing professional might purposely mumble an utterance and see what happens next. To observe a child's use of an expressive repair strategy, the professional might "stack" a series of clarification requests, such as *Huh?, Pardon?,* and *I didn't get that.* The advantage of using elicitation is that a clinician can ensure that a communication breakdown occurs; the disadvantage is that the breakdown is not genuine. A patient might think that the clinician is "teasing" or might grow impatient, especially if communication breakdowns are induced several times during the conversation. Thus, the results may have reduced ecological validity (Lloyd, 1999).

To ensure that communication breakdowns occur during an unstructured interaction, the clinician might use an **elicitation technique** and purposely induce a communication breakdown.

Unstructured conversations can be assessed informally or more formally. At least three ways have been developed to evaluate unstructured communication interactions: transcription analysis, ratings, and *Dyalog.* All three ways typically entail obtaining an audio-videotape recording of the patient engaged in conversation with a communication partner (although sometimes for the rating procedure or *Dyalog,* the analysis is scored on the spot). The partner might be a frequent communication partner, such as a spouse, a child, or a parent; an unfamiliar communication partner, such as a clinician; or a naive communication partner. This latter kind of partner is someone who is unfamiliar to the patient and someone who is also naive about hearing loss. The use of different types of communication partners may indicate how conversational dynamics vary as a function of the familiarity of the partner.

The conversation sample is typically recorded in a quiet room or a room with background noise (e.g., music playing on a radio to induce communication breakdowns). The camera is mounted on a tripod, turned on, and then the camera operator leaves the room so the patient and communication partner can begin to converse. The conversation might be stimulated with the use of "conversation cards" that list topics to talk about. For example, topics might consist of the following:

- What did you do last weekend?
- Where are you going this summer?

- What's your favorite restaurant?
- Do you have any hobbies?
- Tell me about your family.

In the transcription analysis method of evaluation, the conversation is transcribed word for word, and then analyzed. The analysis might reveal information such as the number of communication breakdowns, the number of turn exchanges required to resolve the breakdowns, the number of interruptions, the number of fillers, mean length turn ratio, and the number of different topics discussed (see Tye-Murray, Witt, & Schum, 1995; Tye-Murray, Witt, Schum, & Sobaski, 1995).

A second way to analyze an unstructured communication interaction is to obtain ratings from trained students or clinicians. The observer watches the sample and then assigns a number from 1 *(poor)* to 4 *(good)* to indicate how smoothly the conversation flows without the need for clarification (Erber, 1996). This kind of rating gives a gross assessment of overall fluency and has proven to be a reliable measure both within and between raters.

Finally, a computer-based technique called *Dyalog* (Erber, 1998) permits relatively fast analyses of unstructured communication interactions. It is a software package that loads onto most computers. The clinician watches the conversation from one (Erber, 1998) to three times (Tye-Murray, 2003), depending on how much information is desired. In the three-times version, the clinician first watches it for the purpose of recording talk time for the patient. Every time the patient begins talking, the clinician presses the space bar of the computer keyboard. When the patient stops talking, the clinician releases the space bar. In the second viewing, the clinician records the intervals in which the communication partner talked. Finally, for the third viewing (and the first viewing if only watching one time), the clinician, who by now is well familiarized with the interaction, presses the space bar at the onset of a communication breakdown and releases it at the offset of the breakdown. The program then can be used to compute the following information: mean length turn for the patient, mean length turn for the communication partner, mean length turn ratio, time spent in silence, time spent in communication breakdown, and average length of communication breakdown.

CASE STUDY

A School Boy Opens Up

Anderson and Smaldino (1998) present a case study about how an audiologist used the self-assessment instrument *Listening Inventories for Education (LIFE)* (Anderson & Smaldino, 1998) to gauge the communication difficulties experienced by an 8-year-old boy and then to assess the outcome of intervention. "Jason Roberts" was found during an audiological examination to have a mild sensorineural hearing loss. Jason and his mother did not appear to understand the summary of the audiological test results, so the audiologist decided to administer one of the three inventories that comprise the *LIFE*, the *Student Appraisal of Listening Difficulty*. The audiologist told Jason, "I know you can hear, but not everything and every time. How about if we try to figure out how much that is impacting how you are doing in school? I have a picture book with different situations that most kids experience in school. I'd like to ask you about how well you think you hear and understand. Only you know how things really are, so it's important to be honest with yourself and with me" (p. 76). One picture in the picture book showed a group of children talking around a table, for example.

Jason looked at the pictures and began to open up and describe his difficulties, which included following directions, participating in classroom discussion, and understanding his friends' conversations. "A glimmer came into his eye as he began to realize that his problems in school might be due to hearing loss, and not because he was dumb or unpopular" (p. 76). The audiologist proceeded to tell him about how a hearing aid might be helpful to him, and promised to help his second-grade teacher better understand some of the communication issues that relate to hearing loss. After a telephone call to the teacher, the audiologist sent her a second inventory from the *LIFE*, the *Teacher Appraisal Form*. In this form, the teacher is asked to indicate a student's level of listening difficulty by responding on a 5-point scale (ranging from *always easy* to *always difficult*) to such items as, *Teacher talking in front of room* and *Simultaneous large and small group*. There is an opportunity for the teacher to write comments for each item.

About a month later, Jason returned to the audiological clinic for a post–hearing aid fitting. He and the audiologist together completed the student inventory of the *LIFE* again. He began to realize how much better he could now hear with his hearing aid. Jason's teacher also completed and returned a third inventory from the *LIFE*, the *Teacher Opinion and Observation List*. On this form, she indicated her agreement with such items as *Focus on instruction has improved* and *Improved understanding of answers or comments by peers during discussion*. After talking to Jason and reviewing his teacher's appraisal, the audiologist decided that the boy might benefit from the use of a classroom FM system. After Jason begins to use the system, she plans to ask Jason and his teacher to fill out the *LIFE* questionnaires again to determine the effects of intervention.

FINAL REMARKS

In this chapter, we have considered a variety of ways to assess conversational fluency and the communication difficulties that are associated with hearing-related disability. Each procedure has advantages and disadvantages, and a major challenge for a speech and hearing professional may lie in the optimum selection and use of the measurement procedures. It is not uncommon for clinicians to use a test battery approach and employ more than one type of assessment procedure. This approach can provide a more well-rounded portrait of communication difficulties than the use of a single measure. However, a clinician needs to be careful not to overwhelm patients with assessment procedures. For example, if they spend their entire first class of communication strategies training with assessment, and do not perceive they have benefited by attending, they are not likely to show up for a second class.

KEY CHAPTER POINTS

- Most communication strategies training programs begin and end with an assessment of conversational fluency and hearing-related disability.
- Conversational fluency relates to how smoothly conversation unfolds.
- Hearing-related disability relates to the communication difficulties that arise in daily living activities and includes the psychosocial disadvantages related to the hearing loss.
- Conversational fluency and hearing-related disability are difficult to assess for many reasons. For example, conversational fluency may vary as a function of the communication partner (Is the person familiar? Is the person experienced with talking to people who have hearing loss?) and with the topic of conversation.
- A variety of assessment procedures are available. These procedures include interviews and questionnaires. Each offers both advantages and disadvantages. Often, clinicians opt to use a test battery approach.

TERMS AND CONCEPTS TO REMEMBER

High conversational fluency
Low conversational fluency
Test battery approach
Generous listening
Open- and closed-ended questions
Reactive procedure
Topicon
Elicitation technique

Referential communication
Transcript analysis
Dyalog

MULTIPLE-CHOICE QUESTIONS

1. Which of the following is not one of the reasons why a speech and hearing professional might want to assess conversational fluency and hearing-related disability at the onset of an aural rehabilitation program?
    a. To verify the audiogram
    b. To determine the communication demands placed on an individual during everyday life
    c. To chronicle a person's employment responsibilities
    d. To document the kinds of social activities in which a person is likely to engage

2. What is mean length turn ratio?
    a. The number of years a person has had a hearing loss divided by the person's age in years
    b. The ratio of MLTs of two talkers who are engaged in conversation
    c. The average length of time a person talks during a conversational turn
    d. The ratio between amount of time spent in silence and the amount of time spent in talking during a conversation

3. All but one of the following are reasons that conversational fluency is difficult to measure clinically:
    a. Fluency varies with topic of conversation.
    b. Fluency varies as a function of the communication partner.
    c. Communication difficulties may not arise.
    d. There are no available assessment procedures and/or instruments.

4. If a clinician wanted to informally assess someone's conversational fluency, the most direct way might be to:
    a. Administer a questionnaire
    b. Ask the patient to complete a daily log
    c. Stage a structured communication interaction
    d. Conduct an interview using open-ended questions

5. The term *generous listening* is used to describe:
   a. Instances in which a patient listens as a frequent communication partner talks about his or her frustrations about the patient's communication difficulties
   b. Instances in which a clinician listens while providing positive regard, attention, and acknowledgment
   c. Instances in which a clinician employs an assistive listening device to ensure that the patient can understand what the clinician has to say
   d. A term used to describe a component of conversational fluency

6. One disadvantage of using a questionnaire to assess hearing-related disability is that:
   a. The information is redundant with results from speech audiometry.
   b. It is possible to miss important information about communication difficulties because the wrong questions are asked.
   c. So few are available.
   d. Most are difficult to score.

7. Which procedure requires the patient to repeat the process on several consecutive days?
   a. Interview
   b. Questionnaire
   c. Log
   d. Structured interaction

8. The following item is included on a daily log: "Think about your communication interactions today. Indicate how many times you implemented a facilitative strategy." This item is:
   a. Inappropriate because it contains professional jargon *(facilitative strategy)*
   b. Appropriate because it asks about a specific behavior
   c. Appropriate because it provides information that tells the clinician whether communication strategies training is needed
   d. Inappropriate because the item has active verb tense

9. Three means of assessing conversational fluency or communication difficulties include:
   a. Unstructured communication interactions, the NU-6 Test, and *Dyalog*
   b. Unstructured communication interactions, daily logs, and essays

c. Unstructured communication interactions, structured communication interactions, and bistructured communication interactions

d. Daily logs, questionnaires, and interviews

KEY RESOURCES

THE HEARING HANDICAP INVENTORY FOR THE ELDERLY (HHIE)

(Reproduced with permission by Ventry, I. J., and Weinstein, B. (1982). The hearing handicap inventory for the elderly: A new tool. Ear and Hearing, 3, 128–134.)

Instructions: The purpose of this scale is to identify the problems your hearing loss may be causing. Answer YES, SOMETIMES, or NO for each question. Do not skip a question if you avoid a situation because of your hearing problem. If you use a hearing aid, please answer the way you hear without the aid.

		YES (4)	SOMETIMES (2)	NO (0)
S-1	Does a hearing problem cause you to use the phone less often than you would like?			
E-2	Does a hearing problem cause you to feel embarrassed when meeting new people?			
S-3	Does a hearing problem cause you to avoid groups of people?			
E-4	Does a hearing problem cause make you irritable?			
E-5	Does a hearing problem cause you to feel frustrated when talking to members of your family?			
S-6	Does a hearing problem cause you difficulty when attending a party?			
E-7	Does a hearing problem cause you to feel "stupid" or "dumb"?			
S-8	Do you have difficulty hearing when someone speaks in a whisper?			
E-9	Do you feel handicapped by a hearing problem?			
S-10	Does a hearing problem cause you difficulty when visiting friends, relatives, or neighbors?			
S-11	Does a hearing problem cause you to attend religious services less often than you would like?			
E-12	Does a hearing problem cause you to be nervous?			

continues

	YES (4)	SOMETIMES (2)	NO (0)
S-13 Does a hearing problem cause you to visit friends, relatives, or neighbors less often than you would like?			
E-14 Does a hearing problem cause you to have arguments with your family members?			
S-15 Does a hearing problem cause you difficulty when listening to TV or radio?			
S-16 Does a hearing problem cause you to go shopping less often than you would like?			
S-17 Does any problem or difficulty with your hearing upset you at all?			
S-18 Does a hearing problem cause you to want to be by yourself?			
S-19 Does a hearing problem cause you to talk to family members less often than you would like?			
E-20 Do you feel that any difficulty with your hearing limits or hampers your personal or social life?			
S-21 Does a hearing problem cause you difficulty when in a restaurant with relatives or friends?			
S-22 Does a hearing problem cause you to feel depressed?			
S-23 Does a hearing problem cause you to listen to TV or radio less often than you would like?			
E-24 Does a hearing problem cause you to feel uncomfortable when talking to friends?			
E-25 Does a hearing problem cause you to feel left out when you are with a group of people?			

For clinicians' use only: Total score: _____

Subtotal E: _____

Subtotal S: _____

SELF-ASSESSMENT OF COMMUNICATION (SAC)

(Reprinted by permission from Schow, R. I., and Nerbonne, M. A. (1982). Communication screening profile: Use with elderly clients. Ear and Hearing, 3, 135–147.)

Name _____

Date _____

Raw Score _____ x 2 _____ –20 _____ x 1.25 _____%

Please select the appropriate number ranging from 1 to 5 for the following questions. Circle only one number for each question. If you have a hearing aid, please fill out the form according to how you communicate when the hearing aid is not in use.

DISABILITY

Various Communication Situations

1. Do you experience communication difficulties in situations when speaking with one other person? (for example, at home, at work, in a social situation, with a waitress, a store clerk, a spouse, a boss, etc.)

    (a) almost never (or never)

    (b) occasionally (about $\frac{1}{4}$ of the time)

    (c) about half of the time

    (d) frequently (about $\frac{3}{4}$ of the time)

2. Do you experience communication difficulties in situations when conversing with a small group of several persons? (for example, with friends or family, coworkers, in meetings or casual conversations, over dinner or while playing cards, etc.)

    (a) almost never (or never)

    (b) occasionally (about $\frac{1}{4}$ of the time)

    (c) about half of the time

    (d) frequently (about $\frac{3}{4}$ of the time)

    (e) practically always (or always)

3. Do you experience communication difficulties while listening to someone speak to a large group? (for example, at a church or in a civic meeting, in a fraternal or women's club, at an educational lecture, etc.)

    (a) almost never (or never)

    (b) occasionally (about $\frac{1}{4}$ of the time)

    (c) about half of the time

    (d) frequently (about $\frac{3}{4}$ of the time)

    (e) practically always (or always)

4. Do you experience communication difficulties while participating in various types of entertainment? (for example, movies, TV, radio, plays, night clubs, musical entertainment, etc.)

    (a) almost never (or never)

    (b) occasionally (about $\frac{1}{4}$ of the time)

    (c) about half of the time

    (d) frequently (about $\frac{3}{4}$ of the time)

    (e) practically always (or always)

5. Do you experience communication difficulties when you are in an unfavorable listening environment? (for example, at a noisy party, where there is background music, when riding in an auto or bus, when someone whispers or talks from across the room, etc.)

    (a) almost never (or never)

    (b) occasionally (about ¼ of the time)

    (c) about half of the time

    (d) frequently (about ¾ of the time)

    (e) practically always (or always)

6. Do you experience communication difficulties when using or listening to various communication devices? (for example, telephone, telephone ring, doorbell, public address system, warning signals, alarms, etc.)

    (a) almost never (or never)

    (b) occasionally (about ¼ of the time)

    (c) about half of the time

    (d) frequently (about ¾ of the time)

    (e) practically always (or always)

HANDICAP

Feelings About Communication

7. Do you feel that any difficulty with your hearing limits or hampers your personal or social life?

    (a) almost never (or never)

    (b) occasionally (about ¼ of the time)

    (c) about half of the time

    (d) frequently (about 3/4 of the time)

    (e) practically always (or always)

8. Does any problem or difficulty with your hearing upset you?

    (a) almost never (or never)

    (b) occasionally (about ¼ of the time)

    (c) about half of the time

    (d) frequently (about ¾ of the time)

    (e) practically always (or always)

Other People

9. Do others suggest that you have a hearing problem?

  (a) almost never (or never)

  (b) occasionally (about ¼ of the time)

  (c) about half of the time

  (d) frequently (about ¾ of the time)

  (e) practically always (or always)

10. Do others leave you out of conversations or become annoyed because of your hearing?

  (a) almost never (or never)

  (b) occasionally (about ¼ of the time)

  (c) about half of the time

  (d) frequently (about ¾ of the time)

  (e) practically always (or always)

HANDICAP INVENTORY FOR ADULTS (HHIA)*

Instructions: The purpose of the scale is to identify the problems your hearing may be causing you. Check YES, SOMETIMES, or NO for each question. Do not skip a question if you avoid a situation because of a hearing problem.

		YES (4)	SOMETIMES (2)	NO (0)
S-1	Does a hearing problem cause you to use the phone less often than you would like?			
E-2	Does a hearing problem cause you to feel embarrassed when meeting new people?			
S-3	Does a hearing problem cause you to avoid groups of people?			
E-4	Does a hearing problem make you irritable?			
E-5	Does a hearing problem cause you to feel frustrated when talking to members of your family?			
S-6	Does a hearing problem cause you difficulty when attending a party?			
S-7	Does a hearing problem cause you difficulty hearing/understanding coworkers, clients, or customers?			
E-8	Do you feel handicapped by a hearing problem?			
S-9	Does a hearing problem cause you difficulty when visiting friends, relatives, or neighbors?			

continues

*Reprinted with permission from Newman, C. W., Weinstein, B. E., Jacobson, G. P., et al. (1991). Test–retest reliability of the Hearing Handicap Inventory for Adults. *Ear and Hearing*, 12, 355–357.

		YES (4)	SOMETIMES (2)	NO (0)
E-10	Does a hearing problem cause you to feel frustrated when talking to coworkers, clients, or customers?			
S-11	Does a hearing problem cause you difficulty in the movies or theater?			
E-12	Does a hearing problem cause you to be nervous?			
S-13	Does a hearing problem cause you to visit friends, relatives, or neighbors less often than you would like?			
E-14	Does a hearing problem cause you to have arguments with family members?			
S-15	Does a hearing problem cause you difficulty when listening to TV or radio?			
S-16	Does a hearing problem cause you to go shopping less often than you would like?			
E-17	Does any problem or difficulty with your hearing upset you at all?			
E-18	Does a hearing problem cause you to want to be by yourself?			
S-19	Does a hearing problem cause you to talk to family members less often than you would like?			
E-20	Do you feel that any difficulty with your hearing limits or hampers your personal or social life?			
S-21	Does a hearing problem cause you difficulty when in a restaurant with relatives or friends?			
E-22	Does a hearing problem cause you to feel depressed?			
S-23	Does a hearing problem cause you to listen to TV or radio less often than you would like?			
E-24	Does a hearing problem cause you to feel uncomfortable when talking to friends?			
E-25	Does a hearing problem cause you to feel left out when you are with a group of people?			

For clinicians' use only: Total score: _____

Subtotal E: _____

Subtotal S: _____

CHAPTER 9

Communication Strategies Training

OUTLINE

- Self-efficacy
- Issues to consider when developing a training program
- Getting started
- Model for training
- Short-term training
- Communication strategies training for frequent communication partners
- Communication strategies training for children
- Benefits of training
- Case studies: An increased sense of self-efficacy
- Final remarks
- Key chapter points
- Terms and concepts to remember
- Multiple-choice questions
- Key resources

There are many ways to provide training in the use of communication strategies. Current practices range from simply making printed materials available in the clinic waiting room to presenting a weekly program that may extend several weeks or even months. Training activities may include paper-and-pencil tasks, role-playing, group discussions, and workbook exercises. When possible, the training program is designed to meet the participants' expectations, age, socioeconomic background, lifestyle, and particular communication problems. Often, communication strategies training is one component of a more comprehensive aural rehabilitation program, for instance, as a part of a hearing aid orientation program or an assertiveness training session.

Sensitivity to People's Self-Perceptions

"[Speech and hearing professionals] may find it particularly helpful when working with hard-of-hearing adults and their families to remember that how people perceive communication problems (i.e., their meaning or significance to the people involved) is a very important factor to consider. For example, some hard-of-hearing people believe that, due to their hearing loss, they are a burden on other people, and this belief leads them to withdraw from social contact and also probably leads to depression. As another example, many people believe that hearing aids correct hearing problems to the same degree that glasses correct visual problems. It is difficult for people holding this belief to understand why a person wearing hearing aids does not understand what is being said, and it does not occur to them to think about doing anything else to remedy the situation. So, included in the [communication strategies training] programs I conduct are some ways to help people separate fact from fiction pertaining to hearing loss, and methods for helping hearing-impaired people develop a more realistic appraisal of themselves and their hearing problem" (Trychin, 1994, p. 248).

The content of a communication strategies training program typically concerns problems specifically related to hearing loss and how these problems can be minimized. Content may include training for the two types of communication strategies, facilitative and repair (Chapter 7). Participants typically learn about assertive versus nonassertive behaviors too, and work on developing their skills to deal assertively with communication difficulties (Chapter 10). In this chapter, we will begin with a consideration of self-efficacy and then consider communication strategies training.

SELF-EFFICACY

One goal of a communication strategies training program may be to enhance patients' sense of self-efficacy (Smith & West, 2006). **Self-efficacy** is a belief that one can be successful in performing a task, independent of external odds. It is domain-specific. A person may believe that he or she can swim 100 meters in an Olympic-size swimming pool but not in the open ocean. Self-efficacy may or may not be grounded in a sense of self-worth or in reality. A person may or may not consider oneself a good athlete, and someone who believes that he or she is a great swimmer might sink like a stone in the water.

In aural rehabilitation, self-efficacy refers to the beliefs patients have about their abilities to manage difficult communication situations. One's sense of self-efficacy can influence a patient's willingness to engage in activities and conversations. It can influence the efforts patients will invest into completing an activity and the time that they will devote to an activity or challenging communication situation. The higher the sense of self-efficacy, the more determined and perseverant will be a person in the face of obstacles or challenges. Bolstering self-efficacy beliefs can be accomplished through four types of experiences:

- **Mastery experience:** Direct experience in a successful communication interaction is perhaps the most powerful source of self-efficacy. If a patient practices using a repair strategy many times in a safe and comfortable setting, and often experiences success when doing so, the patient will likely acquire a sense of mastery and high self-efficacy for this task.
- **Vicarious experience:** Direct observation of others succeeding can bolster the patient's belief that he or she too can succeed. If a patient watches two classmates resolve a difficult communication situation effectively, the patient might end up thinking, "Hey, I can do that too."
- **Verbal persuasion:** A clinician might tell or logically explain to the patient that communication difficulties can be managed and that a patient has the tools necessary to manage them.
- **Emotional arousal:** If a patient breaks out into a cold sweat at the very thought of attending a social event, then that patient probably judges his or her self-efficacy to be low. Activities that lower a person's arousal, such as relaxation or breathing activities, might enhance perceived self-efficacy.

Participation in a communication strategies training program may bolster patients' self-efficacy as well as provide patients with concrete means to alleviate communication difficulties.

Self-efficacy is the confidence that a person has for performing a particular task.

To increase self-efficacy with verbal persuasion:

- Use didactic training to explain.
- Provide realistic feedback focused on patient capabilities or effort.
- Encourage the involvement of a significant other.
- Make accurate and convincing comments about the ease of learning the skills.

Quoted in parts from Smith and West (2006, p. 52)

ISSUES TO CONSIDER WHEN DEVELOPING A TRAINING PROGRAM

In developing a training program, one issue to consider is the optimum program length. Some persons will have minimal time to devote to a communication strategies training program, and 1 hour may be all that is available. Standard programs usually require 12 to 40 hours, and are presented in one of two formats. The course may provide intensive instruction during a weekend-long period, meeting 4 to 7 hours per day, or may be spread over an 6- to 15-week period, with each session lasting a couple of hours each week.

Communication strategies training may be provided during a one-on-one class, a couple's session, or in a group. Common wisdom suggests that the most effective means is the group setting, where people interact with other persons who have hearing loss, and also interact with their family members. Defenses and recriminations between a patient and a family member may subside when they recognize that other families share common experiences and when they share solutions with individuals who are in similar situations.

When working with groups, it is important to develop a group spirit and esprit de corps. Table 9-1 presents attributes of a class group where participants receive optimal benefit from participation.

Table 9-1. Attributes of an optimal class spirit.

1. Every class member accepts every other class member with an appreciation of the individual's strengths and a tolerance of the individual's quirks and weaknesses.
2. There is a familiarity of approach among the members of the class, with an awareness of each person's hearing difficulties and backgrounds.
3. Contributions from each class member are encouraged and recognized.
4. Class members can communicate easily with one another, possibly with the use of assistive listening devices.
5. There is acceptance of and conformity to a code of behavior (e.g., "only one person may speak at a time"), usually involving courtesy, mutual respect, and empathy.
6. There is an ability to recognize and use wisely the experiences of individual class members to educate other participants in the class.
7. There is a clear definition of the class agenda and format so each individual knows what to expect.
8. Discussion remains focused, and comments are not made to distract the class.
9. Class members are encouraged to be specific and to use examples.

Source: Adapted from Houle, C. O. (1997). *Governing boards.* San Francisco: Jossey-Bass.

GETTING STARTED

Before the first session, the clinician usually develops a curriculum and collects materials that will be used during the program. Sample curricula include those presented in *Speechreading: A Way to Improve Understanding* (Kaplan, Bally, & Garretson, 1985), *Learning to Hear Again With a Cochlear Implant* (Wayner & Abrahamson, 1998), *Learning to Hear Again* (Wayner & Abrahamson, 1996), and *Active Communication Education (ACE): A Program for Older Persons With Hearing Impairment* (Hickson, Worrall, & Scarina, 2006a). Although a curriculum provides a loose blueprint of what will happen in the class, it should be flexible enough to meet the needs of the class participants. A cardinal rule for a communication strategies training program, or any aural rehabilitation plan, is that it should cater to the specific concerns of the patient(s), experienced at the point of time that he or she engages in the program.

Materials that might be needed to conduct the program may include name tags, handouts, diagrams, whiteboard and whiteboard markers, videotapes, planned communication scenarios for role-playing, FM or infrared system, overhead projector, PowerPoint, snacks, and pencil and paper. The program may include workbooks and homework materials.

A program may begin with setting ground rules for group interactions (e.g., *Only one person speaks at a time. Let us know when you are finished speaking by nodding your head. You have a right to pass on a question. Everything said in this room is confidential.*) It is important to establish a secure and safe environment at the onset of a communication strategies training program so that participants feel comfortable in sharing their feelings and their solutions with one another. The Key Resources presents a class handout for establishing ground rules.

After introductions, for adult patients (and their frequent communication partners, if they are in attendance) a common way to begin a communication strategies training program is to ask participants to identify those situations or predicaments in which they most frequently experience communication difficulties. In a group setting, this may be done by going around the table person by person, asking each one to talk about why he or she is attending the class, and when and where and with whom each experiences communication difficulties. For instance, one person may feel that group meetings at work pose the greatest challenge. Another person may remark that listening to her granddaughter on the telephone is frustrating. These specific examples can be the focus of problem-solving exercises. Participants can brainstorm about how to facilitate communication within specific environments that are problematic for them and how to facilitate communication with specific people they may interact with on a regular basis.

〽 MODEL FOR TRAINING

The model presented in Figure 9-1 provides a framework for conceptualizing the stages of communication strategies training (Tye-Murray, 1992a; modified by Witt, 1997). The first stage entails formal instruction. The second stage centers around guided learning, and the third stage involves real-world practice. In the ideal program, students move through the three stages sequentially, with one stage providing the foundation for the next. Sometimes a student may revisit a previous stage before advancing to the next one, perhaps to review or refresh important concepts.

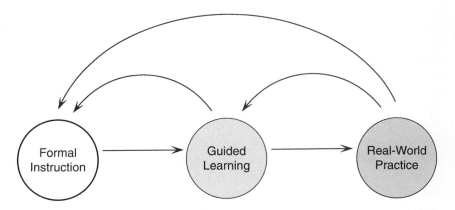

FIGURE 9-1. A framework for conceptualizing the stages of communication strategies training. From S. Witt, 1997, *Effectiveness of an intensive aural rehabilitation program for adult cochlear implant users: A demonstration project.* Unpublished master's thesis, University of Iowa, Iowa City. Reprinted with permission.

Formal Instruction

Formal instruction provides individuals with explicit information about various types of communication strategies and appropriate listening and speaking behaviors; the first stage in a communication strategies training program.

During **formal instruction**, individuals are introduced to the various types of communication strategies and other appropriate listening and speaking behaviors, and they receive examples of each. In a group setting, the speech and hearing professional might ask people to talk about ways they manage their communication difficulties, perhaps in the context of the communication difficulties that the group has just identified. For example, someone in a group might say, "I have difficulty understanding speech in a noisy restaurant. Since I have to eat out a lot as part of my job, this is a big problem." This remark serves as a springboard for a discussion about facilitative strategies. Participants can suggest strategies they have found to be helpful in this specific situation. Their suggestions can lead to a consideration of constructive and instructional strategies. For each solution generated, the group might analyze and evaluate its potential benefits, drawbacks, feasibility, and acceptability. The group leader may also share specific suggestions that were not generated by group members.

Writing participants' ideas and responses on a whiteboard or an oversize hanging notebook can serve to stimulate contributions to an ongoing discussion. Formal instruction usually is most effective when the clinician engages everyone in a dialogue as opposed to making a formal presentation. A long-winded lecture and advice giving will alienate (and anesthetize) participants.

Guided Learning

The purpose of **guided learning** is to encourage people to use conversational strategies in a structured setting. Activities for guided learning include modeling, role-playing, analysis of videotaped scenarios, attention, and continuous discourse tracking. Any number or combination of these activities can be included.

In **guided learning**, the second stage in a communication strategies training program, students use conversational strategies in a structured setting.

Example of a Formal Instruction Training Activity

When sections on passive, aggressive, and assertive behaviors are included in the content of a communication strategies training program, participants must reflect on their own styles of handling communication difficulties and consider alternative, perhaps more effective, styles. Following is a paper-and-pencil exercise from Kaplan, Bally, and Garretson (1985) that asks respondents to identify communication styles exhibited in each situation. Answers and discussion are provided afterward.

A. "Penny entered the office of her boss, the dean. She noticed it was dark and probably it would be hard to speechread. She pushed past the dean's desk (he was sitting at it!) and opened the blinds. Then she sat down and said, 'Let's get this meeting over with.'"

B. "Wilma replaced the battery in her hearing aid and entered the classroom for the course she signed up for, Feminism in the Deaf Community. She immediately noticed that the room was arranged with desk-chairs in a circle. She was relieved to think that this would facilitate speechreading.

continues

Example of a Formal Instruction Training Activity, *continued*

However, when the rapid-fire discussions began, she had difficulty identifying which of the 22 participants was speaking. Although she was really interested in the topic, she dropped the course the next week."

C. "Harry stopped at his instructor's office after the first day of his geometry class. He was feeling really frustrated because he was unable to understand the questions being asked of the instructor by class members in front of him; he couldn't see their lips. The instructor suggested he move to the front row and look back at the questioners. The next day he was back again. 'I still have a problem,' he admitted. 'I can't identify the speaker quickly enough to speechread. Could we ask the questioners to identify themselves by holding up their hands a little bit longer?' Harry was able to follow class discussions after that."

Answers
A. Aggressive. Penny's behavior was both rude and demanding.
B. Passive. Wilma didn't try to solve her problem; she gave up on it.
C. Assertive. Harry recognized his problem and worked it out with his instructor. (pp. 37–38)

Modeling

Modeling is the act of representing or demonstrating a behavior.

Modeling is a technique often used with children and it entails learning by observing. After a formal consideration of effective listening behaviors or communication strategies, a clinician or teacher might demonstrate them through modeling. When modeling, the clinician explicitly points out what is appropriate and inappropriate about the modeled behaviors and does not assume students will automatically recognize this independently. During modeling, the clinician might ask someone in the group or class to help demonstrate the use of a repair strategy. The clinician might pretend to misunderstand a remark spoken by the person and then turn to the group and say, "I didn't understand what she said, did you? I'm going to ask her to tell me what she is talking about." *(The clinician is asking for a key word repair strategy.)* When observing a model, a student might pick up on two kinds of information, (a) information about behaviors or strategies and (b) information about what happens to someone as a result of using these behaviors and strategies; that is, they may experience **vicarious consequences.** By watching vicarious consequences, students might become

When students observe the consequences of a model's behaviors, they experience **vicarious consequences**.

less fearful about implementing communication strategies because they realize that they can use them without incurring negative reactions from others.

Role-Playing

A hypothetical conversational interaction is staged during **role-playing**. Participants practice using communication strategies and other assertive listening behaviors. If possible, the situation parallels one that is relevant to the participants' everyday experiences. Role-playing can heighten patients' sense of self-efficacy in that it provides them with opportunity to experience success in managing communication difficulties.

When the participants are children, a clinician might set up a fast-food restaurant. The student is charged with ordering dinner for the family. The clinician might occasionally speak with inappropriate speaking behaviors, such as mumbling or speaking in profile. The student must respond to the questions, and when necessary, use facilitative and repair strategies to promote communication. At the end of a role-playing interaction, the clinician and classmates review it. They talk about what happened, what worked and what did not work, and what communication strategies were implemented.

Role-playing may involve direct instruction, **prompting**, **shaping**, reinforcement, modeling, and feedback. The following interchange between a clinician and an adult patient illustrates each of these components of role-playing, even though the patient is not told explicitly that he will be engaging in "role-playing" per se. Some adults balk at the idea of role-playing. Such an interaction might occur in a group setting or in a one-on-one situation:

Clinician:	Suppose you're at a group meeting at work. You miss something the boss says and you think it's probably important. What might you say?
Bennet:	I don't know. I haven't ever told him about my hearing loss before, we just don't talk about it, although he probably knows I miss hearing things.
Clinician:	Pretend that I'm your boss and there are two more people at the table here. I've just asked you a question but you didn't understand what I said. What might you say to me?
Bennet:	I'm not very good at this.
Clinician:	This is just practice, go ahead, give it a try. [*prompting*]
Bennet:	(grins a mischievous smile) I think that's a good idea. [*role-playing*]

In **role-playing**, individuals participate in hypothetical real-world situations and interactions.

Prompting serves to inspire a behavior or an utterance; a technique designed to assist an individual in formulating or remembering a remark.

Shaping serves to reinforce those conversational turns that increasingly approximate sought-after behaviors.

Clinician:	You're agreeing with me even though you aren't sure what I said. You might be sorry about that if I said something you don't agree with. [*feedback*] Let's see if we can try using one of the repair strategies that we talked about earlier. [*shaping*] There's no need to bluff. [*direct instruction*] See if you can try something like this: 'I was looking at my handout here and missed the last part of what you asked. Can you say that part again?' [*modeling*]
Bennet:	That sounds okay.
Clinician:	Can you try saying something like this?
Bennet:	Okay, let's see. .I didn't get the first part. . . .
Clinician:	So what would you say?
Bennet:	I missed all of that. Could you please repeat that? [*role-playing*]
Clinician:	Much better. [*reinforcement*] That was a direct request for what you need. [*feedback*]

In this example, the person with hearing loss both has received instruction about how to handle a difficult communication interaction and has practiced implementing the suggestions. Chances are that when the opportunity arises to signal a communication breakdown in a real-world setting, Bennet will be less anxious and less fearful than he would have been otherwise and have a greater sense of self-efficacy. As this example illustrates, role-playing allows a patient to practice feared behaviors without incurring negative consequences.

Attention

The clinician can reinforce formal instruction by focusing group members' attention on both identifying and rectifying environmental problems and on reinforcing appropriate talker behaviors. For instance, a man with hearing loss and his wife with normal hearing might be participants in the class. Before speaking, the wife might flicker her fingers and ensure that her husband has turned toward her and is watching her mouth. The clinician might observe to the group, "That was an effective strategy in helping him to speechread. She got his attention first, before speaking, so he could watch her lips."

Analysis of Videotapes and Computer-Based Interactions

Videotaped scenarios provide examples of communication interactions that can be used to stimulate discussion about communication strategies.

Videotaped scenarios help patients identify and talk about their communication problems by providing concrete examples. Individuals view videotaped scenarios that contrast inappropriate with appropriate use of communication strategies. For instance, one scenario might show a couple in the living room. One person has a hearing loss; the other one does not. The person with normal hearing talks behind a newspaper to the other one. The person with hearing loss accuses the talker of mumbling and leaves the room in anger. The videotape is stopped at this point so that the class can discuss how the person might have effectively implemented an instructional strategy in this context. After the discussion, the class views a second videotape scenario, where the person with hearing loss demonstrates how to use an instructional facilitative strategy appropriately.

Continuous Discourse Tracking

Continuous discourse tracking is another means to provide guided learning. In **continuous discourse tracking** (DeFillipo & Scott, 1978), the clinician or a frequent communication partner plays the role of **sender** and the patient plays the role of **receiver**. The sender reads a selection from a book, phrase by phrase. After each phrase, the receiver attempts to repeat it verbatim. If the receiver cannot recognize it, then he or she must bear the

Continuous discourse training is an aural rehabilitation technique in which the listener attempts to repeat verbatim text presented by a sender.

The **sender** is the participant in a continuous discourse training session who presents the message.

The **receiver** is the participant in a continuous discourse training session who receives the message and attempts to repeat it back.

Example of a Guided Learning Training Activity

After the patient views the picture in Figure 9-2, a clinician will ask him or her to perform a continuous discourse tracking procedure, with the clinician assuming the role of sender and the patient assuming the role of receiver. The following passage corresponds to the picture (Figure 9-2). The sender reads it sentence by sentence, and the receiver attempts to repeat it verbatim. When unable to do so, the sender encourages the receiver to use a repair strategy, and request an alteration of the passage so that it can be tracked correctly.

PASSAGE: At Camp Eagle, children learn how to ride horses. Every morning, they arrive at the barn and saddle their mounts. They fall in line behind their camp counselor. The morning ride lasts about four hours. They ride through the forest. Sometimes they pass a lake. Other times, they ride into the mountains. Halfway through the ride, they stop and eat a hearty breakfast. The camp counselor prepares the breakfast over a campfire.

This is what might happen during a continuous discourse tracking exercise:

Sender: At Camp Eagle, children learn how to ride horses.

Receiver: Something about children and horses.

continues

Example of a Guided Learning Training Activity, *continued*

Sender:	Yes. Children learn how to ride horses.
Receiver:	Children learn how to ride horses.
Sender:	(nods) At Camp Eagle, children learn how to ride horses.
Receiver:	Didn't get that first part.
Sender:	Camp.
Receiver:	Camp?
Sender:	(nods) At Camp Eagle . . .
Receiver:	At Camp Eagle?
Sender:	At Camp Eagle, children learn how to ride horses.
Receiver:	At Camp Eagle, children learn how to ride horses.
Sender:	Every morning . . .
Receiver:	Every morning . . .
Sender:	(Presents rest of the sentence)

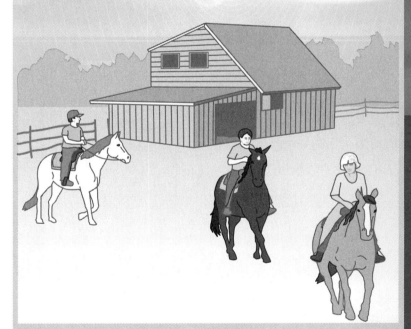

FIGURE 9-2. A picture that provides a context for a continuous discourse tracking task.

onus of repair and be responsible for using a repair strategy. For instance, the receiver may say, "Can you tell me in a different way?" The instructor provides coaching and suggestions in how to select and implement particular repair strategies effectively. In group settings, participants can pair up and practice the activity for a set period of time.

Real-World Practice

The final stage of the training model shown in Figure 9-1 is real-world practice. **Real-world practice** includes activities that students have performed successfully in the classroom and also some activities that require them to communicate in a setting that is highly motivating, such as the office or a social gathering. Individuals can report back to the class about their successes and problems, and they can share ideas of how to handle problems in the future. Instructions for the activity can be provided to the students in written form, in language that is simple and easily understood. The students might have a means to record their experiences and to share them later with their instructor and other members of their communication strategies training group.

An adult might maintain a calendar like that shown in Table 9-2. The days of the week are listed in the left-most column, and the patient's frequent communication partners are listed in the row across the top. The patient's task is to indicate when he or she repaired a breakdown in communication by asking the communication partner for a repair. After 1 week, the group leader or the group as a whole can review the calendar with the patient.

"Therapists often ask me for suitable texts for continuous discourse tracking. My response is always to look at fiction written for older children and teenagers. Books from the *Harry Potter* series are an obvious example. These usually 'read' well when they are spoken, and sound quite natural. Most adult fiction, on the other hand, bears little resemblance to the realities of everyday conversational speech."

Geoff Plant, aural rehabilitation specialist

(Personal communication, June 15, 2007)

In **real-world practice**, students practice a new skill or behavior in an everyday environment.

Table 9-2. A calendar for recording a real-world practice activity.

When Did you repair a Communication Breakdown?

	WIFE	SON	SISTER	CO-WORKER
Monday	At dinner			Eating lunch in cafeteria
Tuesday		Watching TV		Weekly meeting
Wednesday		Watching TV		On telephone
Thursday	On the drive home from shopping			
Friday			In the car	
Saturday				
Sunday				

Example of a Real-World Training Activity

Topic = Listening for Directions

Instructions: Ask a partner to hide an object somewhere in your house. Then ask your partner for directions for finding it. Only listen as the directions are told to you, and ask for clarification if necessary. After finding the object, answer the following questions:

1. Did you understand the directions?
2. Did you ask for clarification about any part of the directions? If yes, what did you say? How did your partner respond?
3. Did you have any problems in finding the object? If yes, did you ask for more information from your partner? What did you say?

SHORT-TERM TRAINING

For many reasons, an extended program such as the one we have considered may not be feasible. A person may not have time to commit to a longer program, or the clinic may not have the personnel available to conduct training. In these situations, short-term approaches are available for providing brief communication strategies training. One approach is to provide materials and self-directed instruction. Another approach is to provide a short tutorial.

Materials Approach

The *materials approach* for providing communication strategies training during a brief time interval includes providing printed and recorded materials to the patient and frequent communication partner about communication strategies. This might be accomplished by means of a clinic library, an audio-videotape station, and printed pamphlets.

The library can be established in a small room adjacent to the clinic waiting room or in the waiting area itself. It might include periodicals and books about hearing loss, communication strategies, speech and auditory training activities, and assistive devices. The materials can be read in the waiting room before or after an appointment, or even checked out and returned by mail. A DVD player also might be placed in the library or waiting room. Individuals can view commercially available videos about hearing loss and communication strategies.

Short Tutorial

Another way to provide a brief communication strategies training program is by means of a short tutorial. **WATCH** is an acronym that Montgomery (1994) coined to describe his short-tutorial communication strategies training program. This program requires about 1 hour to administer. The acronym represents the following concepts:

W = Watch the talker's mouth, not his eyes.

A = Ask specific questions.

T = Talk about your hearing loss.

C = Change the situation.

H = Acquire health care knowledge.

The clinician discusses with the patient each of these concepts in this order.

During the "W" component, the clinician encourages the patient to focus on the talker's mouth for speechreading, as opposed to hand gestures or other items in the communication setting.

During the "A" component, the patient is encouraged to use specific rather than nonspecific repair strategies. A clinician might dramatize this point by speaking with a low voice or slurred speech, and then ask the person to use specific repair strategies.

During the "T" component of the program, the clinician discusses the importance of revealing a hearing loss to one's communication partners. A patient can then manage the communication interaction more effectively and implement instructional strategies.

The clinician asks the patient to identify situations in which communication is problematic during the "C" component. Together, they consider possible ways to overcome these problems.

Finally, the clinician provides information about health care and hearing loss resources during the "H" component of the program.

A short program such as WATCH may not always result in a momentous change in how a patient uses communication strategies. However, much of the program's value lies in the fact that simple ideas have been reviewed. The individual might reflect on these ideas and develop them or even become motivated to enroll in a more extended communication strategies training program.

WATCH is an acronym for an example of a short-tutorial program of communication strategies training.

SPEECH

The acronym SPEECH presents a short tutorial about communication strategies for frequent communication partners (Schow, 2001, p. 20):

- **S**potlight your face and keep it visible. Keep your hands away from your mouth so that the hearing-impaired person can get all the visual cues possible. Be sure to face the speaker when you are talking and be at a good distance (5–10 feet). Avoid chewing gum, cigarettes, and other facial distractions when possible. And be sure not to talk from another room and expect to be heard.
- **P**ause slightly between the content portions of sentences. Slow exaggerated speech is as difficult to understand as fast speech. However, speech at a moderate pace with slight pauses between phrases and sentences can allow the hearing-impaired person to process the information in chunks.
- **E**mpathize and be patient with the hearing-impaired person. Try plugging both ears and listen for a short while to something soft that you want to hear in an environment that is distracting and noisy. This may help you appreciate the challenge of being hard of hearing and it should help you be patient if the responses seem slow. Rephrase if necessary to clarify a point and remember, empathy, patience, empathy!
- **E**ase their listening. Get the listener's attention before you speak and make sure you are being helpful in the way you speak. Ask how you can facilitate communication. The listener may want you to speak more loudly or more softly, more slowly or faster, or announce the subject of discussion, or signal when the topic of conversation shifts. Be compliant and helpful and encourage the listener to give you feedback so you can make it as easy as possible for him or her.
- **C**ontrol the circumstances and the listening conditions in the environment. Maximize communication by getting closer to the person. If you can be 5 to 10 feet away, that is ideal. Also, move away from background noise and maintain good lighting. Avoid dark restaurants or windows behind you that blind someone watching you.
- **H**ave a plan. When anticipating difficult listening situations, set strategies for communication in advance and implement them as necessary. This might mean that at a restaurant you communicate with the wait staff instead of having your hard-of-hearing family member or friend do so.

COMMUNICATION STRATEGIES TRAINING FOR FREQUENT COMMUNICATION PARTNERS

Two parents, Mrs. Ansley and Mrs. Kemp, were asked to instruct their children (cochlear implant users) to perform simple tasks, including unwrapping a mint candy (Tye-Murray, 1994b, pp. 89–90; Tye-Murray & Kelsey, 1993). Each parent and her child sat before a table that held a variety of objects. The goal of the investigation was to determine what would happen in those instances that children misunderstood instructions. Would the parents repeat the message? If so, would these repetitions help their child to recognize the instruction?

In both instances, neither child understood the instruction, *Unwrap the mint,* after their mothers presented it for the first time. Here is what happened next.

After saying it the first time, Mrs. Ansley repeated the original instruction, "Unwrap the mint." Her daughter, Libby, picked up a red block and threw it gently. "Unwrap the mint," Mrs. Ansley repeated again. Libby gave her a puzzled expression. "Unwrap the mint," her mother said again. Libby picked up a cup and set it on a cardboard box. "No, unwrap the mint." Libby shook a sheet of plastic. "Unwrap the mint," her mother said in response. This interchange continued for 1 minute, until Mrs. Ansley gave up trying to convey the instruction.

In this interaction, the repeat repair strategy was ineffective. No matter how many times Mrs. Ansley repeated the instruction, Libby never understood that she was to unwrap the candy.

The second mother, Mrs. Kemp, adopted a different tack. When her son, Tim, did not understand the instruction, she used different words and said, "Take the paper off the candy." When he still did not comprehend the instruction, Mrs. Kemp said, "Tim, where's the candy?" Tim picked up the mint. "Open it," Mrs. Kemp instructed. Tim looked at his mother and started to open the candy. "Mmmm," she said encouragingly, "Open it." Tim then unwrapped the mint.

Unlike Mrs. Ansley, Mrs. Kemp used repair strategies other then repetition. She rephrased the instruction (i.e., "Take the paper off the candy."), she emphasized an important key word ("Where's the *candy?*"), and provided feedback when her son began to understand the message ("Mmmm."). By using a variety of repair strategies, she was able to convey the message successfully.

This investigation, which also included other parents of cochlear implant users, illustrates two important points. First, the repeat repair strategy is not always the optimal strategy to use in repairing communication breakdowns (Chapter 7). Second, frequent communication partners often do not have an implicit knowledge of communication strategies, even if they have lived with a person with hearing loss for many years. This is true of spouses and significant others as well as parents and guardians.

People with whom a person with hearing loss converses frequently also may benefit from receiving communication strategies training. A frequent communication partner may be a spouse, a son or daughter, a close friend, or a health care provider. If the patient is a child, this person may be a parent or guardian. The goals of communication strategies training for frequent communication partners are to foster empathy for the difficulty of the speechreading task, encourage the use of appropriate speaking behaviors, learn how to tailor messages so they are easy to recognize, and learn how to repair communication breakdowns effectively. Table 9-3 summarizes topics that may be reviewed.

Table 9-3. Content that may be included in a communication strategies training program for frequent communication partners.

Appropriate Speaking Behaviors

Frequent communication partners may be encouraged to:

- Speak clearly and slowly.
- Speak with their faces toward the hard-of-hearing individual.
- Avoid putting objects in or near their mouths while speaking.
- Stand away from windows or bright light sources when talking to someone who has a hearing loss.

Empathy

Frequent communication partners may be asked to consider:

- The difficulty of the speech recognition task when one must rely on a degraded audio signal, perhaps with the use of filtered speech samples.
- The difficulty of the lipreading task.
- How stress and anxiety levels may rise when someone has a hearing loss, and how persons with hearing loss often may experience fatigue and desire social withdrawal.

Organized Messages

Frequent communication partners may be asked to:

- Avoid verbosity, and to use concise and syntactically simple sentences. For example, they might say, "Let's go to a movie," rather than "I haven't really thought much about it, but I know we aren't doing much on Saturday, so maybe let's go to a movie."
- Avoid ambiguity by using precise terminology. For example, they may say, "The sweater is Sarah's," rather than, "It's hers."

Comprehension

Frequent communication partners may be encouraged to:

- Ask their partner often if he or she comprehended a message.
- Ask for verification and listen to the person with hearing loss repeat or paraphrase what they have just said.
- Provide feedback about whether the individual correctly recognized the message.

Table 9-3. *continued*

Repair of Communication Breakdowns

The frequent communication partner may receive coaching about how to use repair strategies optimally. Following a communication breakdown, they might:

- Repeat their messages.
- Rephrase their messages, and say it in a different way. For example, the sentence, "I left," might be rephrased as "I went home."
- Repeat a key word to indicate the topic of conversation. For example, if the sentence "Tom fell down" was not recognized, the communication partner might repair the communication breakdown by saying, "Tom. Tom fell down."
- Simplify the message by using fewer words or by using more commonplace words. For example, the sentence, "Jane bought a brown bowler hat" might be simplified to "Jane bought a hat."
- Elaborate, by providing more information and repeating important key words. For instance if the sentence, "I cut the paper" was misunderstood, the frequent communication partner might say, "I have some scissors. I cut the paper with the scissors."
- Build from the known by presenting information that can easily be recognized to establish a context. For instance, the original sentence might have been, "Please put the wallet in my purse." In repairing a communication breakdown, the communication partner might say, "Please put the wallet [and then point to the wallet] in my purse" (with a gesture toward a purse).

Communication strategies training for frequent communication partners often is provided at the same time that the patient receives training, frequently within the same class. In addition to receiving communication strategies training, they also may receive support and counseling from the speech and hearing professional about adjusting to the changes in life quality that occur because of their relatives' or friends' hearing losses.

Hearing Loss Affects More Than the Patient

Frequent communication partners often detect changes in their life quality after the patient incurs a hearing loss (Stephens & Hétu, 1991). Sometimes they report feeling stressed by excessive noise in the home, such as a loud television volume or loud speaking. They may experience annoyance, irritation, or tension as a result of this noise and also as a result of recurring misunderstandings between themselves and the person with hearing loss. Social interactions outside the home may decrease, and feelings of social isolation and loneliness may set in. The frequent communication partner also may have to assume extra tasks

continues

Hearing Loss Affects More Than the Patient, *continued*

as a result of the patient's hearing loss, such as interpreting for the person during group conversations or acting as intermediary for the person's telephone calls. In many cases, communication strategies training, along with counseling, can enhance and accelerate the adjustment process that frequent communication partners may have to undergo.

Spouses of persons who have hearing loss or frequent communication partners can learn how to speak with clear speech. In one study, one spouse received instruction about clear speech, which included a description of clear speech (including a discussion of speech rate, precise articulation, pausing, and key word emphasis) (Caissie, Campbell, Frenette, Scott, Howell, & Roy, 2005). He also listened to demonstrations. He then was provided with an opportunity to practice speaking with clear speech and was given feedback about his performance. He was encouraged to practice clear speech for 1 week with his wife who has hearing loss, and he received an information booklet describing the procedures. A second spouse who participated in the study was merely told to "speak clearly." Recordings of the two men's speech were presented to a group of 15 research participants who had normal hearing and 15 research participants who had hearing loss. The results showed that the utterances spoken by the talker who had received training were significantly more intelligible than those by the talker who had received no training, and this was especially true for the participants who had hearing loss. These results suggest that the aural rehabilitation plan might routinely include clear-speech training for frequent communication partners.

COMMUNICATION STRATEGIES TRAINING FOR CHILDREN

Children with hearing loss also may benefit from communication strategies training. This kind of training is usually appropriate for children in the higher grades of elementary school or in junior high school or high school. Some of the concepts underlying communication strategies training may be too abstract for children in lower grades to understand.

Formal instruction for children might include a review of effective listening behaviors (e.g., *Pay attention, Watch the talker's face, Try to identify key points*) and how to ask talkers to clarify a message (e.g., *When you don't understand a message, ask the talker to say just one word. This will tell you what he or she is talking about.*). During guided learning, children might watch the clinician or classroom teacher demonstrate the desired behavior and then try to imitate it. Teacher-made or commercially available books might be used to provide vicarious consequences. For instance, the drawings in Figure 9-3 present sample pages from a teacher-made story about a young

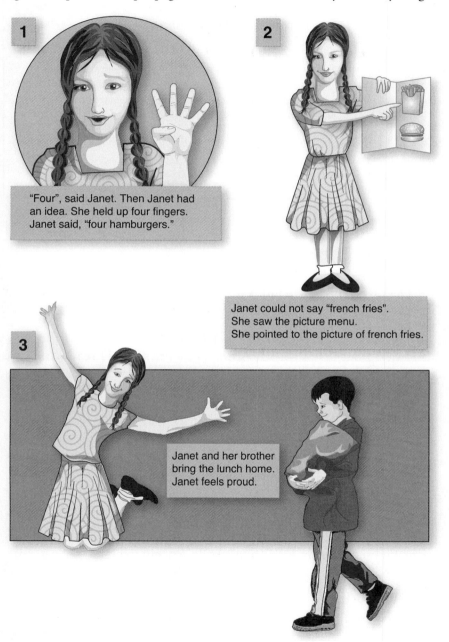

1

"Four", said Janet. Then Janet had an idea. She held up four fingers. Janet said, "four hamburgers."

2

Janet could not say "french fries". She saw the picture menu. She pointed to the picture of french fries.

3

Janet and her brother bring the lunch home. Janet feels proud.

FIGURE 9-3. Sample pages from a teacher-made book about expressive repair strategies. In the story, "Janet," who has a hearing loss, is ordering lunch from a fast-food restaurant.

Table 9-4. Guidelines for developing real-world practice activities for children.

A. Assign a real-world practice activity that the child has performed successfully during guided learning practice.
If the child is to ask someone to repeat a message following a communication breakdown, the youth first should practice asking for clarification in the classroom or clinical setting. Then the child can be asked to attempt the strategy in, for example, art class. Although not necessary, the art teacher can be briefed beforehand that the child will practice repair strategies with her or him.

B. Select a communication situation in which the child will feel motivated to communicate.
For instance, a young child might be asked to use repair strategies when ordering food at a fast-food restaurant.

C. Select an interaction that allows the child to experience some success.
For example, you might ask the child to interact with a familiar teacher before asking the youth to try using repair strategies with an unfamiliar store clerk.

D. Provide instructions for the activity. Present the instructions with simple language and vocabulary.
The purpose of a homework activity might be to listen for the main points of a one-paragraph narrative. The clinician might provide the following written instructions:

This envelope contains a story. Ask your mother to read it to you. Watch and listen carefully. If you do not understand the story, ask questions. Draw a picture about the story.

E. Provide a means for the child to record the experience.
In the activity described in Item D above, the record is the child's drawing.

Source: Adapted from Glennon, S. L. (1990). Homework activities for social skills training. In P. J. Schloss & M. A. Smith (Eds.), *Teaching social skills to hearing-impaired students* (pp. 85–90). Washington, DC: Alexander Graham Bell Association for the Deaf.

girl who used expressive repair strategies successfully while placing an order at a fast-food restaurant. A teacher and her class might review similar materials before a field trip that includes a lunch outing.

Real-world practice activities help children transfer their use of communication strategies to natural settings. Activities should require them to interact with different talkers, in a variety of contexts. Guidelines for developing real-world activities for children are presented in Table 9-4.

In addition to learning how to use facilitative and receptive repair strategies, children also can learn to use expressive repair strategies. Expressive repair strategies may be appropriate to use when the child presents a message, usually with speech, and the communication partner does not recognize it. The child then repairs the communication breakdown, perhaps by trying again using his or her best speech or by adding hand gestures.

Table 9-5 summarizes a five-step training plan of action for teaching children to use expressive repair strategies (Elfenbein, 1994). Formal instruction and guided learning occurs during the first four steps. Real-world practice is provided in the fifth step.

In this plan, children begin by reviewing principles of basic communication processes and consider the sender–message–receiver relationship and the various ways of communicating. Children may create a book about the ways people communicate, tearing pictures from old magazines for

Table 9-5. Five-step plan of action for teaching children to use communication strategies.

Step 1. Understanding Basic Communication Processes
A. Sender–message–receiver relationship
B. Ways to communicate (e.g., speech, sign, writing, mime, gesture)
Step 2. Understanding Communication Breakdowns
A. Definitions and examples
B. Causes of communication breakdown
C. Ways people signal confusion
Step 3. Message Formulation
A. Information to be transmitted
B. Evaluation of the receiver's position (e.g., background knowledge)
C. Evaluation of sender's abilities (e.g., speech proficiency)
D. Environmental constraints (e.g., background noise)
E. Social constraints (e.g., conventions of politeness and etiquette)
Step 4. Introduction of Communication Repair Strategies
A. Receiver's responsibilities
1. Acknowledge confusion
2. Identify causes of breakdown
3. Implement receptive repair strategies
B. Sender's responsibilities
1. Be alert to signals of confusion
2. Identify causes of a communication breakdown
3. Implement expressive repair strategies
Step 5. Practice Using Communication Repair Strategies
A. Move from sheltered environments to the real world
B. Move from transmission of simple to complex more complex messages
C. Discuss feelings associated with communication breakdown

Source: Adapted from Elfenbein, J. (1994). Communication breakdowns in conversations: Child-initiated repair strategies. In N. Tye-Murray (Ed.), *Let's converse: A how-to guide to develop and expand the conversational skills of children and teenagers who are hearing impaired* (pp. 123–146). Washington, DC: Alexander Graham Bell Association for the Deaf.

illustrations. Step 2 entails talking about communication breakdown: What happens when a breakdown occurs? How can you tell that it has happened? Why did it happen? Here, children might generate a list of the ways that people signal a breakdown. In Step 3, the group leader asks the children to consider how best to formulate and transmit their messages. This entails considering the needs of the communication partner, such as how much information the receiver already has. For instance, if the child talks about last summer's vacation, will the receiver recognize the locale? The fourth step introduces expressive repair strategies, and children practice revising their own messages using different words and practice modifying their listening environments (e.g., turning off a radio). One of the most important messages conveyed during this step is that children share responsibility in managing their conversational interactions, and they have a variety of options available to them for rectifying their communication breakdowns. The final step provides practice in using repair strategies. At this time, children might talk about their feelings and responses to communication breakdown. Often, it is reassuring to learn that their classmates have experienced similar frustration and embarrassment following a communication breakdown. In practicing repair strategies, children progress through increasingly difficult settings: role-playing, then sheltered environments, such as talking to the school administrative assistant, then real-world situations.

BENEFITS OF TRAINING

Few experimental investigations have focused on the benefits of communication strategies training. The reason for this is probably because communication strategies training is often packaged together with a hearing aid orientation program or a counseling and psychosocial adjustment class. Rarely does the entire content of an aural rehabilitation program consist of communication strategies training. It is also difficult to gauge changes in communication strategy usage (Chapter 8). Many studies have reported a reduction in perceived hearing-related disability following a counseling- and communication-strategies-based aural rehabilitation program (e.g., Abrams, Hnath-Chisolm, Guerro, & Ritterman, 1992; Benyon, Thornton, & Poole, 1997; Chisolm, Abrams, & McArdle, 2004; Heydebrand, Mauzé, Tye-Murray, Binzer, & Skinner, 2005; Hickson, Worrall, & Scarinci, 2006; Kramer, Allessie, Dondorp, Zekveld, & Kapteyn, 2005; Preminger, 2003; Primeau, 1997). A few have not (e.g., Kricos, Holmes, & Doyle, 1992) and some have reported mixed results (e.g., Brewer, 2001). Brewer (see also Hawkins, 2005) suggests that one reason for this variability in findings may relate, in part, to the use of standardized or non-patient-specific measures of handicap and disability rather than some index of how patients perceive their individual communication challenges.

Research that suggests benefit generally can be categorized as showing (a) good patient participation, (b) change in communication strategies usage, or (c) change in perceived hearing-related disability.

Good Patient Participation

Abrahamson (1991) reported that 89% of the patients who began a 6-week communication strategies training program completed it. Attendance rates at the classes averaged 85%. Their willingness to stay with the program suggests that participants benefited from it. Similarly, Hickson et al. (2006)

provided a program called *Active Communication Education (ACE)* to 96 adults aged 58 to 94 years. The 5-week program (2 hours per week) commenced with a communication needs analysis for each patient (and the patient's frequent communication partner) and then focused on developing individual problem-solving skills, including ways to analyze the source of difficulty, identify potential solutions, and practice communication strategies. More than 50% of the participants reported that the ACE program was "very much worth the trouble" in response to a questionnaire.

Change in Communication Strategies Usage

One investigation showed that patients changed how they used repair strategies after participating in a communication strategies training program that concentrated on repair strategy use (Tye-Murray, 1991). Following training, subjects began to use the repair strategies they found were especially helpful during their training sessions. For example, if during the course of training an individual found that asking for the topic of conversation helped him or her to understand an unrecognized message, then the individual was more likely to begin using that strategy.

Chisolm et al. (2004) also found improvement, on average, in the use of communication strategies (i.e., anticipatory, repair, and constructive) by 53 veterans who had received new hearing aids and who had participated in a 4-week aural rehabilitation program. Measures were obtained 6 months following the program's end. The 53 participants in the control group showed no such improvement.

Change in Perceived Hearing-Related Disability

Benyon et al. (1997) measured "handicap," which relates to hearing-related disability. The researchers showed that 21 first-time hearing aid users who participated in a 4-week program in aural rehabilitation had a larger reduction in perceived handicap as compared to 26 first-time hearing aid users who did not participate.

Benefits for Children

A few investigations have focused on the benefits of communication strategies training for children. In one study, 20 children with hearing loss, who ranged in age between 8 and 11 years, were asked to request an item from a clerk (Elfenbein, 1992). Before participation in the communication strategies program described in detail in this chapter, only three of the children were able to obtain the target object prior to training. They

"This client drove 65 miles and stayed overnight in a motel before each class, reporting that he never knew when he'd be too dizzy to drive and didn't want to miss a class. A year later he reported spending more time with his family. He had avoided them for many years because of his hearing." (p. 47)

Judy Abrahamson, instructor for the *Living With Hearing Loss* program

(Abrahamson, 1991, p. 47)

used a combination of pointing, drawing, and writing. Following participation, 16 of the 20 children met with success. They demonstrated the following changes: "increased responsibility for initiating and managing repair, better matching of strategy to situation, greater variety of strategies used, and improved assessment of partner's viewpoint" (p. 28). In contrast, Baylock, Scudder, and Wynne (1995) selected the *showing* repair strategy from Elfenbein's menu of repair strategies (1994) and provided training for 10 minutes per day, 4 days per week for 4 weeks to 10 children who ranged in age from 4 to 9 years. The children did not use this strategy more than did the 10 children in a control group following training.

CASE STUDY

An Increased Sense of Self-Efficacy

Backenroth and Ahlner (2000) compiled a set of case studies from a group of 30 individuals with moderate to severe hearing loss who had participated in a group aural rehabilitation program. The program included counseling and communication strategies training. In general, consequences stemming from their hearing losses included limited participation in recreational activities, avoidance of social interactions, and recurrent irritations within the family. Following the aural rehabilitation program, a majority reported a "more relaxed relationship with their hearing-impairment" and a sense of having "learned to live with it" (p. 228). Several expressed an increased sense of self-efficacy. The investigators noted a problem that is not atypical. It is often difficult to convince adults with hearing loss to sign up for communication strategies training because they do not appreciate its value. Yet, once they enroll, they realize the benefits.

Case Study 1 was a 54-year-old woman who worked as a counselor. She reported that her hearing loss was linked to communication difficulties at work, at home, and at social functions. When asked of her expectations of the aural rehabilitation program, she responded, "I didn't have any high expectations of the audiological rehabilitation and I was hard to convince. I didn't think I needed any rehabilitation. . . . The audiologist convinced me to participate" (p. 228). After the program, she noted that she had received practical information about how to inform others about her hearing loss. "I now inform colleagues at my work place . . . The main outcomes of the rehabilitation [are] (a) I have become aware of the hearing impairment and allow myself to be fooled less; (b) I now feel more comfortable when using [a] hearing aid; (c) I dare to talk about my hearing impairment and demand more of others; (d) I have gained insight into the reasons for my tiredness; and (e) I generally [feel] supported by people who understand" (p. 229).

Case Study 3, a self-employed 42-year-old male, also expressed reluctance. "I didn't have any high expectations. I was rather skeptical about taking part in a 3-week rehabilitation program, as I run my own business." Although he acknowledged that hearing loss affected his family and social life, he claimed that, "My hearing loss has not affected my work situation." He then went on to add, "I work fewer hours now" (p. 231), suggesting that he had indeed made accommodations because of hearing loss. He expressed satisfaction with the outcome

continues

CASE STUDY, *continued*

An Increased Sense of Self-Efficacy, *continued*

of aural rehabilitation: "I gained further insight into my hearing impairment . . . I think differently. I understand my situation better, for example that I have difficulty in following group conversations. Before I thought I was the only one . . . I gained better self-confidence" (p. 232).

Finally, Case Study 5, a 50-year-old male, credited his spouse for his participation: "I didn't have any great expectations. I was persuaded to participate—my wife 'dragged' me there!" (p. 233). His hearing loss, like the other two case studies, affected his everyday life. "My interactions in groups are influenced," he told the interviewer. "I don't participate at big dinner parties or work lunches. I do not enjoy a good social life as I cannot hear." Following his participation, his sense of self-efficacy had grown. He told the interviewer, "I have increased self-confidence. I have the confidence to remind others about my hearing loss and ask them to make allowances" (p. 234).

FINAL REMARKS

Communication strategies training can empower patients to manage their communication environments more effectively. However, individuals will vary in the willingness to participate and in the extent to which they benefit. Some individuals are incapable of changing their communication behaviors. Some do not have the metacommunication skills to examine their conversational styles and may not be able to monitor how they interact with their communication partners, regardless of the quality or amount of instruction. For example, an elderly woman might not use communication strategies and might deal with communication problems with excessive aggression, but these behaviors are a part of her personality and likely will not change with aural rehabilitation intervention. In these instances, it is critical that individuals who interact frequently with patients receive instruction as well.

KEY CHAPTER POINTS

- A communication strategies training program should be tailored to accommodate a patient's expectations, age, socioeconomic background, lifestyle, and particular communication problems.

- The content of a communication strategies training program centers around problems specifically related to hearing loss and how these problems can be minimized. Training may be provided for facilitative and repair communication strategies. Patients may also consider assertive versus nonassertive listening behaviors.

- One model for a training program includes three stages: formal instruction, guided learning, and real-world practice. A variety of exercises and activities can be used for each stage.

- Modeling, which entails learning through observing, allows patients to acquire information about effective communication behaviors and strategies and to acquire information about what happens to someone as a result of using these behaviors and strategies.

- Role-playing may involve direct instruction, prompting, shaping, reinforcement, modeling, and feedback.

- A communication strategies training program for children can include instruction for the use of expressive repair strategies in addition to the use of receptive repair strategies and facilitative communication strategies.

- Many persons who participate in communication strategies training develop an enhanced sense of self-efficacy in dealing with their communication difficulties.

TERMS AND CONCEPTS TO REMEMBER

Self-efficacy
Class format
Dialogue versus lecture
Modeling
Vicarious consequences
Role-playing
Videotaped scenarios
Continuous discourse tracking
Record of experiences
WATCH
Appropriate speaking behaviors
Expressive repair strategies training

MULTIPLE-CHOICE QUESTIONS

1. When designing a communication strategies training program (select the statement that best applies):

    a. A clinician can implement any one of many available published curricula, which are applicable to almost all patients.

    b. A clinician typically designs a curriculum for patients and another one for frequent communication partners.

    c. A clinician tailors the intervention according to the specific concerns of the patient, experienced at the point of time at program entry.

    d. A clinician decides whether to focus on repair or facilitative strategies.

2. At the beginning of a communication strategies training program, the clinician often reviews rules for group interactions. The reason for this is:

    a. To establish a safe and secure environment where patients feel comfortable in sharing their feelings and their solutions

    b. Because there are always time constraints, to ensure that people do not digress once the class gets going and that the extensive curriculum content is covered in the limited time available

    c. To ensure that frequent communication partners understand their role in the program

    d. To serve as an ice-breaker and an exercise in assertive behavior

3. A clinician stands up at a whiteboard and lectures the group about how to manage the communication environment. During the presentation, slides and overheads are used to supplement the talk. Which statement best describes this technique for formal instruction?

    a. A prelude to real-world practice

    b. A good way to conduct formal instruction because visual aids support the spoken message, and persons with hearing loss can easily follow the lecture

    c. A means to ensure that both the patient and the frequent communication partner share the same information, and hence, start from the same playing field

    d. An ineffective way to convey information to a communication strategies training group

4. Which of the following activities is something that might happen during guided learning?

    a. Patients describe their most difficult listening situations.

    b. Patients practice ordering in a restaurant in a simulated interaction.

    c. Patients take a multiple-choice test.

    d. Frequent communication partners quiz patients on the night before each class about what they learned at the last communication strategies training class.

5. An example of a vicarious consequence is:
   a. A spouse learns about appropriate speaking behaviors because his wife reads an article in a health journal and repeats the information to him.
   b. A person with hearing loss is enrolled into a communication strategies program in lieu of attending a hearing aid orientation session.
   c. A patient watches someone else ask for a key word and then realizes that asking for a key word can lead to successful communication breakdown repair.
   d. A patient engages in continuous discourse tracking with her clinician and then feels more confident about using repair strategies with her frequent communication partner.

6. What is continuous discourse tracking?
   a. A way to track one's use of repair strategies during real-world conversations
   b. An example of a guided learning activity
   c. A way to assess conversational content
   d. A communication strategy in which patients inform their frequent communication partners about what they understood

7. A classroom teacher says to a student, "Mary, you told me what you heard. Now I know what information you missed. I find that helpful in helping to understand what I just said." This is an example of:
   a. Modeling
   b. Role-playing
   c. Formal instruction
   d. Attention technique

8. For real-world activities, students should:
   a. Have a means of recording their experiences so they can later share the results with the group
   b. Select a situation that will be challenging enough to test the limits of their abilities
   c. Never be asked to do something that might lead to an unsuccessful communication interaction
   d. Develop the activity at home, as a homework assignment

9.   Mr. K. lives in a rural town in Illinois. His clinician lives several hours away. The most feasible intervention for Mr. K. might be, at least initially:

    a.   Guided-learning drill activities that he can do at home

    b.   A workbook and set of how-to pamphlets

    c.   A short tutorial

    d.   A correspondence course

10.   One of the key principles that children learn during an expressive communication strategies training program is that:

    a.   The general public does not understand the nature of hearing loss.

    b.   They can take charge in managing their communication difficulties.

    c.   The most effective way to receive a message is to ask people to speak slowly.

    d.   Nonverbal communication entails fewer communication breakdowns than does verbal communication.

11.   The goal of a particular communication strategies program is to increase patients' sense of self-efficacy. If the program is successful in achieving this goal, what might a participant say at its conclusion:

    a.   "I improved my score on the *Communication Profile for the Hearing Impaired (CPHI)* by 20%."

    b.   "I use a greater variety of repair strategies during continuous discourse tracking now than I did at the beginning of the program."

    c.   "I have fewer communication breakdowns at work, thanks to the practice in using facilitative and repair strategies."

    d.   "I can now talk with clients on the phone much better than before."

KEY RESOURCES

GROUND RULES FOR A GROUP AURAL REHABILITATION PROGRAM

1.   Only one person speaks at a time.

2.   Let us know when you are finished speaking by nodding your head.

3. If we are using a group assistive listening device, wait until you have the microphone before beginning to speak.

4. You have a right to pass on a question.

5. Everything said in this room is confidential.

6. There are no "right" or "wrong" answers or remarks. All comments are welcome and respected.

7. Say what you have to say but be sure that everyone has a chance to talk.

8. Be specific and use examples.

9. Indicate when you do not hear or understand something that is said—no bluffing and/or pretending to understand allowed.

CHAPTER **10**

Counseling, Psychosocial Support, and Assertiveness Training

OUTLINE

- Who provides counseling, psychosocial support, and assertiveness training?

- Counseling

- Psychosocial support

- Assertiveness training

- Related research

- Case study: Solving challenging situations

- Final remarks

- Key chapter points

- Terms and concepts to remember

- Multiple-choice questions

- Key resources

Hearing-related **counseling** is a professional service designed to help patients better understand and solve their hearing-related problems.

Hearing-related **psychosocial support** is the means by which speech and hearing professionals help patients achieve long-term self-sufficiency in managing the psychological and social challenges that result from hearing loss.

Hearing-related **assertiveness training** is aimed at teaching patients to express themselves assertively in their interpersonal communication interactions and to state both negative and positive feelings directly.

An individual's awareness of his or her biological or physical self and personality contributes to a person's **self-image**, as does the individual's sense of identity and self-worth.

One goal of an aural rehabilitation plan may be to help persons with hearing loss and frequent communication partners realize the effect of hearing loss on their lives and to develop the skill sets and self-acceptance to carry on conversations with each other, using communication strategies effectively. Another goal may be to help them understand the often permanent nature of the hearing loss and to accept the idea of using appropriate listening devices. Hearing-related **counseling**, **psychosocial support**, and **assertiveness training** are means to achieve these goals.

There is a fine line between hearing-related counseling, psychosocial support, and assertiveness training, and often the boundary between where one begins and the next ends is unclear. Whereas counseling may center only on issues directly related to hearing loss, psychosocial support may dig deeper and delve into the realms of a person's **self-image** and intrapersonal communication patterns. Assertiveness training may focus on conversational behaviors and effective means for interacting with other people. In this chapter, we will consider each one of these components, beginning with a consideration of who provides support.

WHO PROVIDES COUNSELING, PSYCHOSOCIAL SUPPORT, AND ASSERTIVENESS TRAINING?

Speech and hearing professionals often provide counseling to patients and their frequent communication partners. This professional might be an audiologist, speech-language pathologist, or a teacher of children who are deaf and hard of hearing. Sometimes the patient may receive counseling from another health care professional, such as a physician, nurse, psychologist, school counselor, or occupational therapist. Counseling might be provided in the context of an audiological examination or during the development of an individualized family service plan, or it may be provided during times specifically designated for this purpose, such as when a group of adults enroll in a communication strategies training class.

Speech and hearing professionals may also participate in providing psychosocial support. When this happens, the speech and hearing professional may team up with a certified psychosocial therapist or a clinical psychologist. Advantages of a team approach are that patients benefit from receiving the expertise of two types of professionals, and the two professionals can model and role-play desirable behaviors. In cases when the participants have profound losses, and assistive listening devices cannot be used, one professional can write notes on a whiteboard or hanging easel, while the other professional leads the discussion. Disadvantages relate to the cost of labor and the logistics of arranging for the professionals to be at the same place at the same time.

⌒ COUNSELING

Counseling often provides patients with the following benefits (Erdman, 2000):

- Enhanced understanding of hearing loss and its effects on communication
- Better self-disclosure and self-acceptance
- Greater knowledge about how to manage communication difficulties
- Reduced stress and discouragement
- Increased satisfaction with aural rehabilitation services
- Increased motivation to minimize listening problems
- Stronger adherence/compliance with the aural rehabilitation plan, including use of amplification

After a hearing test, an audiologist typically explains the nature and degree of hearing loss to the patient, usually in conjunction with a review of the person's audiogram. The audiologist then reviews the relevant steps in the aural rehabilitation plan. This review may include a discussion of the benefits and limitations provided by a hearing aid and possibly a hands-on demonstration. In this type of interaction, the audiologist provides **informational counseling** (Figure 10-1). The professional instructs, guides, and gives expert information in the format of a give-and-take dialogue. Information provided during this type of counseling may concern the hearing loss itself, listening device technology, community and government services available to persons with hearing loss, and

During **informational counseling**, information is imparted to the patient about the hearing loss and hearing disability and the recommended steps for management.

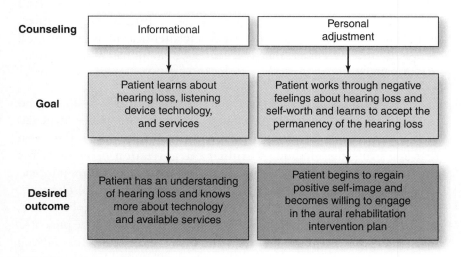

Counseling	Informational	Personal adjustment
Goal	Patient learns about hearing loss, listening device technology, and services	Patient works through negative feelings about hearing loss and self-worth and learns to accept the permanency of the hearing loss
Desired outcome	Patient has an understanding of hearing loss and knows more about technology and available services	Patient begins to regain positive self-image and becomes willing to engage in the aural rehabilitation intervention plan

FIGURE 10-1. Two kinds of counseling provided in the aural rehabilitation setting.

Personal adjustment counseling focuses on the permanency of the hearing loss and on psychological, social, and emotional acceptance.

"The consultation needs to be a dialog in which the clinician listens to the patient as well as the other way around. If the patient's ideas are evaded or inhibited, the patient is less likely to remember important information. Even the clinician's anxiety affects recall. Patients remember less when the information is provided by an overtly anxious clinician. Information presented in a manner that emphasizes its importance is more likely to be remembered than information presented in a matter-of-fact manner."

Robert H. Margolis, Professor and Director of Audiology, University of Minnesota Medical School

(Margolis, 2004b, p. 12)

The method of **explicit categorization**, a way to ensure retention, is an informational counseling technique wherein the clinician enumerates the topics that will be covered and then announces each one before talking about it.

the availability of aural rehabilitation classes, such as speechreading or communication strategies training.

During **personal adjustment counseling** (Figure 10-1), clinicians focus on the permanence of the hearing loss and on the healthy incorporation of hearing loss into a patient's self-image. The acceptance of hearing loss allows patients to accept the realities of their disability and to adjust their values and priorities while still continuing to lead fulfilled and productive lives. An audiologist might introduce the possibility of using a listening device and listen as a patient expresses a reaction. A teacher for children who are deaf and hard of hearing might explore some of the complicated issues that prevent an adolescent from engaging in social activities with peers or from using an FM assistive listening device in the classroom.

Informational Counseling

Informational counseling provides relevant information about the nature of the hearing loss and effective steps to manage the loss. In addition, this type of counseling can inspire the patient and the family to play an active role in the aural rehabilitation plan and to prevent further long-term consequences (such as noise-induced hearing loss). Informational counseling is provided as part of a dialogue, in which the clinician listens to questions and concerns and presents germane information in response. An effective clinician understands what the patient is interested in learning about and the level of understanding that the patient is capable of achieving.

One of the most important goals during informational counseling is to present information in such a way that the patient will both understand what is said and remember the important points. Patients forget as much as 40% to 80% of information immediately after hearing it in a medical setting. Of this percentage, they may remember about half of it incorrectly (Kessels, 2003).

Ways to promote understanding include speaking with easy-to-understand language and supplementing the verbal presentation with graphic materials such as pictures and drawings. Presenting the most important information first and using the method of **explicit categorization** helps to ensure retention. In using explicit categorization, the clinician organizes information into specific categories such as (a) *Explanation of Systems,* (b) *Diagnostic Tests,* (c) *Results,* (d) *Prognosis,* and (e) *Recommendations* (Margolis, 2004a, p. 15). The clinician advises the patient that information will be presented in each of these categories and then announces each one before talking about it. Patients then are encouraged to ask questions within each category before moving on to the next. These and other strategies for ensuring understanding and retention are listed next (Margolis, 2004a, p. 15):

- Advice should be given as concrete instructions. "Use ear plugs when you use your power tools," rather than "Keep your noise exposure to a minimum."
- Use easy-to-understand language.
- Present the most important information first to capitalize on the primacy effect.
- Stress the importance of recommendations or other information that you want the patient to remember.
- Use the method of explicit categorization. Tell the patient, "We are going to go over *recommendations,* then we will talk about your specific hearing problem *(diagnosis),* then we will go over *test results,* then we will talk about how your hearing may change in the future *(prognosis).*" Ask the patient for questions before moving on to the next category.
- Repeat the most important information.
- Don't present too much information.
- Specifically address the patient's reason for seeking a hearing evaluation [or other service].
- Supplement verbal information with written, graphical, and pictorial materials that the patient can take home.

Personal Adjustment Counseling

Personal adjustment counseling occurs less often than informational counseling. For instance, such counseling is rare in audiological practices that dispense hearing aids (Stika, Ross, & Ceuvas, 2002). This rarity may reflect speech and hearing professionals' lack of comfort in providing this type of counseling and/or it may reflect that fact that there is simply not enough time available in many practices for audiologists to provide it. Nonetheless, this kind of counseling may be beneficial for many patients.

Although there are probably as many different approaches to personal adjustment counseling as there are professional counselors, the various approaches can be broadly sorted into three general categories: approaches aimed at modifying thought process *(cognitive),* approaches aimed at modifying behavior *(behavioral),* and approaches aimed at modifying emotions *(affective).* In practice, most counseling entails a combination of all of these approaches. Even an approach that is considered to be primarily, say, cognitive may also entail behavioral and affective elements.

Some of the Issues That Might Be Addressed During Personal Adjustment Counseling:

- How do I prevent friends and coworkers from avoiding me?
- How do I increase my self-esteem?
- How do I gain confidence to behave more assertively?
- How do I deal with feeling isolated?
- How do I deal with the anger I feel because I experience so many communication breakdowns?
- How do I decrease my dependence on others?

(Trychin, 1994)

Cognitive Approach

A cognitive approach to counseling (e.g., Beck & Emery, 1985; Ellis & Grieger, 1977) relies on intellectual means for addressing problems related to hearing loss. In this approach, faulty thought processes are assumed to underlay inappropriate emotional responses to hearing loss and to underlay erroneous assumptions and self-image difficulties. The speech and hearing professional implements logic to direct and redirect individuals' thoughts, belief systems, perceptions, values, ideas, and opinions. This educational experience is designed to increase self-worth and decrease inferiority feelings and discouragement. For instance, a woman with hearing loss may believe she can no longer serve on a charitable board because her hearing loss prevents her from understanding everything that is said during meetings. The clinician might counter this by asking her to consider her experience and expertise, which brought her to serve on the board in the first place, and then by asking her to consider some of the ways she might enhance the communication setting during meetings. Sometimes the clinician is passive in a process like this, and at other times, the clinician might direct a counseling session using didactic questioning that may be both accepting and confrontational at the same time. The goal is to eliminate cognitive distortions and arbitrary assumptions and to replace them with positive thoughts and positive perspectives. Techniques that are used in cognitive approaches include questioning, interpreting, goal setting, creation of contracts, and homework assignments. An example of a homework assignment appears in Figure 10-2, and an example of a contract appears in Figure 10-3.

The **Rational Emotive Behavior Therapy (REBT)** approach, developed by the psychotherapist Albert Ellis, exemplifies a predominantly cognitive approach to counseling. Ellis (2001; Ellis & MacLaren, 1998) describes an

Rational Emotive Behavior Therapy (REBT) is a solution-oriented counseling (or therapy) approach that focuses on resolving specific problems using cognitive, behavioral, and affective elements; key to the approach is the idea that emotions result from beliefs rather than events or circumstances.

---

1. Choose a person at work, a friend or neighbor, or someone in your extended family and tell the person that you have just received a new hearing aid.

2. Explain to this person the benefits and limitations you perceive your hearing aid will afford you.

3. You might use the results of the speech tests that we collected during your appointment today to explain how well you now understand speech.

FIGURE 10-2. A counseling homework assignment.

Personal Contract

Name:_____

Clinician:_____

Before I return to my next appointment, I will:

- Explain to people that I have a hearing loss

- Use repair strategies when I do not understand a spoken message

- Not scold myself when I do not recognize a message

- Remind my wife to use optimal speaking behaviors so that I may understand her, using language that is assertive but not aggressive

Signed: _____

Date: _____

FIGURE 10-3. Example of a contract that might be issued during a counseling session.

A-B-C framework of emotional functioning (Figure 10-4). The A stands for an *activating event* or an *adversity* that a patient confronts. In the context of aural rehabilitation, an example of an activating event might be a young bachelor receiving a diagnosis of hearing loss and a recommendation for a hearing aid from his audiologist. The B stands for the evaluation of the event, which might be *behavioral-affective-cognitive*. For instance, the man might conclude, "Only old folks have hearing loss and wear hearing aids." The C is the *consequence* of the patient's evaluation. In this case, the man may decide that he will never wear a hearing aid because he does not want to be perceived as old by women of his own age. The key to counseling is to help the patient realize that his evaluation of the event, and not

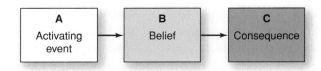

FIGURE 10-4. The A-B-C framework of emotional functioning. A = Audiologist recommends a hearing aid; B = Patient believes potential girlfriends will think that he is too old if he wears a hearing aid; C = Patient declines to participate in a hearing aid evaluation.

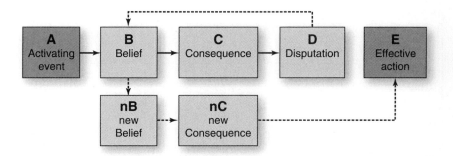

FIGURE 10-5. An example of a cognitive approach to counseling. A = Audiologist recommends a hearing aid; B = Patient believes potential girlfriends will think that he is too old if he wears a hearing aid; C = Patient declines to participate in a hearing aid evaluation; D = Audiologist disputes belief (B) by naming several prominent musicians who wear hearing aids; nB = Patient revises his original belief, that is, develops a new belief; nC = Patient agrees to a hearing aid evaluation, that is, has a new consequence; E = Patient wears hearing aid in everyday situations and becomes a more effective communicator.

the activating event itself, is the cause of the undesirable consequence. By obtaining a more rational view of hearing loss and of other people (e.g., women do not necessarily equate hearing aids with aging), patients are more likely to react to adversity in a more self-serving and adaptive manner. Some clinicians include a D and E component when applying Ellis's model. D stands for *dispute* and E stands for *effective action or philosophy.* In the present example, the audiologist would implement the D component by helping the young man dispute his evaluation of hearing loss and hearing aids; that is, the B of this particular A-B-C-D-E sequence. This might be accomplished by asking the young man to provide evidence for his belief or by asking him to consider what would happen if he abandoned this belief. The result of abandoning or replacing the irrational belief with a rational one results in an effective course of action (the E component); in this case, the use of an appropriate hearing aid. Figure 10-5 presents the stages in the A-B-C-D-E process.

Behavioral Approach

Skinnerian learning theory (Skinner, 1953, 1971) forms the basis for many behavioral approaches to counseling. A fundamental tenet is that maladaptive behavior is learned, and as such, it is possible to "unlearn" it. This approach often focuses on observable and measurable behavior foremost, with the idea that changes in cognitive and emotional adjustment will follow behavioral changes. For example, a businessman might hyperventilate before major meetings because he fears he may not understand the other participants' remarks. The clinician may implement a **desensitization** process, which is a strategy to help someone reduce excessive anxiety or

Desensitization is a way to reduce a patient's negative reactions in specific situations by means of repeatedly exposing the person to them in mild form, either in reality or in role-playing or imagination.

Right before a major meeting, I worry that I will not understand what is said at the conference table. I experience the following physical symptoms of stress:

My head pounds.

My palms sweat.

My heart beat races.

My stomach churns.

I feel short of breath.

My neck aches.

I feel dizzy as I walk toward the conference room.

My mouth goes dry.

After the meeting, I think about my performance. Once I get home, I feel the following emotions:

Depression

Anxiety

A sense of being on edge

Anger

FIGURE 10-6. A behavioral approach to counseling. A businessman who has hearing loss is asked to identify his stress reactions to business meetings.

fear that occurs in specific situations. The clinician might first ask him to identify those physical symptoms he experiences in response to stress (Figure 10-6), and then introduce him to relaxation techniques, such as that described in Figure 10-7. Behavioral techniques such as this work directly on the physical response to stress.

Affective Approach

An affective approach (e.g., Rogers, 1980) centers on feelings and on fostering emotional adjustment to hearing loss. The clinician creates an empathetic, accepting environment in which patients can evaluate self-concepts and their reactions to hearing loss. The goal is phenomenological: Patients change how they view themselves and their place in the world,

What the Patient Might Really Be Saying When Asking Whether a Hearing Loss Is Permanent:

- "This is worse than I thought, I was hoping it was nothing serious."

- "I'm worried about the future, how am I going to manage this with so much else going on in my life?"

- "I know it sounds silly, but this makes me feel old."

(Clark & English, 2004, p. 76)

- **Focus on point one inch below navel, in the middle of your body**

- **Breath deeply**

- **Expand lower abdomen as you breathe in**

- **Flatten abdomen as you breathe out**

- **Perform exercise for 10–20 minutes**

FIGURE 10-7. Relaxation techniques to reduce stress responses. These techniques may be reviewed in a behavioral counseling approach (Hogan, 2001).

even though their circumstance may remain the same. By receiving unconditional positive regard from the clinician, the person with hearing loss develops a sense of being loved and cared for because the person is who he or she is. Central tenets of Rogers's affective approach are congruence with self, unconditional positive regard, and empathetic understanding. Although these tenets are hallmarks of an affective approach, they likely should be a part of any counseling interaction between a speech and hearing professional and a patient (or patient's family member).

Congruence with self means that clinicians act as themselves and do not assume an imposing facade of professionalism. They relate to patients honestly and sincerely. Instead of saying to a first-time patient: "Your audiogram indicates a mild-to-moderate sensorineural hearing loss bilaterally with a conductive component," a pronouncement replete with professional jargon, an audiologist might instead say, "I know you are worried about your hearing. My tests seem to agree with your impression that you are not hearing as well as you used to hear. I'd like to answer your questions." With the former statement, the audiologist might inadvertently increase the patient's anxiety. With the latter approach, the audiologist has validated the patient's own opinions and allowed the patient to share the lead in discussing the test results. The audiologist has set the stage for the patient to take responsibility and participate in the aural rehabilitation plan.

A second tenet is **unconditional positive regard**. The clinician assumes that patients know best and that they have the inner resources to overcome their communication difficulties. The professional accepts persons with hearing loss as human beings of stature; respects them regardless of their employment or social status; and brings appropriately placed empathy, sincerity, and caring to the interaction. Unconditional positive regard engenders a nonthreatening context for patients to express their concerns about their hearing losses, their painful or defensive feelings about their communication difficulties, and their apprehensions about using a listening device.

Congruence with self is the first tenet of person-centered counseling in which clinicians act as themselves in interactions with patients and do not assume a facade of professionalism.

In **unconditional positive regard**, the second tenet of person-centered counseling, clinicians assume that patients know best and assume that they have the inner resources to overcome their conversation difficulties.

Rogers's third tenet is **empathetic understanding**. The clinician listens carefully as patients perhaps rationalize or deny their hearing difficulties, as they talk about their concerns and feelings, and as they express their ideas and solutions. The professional establishes the patient's viewpoints, often through techniques of **reflection** and **clarification**, and tries to appreciate the patient's situation from the patient's point of view. For example, a person might cite the soft presentation level as a reason for poor performance on a word recognition test. In this instance, the audiologist would probably not say, "I presented the words at a normal conversational level, Mr. Smith. There is no doubt you have a word recognition problem." Instead, in order to show empathy and respect for the patient's feelings, the audiologist might respond, "I know the words were not very loud for you. Are there occasions during your typical day when speech seems too soft to hear?" With this remark, the patient's impressions are acknowledged, and the test results are related to situations that are relevant.

Targeting Counseling

As speech and hearing professionals develop aural rehabilitation strategies and implement aural rehabilitation plans, they will want to consider how best to target counseling for particular concerns. For example, one patient, Candice Brown, commented to her audiologist, "I worry that I can't be there for my 17-year-old daughter the way I want to be. It's too much of an effort for her to talk to me, she says. Lately, she just tunes me out." She noted that she felt a low-grade anxiety throughout many of her waking hours. In this case, the aural rehabilitation plan might include the following counseling tactics:

- Provide informational counseling by talking to Candice about a group communication strategies training program. An audiologist might give her a program's brochure and answer her questions about program content. The audiologist might also provide an overview of some of the communication strategies that are typically included in such a program.
- Provide personal adjustment counseling, and help Candice understand that communication between a teenage daughter and her parent is universally problematic and not just an issue for a mother who has hearing loss. During this process, a speech and hearing professional might follow the steps in the A-B-C-D-E model depicted in Figure 10-5, beginning by identifying an activating event, such as the daughter's reluctance to talk about school (A), then Candice's beliefs about the event, that is, that she's "not there" for her daughter (B), and third, the consequences of these beliefs,

Empathetic understanding is the third tenet of person-centered counseling. The counselor listens to the patient's concerns and feelings about the hearing problem, reflects them back to the patient, and helps the patient identify solutions.

Reflection is a counseling technique whereby clinicians paraphrase or summarize what their patient has just said. By this means, clinicians demonstrate that they are listening carefully and accurately and also provide their patients with an opportunity to examine their own views or feelings by hearing them expressed by another person.

Clarification is a counseling technique whereby clinicians abstract the essence of a patient's remarks and summarize them back to their patient.

Ways to enhance empathy:
- Listen without interruption.
- Express empathy and concern by "getting into the other person's movie."
- Involve the client in the decision-making process.
- Talk openly.
- Ask open-ended questions.

(Moore, 2006, referencing Rebecca Shafir in The Zen of Listening)

Components That, Taken Together, Determine Psychosocial Reaction to Hearing Loss:

Emotional: May include shame, guilt, anxiety, anger, frustration, embarrassment, depression.

Cognitive: May include inattentiveness, reduced concentration, low self-esteem, low self-confidence, increased effort required for listening comprehension.

Interpersonal: May include bluffing, social withdrawal, dominating conversations, a loss of intimacy.

Behavioral: May include a limitation of activities or social isolation.

Physical: May include fatigue, muscle tension, headaches, stomach problems, sleep problems.

(Preminger, 2007, p. 114)

which for Candice is increased anxiety (C). The speech and hearing professional might question Candice's beliefs (D) with the goal of stimulating more effective action on Candice's part (E).

- Continue personal adjustment counseling. Once Candice has enrolled in the communication strategies training program, the daughter might be encouraged to attend, so both will have an opportunity to share their frustrations, feelings, and ideas for solutions. Desensitization might be provided by allowing them to role-play solutions for difficult communication situations, such as talking on the telephone.

PSYCHOSOCIAL SUPPORT

Counseling may be expanded to include psychosocial support in some instances. Psychosocial support is particularly valuable when patients' emotional responses to hearing loss are negative and when they have experienced communication failure and other people's disapproving attitudes. The goal of the support is to facilitate emotional adjustment in the context of the aural rehabilitation plan. The outcome is increased self-acceptance, increased self-confidence, and more effective use of communication strategies.

Psychosocial Consequences for Persons with Hearing Loss

Losing one's hearing can be devastating, particularly if the loss is severe enough to result in isolation from society. The loss, and concomitant changes in how the person with hearing loss relates to family, friends, and coworkers, can decrease one's self-confidence and foster a negative self-image, which may be reinforced by others' reactions, including their stigmatization. Because acquired hearing loss may cause a restriction in one's activities and create unsatisfactory interactions, depression may follow. For example, Knutson and Lansing (1990) showed that adults with profound hearing loss were likely to be depressed, introverted, and lonely and to experience social anxiety, particularly if they had inadequate communication strategies. Hétu and Getty (1991) found a prevalence of a negative self-image among individuals with hearing loss.

Hearing-related stress includes the stress of adjusting to a new self-concept, the stress of living with an impaired sensory system, and the stress of living with the reactions of society to people who have a disability and who experience communication difficulties.

Hearing loss also may create **hearing-related stress**, which is an individual's response to either an acute or chronic strain. Stress in turn may create feelings of frustration, anger, and even despair (Clark & English, 2004, p. 130). Adults with hearing loss may experience a three-pronged stress: (a) having to understand speech with impaired hearing, (b) having to adjust to a new self-concept, that of a person with hearing loss, and (c) having to adjust to society's reactions to self-as-hearing-impaired.

Individuals who suffer a hearing loss, whether it is sudden or gradual, often develop a sense that they have gone from being "able-bodied" to being "abnormal." They no longer are able to communicate as easily as they once did, and they may no longer be able to perform their professions and daily responsibilities as effectively because of hearing loss (Clark & English, 2004; Dannermark & Gellerstedt, 2004). Their social and emotional interactions may be less rewarding than before, and they may have a lost or diminished sense of independence and self-sufficiency. One woman, when asked how she was different now that she had a hearing loss, responded, "I feel like the world dumped on me." A man, asked the same question, responded, "I feel like I'm a piece of driftwood drifting away." Hearing loss may lead to feelings of insecurity, because patients no longer trust their ears. They may begin to wonder whether they are responding appropriately in any given situation (Siemens Audiologic Group, 2000).

Individuals who are born with hearing loss, or who acquire hearing loss early, may also experience isolation and a negative self-image, especially as they begin to realize they are in some ways different from others in their social and school environments (Harvey, 2003). The individual may develop a self-image of being less capable than others. Their self-esteem may suffer as they experience difficulties in socializing with their peers who have normal hearing or difficulties in learning academic material. Preadolescents and teenagers who are mainstreamed into hearing classrooms, in particular, may experience adjustment issues and a sense of rejection.

Creating a Dialogue with Children

Children who have hearing loss may sometimes experience difficulty in talking about their psychosocial issues. Clark and English (2004) suggest the following two techniques for helping children to express their concerns:

- *I start, you finish:* Ask the child to complete a set of open-ended statements that encourage self-expression. Examples of these statements include, "I am happy when . . ."; "I am sad when . . ."; "Because I have a hearing problem . . ."; "I'm afraid to . . ."; "One thing I do well is . . ." The child should understand that this activity has no right or wrong answers but is a way for the child to help the clinician understand "what it is like to be me."

continues

Creating a Dialogue with Children, *continued*

• *Play a game of "Dreams and Maps":* Ask the child to describe a short-term goal (a "today" dream) and a long-term goal (a "tomorrow" dream). A short-term goal may be for a girl to learn how to play soccer so she will not feel excluded during gym class. A long-term goal may be for the youth to attend a particular university. Next, consider along with the child how to accomplish a "today" dream, step-by-step. As brainstorming ensues, write down the suggestions and ideas and organize them into a beginning, middle, and end. For example, learning how to play soccer may entail acquiring a rule book, watching games on television, and practicing with a sibling at home. After several "today" dreams have been achieved, the child may be ready to tackle a "tomorrow" dream.

Because hearing loss has a deleterious impact on interactions with others, the individual with hearing loss may have a psychological experience that is closely related with the social consequences of the disability. These consequences may include being ostracized by peers, loss of job opportunities, changes or limitations in everyday roles (e.g., as a spouse, a parent, a friend), and attendant levels of stress, anxiety, isolation, and fatigue (Getty & Hétu, 1991; Hétu & Getty, 1991; Hogan, 2001). A psychosocial feedback loop may develop, where the impaired social, vocational, or academic function related to the hearing loss stimulates a negative self-image (e.g., "I'm inadequate."). A person's coping responses may in turn deteriorate or not develop, and the person may experience limited confidence and feelings of helplessness and unworthiness (Heydebrand, Mauzé, Tye-Murray, Binzer, & Skinner, 2005; Hogan, 2001).

Psychosocial Consequences for Frequent Communication Partners

Not only must patients adjust to hearing loss, but so too must their family members. Communication, which is the centerpiece of intimacy, invariably suffers when a member of a marriage or partnership has hearing loss. Social and emotional issues that may arise include frustration over communication difficulties, impatience over the difficulties of communication (e.g., "Forget it, it's not worth repeating"), anger (e.g., "What am I supposed to do about your problem?"), guilt, a sense of incompetence for not knowing how to minimize the listening problems for the patient, pity, and anxiety. Communication difficulties might be mistakenly attributed to lack of concentration, an unwillingness to communicate, or disinterest. Other difficulties might be that for some, the relationship is less personal, with less small talk and joking, and it may lack spontaneity.

In a now classic examination of this topic, Hétu and his colleagues (Hétu, Riverin, Lalande, Getty, & St-Cyr, 1988; see also Hétu, Jones, & Getty, 1993; Hétu, Lalonde, & Getty, 1987) interviewed men with noise-induced hearing loss and their wives. Couples reported that the presence of hearing loss in the family had led to a restricted social life, "effortful" communication patterns, and increased anxiety and stress. The spouses reported being bothered by elevated television volume levels, the need for continual repetition, having to serve as an interpreter during group conversations, and having to answer all telephone calls.

> "Spouses play [an important role] in initiating aural rehabilitation . . . and may become so frustrated with their partners' hearing loss that they are often the primary reason why the person [with hearing loss] presents for audiological services."
>
> Nerina Donaldson and colleagues, researchers at the University of Queensland in Australia
>
> (Donaldson, Worrall, & Hickson, 2004, p. 30)

Eye-Witness Accounts

We once posed the following question to a group of persons married to persons with significant hearing losses: "What are some of the most difficult aspects of living with a deaf family member?" Here are some of the responses:

Rhonda: I'll list some of them: (1) anger—communication is often difficult that he's "not the same"; (2) concession—everyone has to change what it is he or she is doing or the way they do them (i.e., talking, listening to the TV); and (3) frustration—things have to be done his way to accommodate his hearing loss. It is just simply a whole new way of life. He has to deal with the fact that he is hearing impaired and being his family and loving him as we do, we deal (well or not) with all of the changes too.

Gerald: I cannot communicate with her by phone when she is alone. I once called a next-door neighbor to tell her of a tornado warning—she is so damn independent she was upset about my doing that.

continues

Eye-Witness Accounts, *continued*

Mike: Communication with a family member [who has hearing loss] requires patience and determination. I'm sure the frustration is equally disturbing to my wife. Tempers sometimes flare as one or both attempt communication and fail. Oftentimes communication is abandoned by one or both parties, leaving both equally frustrated.

Jan: We have a captioning device on the TV and the kids sometimes get mad when he wants to see the news captioned and they may go to another TV—poor kids, hah!

Anna: I have to move and make sure he can see my face when I speak to him. And we less and less enjoy "small talk" together. Hearing aids have helped but we have finally reached the point where we cannot talk to each other without extra effort.

Pam: Trying to do business and explain to him what's going on. Especially if someone else is around, he gets real rude and frustrated at me because he can't hear or understand.

Psychosocial Support Intervention Paradigm

For many persons with hearing loss, the stress that results from their communication difficulties and their perceived inabilities is debilitating. One reason they may seek psychosocial support is to understand who they are and what has happened to them, and to get their lives moving forward. Raymond Hétu and Louis Getty at the University of Montreal performed some of the seminal work on developing a psychosocial support paradigm for adults who have hearing loss (Getty & Hétu, 1991; Hétu & Getty, 1991). Their approach (sometimes referred to as *The Montreal Method*) was based on two principles:

1. Knowing that hearing disabilities affect not only the victims themselves, but also anyone with whom they interact, rehabilitative help must consider several levels of coordinated interventions in order to reach the target individuals, families, social networks and institutions.

2. In order to facilitate the interaction between victims of [hearing loss] and others, a change in attitudes and behavior is required (Hétu & Getty, 1991, p. 306).

Their objectives were threefold:

1. To offer a psychosocial support to help affected [patients] and their [frequent communication partners] to better deal with the effects of hearing loss.

2. To allow the [patients] and their [frequent communication partners] to understand the nature and the consequences of the hearing problem.

3. To develop new skills that will help in coping with the effects of hearing loss (Getty & Hétu, 1991, p. 318).

Others who have built on this work include Hallberg (1996, 1999) (working in Sweden), Hogan (2001; Pedley et al., 2005) (working in New Zealand, Australia, and the United Kingdom), Stephens (1996) (working in Great Britain), and Heydebrand et al. (2005) (working in the United States). In common practice, psychosocial support is typically incorporated into communication strategies training. Psychosocial support helps patients recognize:

- The impact of hearing loss on their lives and self-image
- How they may have internalized negative perceptions about hearing loss
- How these negative perceptions limit their living a full and satisfying life
- How new attitudes about themselves and others may allow them to live life in a new and proud fashion, where pride can be defined as made up of "self-confidence, ability, self-esteem, security, a sense of the future, and a sense of where I fit in the world" (Hogan, 2001, p. 18)

Psychosocial support is usually provided in small groups of three to eight persons. Often, the participants' frequent communication partners are encouraged to attend the sessions, because they play a profound role in shaping the participants' self-image and self-confidence and may also have their own psychosocial issues to address. The support may be provided in intensive sessions over 2 or 3 days for 8 hours a day, or might be provided in shorter sessions over the course of several weeks. A sample curriculum for a 2-day program is presented in the Key Resources. This curriculum was adapted from Hogan (2001), which in turn drew heavily from Getty and Hétu (1991).

Problem-Solving Framework

The framework for psychosocial support is a problem-solving model (Figure 10-8). Through a series of activities or exercises, participants learn to identify the kinds of problems they are experiencing, understand the nature and effect of these problems, and then generate effective solutions for resolving them.

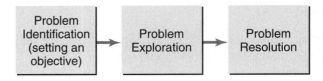

FIGURE 10-8. A problem-solving framework for psychosocial support.

Problem Identification

During problem identification, the participants turn the spotlight on the issues. Problem identification can begin by asking the participants in a psychosocial support group, "What's the worst thing about living with a hearing loss?" (Hogan, 2001). Both the person with hearing loss and the person's frequent communication partner respond to this question. Answers can be written on a whiteboard or a hanging easel. Figure 10-9 presents an array of responses that might be elicited during this activity. As this figure demonstrates, the worst thing might range from specific situations that might be easy to address, such as an inability to hear the doorbell, to more general and more

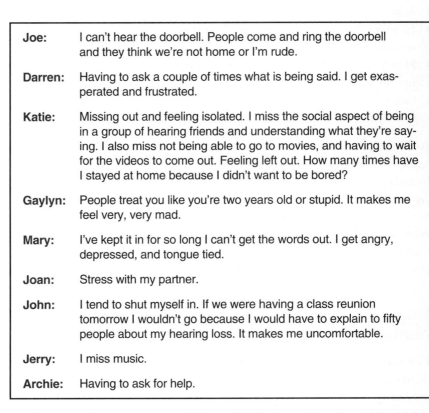

Joe:	I can't hear the doorbell. People come and ring the doorbell and they think we're not home or I'm rude.
Darren:	Having to ask a couple of times what is being said. I get exasperated and frustrated.
Katie:	Missing out and feeling isolated. I miss the social aspect of being in a group of hearing friends and understanding what they're saying. I also miss not being able to go to movies, and having to wait for the videos to come out. Feeling left out. How many times have I stayed at home because I didn't want to be bored?
Gaylyn:	People treat you like you're two years old or stupid. It makes me feel very, very mad.
Mary:	I've kept it in for so long I can't get the words out. I get angry, depressed, and tongue tied.
Joan:	Stress with my partner.
John:	I tend to shut myself in. If we were having a class reunion tomorrow I wouldn't go because I would have to explain to fifty people about my hearing loss. It makes me uncomfortable.
Jerry:	I miss music.
Archie:	Having to ask for help.

FIGURE 10-9. Responses generated during an identification activity to the question, What is the worst thing about living with hearing loss? Respondents are adult cochlear implant users.

difficult-to-address responses, such as depression, stress, anger, and feelings of stupidity. This exercise can be emotionally wrenching for some because it may be painful for participants to verbalize their difficulties to others or to consider how their lives have been affected by the presence of hearing loss. In some cases, the group leader may realize that the psychosocial issues of a particular individual may require referral for more in-depth **psychotherapy**.

Often, the problem identification segment of the program includes establishment of objectives, which helps make a problem manageable. For example, one woman identified her problem as, "Because I have a hearing loss, my husband and I never talk anymore." To tackle this issue in every conversational setting and at every time of day might be overwhelming. However, if the woman were to identify the problem, then establish a well-defined objective, problem solving could be targeted in a concrete manner. For instance, in this case, the woman was asked to identify those times when conversation was most important to her. She responded, "Before I begin to fix dinner; after I get home from work." The objective for this woman and her husband then became, "I would like to converse effectively with my husband for 30 minutes every night before I begin to fix dinner." Solutions were then generated to meet this objective (problem exploration, described next) and included, *sit together in a quiet place before dinner, turn off the television for 30 minutes,* and *refuse to take phone calls during this time.*

The difficulties identified during this stage will help guide the remainder of the program. For example, if stress seems to be a common theme in the responses, then the participants can discuss ways of managing stress and practicing relaxation techniques. If managing communication breakdowns seems to be the prevailing theme, then the group can focus on using repair strategies effectively.

Psychotherapy is a treatment for an emotional or behavioral problem in which a mental health expert (e.g., psychiatrist, psychologist, counselor) discusses feelings and problems with a patient, with the goals being the relief of symptoms, changes in behavior leading to improved social, emotional, and vocational functioning, and personality growth.

Move the Flowers?

In an exploration scenario, the group leader set up the following situation:

I'm your wife/husband's cousin. I am having a pretty big dinner party. I want you to meet some of the other people at my party so I am not going to sit you next to your partner. The flowers are in the center of the table. Would you ask me to move the flowers?

continues

Move the Flowers?, *continued*

Here is the dialogue that ensued:

Jim:	I would explain the situation. I might say, "It would help me to read lips and participate in conversation if you move the flowers."
Group Leader:	Is that explaining part hard to do?
Jim:	Yes. Admitting a problem is hard to do.
Sue:	It's hard. It's not fair that we always have to come up with a solution or that we have to explain things.
Mary:	When you're a guest in someone's home, you hate to impose on them. After all, it's their house so why should you be telling them what to do?

Notice that during this exercise, some of the emotional underpinnings that prevent people from using facilitative strategies are revealed. Jim is embarrassed to tell people that he has a hearing loss. Sue resents that the onus of managing the communication environment always falls on the person who has hearing loss. Mary feels she does not have the right to impose on others.

Problem Exploration

Once problems are identified, they can be explored in more depth. During problem exploration, the group focuses on the personal and social impact of hearing loss. In so doing, they address the social realities of hearing loss, the impact on the conversational partner of living with a person who has hearing loss, and the difficulty of seeking accommodations to hearing loss from other persons. For example, asking a person to turn off the background music requires self-confidence and a healthy self-image (e.g., "I have the right to communicate as effectively as I am able at this gathering"), trust in the communication partner (e.g., the partner could become annoyed or the partner could develop a negative perception of the person with hearing loss as a result of the request), and a willingness to be rejected (e.g., the partner could say no). Often, during periods of exploration, participants in a group will realize they do not manage their communication problems effectively because they do not want to draw attention to their hearing loss, they are fearful of others' reactions, or they want to take the easiest course of action.

Two means of engaging in problem exploration are through creating scenarios and compiling self-profiles. In creating a scenario, the group leader might describe a hypothetical situation:

I'm inviting you to my party. There will be lots of people out there. We are going to cook hamburgers and hotdogs out on the grill. The party will be at night, so I'll have a few lanterns burning. And oh yes, I'm going to have some great music. My brother is lending me his boom box. What would keep you from joining us?

The responses to this kind of scenario might range from, "I won't be able to speechread anyone," and "The music will be too loud to hear anything," to "No one will talk to me because I'm deaf," and "Parties are boring, I just stand off by myself."

As they speak about their reasons for avoiding social situations, the group can explore why they might behave in the ways they predict (e.g., "I don't want to burden people"; "It's not fair to my wife to have to interpret everything for me") and what their options are for dealing with difficulties.

In compiling a self-profile, the participants are asked to describe themselves to each other. This might entail them pairing off and taking turns talking to one another, or drawing a picture of themselves, or creating a collage using pictures torn from magazines. For instance, in one session, participants were divided into groups of three and asked to construct a collage using pictures cut out from a stack of old magazines. One group included a picture of a woman falling out of her high heel shoes and another picture of a woman with her back to the camera, holding a telephone receiver to her ear. When describing their collage to the others, the group members noted that the woman falling out of her shoes conveyed their sense of feeling off balance in a hearing world. The woman with her back to the camera conveyed their feelings of being ignored and excluded in everyday events.

Problem Resolution

Problem resolution is the third stage of the process. Some of the techniques described in Chapter 9 can be employed during this stage, particularly if managing communication problems and difficult listening situations have been cited during problem identification and exploration.

In developing ways to resolve problems, individuals may engage in self-examination and ask themselves such questions as: What are my rights as a person with hearing loss?; What are the consequences of not managing my problems effectively?; and How will I feel if I successfully overcome this difficulty?

Gagné and Jennings (2000, p. 569) present a step-by-step process for problem solving. First, they suggest that the group or an individual sets an

Responding to the Patient

"If a patient requests information, the response [of the audiologist or speech and hearing professional] should provide information, and if the patient expresses an emotion, the response should let the patient know that the emotion was acknowledged and respected."

(English, Mendel, Rojeski, & Hornak, 1999, p. 35)

objective and defines a desired outcome. For example, an objective might be, "Mr. Smith will use repair strategies during his weekly card game. As a result of his participation in this class, he'll be able to understand messages intended for him after using one or two repair strategies." Step 2 in this problem-solving process is to identify possible solutions. For each of the solutions, the implications of using it (e.g., its feasibility, acceptability, potential advantages and disadvantages) are considered. The third step in problem solving is to select a solution and to try it out. Finally, the benefits of applying the selected solution are considered, as well as the factors that facilitate or hinder its implementation.

Example of the Problem Identification-Exploration-Resolution Framework

In an actual session, Mary, the wife of a man with hearing loss, said that the most difficult aspect of living with someone who has hearing loss was as follows: "I'm working in the kitchen and John is in the living room reading. It takes a very, very, very long time for him to respond to me. He hears talking but he doesn't respond."

After identifying this problem, the participants in the group explored it. They asked the couple about other times when this kind of communication difficulty occurs. They discussed who has control of the situation and who has responsibility. The group leader asked whether the situation could be changed. What core beliefs may get in the way of thinking about the possibility of change? During this discussion, Mary noted ruefully, "If you say something he wants to hear, he'll respond."

This remark prompted another member of the group to observe, "You can't jump to conclusions. I just make sure my mother hears what I say and then I wait for a response."

Later in this discussion, some of the emotional undercurrents of the couple's communication problem emerged:

Mary: I enjoy talking and he doesn't. Finally, I have to just cut it off. There is no point aggravating myself. He doesn't talk anymore, but when I want an answer, I get it.

Ben: This is kind of frustrating or aggravating. Hearing loss is a frustrating situation because now you cannot achieve what you would like regularly. I would love to communicate with her. I would like to talk on the phone, listen to music, and not just noise. A hearing problem is very frustrating.

Example of the Problem Identification-Exploration-Resolution Framework, *continued*

During the resolution phase of this issue, the group leader asked the participants to generate a list of possible solutions. Here is what they came up with:

- Mary, go over to Ben and wave.
- Mary, yell.
- Mary, throw something at Ben to get his attention.
- Mary, repeat.
- Mary, tap him.
- Ben, read the paper in the kitchen.
- Ben, help prepare dinner.
- The couple should sit together in a quiet, well-lit room for 20 minutes every night before Mary starts to prepare dinner. Communicate then, when conditions are optimal.

The group leader suggested that the couple pick one, try it, and then review its effectiveness.

"Tell me and I will forget.

Show me and I may remember.

Involve me and I will understand."

McCameron Archer, Principal of Toccal College

(Anthony Hogan, personal communication, February, 2008)

ASSERTIVENESS TRAINING

Although some people who have hearing loss are comfortable with using communication strategies in a secure clinical setting, or even in home situations with familiar communication partners, many often have difficulty using them in other environments. These persons might benefit from assertiveness training. The goal of assertiveness training is to increase the cooperativeness between the person with hearing loss and his or her communication partners, while still maintaining equality among the participants who engage in a conversation (e.g., Trychin, 1988; Trychin & Wright, 1989). Patients develop neutral, nonaggressive behaviors that allow them to maintain their self-esteem without encroaching on the rights of others and that allow them to engage in satisfying conversational interactions. Key elements of assertiveness training entail learning:

- Ways to indicate a hearing loss (e.g., "I have a hearing loss. I may not understand everything you say to me.")
- Means to request a change in the communication environment (e.g., "The light in here is dim. I'm having difficulty reading your lips. May we walk over to another room?")

Issues That Might Be Addressed with Assertiveness Training:

- How do I tell others what to do so that I can better understand their speech?
- How do I improve my communication partner's speaking habits?
- How do I keep someone from speaking too loudly just because I have a hearing loss?

(Trychin, 1994)

- Ways to suggest how the communication partner can facilitate the patient's understanding of spoken messages (e.g., "It helps me to understand you if I can clearly see your face.")
- Means to provide positive feedback to communication partners to reinforce desirable behaviors (e.g., "I appreciate your coming into the room to talk to me. Thank you.")

During assertiveness training, emphasis is placed on choice of language and on the consequences of behaviors. For example, patients may compare the consequences of using language such as, "You never speak clearly when I try to talk to you on the phone even though you know I have a hearing loss!" to those resulting from a statement such as, "It helps me to understand what you are saying when you speak at a slow but not too slow speaking rate." Whereas the former statement is accusatory and puts the communication partner on the defensive, the latter is a neutral statement that provides explicit guidance about how the communication partner can foster understanding.

Assertive behaviors are typically situation-specific. That is, assertive behaviors are not always desirable or adaptive. For instance, it may not be appropriate for a man with hearing loss to remind his supervisor to speak clearly during a conference presentation. Part of the training should include a consideration of the consequences of using assertive behaviors in various situations.

RELATED RESEARCH

Research suggests that these interventions are effective and that people want these services. For example, patients who do not receive counseling are less likely to use their hearing aids than patients who receive counseling. Counseling reduces the amount of hearing-related difficulties perceived by persons who have hearing loss (Brooks, 1979; Taylor & Jurma, 1999), increases their knowledge about hearing-related issues (Backenroth & Ahlner, 2000; Borg, Dannermark, & Borg, 2002; Elkayam & English, 2003), and enhances their abilities to use coping strategies (Backenroth & Ahlner, 2000). Elkayam and English reported that 80% of their 20 adolescent participants derived benefit from participating in counseling, agreeing that it was "helpful" to talk about the hearing-related problems. However, only four reported changes in the management of their problems. After a psychosocial-based communication training program, workers with noise-induced hearing loss were more confident in dealing with their hearing difficulties (Getty & Hétu, 1991), and persons with occupational hearing loss realized at least short-term gains (Hallberg, 1996). Adult cochlear implant users spent significantly less time in communication breakdowns during conversations with an unfamiliar communication partner following their participation in an intensive 2-day psychosocial workshop (Heydebrand et al., 2005). They also reported fewer maladapted behaviors, such as withdrawing, as measured by the CPHI.

In contrast, Borg et al. (2002) did not note a change in measures of conversational fluency on average among their 13 participants and their frequent communication partners, including the frequency of communication breakdowns (although 2 of the 3 participants with the most frequent rate of breakdowns decreased the frequency post intervention), and no change in the use of specific versus nonspecific repair strategies. Their program is a departure from those described in this chapter in that the patients only participated in counseling and psychosocial support, and then they were responsible for addressing the communication problems of their frequent communication partners. The investigators did find, during interviews conducted 1 month following the intervention, that participants reported increased understanding and insight regarding hearing loss and felt increased self-esteem. For communication partners, irritation for the person with hearing loss had decreased.

Patients and their families want these services. As just one of many possible examples, Sweetow and Barrager (1980) found that 20% of parents did not feel comfortable asking their audiologists questions. Over one third of them believed their audiologist did not provide them with adequate emotional support and they wanted more counseling.

CASE STUDY

Solving Challenging Situations

In assessing the effects of an intensive 2-day psychosocial workshop for cochlear implant users and their spouses, we developed a before-and-after measure. The "before" question asked them to describe a common situation where it was difficult for them to manage hearing another person. Then in a series of "after" questionnaires, we asked them to revisit their "before" answer (we provided them with a photocopied version of their remarks) and determine whether they were managing the situation differently. Here are the responses of Diane, a 39-year-old woman who had used a cochlear implant for 2 years.

Baseline Challenging Situation

[Diane wrote,] "Conversations in groups of three or more in a dark or noisy environment are most difficult, especially if my friends are talking about something exciting. By the time I figure out who is talking, I've missed half of what was said, and then another person starts talking and I have to locate them."

continues

CASE STUDY, *continued*

3-Month Challenging Situation

"I am more assertive in asking friends to repeat what I've missed using appropriate strategies. Sometimes if the conversation is going too fast, I will raise my hand, ask for a time-out, explain to everyone that I can understand them better if they speak slower or one at a time or if they raise their hand before talking—depends on if we are in a meeting or a social gathering. Occasionally, I may quietly ask someone next to me a small part of what I missed . . . rephrasing what I heard and having them fill me in to catch up on the conversation."

6-Month Challenging Situation

"Really no change from 3 months ago, although I guess I'm feeling a little more confident these days. I continue to stop and ask friends to repeat or fill me in on conversation. If I get a key word, I may paraphrase it silently to someone next to me in order to catch up. I am doing well and have made significant progress."

12-Month Challenging Situation

"Managing well. I usually ask the group to speak one at a time and at a slower pace. Sometimes they forget and the topic is 'heated' or very fast paced and I will stand up and make a Big 'T' and say, 'Time out please; I'm having a hard time keeping up with the conversation, can we slow it down so I can hear and understand what is going on?' I sometimes have to do this two or three times but I've noticed over time that another member of the group will take the time to slow things down and remind others. It just takes repetition and I've gotten *much* better."

FINAL REMARKS

Hearing aids and other listening devices do not always address the problems that patients with hearing loss experience. They may continue to struggle with the changes hearing loss has wrought in their world. When persons experience a catastrophe in their lives, it is not unusual for the educational and health care systems of many countries to provide emotional and psychological support. Certainly, hearing loss should be afforded the same status as other negative life events.

KEY CHAPTER POINTS

- Counseling provides many benefits to patients and their families, including better self-acceptance and reduced stress and discouragement. A clinician might provide informational counseling and personal adjustment counseling.

- During informational counseling, the clinician strives to ensure understanding and retention using such techniques as explicit categorization and repetition of important information.

- Personal adjustment counseling approaches are often categorized as cognitive, behavioral, or emotional, or a combination of any of these three.

- Rational Emotive Behavior Therapy (REBT) is a cognitive approach to counseling and, in the aural rehabilitation setting, entails questioning erroneous beliefs about hearing-related issues.

- Desensitization is a technique used in a behavioral counseling approach that aims for a patient to "unlearn" a learned behavior.

- Three tenets of Rogers's affective approach to counseling are congruence of self, unconditional positive regard, and empathetic understanding.

- Individuals who suffer a hearing loss, whether it is sudden or gradual, often develop a sense that they have gone from being able-bodied to being abnormal. Some of these individuals might benefit from psychosocial support.

- Psychosocial support aims to facilitate emotional, psychological, and social adjustment to hearing loss. The outcome is increased self-confidence, increased self-acceptance, and more effective use of communication strategies.

- In a problem-solving approach, patients learn to identify the kinds of problems they are experiencing, understand the nature and effect of these problems, and generate effective solutions for resolving them.

- During assertiveness training, individuals learn to increase cooperativeness with their communication partners and to develop neutral nonaggressive behaviors that allow them to maintain their self-esteem without encroaching on the rights of others.

- During assertiveness training, emphasis is placed on choice of language and on the consequences of behaviors.

- Sometimes losing one's hearing constitutes a catastrophic life experience. Individuals require and deserve adequate emotional and psychological support.

TERMS AND CONCEPTS TO REMEMBER

Informational counseling
Explicit categorization
Personal adjustment counseling
Cognitive approach
Rational Emotive Behavior Therapy (REBT)
A-B-C-D-E
Behavioral approach

Desensitization
Affective approach
Unconditional positive regard
Empathetic understanding
Self-image
Problem identification-exploration-resolution
Situation-specific behaviors

MULTIPLE-CHOICE QUESTIONS

1. An intervention that focuses on conversational behaviors and effective means for interacting with others can best be described as:

    a. Assertiveness training

    b. Personal adjustment counseling

    c. Psychosocial support

    d. Empathetic understanding intervention

2. Someone who behaves in a genuine fashion and who does not assume a facade of professionalism is said to have:

    a. Unconditional positive regard

    b. Empathetic understanding

    c. Congruence with self

    d. Rational self acceptance

3. Mrs. Greenfield has just been told that she has a hearing loss. She does not know much about the anatomy of the ear, hearing loss, hearing aids, or assistive listening devices. At this point, the clinician is most likely to provide:

    a. Informational counseling

    b. Personal adjustment counseling

    c. Desensitization

    d. Communication strategies counseling

4. An audiologist has performed an audiological evaluation on Mr. Thompson. The audiogram reveals a noise-induced hearing loss. The audiologist starts the informational counseling session by saying, "I'll first talk about the ear and about hearing, then I will

talk about today's test results, and then about what might happen next. We will also talk about ways to protect your ears against noise." This introduction is an example of:

    a. Focused attention

    b. Problem identification

    c. Explicit categorization

    d. Taking advantage of the primacy effect

5. The stages of a problem-solving approach in psychosocial support are:

    a. Problem exploration, research, solution

    b. Problem identification, exploration, resolution

    c. Problem resolution, practice, review

    d. Problem exploration, identification, management.

6. Psychosocial support typically focuses on all of the following except:

    a. The impact of hearing loss on self-image

    b. The spouse's ability to deal with the effects of hearing loss

    c. Understanding the time course of hearing loss over time

    d. Negative attitudes about self and others

7. Creating a scenario is one means of initiating:

    a. Counseling

    b. Self-profiling

    c. Exploration

    d. Problem identification

8. Patients' frequent communication partners are often encouraged to attend psychosocial support sessions for many reasons, but especially because:

    a. They need to understand the effects of hearing loss on speech recognition.

    b. Research suggests that patients are more likely to attend intervention sessions if they are accompanied by their spouses.

    c. They too can learn assertive conversational behaviors.

    d. They play an influential role in shaping patients' self-images and self-confidence.

9. A woman believes that she did not receive a promotion at work because she has a hearing loss. The audiologist uses the following approach to challenge this belief:

    a. Clarification

    b. Reflection

    c. Problem-solving framework

    d. REBT, where her evaluation of the event is disputed

10. Assertiveness training may include the same three stages as:

    a. Informational counseling

    b. Personal adjustment counseling

    c. Communication strategies training

    d. Behavioral counseling

KEY RESOURCES

The curriculum for the St. Louis Psychosocial Hearing Rehabilitation Workshop (Heydebrand, Mauzé, Tye-Murray, Binzer, & Skinner, 2005). Persons who use cochlear implants and their frequent communication partners attended this 2-day workshop.

Day 1

9:30–9:45 Introduction

Fitting of Group FM assistive devices

Outline of group

- About communication strategies (and why it may be hard to use them)
- Problem identification
- Problem exploration
- Problem resolution

Ask group to generate rules of group communication:

- Right to pass on responding to a question.
- Mutual respect.
- One at a time.

- Confidentiality.
- "I" statements.
- Speak as you want others to speak to you—"clear speech."
- When you finish speaking, signal.

Goals

What do you expect from the group? What do you hope to gain by the end of this workshop? [Have participants write down individual goals.]

9:45–10:30 Ice breaker: Spondee exercise: Select one of the spondee cards (e.g., "base" or "ball") and introduce yourself to the person who has the other half of your word. Take time to talk about when you developed a hearing loss and how it has affected your everyday routines.

10:30–10:40: Break

10:40–11:15 What's the worst thing about living with a hearing loss? For example: What do you miss? If you could change something, what would you change? What frustrates you or upsets you the most?

This group workshop is designed to:

- Help you better understand the problems you face.
- Identify strategies for dealing with these difficulties.

11:45–12:00 Susan's dinner party (schematic of the living room where the party is being held is included in your materials folder)

- Would you come to Susan's party? Why or why not?
- Will you have a good time? Why or why not?
- What might your partner do?
- If you don't do anything, why?
- What does it feel like?
- If you don't come, what would you say to Susan?

Introduction to choices, what is hard/easy about this?

Choices on a continuum, from doing nothing and being passive to being aggressive; brainstorm choices as a group.

General discussion

[Problem identification and exploration]

Which situations do you (or would your partner) find difficult?

What would you do in each situation? What might your partner do? If you don't do anything, why? If your partner would do nothing, why?

[Problem resolution]

Strategies (categories)

- Eliminate the problem.
- Assert your needs.
- Negotiate a better environment.
- Situate yourself away from the noise.
- Put up with it.
- Stay home.

12:00–2:00 Lunch

1:00–2:00 How do you identify yourself? Are you deaf, hard of hearing, impaired, disabled?

- How do you think of yourself?
- Are you happy with how you explain your problem to others?
- Are you comfortable with it?
- Do you see yourself in the hearing world or the Deaf world?
- How do others see you?

Break into groups of four and build a collage, using pictures from magazines, to show the world who you are.

2:00–2:10 Break

2:10–3:00 Exploration of passive, assertive, and aggressive communication behaviors

Marian's social gathering

Identify strategies as passive, assertive, or aggressive

3:00–3:30 The effects of deafness on the body—stress, what is the connection?

- How do you know if you are stressed? (brainstorm)
- What can we do about it? (brainstorm)

Relaxation exercise

3:30–4:00 Wrap-up, anticipate possible emotional reactions to what we have done today

Day 2

9:30–10:00 Review of previous day

How was yesterday's experience for you?

10:00–10:30 Changing roles—participants meet with one clinician, frequent communication partners meet with the other clinician.

- How has your role changed since the onset of the hearing loss? Since the receipt of a cochlear implant?
- How do you feel about your role?
- What style of communication do you use? Why?
- Can you help your frequent communication partner become more assertive? How?

10:30–10:45 Break

10:45–12:00 Explore role changes together.

- Being helpful versus taking over.
- What it is like to be a "partner"/dependent.
- Finding the balance.

Partner issues

- Being helpful versus taking over.
- "Rescuing" and dependency.
- What it's like to be a "partner."
- What has changed since the hearing loss?
- Finding the balance.

12:00–1:00 Lunch

1:00–2:00 How to be assertive

- Role-play difficult situations; discuss communication style and use of communication strategies within the context of each role-playing scenario. For example, at the bank or in the doctor's office, are behaviors assertive, aggressive, or passive? Are they effective?

2:00–2:10 Break

2:10–2:45 Individual goals and contracts

Set realistic goals (examples).

What do you want to change?

What are you in control of?

Focus on step-by-step progress.

Keep a journal?

2:45–3:00 Relaxation exercises

3:00–3:45 Evaluation/debriefing

- What was the most important thing you learned during this workshop?
- What was the least useful?
- Will what you have learned help you in your everyday life?
- Has your partner's presence changed anything in how the workshop went for you? What made you decide to come?

PART 3

Aural Rehabilitation for Adults

CHAPTER 11

Adults Who Have Hearing Loss

OUTLINE

- Prevalence of hearing loss among adults

- A patient-centered approach

- Characteristics of adult-onset hearing loss

- Who is this person?

- Where is the person in terms of adjustment to hearing loss?

- Case studies: One size doesn't fit all

- Final remarks

- Key chapter points

- Terms and concepts to remember

- Multiple-choice questions

- Key Resources

- Appendix 11-1

This chapter concerns persons who are between the ages of 17 and 60 years. Many individuals in this age bracket are highly involved in family, community, and work situations, and many lead active social lives. A major goal of an aural rehabilitation plan will be to promote effective communication with family members, friends, and coworkers. Although much of what we review will be applicable to the entire adult population, Chapter 13 is devoted to special considerations for older adults, individuals who are over the age of 60 years. In this chapter, we will consider who is this patient and where is the patient in terms of adjustment to hearing loss. In Chapter 12, we will consider aural rehabilitation intervention plans for adults.

PREVALENCE OF HEARING LOSS AMONG ADULTS

Prevalence is the percentage of a population that experiences a particular health problem at a point in time.

A **noise notch** is a pattern of audiometric thresholds characterized by a dip in hearing sensitivity at 4,000 Hz and is often found in someone who has a history of noise exposure.

Causes cited for hearing loss by adults who report having one:

- 51% cite exposure to loud noises, either on the job, from recreational activities, or from both.
- 37% cite age.
- 18% cite a medical condition.

(Prince Market Research, 2004, p. 8)

Although a common perception is that adult-onset hearing loss occurs primarily in older persons, individuals in their 40s and 50s are increasingly experiencing hearing loss. Clarity, a supplier of amplified telephones, in conjunction with the not-for-profit Ear Foundation, sponsored a survey of 437 individuals across the United States in the age range of 40–59 years. Almost half (49%) of the participants believed that they have difficulty in hearing (Prince Market Research, 2004). One in three reported that they had obtained a hearing test and about one in six (15%) reported that they had been medically diagnosed as having a hearing loss. Men in this age bracket appear to be at higher risk than women.

A longitudinal, population-based study of adults in Beaver Dam, Wisconsin, found that the **prevalence** of hearing loss was 19% for men between the ages of 48 and 59 years and 7% for women. If an individual, male or female, in Beaver Dam had been identified as having had a hearing loss 5 years earlier (Cruickshanks et al., 1998), then they had a better than 50% chance of having had their hearing worsen over the half-decade interval (Cruickshanks et al., 2003).

Even young adults are at risk for hearing loss in this era of iPODs, loud music, power engines, recreational vehicles, and personal sound systems (Figure 11-1). A group of researchers analyzed the yearly rates of hearing loss among adults between the ages of 17 and 25 years who were starting jobs at a U.S. corporation between the years of 1985 and 2004. About 16% of the participants presented a high-frequency sensorineural hearing loss and 20% presented a characteristic audiometric **noise notch** (i.e., a dip in hearing sensitivity at 4,000 Hz). This audiometric configuration, shown

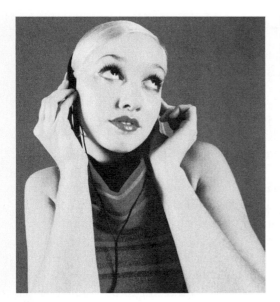

FIGURE 11-1. Noise exposure and hearing loss. Many adults under the age of 60 years have experienced a lifetime of noise exposure. *Copyright Photodisc/Getty Images.*

"Baby boomers are the first generation to be exposed to electronically amplified sound. Today, we know that prolonged exposure to loudly amplified music over 85 dB [SPL] can cause permanent hearing loss. Many cases of hearing loss among baby boomers can be traced to their youth when they listened to rock bands or played in them. Additionally, baby boomers are the first generation to experience prolonged exposure to loud sounds from electric blenders, lawn care equipment, power tools, recreational vehicles, jet airplanes and even electric tooth brushes."

Randy Wohlers, President of HearPod, Inc., which specializes in treating hearing loss in adults.

(PRWebRelease Press Release, February 22, 2006)

in Figure 11-2, is considered to be a hallmark of noise-induced hearing loss. The good news is that the levels of hearing sensitivity appear to have remained stable during the two decades during which the study was performed (Rabinowitz, Slade, Galusha, Dixon-Ernst, & Cullen, 2006).

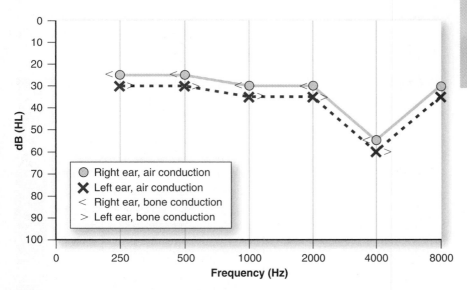

FIGURE 11-2. Audiogram for someone who has a noise-induced hearing loss. It is characterized by the "notch" at 4,000 Hz.

A PATIENT-CENTERED APPROACH

The guiding theme of this chapter is as follows: Any successful aural rehabilitation plan must be founded on a patient orientation.

A **patient orientation** to aural rehabilitation designs and delivers rehabilitation services based on the patient's background, current status, needs, and wants.

This is a simple idea that is the essence of a service practice. A **patient orientation** holds that the most successful aural rehabilitation program is one that best determines individuals' backgrounds, current status, needs, and wants and then accommodates them through the design and delivery of appropriate interventions. The objectives of speech and hearing professionals entail more than arriving at a correct diagnosis of hearing loss and fitting appropriate listening aids. The professionals allow space for their patients to articulate their concerns, they help them to identify their specific communication difficulties and their expectations, and they work to devise solutions, while showing a "human face" (Borrell-Carrio, Suchman, & Epstein, 2004, p. 578). This patient-centered approach is in contrast to a **sales orientation**, in which the emphasis is on telling or persuading people that they need certain aural rehabilitation services or listening devices and that your practice is better than the competition at providing them.

A **sales orientation** to aural rehabilitation emphasizes persuading the patient to pursue and procure services, interventions, and listening devices.

This philosophic orientation does not mean that speech and hearing professionals must begin with a blank slate with every new patient. Rather, certain aural rehabilitation offerings may be more appropriate for some persons than for others, and variable parameters of those services can be adjusted to meet a targeted individual need. A person who has minimal residual hearing may not receive auditory training, but rather, communication strategies and speechreading training. An individual with a mild hearing loss may receive only a hearing aid and counseling.

Who Knows Best?

In an article about why 21 million people in the United States do nothing about their hearing loss (roughly, 80% of persons with hearing loss), Taylor and Hansen (2002) suggest that professionals in the hearing health care field might change the way they counsel potential patients. Instead of focusing on the selling of products and services, we should instead focus on the patient: What triggered his or her visit to the clinic and what is the best way to move the patient toward taking ownership of the hearing difficulties? In discussing this premise, Taylor and Hansen note:

> We have been taught that we "know what is best for the patient." Unfortunately, reluctant patients are not "getting" our

Who Knows Best? *continued*

message. It is even more unfortunate that hearing care professionals aren't getting the message either. *The answer to reluctance resides in the patient, not in the hearing professionals.* One cannot tell, advise, or cajole the reluctant patient into understanding and accepting their disability. If telling, advising, or complaining about the patient's hearing impairment worked consistently, the "nagging" spouse, friends, and loved ones would have succeeded years ago in persuading throngs of people to positively address their disability. . . .

So often in the hearing health care field, professionals are consumed with "The Close." This is not to imply that we're obsessed with selling products or services; rather, there is a tendency to jump forward to the conclusion before allowing the patient to come to that conclusion for him/herself. In short, we need to see our role as a hearing care professional differently. We need to become more interested in the *opening* of the patient. Nothing can be closed if it is not opened first. *It is a monumental occurrence that the reluctant, frightened, anxious, nervous, angry patient that you regularly see has come to the office in the first place.* We need to find out what trigger has finally caused the person to come in after putting off the visit for 7–10 years. There is a great need to move the patient toward **ownership** of their visit to the clinic, and not allow the patient to delude him/herself by blaming their visit on some external force like their spouse. (pp. 32–33)

Ownership refers to the feeling of responsibility and need to manage or oversee.

CHARACTERISTICS OF ADULT-ONSET HEARING LOSS

Most adults lose their hearing gradually over time. The largest segment of adults who have hearing loss has mild or moderate sensorineural hearing loss. Typically, thresholds for the mid and high frequencies are poorer than those for the lower frequencies, regardless of the patient's age (Davis, 1994). Figure 11-3 presents the averages of audiometric thresholds for the frequencies 500, 1,000, 2,000, and 4,000 Hz (obtained in the worse ear) for two groups of individuals, those between the ages of 15 and 50 years and those between the ages of 51 and 60 years, and for two countries,

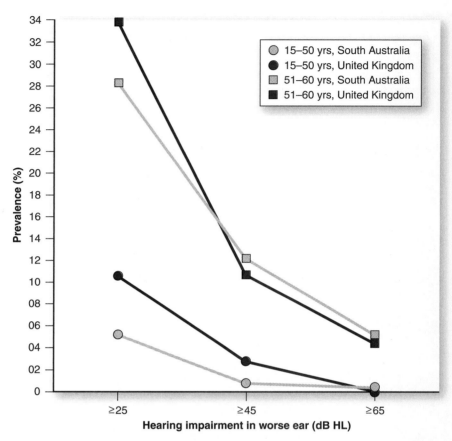

FIGURE 11-3. Prevalence of hearing impairment (averaged over 500, 1,000, 2,000, 4,000 Hz) in the worse ear for a South Australian population (*n* = 926) and a United Kingdom population (*n* = 2662), for participants between the ages of 15 and 50 years and between the ages of 51 and 60 years.

Australia (Wilson et al., 1999) and the United Kingdom (Davis, 1989). This figure reveals a higher prevalence of mild, moderate, and severe hearing loss for the two older groups than for the two younger groups. Whereas the younger groups had a prevalence of moderate hearing loss ranging between 0.8% and 2.8%, the older group had a prevalence ranging between 10.7% and 12.2%.

Adults who have hearing loss may perceive conversational speech as too soft and as sounding mumbled. The greater loss of sensitivity in the higher frequencies compared to the milder loss in the lower frequencies often results in reception of the low-pitched acoustic segments associated with vowel sounds but not the high-pitched segments associated with consonant sounds. Hence, a commonly heard complaint is, "I can hear people talk but I can't understand what they say." The presence of background noise exacerbates this problem because it can further mask the high-pitched consonant sounds that are difficult to discriminate even in quiet. Similarly, females or children may be more difficult to understand than males, due to their characteristically high-pitched voices and softer speaking levels.

WHO IS THIS PERSON?

In addressing the question, "Who is my patient?" a speech and hearing professional might consider a number of variables, including a patient's stage of life, life factors, socioeconomic status, race and ethnicity, gender, psychological adjustment, home, social, and vocational hearing-related communication difficulties, other hearing-related complaints, and whether the patient identifies him or herself as being hard of hearing or Deaf (Figure 11-4). Each one of these variables will be considered one by one.

> "None of us protected our ears at all . . . I'm still a junkie, I still want it so loud . . . [yet when the dishwasher is running] I can't hear any conversation at all."
>
> Pat Benatar, age 54 years, rock singer and guitarist, and spokeswoman for Hearing Education and Awareness for Rockers (HEAR)
>
> (Rosenbloom, 2007, p. E6)

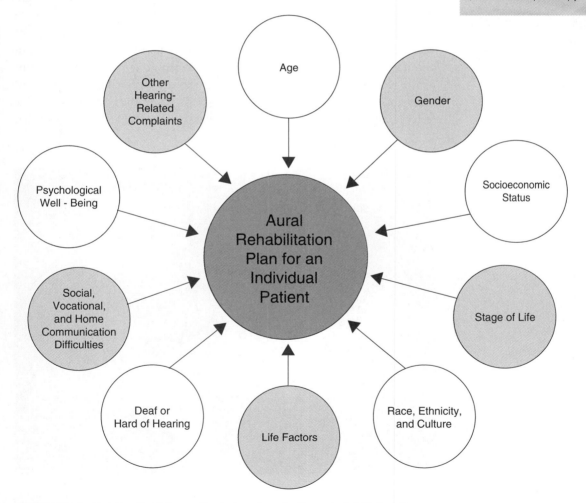

FIGURE 11-4. Variables that influence the design of a patient's aural rehabilitation plan.

Stage of Life

Jim Lawson and his 20-year-old son Kevin were in a car accident. Both received head trauma and, as a result, incurred irreversible bilateral hearing losses (Figure 11-5).

For both Lawsons, life with hearing loss will never be like it was before the accident. However, the impact differs somewhat because the two men are in different stages of life.

Jim Lawson owns a small advertising firm, which he started after college graduation. After many years of long hours and hard work, the firm is well-established and successful.

The accident has left Jim filled with bitterness. He believes life has dealt him a blow just when he was experiencing decreased responsibilities and more freedom to pursue leisure activities. He now contemplates early retirement because his hearing loss interferes with his ability to interact with clients, but also has misgivings because he had hoped to have a larger savings account before retiring. Jim no longer socializes at executive meetings and plays less tennis because he cannot converse easily with his friends on the court. He feels old and frequently is saddened by passing thoughts, such as the fact that

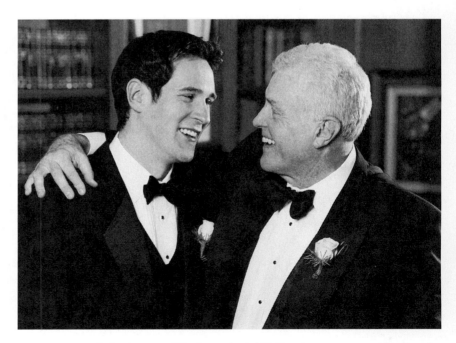

FIGURE 11-5. Patient's stage of life. An aural rehabilitation plan may vary as a function of a patient's stage of life.

he will never hear the voices of his grandchildren. Increasingly, he depends on his wife for communication with the outside world.

Jim's son is a junior in college with a major in public relations. Prior to the accident, Kevin Lawson participated in several extracurricular activities and dreamed of creating a public relations empire.

The hearing loss has left Kevin deflated. Because public relations entails communication, he wonders whether he should complete his college program. He feels embarrassed by the use of a professional note taker in class, but fears that asking classmates to share notes might elicit pity. Kevin spends hours alone in the gym lifting weights, bedeviled by concerns for his future.

Table 11-1 summarizes **life stages** and indicates how hearing loss may have an impact (Van Hecke, 1994). Adults who have hearing loss often experience

Life stages are age ranges in which a hearing loss may have a different impact.

Table 11-1. Life stages and the impact of hearing loss (see Van Hecke, 1994).

STAGE	EVENTS ASSOCIATED WITH STAGE	IMPACT OF HEARING LOSS
Young adulthood	Develop intimate relationships with others Accept financial responsibility for self Develop a vision of one's future life and begin to pursue dreams	Begin to reassess dreams Experience self-doubt about finding life partner
The thirties	Reassess life decisions (e.g., Is this the right job?) Career consolidation Modify life structures or reverse decisions that now seem inappropriate Invest self in job, family, and friends	Energy is not invested in reassessment Hesitation about change arises
Middle adulthood	Begin to consider own mortality Note clear signs of physical aging in self May feel that this is last chance to make life changes	Upward mobility may cease Uncertainty about goals and ability to achieve them may increase
The fifties	Children may have left home Career may be well-established Time is available to pursue leisure activities	May consider early retirement Fears of aging intensify Withdrawal from leisure activities may occur
Late adulthood	Deterioration occurs in health, physical attractiveness, and strength Friends and family are lost through death or relocation as a result of retirement One begins to review one's life and reflect on its meaning	Other problems related to aging are intensified (e.g., loneliness) Overall sense of loss is exacerbated

similar emotions such as frustration, and they experience common difficulties such as communication breakdown. However, as the example of the Lawson family illustrates, the impact of hearing loss relates to an individual's *stage of life,* that is, whether the individual is in young adulthood, in the 30s, 40s, 50s, or in the later years. Physically, cognitively, and socially, individuals at age 55 differ from their 25-year-old selves. Depending on their life stage, patients will confront different issues. Adulthood is a lifelong journey that is multidirectional and multidimensional, historically embedded, and contextual. By being sensitive to where patients are in the life span, a speech and hearing professional will gain additional insight into their concerns and aural rehabilitation needs.

Life Factors

By adulthood, most people have achieved socialization. They have established relationships with others, embarked on a vocation, and developed a personality and a personal view of the world. **Life factors** are in place. These factors may be socially and culturally determined, controlled by the individual, fixed, determined by the environment, or influenced by other qualities of the individual and his or her life situation. As with demographic factors, life factors influence the ways in which people cope with the advent of hearing loss. For instance, an individual with a heart problem and an extended family may not be as concerned about a subsequent mild or moderate hearing loss than someone who has been taking antidepressants and who has recently lost a job. Someone who holds prejudices about hearing loss beforehand may suffer from a negative self-image and self-stigmatization afterward.

Life factors are conditions that help define one's life, such as relationships, family, and vocation.

Figure 11-6 presents a model of the life factor influences that have an impact on how a male patient might view hearing loss, factors that also have an impact on the patient's aural rehabilitation needs. The figure is comprised of concentric circles corresponding to self, home, work, recreation, and community. First, there is the innermost circle of self. Prior to hearing loss onset, this person viewed himself as competent and independent. Hearing loss may have at least one of two effects on his perceived role and self. He may come away with the belief of, "I can handle my hearing difficulties; I've tackled tougher obstacles before." Alternatively, the onset of hearing loss may pull the rug out from under who he thinks he is and fill him with a sense of loss of self. The next ring of influence is the home. In this venue, the patient may fill the roles of husband, father, and principal wage earner. He may believe that hearing loss undermines his ability to fulfill these roles, especially if his wife and children believe likewise and hold negative stereotyped images of persons who have hearing loss. At work, the hearing loss may hamper the person's ability to manage employees and interact with colleagues during group meetings.

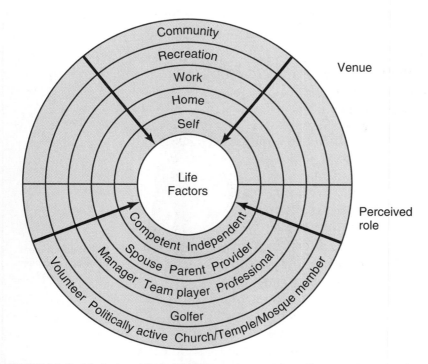

FIGURE 11-6. Life factors. Life factors influence how a patient will react to the onset of hearing loss and will affect the content of an aural rehabilitation intervention plan.

This scenario may be especially true if he is the first person in his company to present significant hearing loss and if his workplace is unfamiliar with accommodating his listening needs. On the golf course, he may become the object of subtle teasing from his golf partners, whereas in the community, he might encounter ignorance and prejudice about disabilities. Such reactions from the community, recreational venues, and even the workplace, may result in the patient withdrawing into himself and succumbing to feelings of uncertainty and isolation. The constricting arrows in Figure 11-6 reflect a common tendency of persons with hearing loss to withdraw and to cope ineffectively with hearing loss.

The influence of community is furthered detailed in Figure 11-7. Here, the person with hearing loss is represented as a jigsaw puzzle who might be rearranged according to the surrounding community norms, services, and mores. The person will live in a world that has definite notions about who is an ideal citizen and to what extent a disability removes a person from achieving this ideal. He may live in a community that views hearing loss as a tragedy, a social problem, or a medical problem. The community, and its prevailing viewpoints, will determine what support services and technologies are available, and what expectations are placed on the patient about how he or she should

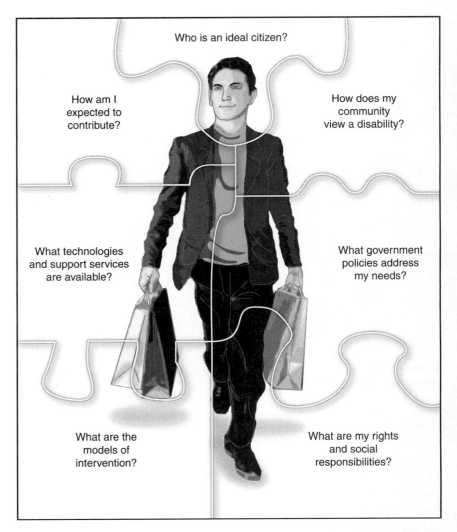

Who is an ideal citizen?

How am I
expected to
contribute?

How does my
community
view a disability?

What technologies
and support services
are available?

What government
policies address
my needs?

What are the
models of
intervention?

What are my rights
and social
responsibilities?

FIGURE 11-7. The community. The community will affect how well a patient functions with hearing loss.

lead his or her life. The community will help him answer such questions as: What kind of help do I need and where will I get it?; How am I to live my life as a person with hearing loss?; What kind of financial and technical support might I expect?; and How am I to contribute to the world around me and live my life?

Socioeconomic Status

In addition to stage of life and life factors, one's socioeconomic status can affect the impact of hearing loss and the design of an aural rehabilitation plan. Social scientists have defined at least six socioeconomic classes in American society. One's classification within this schema is based on a consideration of income, occupation, educational level, and dwelling type. These six classes are:

- high uppers
- low uppers
- high middles
- low middles
- high lowers
- low lowers

In general, persons with lower incomes (below $20,000 per year) and less education (no high school diploma) are more likely to have hearing loss than persons with higher income (over $50,000 per year) and a high school diploma (National Council on Aging, 1999).

Ways in which socioeconomic status may affect the management of hearing loss are illustrated in the following examples:

- Financial status may relate to whether an individual can afford binaural hearing aids or assistive devices.
- Educational history may determine how much background knowledge someone has about the anatomy of the ear and its possible disorders and may dictate how the problem is discussed.
- Work schedule and level of employment may determine whether someone is able to attend aural rehabilitation classes scheduled during a weekday.

Race, Ethnicity, and Culture

Health researchers recognize the multidimensional nature of race and ethnicity. Race is a confluence of biological factors, geographic origins, **culture**, and economic, political, and legal factors (Williams, 1996). None-theless there appears to be a general consensus that socioeconomic status is closely linked with racial/ethnic status (Hayward, Crimmins, Miles, & Yang, 2000). In the United States, African Americans, Hispanics, and Native Americans tend to have lower levels of income, education, wealth, and occupational status than do Whites. Not only will socioeconomic status affect the management of hearing loss, but it will have other ramifications as well. For instance, some adults of a minority may have experienced economic hardship and inadequate medical care growing up. Some may be inexperienced with interacting with health care professionals or may be distrustful of them. Some members of minority groups may hold jobs that do not offer health care benefits or they may be unemployed, so they may not have access to the best health care possible. They may live in poorer,

Culture is a conglomeration of the thoughts, communications, actions, customs, beliefs, values, and institutions of racial, ethnic, religious, or social groups.

less sought after neighborhoods (even if they share the same level of income as their White counterparts), and the health care services may not match the quality, availability, and affordability of those available in more affluent neighborhoods. For instance, closures of hospitals and health clinics happen more often in low-income and minority neighborhoods (Caesar & Williams, 2002). Older African Americans with hearing loss are less likely to use hearing aids than their White peers (Bazargan, Baker, & Bazargan, 2001), as are Hispanic adults (Lee, Gómez-Marín, & Lee, 1996).

The last U.S. census revealed that our diversity has increased significantly during the past 10 years and will continue to do so. If current trends continue, by the year 2050, 50% of the population will be ethnically or racially diverse. Figure 11-8 reflects how the general makeup of the United States has changed between the years 2000 and 2006.

Although the U.S. Bureau of Census has identified standardized categories for identifying race or ethnicity, each category contains diversity. For instance, the category of *Hispanic* includes individuals who describe themselves to be of Mexican, Puerto Rican, Cuban, and Central American origins.

With this caveat, it is still valuable to consider the general makeup of the U.S. population according to broad categories so as to gain an appreciation of the diversity of potential adult patients. Figure 11-9 illustrates the race

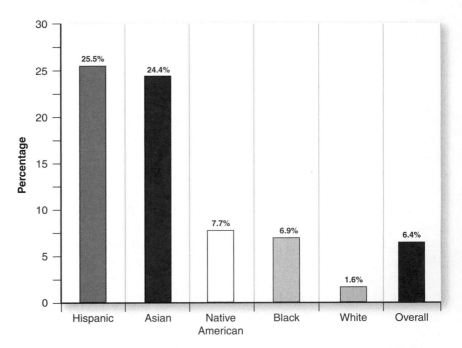

FIGURE 11-8. U.S. population growth from 2000 to 2006 according the U.S. Census Bureau. Modeled after El Nasser and Overberg (2007).

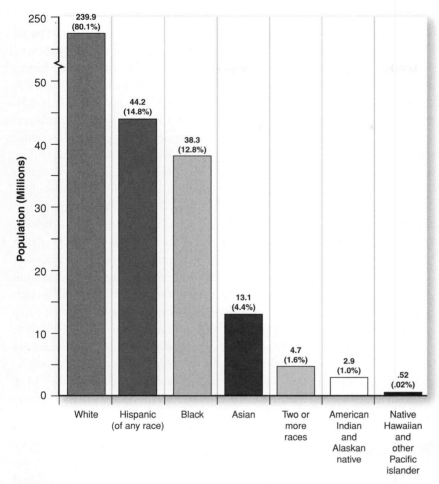

FIGURE 11-9. The race and ethnic composition of the United States as reported by the U.S. Census Bureau (2006).

and ethnicity composition of the United States. About 80% of the respondents describe themselves as White whereas the remaining 20% describe themselves as Hispanic of any race, African American or Black, Asian, Native American or Alaskan Native, or Native Hawaiian or Pacific Islander.

Hand in hand with the growing racial and ethnic heterogeneity within the United States is a growing cultural and linguistic heterogeneity. For every 1,000 Americans, 173 speak a language other than English at home. Many speech and hearing professionals will have to learn to work with patients of different cultural and linguistic backgrounds. Occasionally, they may be required to work with an **interpreter** or a **translator**. The Key Resources presents an English–Spanish list with some key audiological terms.

TRIBUTE

Treat each patient as having unique personal and hearing needs.

Respect cultural differences through both your verbal and non-verbal behaviors.

Identify the personality and learning preferences of each patient.

Begin by learning some basic information on cultural difference through formal learning in courses and worships. Supplement this information with your own informal learning experiences in the workplace and in the community.

Use language and cultural [interpreters] to keep intended messages clear between you the patient.

Tell your patients about their hearing loss and hearing needs in plain language, avoiding audiologic jargon.

Explain that adjusting to hearing loss is a family event, and include family members whenever possible in the rehabilitation process.

(Dancer, 2006, p. 26)

An **interpreter** is a person specially trained to translate oral or signed communications from one language to another.

A **translator** is a person specially trained to translate written text from one language to another.

Despite the increasing diversity (and the complexity of that diversity) of their patient population, many speech and hearing professionals feel unprepared to serve multicultural populations. An ASHA 2001 Omnibus Survey showed that 31% of its members felt only "slightly qualified" to provide services to multicultural populations, whereas 14% felt "not at all qualified." Only 10% considered themselves to be "very qualified" (*ASHA Leader,* 2002, p. 32). Many speech and hearing professionals will find it valuable to acquire **cultural and linguistic competence**, and to learn more about the people they serve, through developing relationships with people who can act as cultural informants, by attending cultural events in their communities, and by learning how a patient's linguistic and cultural background might influence the clinical decision-making process (Tomoeda & Bayles, 2002, p. 17). Racial, ethnic, and cultural and linguistic groups often have distinctive customs, beliefs, and service preferences, and these should be considered when customizing an aural rehabilitation program. For example, some cultures value expressing emotions whereas others do not. Some cultures have concepts of **clock-time** whereas others have concepts of **event-time**. Some cultures may hold health care professionals in high esteem whereas others may not. Some cultures adhere to alternative healing systems such as acupuncture (e.g., Chinese), Ayurvedic medicine (e.g., Asian-Indian), and religious/spiritual ceremonies (e.g., Laotian Hmong) (Moxley et al., 2004). Some individuals may be unaware of Medicare services and other health care systems. Appendix 11-1 summarizes some of the knowledge and skills needed by speech and hearing professionals to provide culturally appropriate services.

Cultural and linguistic competence is a set of congruent behaviors, attitudes, and policies that come together in a system, in an agency, or among professionals that enables effective work in cross-cultural situations.

Clock-time orientations are driven by the clock and are characterized by an adherence to time as a factor in determining the length of an interaction or the time-course of an intervention.

Event-time orientations are process-driven and conclusions are pursued to their natural conclusions no matter how long that might take.

LEP is an acronym for *limited English proficiency,* and is used in reference to persons who are limited in their English proficiency.

Executive Order 13166

In August 2000, President Bill Clinton signed Executive Order 13166, *Improving Access to Services for Persons with Limited English Proficiency* (**LEP**). The order mandated that "each Federal agency shall examine the services it provides and develop and implement a system by which LEP persons can meaningfully access those services consistent with, and without unduly burdening, the fundamental mission of the agency." In conjunction with this order, the U.S. Department of Justice issued a Policy Guidance Document, *Enforcement of Title VI of the Civil Rights Act of 1964—National Origin Discrimination Against Persons with Limited English Proficiency.* This document set forth the compliance standards that recipients of federal funding must follow in order to ensure that their programs and services that are typically available in English are accessible to persons with LEP, and to ensure that such persons are not discriminated against on the basis of national origin.

Gender

Patients' gender may influence the content of their aural rehabilitation program (Figure 11-10). For example, in a traditional family structure, an adult female may fear that hearing loss decreases her ability to nurture her children, and she may experience a loss of self-esteem and sense of desirability. A male may worry that he has lost his means to provide financially for his offspring and believe that he has become less manly or less vigorous in the eyes of his friends. In these two examples, counseling will have to be tailored to suit individual concerns.

Gender effects on the aural rehabilitation needs of patients have not been well studied by researchers, although a few investigators have tackled the issue, especially with regard to the older population. In middle and older adulthood, studies have shown that men have poorer speech recognition abilities than do women, even after controlling for differences in audiometric thresholds (e.g., Dubno, Lee, Matthews, & Mills, 1997; Wiley et al., 1998). Garstecki and Erler (1999) found that older females are more reliant on nonverbal repair strategies than are older males (as determined by the CPHI; see Chapter 8), and that women place a greater importance on being able to communicate in social situations. Older women also appear to be more likely to experience negative feelings (such as annoyance, anger, and aggravation) and stress during everyday communication and are more sensitive to the negative reactions of families and friends. In their study, females were more likely to report acknowledging

Cultural competency

"Gaining knowledge of salient cultural features also includes learning about social organization and communication styles. Does the culture have an individual or collectivist orientation? Is the focus on the nuclear or extended family? Is the communication style implicit or explicit?"

(Moxley et al., 2004, p. 7)

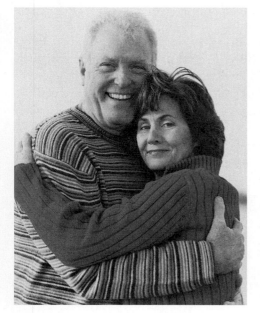

FIGURE 11-10. Gender. Gender may influence the design of an aural rehabilitation plan. Women and men may vary in their financial resources, their physiological responses to hearing loss, and their everyday listening demands.

a hearing loss than were males, and they were more likely to report actively reducing their communication difficulties (e.g., seeking favorable seating at a lecture hall).

Some women use a variety of strategies according to the "emotional temperature" of the communication situation, using repair strategies in a "friendly" situation and bluffing in an "unfriendly" situation (Hallberg & Jansson, 1996), whereas men are more apt to bluff in general (Hallberg, 1999). These findings suggest that men may use a smaller corpus of repair strategies to rectify or prevent communication breakdowns and that they might be less willing to admit communication difficulties. As such, an aural rehabilitation plan for men might include problem-solving techniques and an emphasis on expanding their repertoire of repair strategies. It might also entail counseling to accelerate and promote acceptance of hearing loss (Helfer, 2001). An aural rehabilitation plan for women might be aimed at reducing the negative impact of hearing loss, such as by use of stress management exercises and relaxation techniques (Garstecki & Erler, 1999).

As is the case with race, ethnicity, and culture, gender can be divided into subcategories. For instance, females can be divided into subsegments of "homemakers" and "workers." The latter group can be distinguished further; for example, two categories are clinical-technical and management professionals. As a function of their subsegment, individuals will require different aural rehabilitation interventions. A homemaker may be interested in obtaining a baby-cry alerting assistive device, whereas a business executive may inquire about group amplification systems.

The age of female patients may also affect the aural rehabilitation intervention. Erler and Garstecki (2002) found that younger women (those between the ages of 35 and 45 years) viewed hearing loss and the use of hearing aids more negatively than did older women (those between the ages of 75 and 85 years). One reason is that hearing loss may pose a greater communication barrier for younger women. They tend to be engaged in child rearing, work, and situations that require effective communication. Another reason is that older women usually have more friends and relatives who have hearing loss and who use hearing aids, and thus, hearing loss and the use of amplification are not as foreign to them as they might be to younger women.

Psychological Well-Being

As noted in the last chapter, adults who have hearing loss may be more likely to suffer from feelings of loneliness than their counterparts who have normal hearing and more likely to experience decreased self-esteem and other emotional difficulties, including embarrassment, shame, and uncertainty about one's social identity. They may feel isolated both socially and emotionally. Depending upon a patient's psychosocial well-being, the aural rehabilitation may be tailored to including psychosocial support and counseling.

Home, Social, and Vocational Hearing-Related Communication Difficulties

How individuals spend their time each day will factor into the development of an aural rehabilitation plan. The needs of a man who spends most of his free time playing computer games will differ from those of a man who spends most of his free time socializing with friends. Figure 11-11 illustrates how the average man and woman in the United States spends a typical day. These statistics were compiled by the *Bureau of Labor Statistics American Time Use Survey*, which asked 13,000 household respondents to describe how they lived

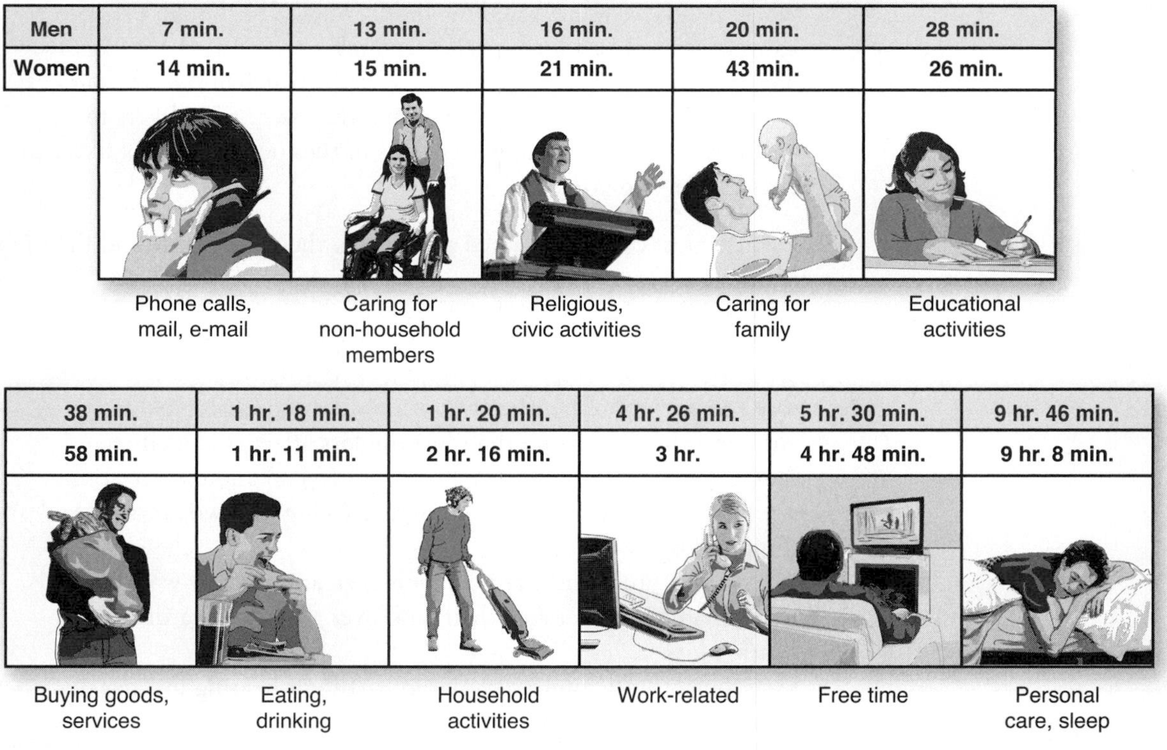

"Besides reduced ability to enjoy music and other sounds that we appreciate, hearing loss may produce social isolation, distorted communication, and, in some cases, stigmatization, all of which can affect mental health and quality of life."

Kristian Tambas, Researcher at the Norwegian Institute of Public Health

(Tambas, 2004, p. 776)

Men	7 min.	13 min.	16 min.	20 min.	28 min.
Women	14 min.	15 min.	21 min.	43 min.	26 min.
	Phone calls, mail, e-mail	Caring for non-household members	Religious, civic activities	Caring for family	Educational activities

38 min.	1 hr. 18 min.	1 hr. 20 min.	4 hr. 26 min.	5 hr. 30 min.	9 hr. 46 min.
58 min.	1 hr. 11 min.	2 hr. 16 min.	3 hr.	4 hr. 48 min.	9 hr. 8 min.
Buying goods, services	Eating, drinking	Household activities	Work-related	Free time	Personal care, sleep

FIGURE 11-11. How American men and women spend their time each day (min = minute; hr = hours). Modeled after Dykman (2006).

a single day in the year 2005 (Dykman, 2006). Besides time for personal care and sleep, the majority of the 24-hour day appears to be devoted to work-related activities and free time. The survey found that the most common free time pastime was television viewing, between 2 hours and 41 minutes and 3 hours and 28 minutes, on average, for women and men respectively. These findings imply that instruction about closed-caption use and provision of television-related assistive listening technology might be included in many patients' aural rehabilitation plans. Solutions for work-related communication difficulties may be at the top of many patients' wish lists.

A survey conducted by Prince Market Research (2006) focused on hearing-related difficulties experienced by adults between the ages of 41 and 60 years. The organization conducted interviews with 458 individuals across the United States. The responses obtained are representative of the kinds of problems that patients might report experiencing. Difficulties affecting home and social life were as follows (p. 9):

- Two thirds of those interviewed reported some difficulty in hearing the television.
- Three quarters said that they often found themselves in situations where people were not speaking loudly or clearly enough or where the television wasn't loud or clear enough.
- The participants in the survey, when asked which areas were most affected by their hearing loss, said that they were most likely to avoid watching television with others in the room and most likely to avoid social gatherings.

The issues most commonly cited as affecting their workplace and their jobs were as follows (p. 10):

- One fourth of those interviewed reported that hearing loss affects their work, including 67% of respondents who have severe hearing loss and 42% of respondents with a moderate hearing loss.
- Amongst those who said their hearing loss affects work either "somewhat" or "quite a bit," phone calls (64%) and conversations with coworkers (61%) were reported as being the two areas most impacted by hearing loss.
- Despite the problems that hearing loss creates in their workplace, fewer than 5% have asked their employer for help regarding their hearing loss.
- One fourth of the sample pool said that their hearing loss has decreased their earning potential.

Other Hearing-Related Complaints

Some patients will experience other impairments related to their hearing loss, the most common of which is **tinnitus**. The word *tinnitus* is a derivative of the Latin word *tinnire,* which means to ring or tinkle. Tinnitus often accompanies adult hearing loss, with about 70% to 80% of patients who report tinnitus also reporting "significant hearing difficulties" (Vernon & Miekle, 2000), although individuals with normal hearing also experience it. Most tinnitus is subjective, meaning that it is a phantom sound sensation. A minority of patients have tinnitus that relates to an internal sound source, such as a pulsing blood vessel, or other vascular, muscular, or respiratory origins. This latter type of tinnitus can sometimes be ameliorated by medical intervention (Eggermont, 2005).

Tinnitus is the perception of sound in the head without an external cause.

Common descriptors of tinnitus include leaves rustling, the ocean roaring, crickets chirping, a radio playing off-station, a siren blasting, or a telephone ringing. The quality of sound might be crackling, pulsing, pounding, hissing, humming, musical, throbbing, whistling, popping, or whooshing. A person might perceive sound in the right ear, left ear, both ears, or inside or outside of the head.

The prevalence of tinnitus in the general adult population has been estimated to be between 10% and 15% and the prevalence rate rises with increasing age (Hoffman & Reed, 2004). British epidemiologists suggest that 5% of the United Kingdom's adult population experience tinnitus that can be described as a "problem" (Davis & Rafaie, 2000). In Sweden, 3% of the population describe tinnitus as a "severe problem" (Axelsson & Ringdahl, 1989). Tinnitus is correlated with degree of hearing loss, with those who have greater hearing loss also having a greater complaint of tinnitus. The presence of tinnitus may greatly influence, and even determine, the aural rehabilitation intervention.

As Table 11-2 indicates, etiologies of tinnitus are varied. The data reported in this table were collected from 2,369 patients at the Oregon Tinnitus Clinic. Forty percent reported that they could not identify a cause. Of the remainder, etiologies reflected four general categories: (a) noise-related, (b) head and neck trauma, (c) head and neck illness, and (d) other medical conditions, illness, drugs, stress (such as bereavement and loss of employment), and surgery.

Ménière's disease is an inner ear disorder that is related to idiopathic endolymphatic hydrops and may cause vertigo, hearing loss, tinnitus, and the sensation of fullness in the ear.

Some illnesses associated with tinnitus are **Ménière's disease**, **acoustic neuroma**, and head and neck injuries, such as whiplash. Some tinnitus-inducing agents include aspirin, salicylates, quinine, aminoglycoside antibiotics, and cisplatin. These kinds of drugs may cause either transient or chronic tinnitus.

An **acoustic neuroma** is a tumor of the auditory or eighth nerve, usually benign, that may cause gradual hearing loss, tinnitus, and dizziness.

Table 11-2. Conditions that have been associated with tinnitus, as reported from 2,369 patients from the Oregon tinnitus clinic (adapted from Henry, Dennis, & Schechter, 2005, p. 1210).

CATEGORY OF ASSOCIATED CONDITION	CAUSE	% (AS SINGLE CAUSE)	TOTAL % AS SINGLE CAUSE	TOTAL % AS ONE OF MULTIPLE CAUSES
Noise related			18%	22%
	Long-duration noise	10%		
	Explosion	5%		
	Brief intense noise	3%		
Head and neck trauma			8%	17%
	Head injury	4%		
	Whiplash/cervical trauma	3%		
	Concussion	<1%		
	Skull fracture	<1%		
Head and neck illness			8%	10%
	Ear infection, inflammation	3%		
	Cold, sinus infection	3%		
	Other ear problems	2%		
	Sudden hearing loss	<1%		
	Allergies, hay fever	<1%		
Other medical conditions			7%	13%
	Other illnesses	2%		
	Drugs, medication	2%		
	Stress	<1%		
	Surgery	<1%		
	Possible temporomandibular syndrome	<1%		
	Barotrauma	<1%		

Barotrauma occurs to divers and snorkelers and relates to water pressure.

Diet may exacerbate tinnitus. For example, salt has been found to aggravate tinnitus, especially in patients who have high blood pressure, because it restricts blood vessels, raises blood pressure, and impedes blood circulation (Keate, 2006).

The heterogeneity of etiologies and experience of tinnitus is so great that it is likely that no one agent or treatment will be appropriate for all patients (Baquley, Davies, & Hazell, 2003). However, many investigators believe that tinnitus problems emerge from an interplay of physical and psychological factors. For instance, an abnormality at the level of the cochlea may lead to the generation of a weak neuronal signal. The signal may be detected on the conscious level as sound and, with continued occurrences, may become irritating to the patient and lead to a heightened cognitive awareness of the phantom signal. Subsequently, greater negative emotional reactions may result when the signal is detected, which may in turn lead to even greater awareness (Jastreboff, 1990, 2001). As we shall see in the next chapter, a number of interventions focus on reducing the psychological factors that contribute to a patient's tinnitus experience.

For some people, tinnitus is a minor annoyance that is bothersome only in quiet situations, such as when trying to go to sleep. For a significant number, however, tinnitus is debilitating, the cause of frustration, depression, hopelessness, and even thoughts of suicide. Tinnitus can result in an inability to concentrate (Hallan, McKenna, & Shurlock, 2004; Rossiter, Stevens, & Walker, 2006), increased difficulty in listening because it can mask the speech signal, and loss of sleep. It also can lead to a reduced quality of life (Nondahl et al., 2007).

Tinnitus Can Be Debilitating

In some people, there is an association between tinnitus and psychopathological characteristics such as depression, anxiety, hysteria, and hypochondria. Though it is not possible to establish a clear cause and effect between tinnitus and such disorders, it appears that tinnitus can impose severe consequences on patients' ability to function in everyday life (e.g., Holgers, Zöger, & Svedlund, 2005; Marciano et al., 2003).

Actor William Shatner, star of the *Star Trek* television series and movies, has experienced tinnitus for almost a decade. As the following excerpt demonstrates, he experienced desperate moments before finding some relief through a therapy offered by Dr. Pawel Jastreboff (Shatner, 1997):

> Over the years I tried herbal remedies. I tried eardrops. I bought masking devices to avoid the silence, and tapes and records of soothing sounds—Japanese music, running water. And inside my house is a little waterfall. The sound of the water is very soothing.

continues

Tinnitus Can Be Debilitating, *continued*

Getting through the nights—that was always the worst. Sometimes I paced the halls. I often turned to writing and exercise, and fatigued myself to sleep. I'd have the television on all night. It affected my marriage; if one person needs noise and the other person is sensitive to it, it can lead to separation . . . I could not sleep without sound. In my darkest moments I thought to myself, "Will it be this way for the rest of my life, the way I am tormented by it now?" I began to think, "What are the ways to take my life? How does one kill oneself?" I went so far as to start making plans. (pp. 154–155)

Mr. Shatner's essay ended on a somber note. He related, "Recently I made a call to somebody in California who had promised Dr. Jasterboff money, and when I called, his wife answered and said he was dead. He had committed suicide because of tinnitus" (p. 155).

The Deaf Culture

The **Deaf culture** is a subculture that shares a common language, American Sign Language (ASL), beliefs, customs, arts, history, and folklore, primarily composed of individuals who have prelingual deafness.

The **Hearing culture** is the mainstream culture in the United States and includes auditory experiences in addition to or in lieu of visual experiences.

Membership in a the Deaf culture may affect the aural rehabilitation plan. Adult members of the **Deaf culture** are individuals who lost their hearing early in life. They rely on sign language for face-to-face communication, and many believe they are culturally and linguistically distinct from hearing society. Members of the Deaf culture use a capital *D* in the term *Deaf* to distinguish themselves from the audiologic condition of hearing loss. Membership in the Deaf culture is not determined by one's degree of hearing loss, but rather, by one's identification with Deaf people. For example, two individuals may have identical severe bilateral hearing losses. One of them may use powerful hearing aids and feel a part of the **Hearing culture**, whereas the other may socialize primarily with Deaf people.

In some ways, members of the Deaf culture have different problems than individuals with adult-onset hearing loss. For instance, some members of the Deaf culture have limited or nonexistent speech production skills. Unlike many adults with adventitious hearing loss, many Deaf adults do not experience being cut off from the life they have known as a result of hearing loss. They can communicate with fellow signers, they have comfortable companionship with their family and require no extraordinary patience or accommodation, and they are free of many of the anxieties associated with attempts to function in a hearing world.

Table 11-3 presents a chronology of significant events in the recent history of the Deaf culture. As this table illustrates, the last several decades have resulted in many advances and challenges for members of the Deaf culture. Two major forces that have affected Deaf adults during this time period are the growth and expression of Deaf pride and advances in medical technology, the cochlear implant in particular (Figure 11-12). These two forces sometimes collide in purpose. Some Deaf adults reject the infirmity model of deafness implied by the use of cochlear implants (i.e., "there's something broken here so let's fix it with surgery"). Some fear that use of cochlear implants may erase their culture, especially because postimplant rehabilitation for children often includes an emphasis on speech and listening skills

Table 11-3. Some significant events in the Deaf culture movement since the 1960s.

1960s	Civil rights movement becomes visible in mainstream America: Deaf people became aware of their own ethnic possibilities.
	The largest worldwide rubella epidemic in recorded history results in a great influx of children with significant hearing loss into the public school systems from 1964 to 1965, while there is a concurrent decline in the number of children with normal hearing.
1970s	Congress passes Public Law 94-142, the Education for All Handicapped Children Act, in 1975, which mandates public education of children with disabilities within the public school system, and subsequently contributes to declining enrollments in public residential schools and increasing enrollments in public day classes.
	A general consensus emerges among linguists that ASL is an official language.
	Congress passes the Rehabilitation Act of 1973 (Section 504), which prohibits federally supported programs or activities from discriminating against qualified people with disabilities.
1980s	A "Deaf Pride" movement grows rapidly among young deaf adults.
	In 1988, I. King Jordan becomes the first Deaf president of the country's oldest institute of higher learning for the Deaf, Gallaudet University, after students stage a demonstration protesting the appointment of a hearing president.
	Harlan Lane, a professor of psychology at Northeastern University in Boston, publishes *When the Mind Hears: A History of the Deaf,* a book condemning the history of oral communication in America.
1990s	Schools for Deaf children increasingly hire Deaf teachers and administrators.
	The Food and Drug Administration (FDA) approves multichannel cochlear implants for use in children in 1990.
	The Americans with Disabilities Act (ADA; P.L. 101-336) is passed into law in 1990 and extends civil rights protection to people with disabilities in private and federal sectors.
	The National Association of the Deaf (NAD) presents a position paper, stating that "the NAD deplores the decision of the Food and Drug Administration (to permit cochlear implantation of children) which was unsound scientifically, procedurally, and ethically" (Broadcaster, 1991).
	In 1994, some members of the Deaf culture accuse Heather Whitestone, the country's first Deaf Miss America, of being an impostor because she primarily uses aural/oral communication.
2000s	NAD revises its position paper, stating that cochlear implants are an acceptable listening technology, but should not preclude the use of sign language.
	The FDA approves cochlear implantation for children 12 months and sometimes younger. The young age of implantation means that many more children will learn spoken language and fewer will learn ASL.
	In 2006, Gallaudet University faces a lack of diversity and a declining enrollment; its 4-year graduation rate is 6%. Student protests force president-designate Jane K. Fernandes to step down. Many charge her with not appreciating the primacy of ASL at Gallaudet and in Deaf culture.

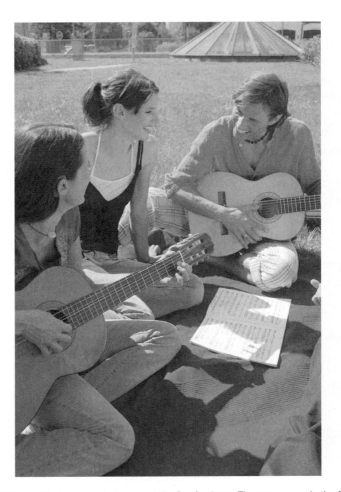

FIGURE 11-12. Cochlear implant use and the Deaf culture. The young man in the foreground is using a cochlear implant in his right ear. Many individuals who received a multichannel cochlear implant after the FDA approved it for children in 1990 are now adults. Some users have become part of the Hearing culture rather than or in addition to the Deaf culture. *Photograph courtesy of MED-EL Corp.*

"Today, 91% [of children who are deaf and hard of hearing] are in public schools . . . The shift away from deaf schools poses a threat to Deaf culture."

Jane K. Fernandes, former president-designate of Gallaudet University

(Boswell, 2007, p. 14)

and a de-emphasis on the use of ASL. Deaf pride, personified by the 1988 protests at Gallaudet University, leads to a celebration of cultural difference. From the perspective of Deaf pride, significant hearing loss is an entryway into a minority community with shared mores, language (ASL), art forms, and traditions.

Adult members of the Deaf culture often do not solicit the kinds of services from speech and hearing professionals that are sought by adults with adult-onset hearing loss. They may not seek hearing tests, they may not use hearing aids or cochlear implants, and they may not be interested in communication strategies training. Some of the professional services they may utilize include sign interpreting, note-taking services, provision of assistive devices, and academic and vocational counseling. Deaf persons who use speech may also seek additional services. Some individuals may want to polish their speaking skills, especially if they have not received speech training for many years. They also may want an assessment of their speech, so that they can better anticipate communication difficulties. Some individuals may also desire training in the use of expressive and receptive communication strategies.

Sign Interpreters

A **sign interpreter** is a professional who translates the spoken signal into a form of signed English or ASL, or vice versa. The interpreter does not participate in the dialogue, but simply conveys messages from one communication partner to the next. Examples of occasions in which a sign language interpreter might be utilized include one-on-one communication situations between a Deaf individual and an individual who does not know sign language, meetings, and lectures. Interpreters often accompany Deaf persons to medical, legal, and educational settings.

Professional interpreters may receive certification from the Registry of Interpreters for the Deaf (RID) or through other statewide screening programs. They are expected to adhere to a set of professional guidelines established by the RID. Scheetz (1993) summarizes the RID code of ethics:

- Interpreters shall keep all assignment-related information strictly confidential.
- Interpreters shall render the message faithfully, always conveying the content of the message and the spirit of the speaker, using language most readily understood by the person(s) whom they serve.
- Interpreters shall not counsel or advise those whom they serve, or interject personal opinions.
- Interpreters shall accept assignments using discretion with regard to skill, setting, and the consumers involved.
- Interpreters shall request compensation for services in a professional and judicious manner. (p. 274)

A **sign interpreter** is a professional who translates the spoken signal into a form of signed English or ASL, or vice versa.

🔊 WHERE IS THE PERSON IN TERMS OF ADJUSTMENT TO HEARING LOSS?

The question of who is this person is followed by the question of where is the person in terms of adjustment to hearing loss. The framework developed by Jones, Kyle, and Wood (1987) presents four phases in the time course of acquired hearing loss: prehearing loss, onset of hearing loss, diagnosis, and adjustment (Figure 11-13). Where a person is in terms of this framework will influence the introduction and development of an aural rehabilitation plan.

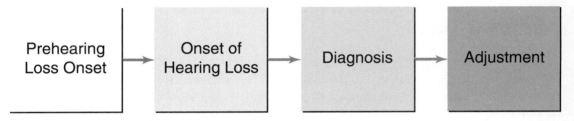

FIGURE 11-13. Four phases in the time course of acquired hearing loss.

Phase 1: Prehearing Loss

Prior to incurring hearing loss, patients will have achieved a certain socio-economic status, personality, and worldview. Life factors are in place. With few exceptions, as in the case of adults who have a family history of hearing loss, few individuals ever anticipate they will suffer from hearing loss, especially while still younger than 65 years of age. Thus, when hearing loss begins, it usually takes a person by surprise.

Phase 2: Onset of Hearing Loss

Phase 2 is the time span stretching between the onset of hearing loss and diagnosis. Often, onset of hearing loss goes undetected. If asked when the loss began, a person may not know. As Hétu (1996) noted:

> It takes a rather striking invalidation of one's perceptual experience to start suspecting that one's sense organs no longer work properly. When hearing loss is progressive and symmetrical, there is no internal reference by which to measure the decrease in one's hearing capabilities. Furthermore, a comparison with others' hearing capabilities is very limited. (p. 17)

The advance from mild loss to awareness might last anywhere from a few days to many years. Situations that often alert people to a problem include having to turn up the television or radio volume, having to ask people to repeat their messages, not hearing a doorbell or someone calling their name, and missing out on conversations that occur in the home. One man, reflecting on this phase, noted ruefully, "For about 2 years, I was snapping at my wife for talking too soft. Then I began to think that other people were mumbling too. It wasn't until my little grandson accused me of not paying attention that I thought to myself, maybe it's my hearing."

Other, less frequently cited indicants include complaining about bad telephone connections, believing that people mumble, and not knowing where sounds are coming from. Family members and others may remark about a patient's coping behaviors and rationalizations.

Phase 3: Diagnosis

Phase 3 is a time when the hearing loss is identified by a professional and the extent of the problem is revealed. An individual may seek out the family doctor first, an otolaryngologist, or go directly to an audiologist. At this point, the individual might expect the hearing professional to provide a rapid solution, and he or she may expect a treatment and complete cure. After her audiologist diagnosed a moderate bilateral sensorineural hearing loss, one patient responded, "My son had a hearing loss when he was 2 years old and the ear doctor gave him tubes. Now he's fine. You think surgery can help me?"

On realizing that hearing loss is here to stay, many people succumb to anxiety. They may worry about possible outcomes, such as decreased professional options, loss of independence, rejection by friends or family members, and altered social status. The magnitude of a person's anxiety may be mollified by what has occurred in Phase 2. For example, if someone has long suspected a hearing loss, then diagnosis may be less traumatic.

During the diagnostic process, the person's type and degree of hearing loss are determined, and the extent to which social, vocational, and educational activities are affected is explored. Typically, an audiologist will obtain a pure-tone audiogram and administer speech recognition tests. The audiologist may then administer a self-report survey or questionnaire aimed at assessing activity limitations and participation restrictions and conduct an interview. The results will indicate how hearing loss interferes with everyday communication in the home, work, and social environments, and reveal related psychological difficulties.

The **Americans with Disabilities Act (ADA)** is a civil rights law that prohibits discrimination on the basis of disability in employment and in services and activities of federal, state, and local government agencies, as well as in goods, services, facilities, advantages, privileges, and accommodations of public places.

The Americans with Disabilities Act

As adults adjust to their hearing loss, they may take advantage of some of the provisions included in the 1990 **Americans with Disabilities Act (ADA)**. This key legislation forbids discrimination against persons with disabilities and requires that "reasonable accommodation" be made in public accommodations, including employment and transportation. The law applies to programs and services of federal, state, and local government agencies, and applies to goods, services, facilities, advantages, privileges, and accommodations. Table 11-4 presents key features of the ADA.

Table 11-4. Key features of the Americans with Disabilities Act as it pertains to individuals with hearing loss (adapted from *Self-Help for Hard-of-Hearing People*, 2004, p. 15).

TITLE	KEY FEATURES
I	Ensures that people with hearing loss have the same opportunities to employment as people without hearing loss and that employers (with 15 employees or more) provide reasonable accommodations to allow them to perform their job. The law does not ensure jobs, but rather, prohibits discrimination for people who are qualified to perform the "essential" functions for a specific job.
II	Requires that state and local government agencies, including transportation programs, make their programs accessible to people with hearing loss. Effective communication must be ensured with auxiliary aids such as assistive listening systems, qualified interpreters, text displays, captioning, provision of TTYs and amplified telephones, and transcriptions of audio programs.
III	Requires public places (operated by private entities) including businesses, professional offices, and nonprofit organizations to provide communications access. These entities include hotels, restaurants, movie theaters, stadiums, concert halls, retail stores, transportation terminals, museums, senior centers, and swimming pools. Required accommodations include all of the aids listed above under Title II as well as television decoders and visual alerting devices (in hotel rooms).
IV	Requires that all telephone companies provide relay services throughout the United States on a 24-hours-per-day/7-days-per-week basis free of charge.

Phase 4: Adjustment

In the final phase, adjustment to hearing loss, Phase 4, individuals begin to adapt to hearing loss. During Phase 4, a person may receive any or all of the following rehabilitation services: counseling, psychosocial support, assertiveness training, hearing aid(s), assistive devices, and formal speechreading, listening, or communication strategies training. Aural rehabilitation is focused on minimizing or solving the communication problems identified in Phase 3.

A study conducted by Kerr and Cowie (1997) provides a general statement about the adjustment, or equilibrium state, that many people achieve. These researchers administered a questionnaire to and interviewed a group of adults who were deaf and hard of hearing and who were under the age of 70 years old. They lived in the Belfast, Ireland, vicinity. In terms of the overall effect of hearing loss, almost 40% of the participants reported that hearing loss had restricted their life at least badly, and 10% of these people felt that the hearing loss had almost destroyed their lives. These results are summarized in Figure 11-14. Factors that contributed to the experiential dimensions of deafness were communicative deprivation and a sense of restriction. Those who believed that their lives were either badly or very badly affected by hearing reported that (p. 181):

- They long to hear particular sounds.
- They must "hear" people speak to them through someone else.
- Someone in the family or a close friend takes over things they would do if they could hear properly.

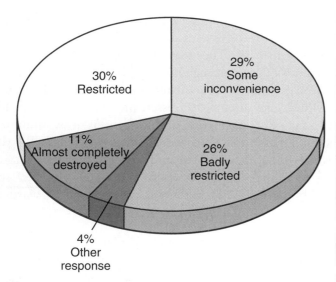

FIGURE 11-14. General effects of hearing loss on patients' lives. Based on data presented in Kerr and Cowie (1997).

- They find themselves spending more time at home because of their deafness.
- People who have normal hearing ignore them in conversation.
- Someone goes with them to a medical or business appointment to help out in case their hearing makes things difficult.
- Their hearing loss holds them back from the kind of work they would like to do.
- They feel that their hearing loss places a strain on relationships with their family.
- They feel as if their hearing loss is like a glass case separating them from the world.

Psychosocial Adjustment

Psychological reactions that some individuals with hearing loss experience when learning of and adapting to a hearing loss may correspond to those experienced by terminally ill patients, although their emotions may be muted by comparison with sick persons. Where they are in terms of psychological adjustment will influence the kinds of aural rehabilitation services that are appropriate at any point in time.

Psychological responses to hearing loss may begin as shock and disbelief, followed by depression, then anger and guilt, and finally, acceptance. Some feel numb or disorganized when the audiologist describes their test results. They then may deny a problem exists and may blame their listening problems on other factors.

Dissonance theory concerns situations in which one's self-perception does not coincide with reality.

A milder version of shock and disbelief relates to **dissonance theory**. Most people do not want to receive messages that run counter to their own self-perception and self-image. They may object to audiological findings that do not fit well with their own cognitions. "Hey, I can't have a hearing loss," a young person may think. "I run marathons—my body is in great shape." Some individuals may attempt to reassert their views of the world either by searching for a disconfirmation of the diagnosis or by minimizing the importance of it. For instance, one woman made a point of telling a family member whenever she heard a noise in the next room, "See, I heard that!" Others may dismiss the hearing loss as being insignificant. "Yes," someone might say, "I miss some things, but most of what I miss isn't worth hearing anyway."

Depression may follow denial, or a mourning for what has been lost (e.g., the loss of hearing, the loss of effortless conversation) and for what may lie ahead (e.g., a continued decrease in hearing, an increase in feelings of powerlessness). Persons may feel isolated from friends and family as they miss out on casual conversational exchanges. They may need to depend more on others for navigating communication with the outside world, and they may experience a concomitant decrease in self-esteem. An inability to hear environmental and body sounds, such as leaves rustling or their footsteps on the pavement, may intensify feelings of loss, as may a decreased ability to enjoy music. One woman reported,

> For a while I felt tired and disinterested all the time. My daughter would ask me to go shopping and I'd say "no." Someone would say the sun was going to shine that day and I'd say "so what?" I had a weight in my heart. I never felt elation and I never felt disappointment. It took me months to realize that I was depressed, and that the depression was related to my hearing loss.

Anger and guilt may follow depression, as patients realize that their lives have been inalterably changed. "Why me?" they may ask, or "What did I do to deserve this?" There may be a perception of unfairness, and a person may protest, "But I am too young to be going deaf!"

Over time, acceptance of the hearing loss occurs. The intensity of feeling stemming from depression, anger, and anxiety cannot be maintained, and a sense of normality returns. The realization emerges that life goes on, albeit differently than before.

Costs

The adjustment phase extracts numerous costs from patients, both monetary and nonmonetary (Figure 11-15). For example, in the course of pursuing an audiological appointment, an individual may lay out money for transportation, the appointment itself, lost wages for the time spent during the appointment, payment for a babysitter if he or she has young children, parking fees, hearing aid molds, hearing aids, and so forth.

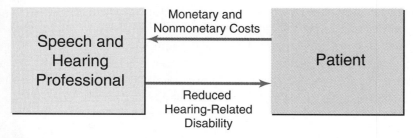

FIGURE 11-15. Costs and benefits associated with seeking aural rehabilitation services.

Psychological costs are nonmonetary costs that relate to a person's psychological well-being.

Perhaps less obvious and often overlooked are the nonmonetary or **psychological costs** of seeking services and adjusting to hearing loss. Such costs for people may include any of the following:

- Acceptance within themselves that they have a hearing problem
- Anxiety that they may be getting old
- Awkwardness for having to ask for time away from work and having to explain the reason for the request
- Worry that the hearing aid may cost too much or that the audiologist will take advantage of them
- Fear that nothing can be done to alleviate the communication difficulties
- Embarrassment for entering a hearing clinic

Often, a primary goal of the experienced speech and hearing professional is to maximize the benefits in exchange for real and perceived monetary and nonmonetary costs.

CASE STUDY

One Size Doesn't Fit All

Many persons who seek the services of a speech and hearing professional will benefit from the use of a hearing aid or other listening aid. However, aural rehabilitation is not a profession of "one size fits all." Patients will vary greatly in the services and support they need before and after they receive a listening device. In this section, three people with differing needs are described.

Doug Kammer has just lost his job as a middle manager because his company merged with another. He is preoccupied with anxieties over his future: Will he get a new job? Does he no longer have the youthful look that employers are looking for? Will his savings tide him over during the interim period of unemployment? He knows at some level that he has a hearing loss and that if he is to be an effective member of a work team, he must be able to communicate effectively. Even so, accepting his hearing loss, taking ownership of his hearing problems, and pursuing a comprehensive aural rehabilitation plan are foreign ideas at this point in his personal turmoil.

Every morning, Mary Saunders starts her day with a flurry of activity—getting children ready for school, making lunches, driving carpool, and cleaning breakfast dishes. All this happens before she heads off to work as an office manager for a small law firm. Life as a single mother and sole breadwinner of two girls seems to be whizzing by her at 100 miles per hour. Some days, she feels like the day has turned into night, without ever providing her with a moment to herself. Lately, she has seemed detached from her surroundings. Her children accuse her of not listening and her coworkers tease her for being absentminded. Is she just overstressed or is something else going on? A few days ago, she realized that she could not hear the high-pitched beeping tone of the office fax machine.

CASE STUDY, *continued*

One Size Doesn't Fit All, *continued*

Carl King lost his wife last year. Since then, the new retiree has been struggling to get on with his life. His grown children come by his house several times a week, concerned about his psychological well-being and determined not to let him isolate himself inside his house. His daughter has talked him into going for a hearing test. She thinks one reason her father is withdrawing into himself is that he cannot hear in groups, and he cannot follow family conversations at the dinner table. Carl figures he will go to the hearing clinic to appease his daughter, but that is all he will do. Why get a hearing aid, he asks himself, when he lives alone with no one to talk to?

All these people could benefit from using a hearing aid and from receiving aural rehabilitation services before and after receiving one. Doug, Mary, and Carl live different lives, experience different demands, and harbor different hopes and expectations. Their aural rehabilitation plans must accommodate their differences. Doug needs to come to grips with the presence of his hearing loss and what having a hearing loss means in terms of his self-image. He might develop strategies for managing his hearing loss, both during his search for a new job and then in adjusting and accommodating to a new work setting. Mary might educate her children and coworkers about her communication difficulties and find time in her busy schedule to receive adequate hearing health care. Carl will have to develop the motivation to participate in everyday conversations, which may require him to expand his social network and to take a greater interest in the comings and goings of his children and grandchildren. These people will require many of the same aural rehabilitation services, but these services must be adjusted to accommodate who they are and where they are in terms of adjustment to hearing loss.

FINAL REMARKS

Aural rehabilitation begins with a solid understanding of the patient population. In this chapter, we have considered how adults with hearing loss differ in their cultural orientation, their demographics, their reactions to hearing loss, their communication needs and problems, and many other factors. We also have considered the four phases of adjustment to hearing loss. This information lays the groundwork for providing aural rehabilitation services to adults. In the next chapter, we consider the development of aural rehabilitation plans.

KEY CHAPTER POINTS

- A patient-centered approach holds that the most successful aural rehabilitation plan is one that best determines a patient's background, current status, needs, and wants and then accommodates these through the design and delivery of appropriate interventions.

- Many baby boomers, and even younger adults, experience hearing loss, in part, because we live in a modern world replete with loud environments.

- Most adults lose their hearing gradually over time. Typically, the loss is greatest in the high frequencies and least in the low frequencies.

- In following a patient-centered orientation, a speech and hearing professional will determine "who the patient is," and consider non-hearing-related variables such as stage of life, socioeconomic status, culture, and psychological adjustment. These variables may affect the aural rehabilitation plan.

- Life factor influences pertain to self, home, work, recreation, and community. For instance, the norms, services, and mores that are present in the surrounding community will help the patient answer such questions as "What kind of help do I need and where will I get it?" and "How am I to contribute to the world around me and live my life?"

- Socioeconomic status is related to racial/ethnic status. Some members of minority groups may be inexperienced with interacting with health care professionals and some may be distrustful of them. Some minority members may not have access to quality care due to financial limitations or their location.

- Members of varying cultural backgrounds may respond differentially to incurring hearing loss, to interacting with health care professionals, and to an aural rehabilitation plan. It is incumbent upon speech and health professionals to respect a patient's traditions, customs, values, and beliefs related to the aural rehabilitation plan.

- Women are more likely to acknowledge a hearing loss than are men, and women are more likely to actively reduce their communication difficulties. Women are also less likely to incur a loss.

- Adults who are hard of hearing may have more psychosocial and vocational difficulties than adults who have normal hearing. They may suffer from feelings of loneliness and decreased self-esteem.

- Tinnitus can be debilitating.

- Adult members of the Deaf culture lost their hearing early in life. They rely primarily on ASL for communication.

- There are four phases in an adult's adjustment to hearing loss: prehearing loss, onset of hearing loss, diagnosis, and adjustment. Aural rehabilitation often starts in the third phase. During this phase, a speech and hearing professional will want to identify a patient's particular communication problems at home, socially, and vocationally and begin to formulate solutions.

- Psychological responses to hearing loss may include the following stages: shock and disbelief, depression, anger and guilt, and, finally, acceptance. A milder form of shock and disbelief relates to dissonance theory ("this diagnosis runs counter to my self-image").

- Adjustment to hearing loss extracts both monetary and nonmonetary costs. Psychological costs include acceptance within one's self that there is a hearing problem and anxiety of aging.

TERMS AND CONCEPTS TO REMEMBER

Prevalence

Noise notch

Patient orientation

Sales orientation

Adult-onset hearing loss

Life factors and life stages

Culture

Cultural and linguistic competency

Limited English Proficiency (LEP)

Tinnitus

Deaf culture

Hearing culture

Sign interpreter

Americans With Disabilities Act (ADA)

Dissonance theory

MULTIPLE-CHOICE QUESTIONS

1. A patient-centered approach means that:

   a. The most successful program is one that best determines a patient's background, current status, needs, and wants and then accommodates them through the delivery of a customized aural rehabilitation plan.

   b. The most successful program is one that persuades patients to procure services.

   c. The most successful program is the one designed to accommodate the background, current status, needs, and wants of the typical patient and packages this program in a financially economical fashion.

   d. The most successful program assumes that every patient is unique, and that every plan must begin from a blank slate.

2. A 40-year-old farmer arrives at an audiological clinic. He is most likely to have what configuration of hearing loss?

   a. A sloping mild to moderate hearing loss

   b. A hearing loss with a 4,000 Hz "notch," so that hearing is poorer at 4,000 Hz than at either 2,000 Hz or 8,000 Hz

   c. A flat hearing loss

   d. An asymmetrical hearing loss

3. Marie Remez speaks Spanish and very little English. She has contracted a professional translator to perform a service. This service is most likely to be to:

   a. Accompany her to an audiological appointment and explain to her in Spanish what the audiologist says in English

   b. Accompany her to an audiological appointment and convey the audiologist's words to her using ASL

   c. Accompany her to an audiological appointment and translate the English words of a speech recognition test into Spanish during speech recognition testing

   d. Translate a pamphlet about hearing aid use from English into Spanish

4. Which of the following statements about tinnitus is false?

   a. Most tinnitus has a medical origin, such as temporomandibular joint disorder or respiratory and vascular conditions.

   b. There is not likely to be a single intervention that is appropriate for all sufferers.

   c. Individuals who have a history of noise exposure often suffer from tinnitus.

   d. Eating too many pretzels or potato chips may exacerbate the experience of tinnitus.

5. Which individual is most likely to be considered a member of the Deaf culture?

   a. Jan, who was born with a severe-to-profound hearing loss and learned to speak and listen. She does not use sign language, because her friends who have hearing loss also speak and listen.

   b. Tom, who attended a residential school for the deaf and married his high school sweetheart.

   c. Steve, who went completely deaf at the age of 21 years.

   d. Jean, who lost her hearing at the age of 35 years and learned sign language so she could communicate with other members of the Deaf culture.

6. A patient with LEP arrives at a public hospital for an appointment. Since the hospital receives federal funding, what is likely to be available when she arrives?

   a. A social worker, who will help her to understand her treatment plan and help her implement it in the home environment

   b. A Medicare form with her claim number

    c. Pamphlets, because she has hearing loss

    d. An interpreter

7. What services will an adult from the Deaf culture likely not seek from a speech and hearing professional?

    a. Interpreting services

    b. ASL instruction

    c. Communication strategies training before a job interview

    d. Provision of assistive devices for the home

8. Aural rehabilitation typically begins during which phase in the time course of acquired hearing loss?

    a. Preheating loss onset

    b. Onset of hearing loss

    c. Diagnosis

    d. Adjustment

9. Mrs. Davidson has anxieties about aging. For this reason, she is reluctant to visit an audiological clinic and have her hearing loss confirmed by an audiologist. This fear is an example of:

    a. Communication handicap

    b. Psychological consequence of hearing loss

    c. Life factor influences

    d. Nonmonetary costs of seeking aural rehabilitation services

10. One way in which a speech and hearing professional can better serve his or her patient case load is to:

    a. Attend cultural events in the community and develop a relationship with a person who can serve as a cultural informant

    b. Adopt a sales orientation

    c. Learn how to better serve those members of the Deaf culture who receive cochlear implants

    d. Become a certified interpreter

KEY RESOURCES

Audilogical terms that might occur during an audilogical visit and their Spanish equivalents. This list can be shared with an interpreter (adapted from Brisy Northrup, northrup@utdallas.edu, accessed October 31, 2006).

ENGLISH	SPANISH
Air conduction	Conduccion o via aerea
Assistive devices for persons who have hearing loss	Aparatos de asistencia para personas Hipoacusicas o sordas
Assistive technology	Tecnologia de asistencia
Audiogram	Audiograma
Audiologist	Aduiologo
Audiometer	Audiometro
Auditory training	Entrenamiento auditivo
Aural rehabilitation	Reeducacion auditiva
Battery	Pila
Battery door	Portapilas
Beep	Bip
Bilateral	Bilateral
Bone conduction	Conduccion o via osea
Bone oscillator	Vibrador
BTE	Retro-auricular
CIC	Minicanal
Cochlear implant	Implante coclear
Conductive hearing loss	Sordera conductiva
dB	Decibelio
Deaf	Sordo
Deafness	Sordera
Direct audio input	Sistema de bucle inductivo, entrada audio
Disability	Discapacidad
Dizziness	Mareo, vahio
Ear/hearing protection	Proteccion auditiva/del oido
Ear canal	Canal auditivo
Ear drum	Membrana timpanica, timpano
Ear hook	Codo, gancho plastico
Earmold	Molde de oido
FM system	Sistema FM
Frequency	Frecuencia

continues

continued

ENGLISH	SPANISH
Gain	Ganancia
Hearing aid	Audifono, aparato de oir protesis auditiva, auxiliar auditivo
Hearing aid fitting	Adaptacion de audifonos
Hearing loss	Perdida auditiva
Infrared system	Sistema de rayos infra-rojos
Insert earphones	Insertos
ITC	Intra-canal
ITE	Intra-concha
Lipreading/speechreading	Lectura labia/del habla
Monaural	Monaural
Oral communication	Comunicacion oral
Otoacoustic emissions	Emisiones otoacusticas
Otoscope	Otoscopio
Phonemes	Fonemas
Presbycusis	Presbiacusia
Sensorineural hearing loss	Sordera neurosensorial
Sign language	Lenguaje manual/de seónas
Sound booth	Cabinas audiometricas
Speech audiometry	Logoaudiometria
Speech-language pathologist	Fonoaudiologo/a
SPL	Nivel de presion acustica
Spondee threshold or SRT	Umbral de captacion o recepcion
T-coil	Bobina telefonica
TDD/TTY	Ayudas de telecomunicacion para personas sordas
Telephone amplifier	Amplificador telefonico
Threshold	Umbral
Tinnitus	Acufeno, zumbidos en el oido, tinitus

APPENDIX 11-1

Cultural Competence Needed to Provide Culturally and Linguistically Appropriate Services to Persons Who Have Hearing Loss (adapted from ASHA, 2004, p. 153)

The speech and hearing professional shall have sensitivity to cultural and linguistic differences that affect the identification, assessment, treatment, and management of hearing loss in patients. This includes knowledge and skills related to:

- Influence of one's own beliefs and biases in providing effective services.
- Respect for a patient's race, ethnic background, lifestyle, physical/mental ability, religious beliefs/practices, and heritage.
- Influence of the patient's traditions, customs, values, and beliefs related to the patient receiving services.
- Impact of assimilation and/or acculturation processes on the identification, assessment, treatment, and management of hearing loss.
- Recognition of the speech and hearing professional's own limitations in education/training in providing services to patients from a particular cultural or linguistic community.
- Appropriate intervention and assessment strategies and materials that do not violate a patient's values or home culture.
- Appropriate communications with patients and family members so that the values imparted in the counseling are consistent with those of patient.
- The need to refer or consult with other service providers with appropriate cultural and linguistic proficiency, such as a cultural informant.
- The importance of advocating for and empowering patients, including advising them of resources for their particular community and the impact of regulatory processes on service delivery to communities.

CHAPTER 12

Aural Rehabilitation Plans for Adults

OUTLINE

- Assessment
- Informational counseling
- Development of an aural rehabilitation plan
- Implementation
- Outcomes assessment
- Follow-up
- Case study: A road map for success
- Final remarks
- Key chapter points
- Terms and concepts to remember
- Multiple-choice questions
- Key resources
- Appendix 12-1
- Appendix 12-2
- Appendix 12-3
- Appendix 12-4
- Appendix 12-5

n this chapter, we consider a general strategy for designing a patient-centered aural rehabilitation plan for adults. The aural rehabilitation process usually requires the orchestration of a number of interventions, and these services often can be integrated in such a way as to achieve maximum benefit for the individual.

Services are often affected by a number of variables, including the country or state where delivery occurs and the way that health care is funded, structured, and delivered. For instance, in the United States, aural rehabilitation services are largely privately paid whereas in Scandinavia, services are more likely to be government funded (Gatehouse, 2003). Some U.S. insurance plans provide partial or full coverage for, say, hearing aids, whereas others provide no coverage. Despite the diversity of settings and delivery service models, it is possible to categorize the components of an aural rehabilitation plan into six general categories (Figure 12-1): (a) assessment, (b) informational counseling, (c) development of a plan, (d) implementation, (e) assessment of outcome, and (f) follow-up.

ASSESSMENT

The first stage in the aural rehabilitation plan entails assessing a patient's (a) hearing impairment, (b) hearing-related difficulties, and (c) individual factors. As noted in the last chapter, this evaluation will include a consideration of who this person is (e.g., What are the individual's culture and gender; what is the person's stage of life?), the individual's audiological and conversational needs (e.g., Is this person a candidate for a hearing aid?), and the individual's ecological concerns (e.g., Does the person work? If so, what are the communication demands associated with the workplace?). Topics to be evaluated also will include economics and psychosocial adjustment. For example, can the individual afford hearing aids? Is the person motivated to use them?

One way to conceptualize the evaluation stage is illustrated in Figure 12-2 (in the spirit of Hyde & Riko, 1994). This figure presents a decision tree, which outlines the decisions that might be made in the initial stages of an aural rehabilitation plan. The squares in this decision tree indicate that a decision must be made at this time. For instance, an audiologist might recommend that the patient receive an audiogram and take a battery of speech recognition tests (moving from left to right, this is the first square in the temporal flow of the decision tree). The circles in the decision tree indicate points that may not be under the clinician's control, such as the patient's performance on a hearing test or the outcome of a particular intervention. The outcome of the assessments will point the

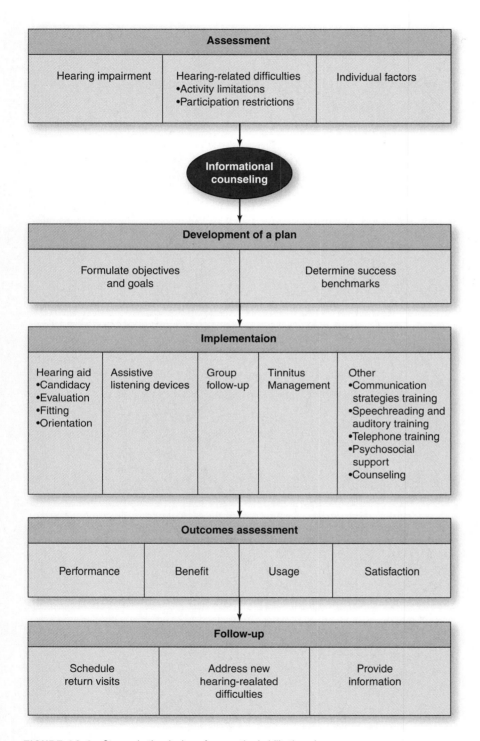

FIGURE 12-1. Stages in the design of an aural rehabilitation plan.

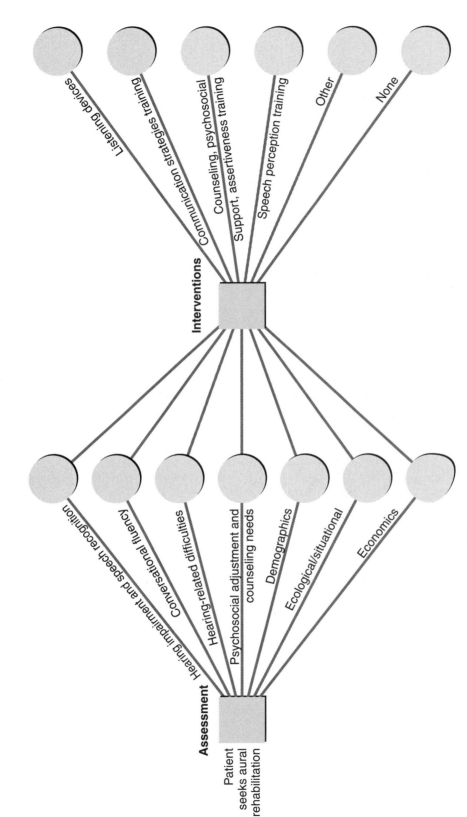

FIGURE 12-2. A decision tree for the initial stages of an aural rehabilitation plan. Squares denote a point in time where a decision is made. Circles indicate points in the temporal flow of the plan that may be beyond the control of the clinician.

way to particular interventions (or no intervention) being selected. The interventions will be determined by the results of the assessment of hearing and speech recognition, conversational fluency, hearing-related disabilities, and psychosocial adjustment and counseling needs, and by what the patient reports about his or her demographic variables, ecological/situational communication circumstances, motivation, expectations, and economic wherewithal.

The Hearing Impairment

The degree, onset, progression, and causation (i.e., sensorineural, conductive, mixed) of the hearing impairment will be determined early on. This step of the assessment will include obtaining an audiogram and performing speech testing. The speech tests may indicate how well a patient can recognize speech stimuli in an audition-only, vision-only, and audition-plus-vision condition and may also include testing in both quiet and noise. If warranted, other kinds of tests may be administered to distinguish between a cochlear from a retrocochlear involvement, to assess middle ear function, to assess vestibular function, and/or to assess central processing. The recommended components of an auditory assessment are as follows (American Academy of Audiology, 2006, p. 33):

- Comprehensive case history
- Identifying type and magnitude of hearing loss via pure-tone and speech audiometry as well as **immitance**
- Measuring loudness discomfort levels (LDLs)
- Otoscopic inspection and cerumen management
- Determine need for treatment/referral to physician or need for further tests (ABR, vestibular, etc.)
- Counsel patient, family, caregiver on the results and recommendations
- Assess candidacy and motivation toward amplification
- Determine medical clearance as determined by FDA

Immitance is a term that refers to the energy flow through the middle ear, and includes admittance, compliance, conductance, impedance, reactance, resistance, and susceptance.

Hearing-Related Difficulties

In Chapter 1, we considered the World Health Organization's (WHO) International Classification of Functioning, Disability, and Health (ICF; World Health Organization, 2001). According to the WHO-ICF, the negative consequences of adult-onset hearing loss include more than the limitations imposed by the auditory impairment; for instance, limitations in the ability to discriminate pitch and loudness or to identify speech sounds. Adult-onset hearing loss may also impose activity limitations and participation restrictions. During assessment, hearing-related difficulties that result in activity limitations and participation restrictions will be identified, and these will provide impetus for the aural rehabilitation objectives.

Hearing-related difficulties might be assessed by means of structured or unstructured interviews, questionnaires and other self-report measures, and structured and unstructured communication interactions. One goal of assessment is to determine the kind and magnitude of hearing-related difficulties that a patient might experience in the home, work, and community environments, and to determine how hearing loss causes activity limitations and participation restrictions in daily life. Another goal is to identify those concerns that the patient believes to be most pressing. The hearing-related difficulties may include poor conversational fluency, psychosocial adjustment issues, and situation-specific listening problems, such as telephone communication. In the course of identifying hearing-related difficulties, a clinician will probe the **significance** of each one to the patient and the patient's **expectations**.

Sometimes the most efficient and effective first step toward formulating an aural rehabilitation plan is to ask a patient for information. A primary goal is to identify the problems that the patient believes are important to resolve and then to make those problems the target of intervention. Through the process of conducting an initial interview, the clinician can determine a patient's level of enthusiasm to participate in an aural rehabilitation program. The interview may also serve to heighten the patient's awareness of his or her communication problems and begin to create motivation within the patient to address them.

The interview may be unstructured or structured. Examples of unstructured questions include:

- What kinds of communication difficulties are you experiencing at home/work/social encounters?
- Have other people commented about your hearing difficulties? What can you recall about what they've said?

Examples of structured questions include:

- Do you need to use the telephone? On what occasions?
- Do you have difficulty in detecting or identifying warning signals (e.g., telephone ringing, doorbell, alarm clock, a baby's cry)?

The clinician might want to organize questions by category, so that information is obtained about communication difficulties experienced in the home, work environment, and recreational and community activities. For instance, when asking about the home environment, an audiologist may

Significance reflects how relevant a specific hearing-related difficulty or communication situation is for a patient.

Expectation describes the patient's attitude about the benefit that will be provided, such as with a hearing aid.

gain an idea of with whom an individual communicates, what his or her specific communication problems are, and whether assistive listening devices might be appropriate. In some instances, it is helpful to classify answers by asking the patient to choose among options. For example, to the question, "Is watching television difficult for you because of your hearing loss?," the patient might be asked to choose from the answers of "always," "sometimes," "rarely," and "never."

When exploring the work environment, questions might be asked about the physical environment of the workplace, specific work tasks performed by the individual, and current hearing-related problems. This information will be important for considering appropriate listening devices, the need for noise protection, and the need for employer/employee education. Example questions about the work environment include: Where do you work (e.g., a factory, an office, construction, in sales)? What is your physical work environment like (e.g., noisy, open space, quiet, small office)? Do you think you have difficulties using the telephone?

As with any group of adults, persons with hearing loss vary greatly in their predilections for social activities. Some people engage only in quiet, one-on-one activities; others interact in groups and attend social events such as concerts or lectures. For those who are more reclusive, an audiologist may explore whether they avoid social activities because they do not enjoy them or because they experience so many communication difficulties that the activities are unsatisfying. If the latter is the case, then there is a specific direction in which to target aural rehabilitation efforts. Example questions concerning the social environment include: What do you do in your free time (e.g., go to movies, attend dinner parties, play bridge)? and Do you remember times when your hearing difficulties have cause you to skip a social event?

An experienced interviewer can probe for information while managing to put the patient at ease. For instance, a person might say, "I don't know if my hearing has affected much about what I do at work or not." The interviewer might follow this remark with, "Tell me about the last time you misunderstood someone at the office." By asking questions with phrases like, *Do you recall* and *Do you think,* the interviewer encourages detailed, thoughtful answers without implying that there is a right or wrong answer to the question.

In addition to interviews, structured-inquiry methods have proven to be effective means for identifying listening circumstances and communication difficulties that a patient considers to be of significance and of high priority. An example of a structured-inquiry instrument is the *Client Oriented Scale of Improvement* (*COSI;* Dillon et al., 1997; presented in the Key Resources at the end of this chapter). Originally developed as an assessment instrument, the COSI can also be used to guide the overall aural rehabilitation plan. At the onset of intervention, the patient nominates up to five situations in which the patient would like to communicate better or to cope with better. The patient is encouraged to be as specific as possible when writing down the situations. The five situations are listed in order of importance. At the end of the intervention, the patient reviews the original descriptions. For each one, the patient indicates (a) how much better or worse the situation is now relative to before aural rehabilitation began, and (b) what is the absolute ease of communication following intervention.

One patient wrote in the first row of the COSI form, "My most common challenge is to understand and be understood in a noisy room." The clinician encouraged him to be more specific, so the patient added, "I want to hear at clubs, because I enjoy going to clubs. Especially I like going to Maxwell's on Friday nights after work." Specificity pinpoints the intervention and better permits the assessment of outcome. On the second row, the patient wrote, "I have trouble hearing people over the telephone, especially when I'm at work and there are people talking all around me." By completing this form, the patient established that there are specific situations in which he would like to communicate more effectively; that is, he acknowledged that a disability related to his hearing loss exists. Second, he conveyed to the clinician the order of importance of his communication needs. After intervention, and after an appropriate adjustment period (about 3 months), the patient revisited his original responses. The use of two ratings, that of "improvement" and that of "final ability," indicated the effectiveness of the aural rehabilitation intervention and potential areas for continued attention. Important to note, the patient developed a sense of having received an individualized intervention program. Another instrument that has been used for structured inquiry is the *Glasgow Hearing Aid Benefit Profile* (*GHAB;* Gatehouse, 1999), which offers a similarly structured approach for identifying patient priorities.

Individual Factors

A case history and an interview may yield information about individual factors such as a patient's age, psychological well-being, other hearing-related complaints, and life factors. The American Academy of Audiology (2006) presents guidelines for nonauditory needs assessment, suggesting that it might include "cognition, patient expectations, motivation, willingness to take risks, assertiveness, manual dexterity, visual acuity, prior experience with amplification, general health, tinnitus, occupational demands, and the presence of support systems" (p. 34). Although this information will first be explored during the assessment stage, such factors will again be considered during the development of the plan and its implementation.

INFORMATIONAL COUNSELING

Informational counseling (Chapter 10) is ongoing and occurs throughout the aural rehabilitation process. Whether a patient is learning how to operate a hearing aid or whether the patient is about to undergo an audiological examination, the individual will receive relevant information about what is happening and why, and information related to listening and communication as it relates to the particular stage of the aural rehabilitation plan.

Although counseling is ongoing, usually a block of time is set aside for informational counseling, usually after (but sometimes before) the assessment and then again, before and/or after a listening device is fitted. The topics covered in the initial counseling session may include a summary of the assessment, discussion of expectations, attitudes, and motivation, and consideration of listening devices, commitments, costs, and nontechnological interventions, such as speech perception and communication strategies training. Figure 12-3 presents a schematic representation of how an informational counseling session might progress, from a discussion of

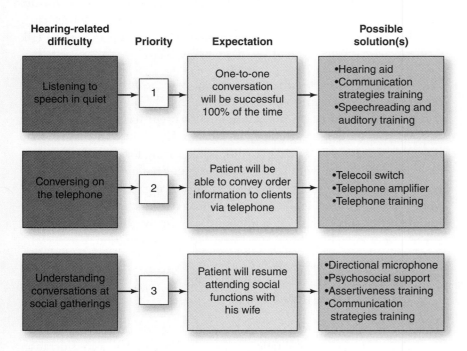

FIGURE 12-3. A schematic representation of how an informational counseling session might progress. *Modeled after Gatehouse (2003, p. 2S79).*

a patient's hearing-related difficulties to possible management solutions. It is often during this session that a clinician will gain a sense of a patient's priorities, willingness to engage in an aural rehabilitation plan, and expectations. For instance, if a patient harbors unrealistic expectations about the benefits of amplification—and this is not uncommon—then the patient may well be at risk for a poor outcome.

During initial informational counseling, the clinician explains the results of the hearing and speech recognition tests and talks about the options available for solving specific communication problems. How a clinician goes about counseling will depend in part on what the professional has learned about the patient from the case history, the interview, the COSI, or other self-assessment instrument if administered, and what the professional perceives about the patient's level of knowledge and the patient's personality. For example, if during the case history the patient has said he or she suspects a hearing loss, then an audiologist might begin a counseling session by confirming this suspicion. The language used in explaining an audiogram to an electrical engineer will differ from that which will be used if explaining it to a fiction writer. There are some patients who will want closure as quickly as possible (e.g., "So, what do we do about it?" a patient might say upon learning about the magnitude of a hearing loss), and others who will want to mull over the information and who will need further explanation (e.g., "This is so much to think about. Let me come back later, after I've had a chance to read this pamphlet you gave me and after I talk to my daughter. What kind of loss did you say I have?").

It is important not to bombard the patient with professional jargon, nor provide the patient with more information than he or she can process or may want at that time. In the case where a patient has been reluctant to come in, an audiologist will likely not turn to the spouse and say, "You're right, Mr. Jones. Your wife has a whopping hearing loss." Rather, the audiologist might begin with sensitivity: "I can understand, Mrs. Jones, why you think people mumble all the time. Your hearing test suggests that you can tell when someone is talking, but you may not hear many of the speech sounds being said." Then the audiologist will likely go on to explain the effects of a sloping high-frequency loss on speech recognition.

DEVELOPMENT OF AN AURAL REHABILITATION PLAN

The next stage is to develop a broad strategy to guide the aural rehabilitation efforts. An aural rehabilitation strategy will be based on a consideration of an individual's needs, the availability of offerings within the particular practice, and the individual's ability or willingness to comply with the specifics of the plan. In developing a strategy, as well as in implementing the plan, an audiologist will develop an active partnership with the patient.

> [Both will be involved in] the recognition, identification, and description of the difficulties experienced; the negotiation and definition of the objectives of the rehabilitation program; the identification, evaluation, selection, and implementation of the intervention strategy itself; the definition of the desired outcome including the criteria used to evaluate the outcome of the program; the identification of the positive and negative factors that contributed to the outcome; and the evaluation of the effects, impacts, and consequences of the rehabilitation program on the person's activities outside the clinical setting. (Gagné, McDuff, & Getty, 1999, p. 48)

Through the development of this partnership, and the implementation of what Gagné et al. call a solution-centered, problem-solving strategy, patients will alleviate those listening challenges that motivated them to seek professional help in the first place. Developing and implementing an aural rehabilitation plan will entail developing specific objectives. Defining the objective serves to identify strategies to solve the listening problem and also provides a standard by which the effectiveness of intervention may be assessed.

Following McKenna (1987), Gagné et al. (1999) present the following guidelines for formulating aural rehabilitation objectives:

> The specific objective should be formulated in a way that identifies:
>
> - all of the individuals involved in the pursuit of the objective;
> - the role of and responsibilities of each person involved in the intervention program;
> - the conditions under which the personalized and customized objective will be accomplished while taking into account the expressed needs, willingness, and capabilities of all of the participants;
> - the criteria that will be used to evaluate whether or not the objective has been reached;
> - a time frame within which the objective should be reached. (p. 49)

The objectives set will be in direct response to the patient's particular problems. For example, if a patient has difficulty listening at professional meetings that are conducted at a rectangular table, an FM system might be recommended. On the other hand, if the patient rarely attends meetings, and complains primarily of experiencing problems in conversing during one-on-one interactions, a hearing aid might serve to alleviate the listening difficulties. The plan will also entail establishing success benchmarks and means for assessing them.

IMPLEMENTATION

In this section, we will review implementation of aural rehabilitation plans that include provision of a hearing aid, provision of assistive devices, tinnitus management, and telephone training. Information about plans that include communication strategies training, psychosocial support and assertiveness training, and auditory and speechreading training appears in previous chapters (i.e., Chapters 4, 6, 9, and 10).

Hearing Aids

When determining whether to include provision of hearing aid(s) in an aural rehabilitation plan, an audiologist first determines whether an individual is an appropriate candidate. If the patient meets the audiological criteria, the audiologist will perform a hearing aid evaluation and provide a hearing aid fitting and orientation. Establishing an appropriate use pattern will be a prominent goal in the aural rehabilitation plan.

Candidacy

Motivation to use a hearing aid is an important but often overlooked issue when determining candidacy. Many people who have hearing loss are not interested in obtaining a hearing aid, although there has been an increasing acceptance of hearing aid use during the past few decades (Figure 12-4). Only about 24% of the approximately 31.5 million persons in the United States who have hearing loss currently own hearing instruments (Kochkin, 2005a). Factors that commonly influence persons to obtain a device include:

- Perception that their hearing loss is getting worse
- Encouragement of family members
- Direction from a medical professional, usually their audiologist or otolaryngologist

In a survey of 2,300 adults 50 years and older, the National Council on the Aging identified barriers to the wearing of hearing aids (National Council

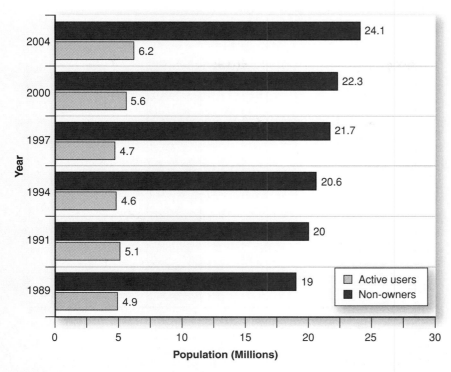

FIGURE 12-4. Population of "active" hearing aid users and non-owners of hearing aids from 1989 to 2004. Kochkin describes an active user as anyone who uses their hearing aid at least once a year. *Modeled after Kochkin (2005, p. 18).*

on the Aging, 1999; see also Kochkin, 2007, for similar findings). Half of the respondents cited the expense of purchasing a hearing aid as a roadblock (see Figure 12-5), and about 20% expressed concerns about vanity and the stigma attached to hearing aid use. Interestingly, the most common responses were "My hearing is not bad enough" and "I can get along without one." A third of the respondents reported that "[hearing aids] will not help with my specific problem."

Expectations factor into candidacy. Jerram and Purdy (2001) examined expectations and adjustment to hearing loss and the relationship between these two variables and hearing aid outcome. The results showed that people who use their new hearing aids for more hours a day are more likely to have greater acceptance of their hearing losses, even before receiving their hearing aids, and are more likely to have higher prefitting expectations. Persons who have not accepted their hearing loss and who have lower expectations wear their hearing aids for fewer hours. The predictive influence of acceptance of hearing loss and prefitting expectations on eventual hearing aid use underscores the importance of developing motivation in patients and providing follow-up counseling.

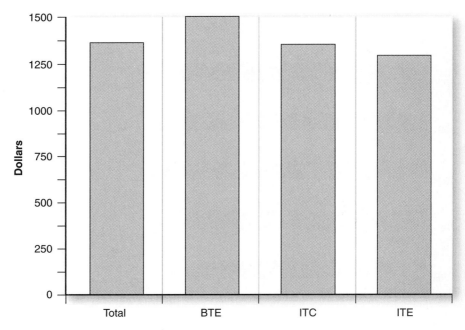

FIGURE 12-5. Average price paid out-of-pocket for hearing aid by patients in the year 2004 (BTE = behind-the-ear; ITC = in-the-canal; ITE = in-the-ear). *Modeled after Kochkin (2005, p. 22).*

What Happens When Hearing Loss Goes Untreated?

Untreated hearing loss leads to both negative social and emotional consequences, including less effective social functioning (Weinstein & Ventry, 1982), diminished psychological well-being (Dye & Peak, 1983), poor self-esteem (Harless & McConnell, 1982), and reduction in quality of life (Dalton et al., 2003). An American Academy of Audiology Task Force (Chisolm et al., 2007) conducted a systematic review of published experiments that have considered how the use of a hearing aid affects **health-related quality of life (HRQoL)**. Such experiments examine the degree to which patients' health status influences their subjective perception of daily functioning and **well-being**. The task force concluded that the use of hearing aids improves HRQoL, and leads to a reduction of psychological, social, and emotional effects of sensorineural hearing loss in adults (see also Kricos, Erdman, Bratt, & Williams, 2007).

Health-related quality of life (HRQoL) refers to the impact of a health condition on the well-being experienced by an individual or a group of people; includes such dimensions as physiology, function, social activity, cognition, emotions, energy, vitality, health perception, and general life satisfaction.

Well-being is an intangible concept that encompasses both a physical aspect (e.g., health, protection against pain and disease) and a psychological aspect (e.g., stress, worry, pleasure); state or condition of being well.

The 10-step hierarchical model presented in Figure 12-6 presents a step-wise process for developing realistic expectations and increasing motivation to use a hearing aid. The 10 steps are grouped into five sets of tasks for the clinician.

Audiologist's Task	Step	Patient Stage
Educate	1.	Understands nature of his/her hearing loss.
	2.	Understands what a hearing aid can and cannot do.
Change Values	3.	Realizes hearing aids are not necessarily a sign of aging.
	4.	Considers using a hearing aid.
Change Attitudes	5.	Learns about appropriate hearing aid styles.
	6.	Perceives that the benefits accrued from using a hearing aid exceed monetary and nonmonetary costs.
Motivate Patient to Act	7.	Understands steps for obtaining a hearing aid.
	8.	Acquires hearing aid.
Establish Use Pattern	9.	Completes trial period with hearing aid.
	10.	Continues appropriate usage.

FIGURE 12-6. A model for developing motivation in adults to use hearing aids for the first time.

1. **Education:** To become successful hearing aid users, individuals must have a clear understanding of the magnitude of their hearing loss and realize that the loss is not medically reversible. They also need to understand their options in managing their communication problems and understand the value and limitations of hearing aids.

2. **Value change:** Individuals must believe that hearing aids will not result in devaluation of them by others. That is, others will not see them as old or as damaged goods. Ideally, they will come to realize

that hearing aids can reduce communication difficulties and that they are relevant to their own lives. This step may entail a discussion of current beliefs.

3. **Attitude change:** The audiologist may discuss appropriate hearing aid styles and ask patients about preferred styles. They may discuss the monetary and nonmonetary costs associated with obtaining a hearing aid. The patient might come to believe that the benefits received from using a hearing aid outweigh the costs.

4. **Action:** The audiologist will describe the steps involved in obtaining a hearing aid. The patient then undergoes a hearing aid evaluation and fitting.

5. **Establishment of use pattern:** Once an individual has obtained a hearing aid, the aural rehabilitation process is not over. The patient will develop a use pattern and will continue to ensure the hearing aid is in good working order.

Hearing Aid Evaluation

Once motivation is established and candidacy is determined, the patient receives a hearing aid evaluation. The audiologist selects the appropriate electroacoustic properties for the hearing aid, commonly by means of a prescriptive procedure. The amount of gain is prescribed, usually so that more gain is provided for the poorer frequencies and less for the better frequencies. The maximum sound pressure level output (SSPL-90) is also determined, after measuring loudness discomfort levels (LDLs).

During the hearing aid evaluation, the audiologist and patient determine the style of hearing aid. This decision is based on a combined consideration of the magnitude of the individual's hearing loss, ear canal size and geometry, ease of insertion and handling, cosmetic concerns, comfort, need for special features such as a telecoil or a directional microphone, and a patient's personal preference. For instance, an audiologist might conclude that a BTE device is most appropriate for a person who has a severe sensorineural hearing loss. However, after discovering that the individual is adamantly opposed to wearing a visible device, the audiologist may recommend an ITE hearing aid instead.

Hearing Aid Fitting and Orientation

Once a hearing aid has been selected, ordered, and received, the patient returns to the audiological clinic for a hearing aid fitting and orientation. An electroacoustic verification of the hearing aid is typically performed before the fitting to ensure that it is in good working order. After the hearing aid is fitted to the patient's ear, performance with the hearing aid is evaluated, often first with real-ear measurements, in which a miniature microphone attached to a plastic tube is placed in the ear canal to measure loudness of sounds, both with and without the hearing aid. Speech recognition performance may also be measured with and without the hearing aid. Finally, the new user is asked about sound quality. The clinician may ask such questions as the following:

- Can you understand my voice? Does it sound natural? Am I too soft or too loud? Do I sound tinny?
- How does your own voice sound? Does it sound hollow? Do you feel like you are talking inside a cave or a barrel?
- How do environmental noises sound? Can you hear the telephone ring? How do your footsteps sound?

Once the hearing aid is introduced, an overview of its operation and maintenance can be presented. This overview includes a demonstration of how to clean it, how to troubleshoot problems, and how to turn it on and off. The new hearing aid user might be given simple printed guidelines for maintaining the device.

If the device has a telephone switch, the patient can practice turning on the switch, placing the telephone handset over the hearing aid, and then conversing on the clinic telephone. If the hearing aid does not have a telephone switch, the patient might practice placing the telephone handset at a short distance from the hearing aid microphone. The patient should insert and remove the device several times, adjust the volume, and practice placing the battery into the battery compartment and taking it out.

During the hearing aid orientation, patients usually receive information about where to purchase batteries, how much they might cost, and how long they should last. Other topics include feedback (what it is, why it occurs, and how it can be minimized), adjustment (one must become accustomed to listening to amplified speech), and how to know when the aid is not functioning normally (what to try at home to fix it and when to return to the audiologist). Appendix 12-1 presents an outline of topics typically covered in a hearing aid orientation session.

Several studies support the value of a comprehensive hearing aid orientation. Patients who receive one are unlikely to return their hearing aids (Kochkin, 1999; Northern & Beyer, 1999). Patients who receive an orientation and counseling session lasting 2 or more hours report high levels of satisfaction (Kochkin, 2002).

When a patient first uses a hearing aid, the patient may feel:

- Self-conscious
- Uncomfortable
- Not his or her "usual" self

Such reactions are:

- Normal
- Part of the "learning curve"
- Transient

(Clark & English, 2004, p. 127)

Establishing a Use Pattern

About 70% of patients who receive a hearing aid are satisfied with the benefits they receive. About 9 out of 10 actually wear it at least once a year. Three out of four patients wear their devices for 4 or more hours each day (Kochkin, 2005b). Reasons that some individuals choose not to wear their devices are that they find a hearing aid uncomfortable to wear or find it difficult to handle. Some are overwhelmed by having to listen in the presence of background noise. Others may have had unrealistic expectations about what a hearing aid can and cannot do, and they may receive less than expected benefit. For some, speech may sound "tinny" or loud. In some instances, patients may have wanted one kind of hearing aid (such as an ITE aid) but the audiologist prescribed another, one that may be more appropriate for the hearing loss configuration (such as a BTE style) (Mueller, Bryant, Brown, & Budinger, 1991). The five most common problems reported by hearing aid users, in order of significance, are as follows: (a) understanding speech at a distance in noise, (b) understanding certain talkers, (c) understanding speech in noise, (d) understanding speech at a distance in quiet, and (e) understanding speech in general (Takahashi et al., 2007). Figure 12-7 presents the results from a survey of

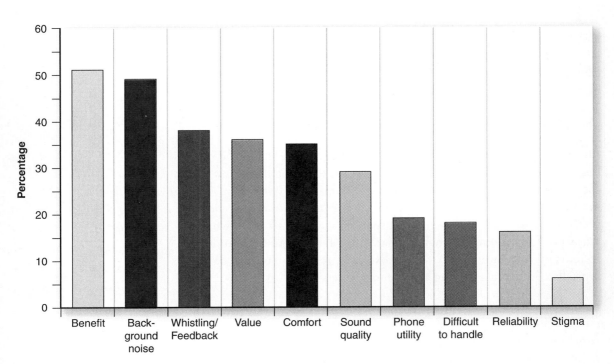

FIGURE 12-7. Common reasons why patients return hearing aids (*n* = 237).

237 individuals who chose to return their hearing aids and the reasons for doing so (Kochkin, 2007).

There are at least three identifiable **hearing aid use patterns** to describe the ways in which adults use hearing aids (Figure 12-8). Those who eventually become full-time users often increase the number of hours per day they use the new hearing aid, so that after several days or weeks it is used during

Hearing aid use pattern refers to the times, situations, and locations in which a hearing aid user wears the hearing aids.

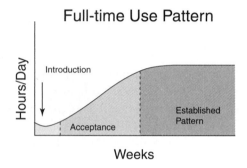

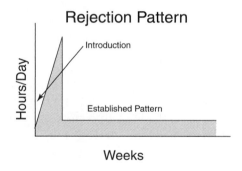

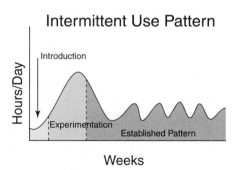

FIGURE 12-8. Patterns of use found in first-time hearing aid users.

almost all waking hours. Commonly, persons who reject their hearing aids either return them to their audiologist or put them away in a drawer, trying them for only a brief trial period of a few days or weeks. Finally, some individuals never achieve full-time use nor do they reject the hearing aid(s). They may try wearing the hearing aid in a variety of situations initially, and then decide they need it only for specific settings. An intermittent use pattern is best established on the basis of experience, so the individual actually tries the device in a variety of situations before deciding when it is and is not helpful, rather than on assumptions made by either the patient or the audiologist.

Group Follow-Up Orientation Sessions

New patients will sometimes participate in a group follow-up orientation program following receipt of a hearing aid. Information about the care and use of the device that was presented during the hearing aid orientation may be reiterated and provision made for supervised practice in handling the device and in using the telephone. Other class topics might include communication strategies, listening, and speechreading. Appendix 12-2 presents an example of a course syllabus for a three-session adult aural rehabilitation group class that has been used by the HEARx network hearing centers in 78 locations and four states (Beyer & Northern, 2000). Each session lasts between 60 and 90 minutes and spouses and family members of the patients are encouraged to attend.

Group follow-up orientation sessions need not be limited to new hearing aid users. Sometimes experienced users require a refresher course, especially if they have received new technology. Appendix 12-3 presents a curriculum for a hearing aid refresher course developed by the Hearing Center at Albany (New York) Medical Center. This center has dispensed more than 8,600 hearing aids during the past 25 years and has experienced a return rate of less than 3% (Wayner, 2005).

Cochlear Implants

The centerpiece of an adult's aural rehabilitation plan may be receipt of a cochlear implant. Adults who have severe-to-profound hearing loss may be considered as candidates for cochlear implantation. A cochlear implant service delivery model usually includes seven components. These components are summarized in Table 12-1. They are: initial contact, preimplant counseling, formal evaluation, surgery, fitting, follow-up evaluation, and formal aural rehabilitation. During these stages, the patient will interact with the members of the cochlear implant team, which typically includes a clinical coordinator, an audiologist, a surgeon, and sometimes, a psychologist (see Pedley, Giles, & Hogan, 2005, for a comprehensive overview about cochlear implants and adults).

Table 12-1. Seven stages of the cochlear implant process.

STAGE	DESCRIPTION	COMMENTS
Initial contact	The clinical coordinator provides the patient with general information about cochlear implants and candidacy; the patient may be scheduled for an appointment at the cochlear implant center	a) Patient may receive an information packet, such as manufacturer's booklets b) Patient learns about alternatives to implantation and receives an overview of the center's procedures and policies
Preimplant counseling	Patient receives specific information about candidacy, benefits, commitments, and costs, usually from the cochlear implant audiologist	a) Patient learns about such topics as sound quality from an implant, success and failure rate, issues related to maintenance b) Patient has an opportunity to see a cochlear implant and learn about how it works
Formal evaluation	Patient receives comprehensive audiological and medical evaluation and sometimes a psychological evaluation	a) Audiological testing typically includes pure-tone audiometry, speech audiometry (including aided speech recognition), otoacoustic emissions b) Otolaryngologic assessment will explore any contraindications to surgery (such as cochlear anomalies or middle ear infection) and typically includes a CT scan of the inner ear and temporal bone c) Psychological assessment will explore concerns such as depression and may establish whether realistic expectations are present
Surgery	The cochlear implant surgeon implants the internal hardware of the cochlear implant	a) Surgery takes about 2–3 hours b) Complications are rare; may include temporary vertigo or tinnitus
Fitting/mapping	The device is fitted to the patient by the audiologist and a map is created; patient receives instruction about care and maintenance	a) Usually occurs after the surgical wound has healed b) The hardware is fitted to the patient and a MAP is established
Follow-up	Any problems are explored, and new developments about cochlear implants are reviewed with the patient	a) Patient is seen a few times during the first year and then at least annually thereafter b) Causes for concern include an intermittent signal, facial stimulation, change in sound quality, cessation of sound, abnormal popping or squeaking
Aural rehabilitation	The patient receives auditory training and sometimes, communication strategies training, speechreading training, and psychosocial support	a) Auditory training is essential as patient learns to interpret new electrical signal b) Psychosocial support may help patient reidentify self as a person with hearing

Receipt of a cochlear implant and follow-up may take upwards of a year. It begins when the patient contacts the cochlear implant center to inquire about candidacy. The patient may have learned about cochlear implants from a physician, an audiologist, a news report, or an acquaintance. The clinical coordinator will provide information to the patient during an initial contact visit.

The counseling session will occur either next or, sometimes, following the formal evaluation. During the counseling session, the cochlear implant audiologist will provide information about the cochlear implant and post-implant management. The audiologist will help the patient to develop realistic expectations by talking about outcomes. For example, many patients will experience great difficulty when listening in noise and some will never learn to appreciate listening to music. There is a wide range of performance levels, and some patients will achieve little more than sound awareness following receipt of a cochlear implant whereas others will be able to talk effortlessly on the telephone.

The formal evaluation will establish candidacy, and will include an assessment of hearing abilities, otologic and general health, and sometimes, psychological status. Once a patient is deemed a candidate, then surgery is scheduled. The surgery typically requires the patient to stay overnight in the hospital and to undergo a 2- to 3-hour surgical procedure. During surgery, the surgeon implants the internal receiver into the mastoid and inserts the electrode array into the cochlea.

The patient returns to the cochlear implant center after the surgical wound heals for the fitting and mapping. The external components are placed on the patient and adjusted so that the patient may wear them comfortably (Figure 12-9). The audiologist adjusts the stimulus parameters of the speech processor, which determine the signals delivered to the electrodes in the electrode array. The components of establishing a map include setting threshold levels, setting comfort levels, and "flagging," or turning off, electrodes that are problematic. The patient will receive instruction about how to handle the device, including how to turn the speech processor on and off, how to change or recharge batteries, how to troubleshoot the device, and how to use the telephone.

After the first year, follow-up visits typically occur on at least an annual basis. The audiologist checks to see that the cochlear implant is working properly and provides any new information about devices.

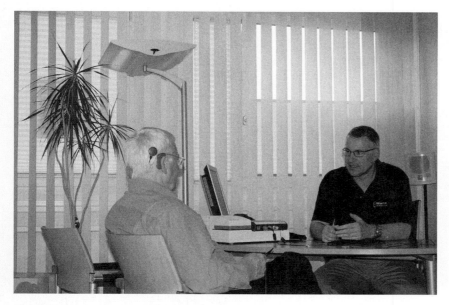

FIGURE 12-9. Cochlear implant fitting. Patients return to the cochlear implant center for the fitting after the surgical wound heals. *Photograph courtesy of MED-EL Corp.*

Aural rehabilitation typically includes formal auditory training, because the patient must awaken auditory memories and learn to associate the new electrical signal with environmental sounds and the speech signal. Auditory training may include both clinic-based sessions and home-based listening exercises, such as listening to books-on-tape with a printed text. Sometimes support counseling is beneficial, as patients learn to reidentify themselves as persons with some (or much) hearing ability. Communication strategies training and group orientation sessions, as well as speechreading training, may also be appropriate.

Assistive Listening Devices and Other Assistive Devices

The aural rehabilitation plan will often include provision of assistive listening devices. Individuals may use assistive listening devices either in addition to or in lieu of a hearing aid or a cochlear implant. The need for various devices relates to a patient's degree of hearing loss, his or her ability to recognize speech in quiet and noise, social and occupational demands, and motivation to use hearing aids or assistive devices. Probably the most common requests for assistive devices pertain to telephone amplification systems and television viewing (Figure 12-10).

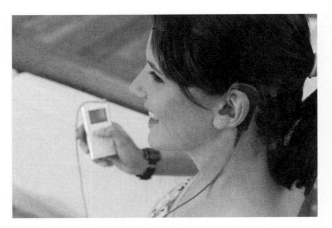

FIGURE 12-10. Assistive listening devices and cochlear implants. Many patients request assistive listening devices that enhance their television viewing. *Photograph courtesy of MED-EL Corp.*

In assessing the need for assistive devices, the clinician might determine those communicative situations for which devices might be indicated. For example, Table 12-2 suggests those circumstances in which alerting, listening, and visual support systems might be appropriate for adults who have severe or profound hearing losses. In this framework, communicative situations are classified as interactive or noninteractive, and warning needs are classified as basic or lifestyle-specific.

Table 12-2. Circumstances in which patients with profound or severe hearing losses may desire assistive listening devices (adapted from Schum & Tye-Murray, 1995).

I. Basic warning signals

  A. Smoke alarms
  B. Doorbell/knock
  C. Telephone ring
  D. Intruders

II. Lifestyle-specific warning signals

  A. Vehicle, such as sirens or horns
  B. Alarm clock
  C. Children/infants
  D. Household appliances, such as microwave or washer/dryer signals

III. Interactive communication

  A. Face-to-face
  B. Telephone conversation
  C. Group
    1. home
    2. workplace
    3. social gatherings
    4. meetings
    5. classrooms

---

continues

Table 12-2. *continued*

---

*IV.***Noninteractive communication**

    A. At home

        1. television

        2. radio

        3. stereo

    B. At work

    C. At public sites

        1. religious services

        2. movies

        3. concerts

        4. dramatic arts presentations

        5. lectures

        6. professional conferences

        7. sports events

        8. airport terminal

To obtain information about a person's need for and current use of assistive listening devices, some clinicians have employed written checklists like those presented in the Key Resources section at the end of this chapter. After a person has had an opportunity to gain experience with a hearing aid or cochlear implant, the audiologist can review this checklist with the patient and ask about situations that still are problematic. As problems are identified, the clinician can refer the individual to the checklist and then demonstrate systems that currently are not used, but that are appropriate for alleviating communication difficulties.

Issues that might be considered as the aural rehabilitation strategy is put together and recommendations for assistive devices are being formulated include (Compton, 1995):

- **Affordability:** How expensive is the device? Especially if an individual has recently purchased a hearing aid or cochlear implant, affordability is an important issue to consider when recommending assistive devices. It may be desirable to have the patient prioritize listening needs, and then to select the most useful/versatile assistive device(s) accordingly.

- **Reliability and Durability:** Will the device work as promised, and will it hold up over repeated usage? Many manufacturers are now producing assistive devices, some of which vary in reliability, quality, and durability. When recommending an assistive device, an audiologist will want to balance the features of a particular device against its cost. Reliability may be of paramount consideration when safety is an issue, as in emergency alerting systems like fire detectors.

- **Operability:** How does it work? The person must be able to manage the device. For instance, he or she should be able to replace the batteries, if applicable, and be able to operate the device. Sometimes formal instruction is necessary; therefore, the patient must have the time and the cognitive (and possibly financial) wherewithal to participate in a training session.

- **Portability:** Can the device easily be transported from one locale to another? In some instances, portability is an issue. If someone travels frequently, for example, then the person will want a telephone amplifier that can easily be transported in a purse or coat pocket. A replacement handset amplifier would be inappropriate in this instance.
- **Compatibility:** Can the device be used with a hearing aid? In many cases, patients wear their hearing aids at all times and will opt to wear the aid with any assistive listening device.
- **Cosmetics:** What does it look like when in use? Some people may be self-conscious about using an assistive listening device. For example, pulling out a wireless FM listening device at a restaurant may be difficult. Counseling and opportunity for practice under the supervision of an audiologist may minimize cosmetic concerns.

In dispensing an assistive listening device, the following steps usually are followed (Sutherland, 1995):

- Demonstrate how to use the device(s).
- Review the advantages and disadvantages of the device and its capabilities and limitations.
- Describe how the devices work and how to install them.
- Demonstrate how to troubleshoot the devices.
- Demonstrate the device to family members.
- Answer any questions.
- Review the Americans with Disabilities Act and talk about patients' legal rights.

Tinnitus Intervention

As noted in the last chapter, tinnitus is a symptom associated with a variety of ear disorders. These disorders include ear infections, excessive cerumen or foreign objects in the ear canal, otosclerosis, Ménière's disease, acoustic neuroma, and acoustic trauma. It often co-occurs with hearing loss, especially noise-induced hearing loss. Tinnitus may also be symptomatic of cardiovascular disease, including anemia, vascular malformations, aneurysm, head tumors, and occlusion of the carotid arteries. Because tinnitus is often symptomatic of medical conditions other than hearing loss, a patient should see an otolaryngologist to rule out medical or surgically treatable ear pathology before entering into a tinnitus management program. A visit to an otolaryngologist is especially important if the tinnitus is unilateral, as that may be symptomatic of an acoustic neuroma. Other members of the tinnitus management team might include a psychologist, psychiatrist, neurologist, pharmacologist, nutritionist, temporal-mandibular-joint specialist, and biofeedback specialist (Sweetow, 2006).

A tinnitus intake interview may be the first audiological step in addressing a patient's tinnitus concerns. During this interview, the audiologist may ask such questions as: What does your most bothersome tinnitus sound like?; Is your tinnitus louder on one side of your head than the other?; Would you please describe the onset of your tinnitus?; and How long have you had your tinnitus? (Henry, Zaugg, & Schechter, 2005, p. 26).

The patient might complete one of the questionnaires listed in Table 12-3. Because tinnitus cannot be measured objectively, it often is difficult to quantify its degree or to understand the magnitude of disability it presents. Some existing questionnaires include open-ended questions (Tyler & Baker, 1983). Some include quantifiable items such as those listed below

Table 12-3. Acronyms, titles, and authors of self-report scales for assessing tinnitus, listed in chronological order of development (adapted from Noble, 2000).

ABBREVIATION	FULL TITLE	AUTHORS
TEQ	Tinnitus Effects Questionnaire	Hallam, Jakes, & Hinchcliffe, 1988
THQ	Tinnitus Handicap Questionnaire	Kuk, Tyler, Russell, & Jordan, 1990
TSS	Tinnitus Severity Scale	Sweetow & Levy, 1990
STSS	Subjective Tinnitus Severity Scale	Halford & Anderson, 1991
TRQ	Tinnitus Reaction Questionnaire	Wilson, Henry, Bowen, & Haralambous, 1991
TH/SS	Tinnitus Handicap/Support Scale	Erlandsson, Hallberg, & Axelsson, 1992
TSI	Tinnitus Severity Index	Meikle, Griest, Stewardt, & Press, 1995
THI	Tinnitus Handicap Inventory	Newman, Jacobson, & Spitzer, 1996
TCSQ	Tinnitus Coping Style Questionnaire	Budd & Pugh, 1996
TCQ	Tinnitus Cognitions Questionnaire	Wilson & Henry, 1998
(none)	The Tinnitus Intake Form	Jastreboff & Jastreboff, 1999

(e.g., Stouffer & Tyler, 1990), presented here with example kinds of questions:

- Location: Is it in the left ear, right ear, or both ears?
- Pitch: On a continuum corresponding to pitch, is it high pitched or low pitched?
- Constancy: Is the tinnitus always present? Is it intermittent? Do you tend to notice it at a particular time of day?
- Composition: Do you hear one sound or more than one sound?
- Fluctuations: Does the tinnitus change from one sound to another? Does it change in pitch?
- Loudness: On a continuum corresponding to loudness, is it loud or soft?
- Conditions that exacerbate the tinnitus: What conditions exacerbate the tinnitus (e.g., drinking coffee, smoking)?
- Annoyance: On a continuum corresponding to annoyance, can the tinnitus be described as not at all annoying, extremely annoying, or somewhere in between?
- Effects on concentration and sleep: Does it have a slight effect? Extreme effect?
- Depression: Does it cause minimal depression? Extreme depression?

The patient may also undergo some of the following audiological and medical procedures prior to entering a tinnitus management regime:

A **tone-decay** test is a test of auditory adaptation during which a continuous tone is presented at about threshold and any change in perception is monitored over a set time interval; an abnormal adaptation may indicate a retrocochlear site of lesion.

- Comprehensive audiological testing, including site-of lesion testing (e.g., **tone-decay testing**)
- Otoscopic examination, because cerumen can be a cause of tinnitus
- Impedance audiometry, to help establish the functional condition of the patient's middle ear, tympanic membrane, and Eustachian tube and to rule out blockage as a source of tinnitus
- Auditory brainstem response testing (ABR), which records the central auditory system's response to sound, to help distinguish between a cochlear and retrocochlear lesion (retrocochlear means the lesion lies between the cochlea and the brain)
- Vestibular and balance tests, such as eletronystagmography (ENG, where the eyeball is recorded in response to balance tests such as tracking, optokinetics, and positional testing), and rotary chair and pursuit tracking tests, to determine whether the vestibular system is involved in the patient's condition
- Head magnetic resonance imaging (MRI), to determine whether a tumor is present in the internal auditory canal
- Vascular studies, such as angiography, to explore the possibility of a cardiovascular cause

An audiologist might administer a tinnitus assessment battery. Using psychoacoustical measurement procedures, the battery typically consists of pitch and loudness matching tasks, perceptual location, minimum masking level, and postmarking effects. For example, when determining the minimum masking level, the audiologist might present white noise to the patient through headphones, gradually increasing the level of presentation. The patient's task is to indicate when the noise is just loud enough to mask the percept of head ringing.

There is no known cure for tinnitus. However, there are a variety of options that provide relief or some control over the sensation of tinnitus. Some of the more common treatments are summarized in Table 12-4. Treatments include masking the tinnitus with an auditory signal, electrical stimulation, relaxation therapy and biofeedback, acupuncture, counseling, herbal extracts and vitamins, and other forms of pharmacological interventions (which include sleep aids and medications to reduce anxiety).

One treatment that has received attention in recent years is tinnitus retraining therapy (TRT), which relies on the natural ability of the brain

> "I would use just about any means available to stifle him [tinnitus], to eradicate him from my life, or just to reduce his overwhelming influence on what I have of a life. . . . Others like me want to say to the clinicians and researchers on the leading edge of audiology research: Give us new weapons in our struggle for liberation. We will try just about anything."
>
> George R. Brown, MD, Chief of Psychiatry, Mountain Home Veterans Administration Medical Center, TN, and tinnitus sufferer
>
> (Brown, 2004, p. 53)

Table 12-4. Summary of a variety of methods available for managing and controlling tinnitus (Vernon & Meikle, 2000; Wilson & Henry, 2000).

METHOD OF TINNITUS TREATMENT	DESCRIPTION
Relaxation training	The patient is taught to decrease muscular tension through a series of exercises, sequentially tensing and relaxing targeted muscle groups. Discussion focuses on tinnitus as a source of stress, and the use of relaxation both at home and in real-life situations to relieve stress and associated tinnitus.
Biofeedback	This method is a form of relaxation training in which changes in a person's muscle tension or skin temperature are reinforced with a simple signal, such as a tone that changes in pitch or loudness. This signal helps the patient control arousal level.
Cognitive therapy and counseling	Patients learn to control where their attention is directed or change the content of their thoughts. For example, they learn to replace maladaptive thoughts with constructive thoughts and learn to direct their attention away from the tinnitus.
Masking devices	The patient wears a masking device (behind the ear) that delivers a sound to the ear that masks the tinnitus, or the patient sets a radio or CD player to make continual sound. The masking sound may be easier to tune out because it is a constant sound, and it also gives the patient a sense of control over the condition because the patient determines whether to hear the masking sound. Often, the pitch of the masking sound is adjusted to match the pitch of the patient's tinnitus.
Tinnitus retraining therapy (TRT)	TRT involves a combination of counseling and sound therapy. During counseling, three main points are considered: (a) Tinnitus is a form of compensation by the auditory system due to damage or dysfunction within the auditory pathways; (b) tinnitus becomes a problem because of emotional and autonomic responses; and (c) the brain can learn to attenuate these abnormal activations (Jastreboff, 2000). During sound training, patients receive constant broadband low-intensity noise, allowing the patient to still hear tinnitus. The noise generators facilitate habituation and reverse the distress experienced as a result of tinnitus.

General counseling points for tinnitus sufferers:

- Avoid noise exposure.
- Reduce stress.
- Get adequate sleep.
- Limit intake of alcohol, caffeine, tobacco, and salt.
- Maintain a constant background of sound.
- Stay busy with meaningful activities to distract you from tinnitus.

(Henry, Dennis, & Schechter, 2005, pp. 1219–1220)

to "habituate" to a signal and filter it out on a subconscious level so it never reaches conscious awareness. Just as persons can habituate external auditory signals such as air conditioner fan noise and a refrigerator hum, they can learn to ignore the sound of their tinnitus. In this neurophysiologic approach, patients receive counseling then listen to broadband white noise for approximately 6 hours a day for 12 to 18 months to habituate themselves to the phantom signal. Eventually, they do not attend to it, nor experience an emotional reaction, even though the tinnitus may still be present. There is some evidence this treatment works for some patients (Berry, Gold, Frederick, Gray, & Stacker, 2002; Jastreboff et al., 1996).

Persons who suffer severe tinnitus often benefit by enrolling in a self-help group. The American Tinnitus Association (ATA) is the umbrella organization for many such groups. The ATA provides patients with information about the problem and current techniques for managing it. The organization sponsors workshops, regional meetings, and seminars, allowing patients to interact with each other and with professionals. They also sponsor self-help groups in the majority of the states in the United States. These self-help groups provide guidance to members and help them relieve distress and regain hope by allowing them to share their experiences and solutions with other individuals with tinnitus. Often an audiologist or other speech and hearing professional serves as the group facilitator who shares professional knowledge (and often personal experiences because they frequently experience tinnitus too). Persons interested in starting a self-help group can contact the ATA (the address is provided in Appendix 12-4 at the end of this chapter) to receive start-up materials (Reich, 2000).

Dancer (2001) reported the top five tinnitus management methods used by audiologists who responded to a survey. In order of popularity, the treatments are counseling (64%), masking (51%), support groups (41%), drug therapy (22%), and herbal extracts and vitamins (21%).

What Every Tinnitus Sufferer Needs to Know:

- Tinnitus is not unique to that one patient.
- Tinnitus is not a sign of insanity or grave illness
- Tinnitus probably is not a sign of impending deafness.
- There is no evidence to suggest the tinnitus will get worse.
- Tinnitus does not have to result in a lack of control.
- Patients who can sleep can best manage their tinnitus.

What Every Tinnitus Sufferer Needs to Know: *continued*

- Tinnitus is real, and not imagined.
- Tinnitus may be permanent.
- Reaction to the tinnitus is the source of the problem.
- Reaction to the symptom is manageable and subject to modification.
- If significance and threat is removed, habituation or "gating" of attention can be achieved.
- Stay off the Internet!

(Sweetow, 2006)

Telephone Training

An aural rehabilitation plan may include telephone training. Patients sometimes express a desire to communicate more effectively on the telephone, even if they have received an assistive device that facilitates telephone conversations (e.g., a telephone amplifier) or if they have a listening device with a telephone adapter. Often, these people are new cochlear implant users who have not used the telephone for a long period prior to receiving their implant. After many years of not using the telephone, some people need assistance in overcoming apprehensions and fears. There are a few training programs available specifically designed to promote success using the telephone (e.g., Castle, 1988; Erber, 1985; Wayner & Abrahamson, 1998).

Telephone training may begin with a discussion of useful tips. For example, a speech and hearing professional might encourage the patient to practice some of these lines (Wayner & Abrahamson, 1998, p. 32):

- I can't listen as fast as you can talk. Will you slow down for me?
- I'm not good at recognizing voices. Who is calling please?
- Let me repeat that back to you to make sure I heard you right.
- I think I could understand you better if you would talk a little softer.
- Did you just say that [for example] the meeting is next Sunday at 7:00?

Initially, the patient will practice speaking on the telephone to familiar persons, such as the clinician or a family member, about familiar topics. The communication partner might read from the newspaper or from a simple passage. With practice, the conversations can become more interactive and less structured. For instance, an audiologist may coach a patient as he or she calls the bank and checks the balance in an account or calls a restaurant to make a reservation.

OUTCOMES ASSESSMENT

After the plan has been implemented, and time has elapsed for the patient to experience benefit, success can be assessed. Common means of evaluating outcome include direct measurement of performance, interviews, observation of performance, self-report scales and questionnaires, and daily logs. The goal of assessment is to determine the extent to which activity limitations and participation restrictions have been reduced and to determine whether additional concerns remain to be addressed. There is no universal agreement as to how best to measure outcome. For instance, Humes (1999) suggests that when a hearing aid is provided, an evaluation should follow a test battery approach, and include measures of aided speech recognition performance, and objective and subjective measures of benefit, satisfaction, and use. Alternatively, Gagné (2003) suggests that a unique set of outcomes measures should be identified for each patient, measures that can capture the changes that might have occurred in an individual's involvement in specific activities that were identified as the target of intervention. An example of an assessment that is consonant with this latter viewpoint appears in Table 12-5. In this functional assessment, information was culled from interviews with both the patient and family members and from objective tests to develop concrete goals of intervention and then again following a hearing aid fitting to obtain specific information about whether these goals had been met (Heide, 2005).

Table 12-5. An example of an assessment of functional outcomes (adapted from Heide, 2005, p. 64). This patient received a hearing aid.

Prefitting

SYMPTOM	ACTIVITY LIMITATION	PARTICIPATION RESTRICTION
Inattention	Is perceived by others to be disinterested	Loss of social interactions
Isolation	Is unable to hear in groups	Does not attend plays or public meetings

Postfitting

ACTION	PERCEPTION	OUTCOME
Engages in conversation and in groups	Is perceived by others to be alert and a good listener	Frequently asked to join others at home for dinner or to play cards
Uses telephone with ease	Is perceived by others to talk easily with them on the phone	Nominated to be in charge of the phone tree for local service club

An outcomes assessment might be fairly unstructured, as when a seasoned clinician determines the extent to which a plan has succeeded by talking with the patient and through observation. For instance, the clinician might consider whether the patient demonstrates successful use of the telephone, listens to the television at a volume that is comfortable for family members as well, or demonstrates good conversational fluency when talking to the clinician, a spouse, or a friend (Heide, 2005, p. 64). Alternatively, an assessment might be highly structured, requiring the clinician to document success by collecting quantitative data. In one survey, only about a third of audiologists surveyed reported routinely using formal outcomes measures (Kirkwood, 1999).

The assessment might include any or all of four domains: performance, benefit, usage, and satisfaction (e.g., Meister, Lausberg, Kiessling, Von Wedel, & Walger, 2003). **Performance** is how well a patient can recognize speech with a listening device (e.g., Cox & Gilmore, 1990), or how well a patient functions in everyday communication interactions after having received other aural rehabilitation services, such as communication strategies training or assertiveness training. Performance might be assessed with speech recognition tests or by means of a self-report instrument, such as the *Gothenburg Profile* (Ringdahl et al., 1998). Although originally designed to be used during the initial contact with a patient, the *Gothenburg Profile* can also be used as an outcomes assessment instrument. Sample questions include: *Are there occasions when you cannot follow a conversation when you are in your home and speak to one person?; Are there occasions when you cannot hear a speaker at a meeting, even if you are well-positioned?; Are there occasions when you hesitate to meet new people because of your hearing difficulties?;* and *Are there occasions when you avoid social gatherings, because it is hard to follow a conversation?* Patients use a 10-point scale in responding, ranging from *never* to *always.*

As noted in Chapter 3, benefit is the improvement gained in an aided as compared to an unaided listening condition, and is typically a differential measure. Benefit might be assessed through speech recognition tests that are administered in an unaided and then an aided condition, or through self-report measures such as the COSI (see Key Resources) or the *Glasgow Hearing Aid Benefit Profile* (Gatehouse, 1999). If the patient has completed the COSI at the outset of the rehabilitation program, then giving it again can determine whether the patient's goals and expectations were met and indicate whether aural rehabilitation should be modified or extended. Several questionnaires exist that ask respondents to consider aided and unaided conditions, such as *The Abbreviated Profile of Hearing Aid Benefit* (*APHAB*; Cox & Alexander, 1995). The APHAB has 24 items that ask patients to consider the amount of difficulty that they experience in communicating in various everyday situations, both when they are wearing their hearing aid and when they

Performance refers to how well a patient can recognize speech.

are not wearing the hearing aid. For example, they are asked to indicate agreement on a 7-point scale with the item, *When I am in a crowded grocery store, talking with the cashier, I can follow the conversation,* first *without my hearing aid* and then *with my hearing aid.* Benefit is calculated by comparing reported difficulty in an unaided with an aided condition.

A patient is unlikely to receive benefit from, say, a hearing aid unless the patient uses the device. Usage, as noted in Chapter 3, relates to both frequency of use and contextual use. For instance, how long does a patient wear a hearing aid during an ordinary day and in what situations? Although listening device usage is typically assessed, the domain of *usage* can be extended to include the use of communication strategies as well. For instance, the daily logs that we considered in Chapter 8 might be appropriate for tracking one's communication behaviors before and after a communication strategies training course.

Mail-In Daily Logs

A simple method to assess usage of a new hearing aid is through the use of daily logs. The audiologist creates seven postcards, each addressed with the audiologist's business address and each with a stamp. On the other side of each card, a date is printed, with the seven cards having seven consecutive dates. Each day, the patient's task is to complete three items printed on the back of that day's card: the time the hearing aid was put on, the time the hearing aid was taken off, and any additional comments. The patient mails a card every day, so the audiologist is assured the cards were not completed on one occasion.

This daily log allows the audiologist to monitor the patient's progress during the initial period of adjustment. The audiologist can determine whether the patient is gradually increasing use time and whether the patient is experiencing any difficulties. For example, one patient commented that her hearing aid squealed on three separate days. Anytime a patient seems to be having difficulty in adjusting to the hearing aid (e.g., if the patient reports a problem on 2 or more days), the audiologist can call the patient and discuss the difficulties, and if necessary, schedule an appointment. In a similar vein, Humes (2004) recommends the use of small pocket calendars during the 30-day hearing aid trial period. New users are asked to record the hours of daily usage and any problems with the device. For patients who use the Internet, a web-based reporting system can be devised.

Satisfaction, which we also considered in Chapter 3, can be included in an outcomes assessment, and reflects a patient's contentment with his or her current situation. Satisfaction is positively correlated with benefit (e.g., Brooks & Hallam, 1998; Dillon et al., 1997), but may also be influenced by the patient's expectations (Cox & Alexander, 2000). An example of a self-report measure that might be used to assess satisfaction with a hearing aid is the *SADL* (Cox & Alexander, 1999), an adaptation of which is included in the Key Resources.

An international group of 15 experts who participated in the Eriksholm Workshop held in Copenhagen, Denmark, generated a brief self-report instrument that they believed to be universally applicable, one that allows comparisons across social, cultural, and health care delivery systems (Cox et al., 2000). The *International Outcome Inventory for Hearing Aids (OI-HA)* includes seven items, together which query the patient about performance, benefit, usage, and satisfaction. An adaptation of the OI-HA is included in the Key Resources.

FOLLOW-UP

The aural rehabilitation plan should be flexible. If new problems arise or the intervention proves unsuccessful, the plan should be adaptable. Patients and their predicaments often change, so the aural rehabilitation plan may require fine-tuning and adjusting as it unfolds. A **predicament** is the sum of the relevant variables affecting the patient, including the hearing loss, situation, attitudes, aptitudes, lifestyles, and communication behaviors. For example, one patient originally sought aural rehabilitation because she could not understand speech in quiet situations. Her audiologist fitted her with a BTE that was equipped with a telecoil. She is delighted with the hearing aid and now finds she wants to use the telephone, something she has avoided using for 3 years. The patient would now like to incorporate telephone training and telephone-related conversational strategies into her aural rehabilitation plan. This situation is an example where the aural rehabilitation plan must be adapted to the changing needs of the patient.

Predicament is the "sum of all pertinent aspects of client state and situation, including disorders, impairments, disabilities, handicaps, environments, demands, resources, attitudes, behaviors, and so on" (Hyde & Riko, 1994, p. 351).

This patient's situation is illustrated graphically in Figure 12-11. Before aural rehabilitation, she desired to converse more effectively in quiet. After her aural rehabilitation intervention, in which she received a hearing aid and communication strategies training, the intervention has had an impact on her lifestyle because she can now talk to friends and family with more success. This impact has given her the desire and confidence to begin using the telephone and the desire to solve her telephone-related communication problems.

During an annual visit, an audiologist can:

- Monitor hearing.
- Make hearing aid adjustments if hearing has changed.
- Examine ear canal for cerumen buildup.
- Review other sources of help (e.g., communication strategies training).
- Clean hearing aids.
- Ensure hearing aids are in good working order.
- Review hearing aid warranty coverage.
- Provide information about new developments (e.g., in federal law).

(adapted from Hampton, 2005, p. 79)

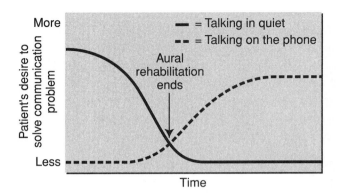

FIGURE 12-11. Flexibility and adaptation. The aural rehabilitation plan may require fine-tuning as patients' predicaments change.

In performing routine follow-ups, the clinician might provide written materials via the mail and occasionally write short letters inquiring about the patient's satisfaction and progress with amplification. Communication through e-mail can be effective, as well as the use of Internet chat rooms centered on hearing loss and aural rehabilitation. Typically, individuals return to their audiologists on an annual basis for a hearing test and a hearing aid (or cochlear implant) check. During these visits, the audiologist can assess whether hearing has worsened and whether the hearing aid is still functioning properly.

Individuals might be encouraged to join self-help organizations. One such organization is the Hearing Loss Association of America, formerly known as Self Help for Hard of Hearing People, Inc. (SHHH). It is comprised of hundreds of local chapters and a national office that disseminates information about hearing loss and communication. Appendix 12-4 presents addresses for this group as well as other self-help organizations. In addition, it lists professional organizations that serve adults with hearing loss and Deaf adults.

CASE STUDY

A Road Map for Success

Heide (2005) recommends using a functional outcomes approach to providing hearing aids, which she describes as the ability of a patient to use a hearing aid in everyday activities. For each patient, she creates a "road map," which has concrete goals toward which to work. To illustrate this approach, she presents a case study of "Mr. Smith." Mr. Smith was unable to converse on the telephone and frequently asked his wife to conduct his phone conversations. He was fitted with a hearing aid that had a telecoil. The following

CASE STUDY, *continued*

A Road Map for Success, *continued*

questions were posed to illustrate how functional outcomes might be measured and recorded, and how direction for further intervention might be clarified (p. 64):

- Can Mr. Smith successfully use the telephone?
- Does he need practice or [additional] intervention?
- Can Mr. Smith listen to the TV at a volume that is comfortable for others in the family?
- Is the patient able to demonstrate use of the telephone with ease?
- Can he hug his friends and family without feedback?
- Can he demonstrate speech understanding at a distance of more than 6 feet?
- Can he demonstrate speech understanding to his satisfaction in restaurants or groups (or simulated backgrounds of noise in a clinic)?
- Can Mr. Smith hear others when in the kitchen or the living room?

In cases such as this, patients receive a copy of their "scorecard" so that they can use it as a baseline for their personal reference. The clinician shares with them the areas that have been positively affected by the aural rehabilitation program to date and those areas that still warrant improvement.

FINAL REMARKS

Technology has opened new vistas for the rehabilitation of individuals who have hearing loss. Sophisticated hearing aids, various assistive listening devices, and cochlear implants have made it much easier for clinicians to alleviate listening difficulties. Ironically, these very advances sometimes make us lose sight of the fact that many adults continue to have problems with communication even after receiving high-technology devices. They still need to receive aural rehabilitation follow-up services.

KEY CHAPTER POINTS

- There are six stages involved in developing an aural rehabilitation plan: assessment, informational counseling, development of a plan, implementation, outcomes assessment, and follow-up. At each stage, the focus will be on customizing the plan for the individual.
- The first stage of an aural rehabilitation plan entails assessing a patient's hearing impairment, hearing-related difficulties, and individual factors.
- The World Health Organization suggests that a hearing impairment leads to both activity limitations and participation restrictions.

> "Create a roadmap for success for each individual by measuring their abilities and providing appropriate training, tools, or intervention until the outcome measured is the outcome desired."
>
> Veronica Heide, AuD., private practitioner in Madison, Wisconsin
>
> (Heide, 2005, p. 65).

- In developing a strategy, and in implementing a plan, a clinician will develop a partnership with his or her patient and develop a solution-centered, problem-solving strategy. The objectives will be influenced by a patient's priorities and expectations.

- Interviews may include unstructured and structured questions and might query about home-, work-, and social-related communication difficulties.

- The COSI is a self-assessment instrument that may be used to guide an overall aural rehabilitation plan and to assess outcome, and in particular can be used to assess hearing aid benefit.

- Motivating a patient to use a hearing aid may entail an education process, a change in the patient's value system and attitude, and establishment of a hearing aid use pattern.

- Hearing aids are available to alleviate a wide range of hearing loss. Candidacy depends on degree of loss and also on a person's lifestyle, occupation, and motivation to use a hearing aid.

- A significant number of adults who receive hearing aids do not use them. There are several reasons for nonuse. For example, some people find the sound unacceptable, and others are disappointed that their hearing aids do not provide greater benefit.

- Issues to consider when recommending an assistive device include affordability, durability, operability, portability, compatibility, and cosmetics.

- A patient who suffers from tinnitus may undergo a variety of medical and audiological tests.

- Although there are no cures for tinnitus, tinnitus retraining therapy (TRT) has been found to be successful in helping many patients manage their problem. Other management strategies include counseling, relaxation therapy, and self-help support groups.

- Some patients will desire telephone training, and a speech and hearing professional may serve as a "coach" for the patient, starting with easy, structured listening tasks to less familiar, more open conversations over the telephone.

- Patients' predicaments change over time, so the aural rehabilitation plan must be fine-tuned and adjusted as it unfolds.

TERMS AND CONCEPTS TO REMEMBER

Priorities
Expectations
COSI
Formulating objectives

Nonuse of a hearing aid
Clear speech for family members
Use patterns
Interactive and noninteractive communication situations
Orientation session
Tinnitus intake interview
Tinnitus retraining therapy
Outcomes assessment
Performance
Benefit
Usage
Satisfaction

 MULTIPLE-CHOICE QUESTIONS

1. Mr. Garcia has arrived for his first audiological procedure. An audiogram has confirmed what he has long suspected: a bilateral moderate sensorineural hearing loss. What would probably not happen on this first visit?

    a. The audiologist would take an impression of his ear for an ITE hearing aid.

    b. The audiologist would provide him information about the irreversible nature of sensorineural hearing losses.

    c. Mr. Garcia would complete a self-assessment instrument.

    d. Mrs. Garcia would receive an explanation about her husband's audiogram.

2. During the assessment phase, the audiologist would most likely consider which of the following variables first as he or she designs an aural rehabilitation plan for an adult patient:

    a. Ecological considerations, the patient's credit rating, and audiogram

    b. Hearing impairment, individual factors, and hearing-related difficulties

    c. The patient's workplace needs, the patient's first language, and family support

    d. The patient's communication mode, educational history, and predicament

3. In a solution-centered, problem-solving framework:

    a. Patients focus on those listening challenges that brought them to the professional to begin with.

    b. One solution may lead to another problem, which in turn may lead to another solution.

    c. The clinician asks the patient to develop a decision tree to address listening problems.

    d. Items a and b.

4. The *Client Oriented Scale of Improvement* (COSI):

    a. Is a multiple-choice self-assessment instrument

    b. Was designed to assess conversational fluency in difficult listening situations

    c. Was originally developed to assess hearing aid benefit, although it can be used to guide the overall aural rehabilitation plan

    d. Was designed to assess performance, benefit, usage, and satisfaction

5. In the context of an aural rehabilitation plan, a *predicament* is best defined as:

    a. An instance in which a patient has a listening difficulty in which the professional can offer little relief, as may happen with a patient who suffers severe tinnitus

    b. A summary of the patient's listening difficulties, and reasons why that person sought services from a speech and hearing professional in the first place

    c. The totality of a patient's state and situation, including disorders, impairments, disabilities, environments, demands, resources, attitudes, and behaviors

    d. The truism that a solution to one problem often creates the onset of another problem

6. Which of the following is an example of an activity limitation?

    a. The patient has a mild-to-moderate bilateral hearing loss.

    b. The patient will not join family and friends for dinner at a restaurant.

    c. The patient cannot engage in one-on-one conversations in the presence of background music.

    d. The patient refuses to participate in a group orientation follow-up session.

7. The following are reasons that patients may choose not to use a hearing aid. Which is probably the most prevalent reason?
   a. They believe their hearing is too good to warrant use of an aid.
   b. They are fearful of new technology.
   c. They realize that hearing aids only make speech louder, not necessarily easier to understand.
   d. Their families are embarrassed about having a family member with a hearing impairment.

8. In developing motivation for hearing aid use, the first step is usually:
   a. Attitude change
   b. Education
   c. Value change
   d. Understanding the steps for acquiring a hearing aid

9. During the hearing aid fitting and orientation, a patient typically learns:
   a. How to change the frequency response of the hearing aid
   b. How to adjust the maximum level sound pressure level
   c. How to troubleshoot problems
   d. How to upgrade the hearing aid if the patient decides he or she wants more "bells and whistles"

10. Once most patients receive a cochlear implant, they engage in all but the following:
    a. Motivational classes to use the device
    b. Auditory training
    c. Annual follow-up visits
    d. Trouble shooting as needed

11. Mr. Rampart comes to an audiologist complaining of unilateral tinnitus. The audiologist:
    a. Recommends that he receive impedance testing
    b. Recommends that he see an otolaryngologist because the tinnitus might be symptomatic of an auditory neuroma
    c. Sends him to a nutritionist for counseling
    d. Sends him to a cardiologist for vascular studies because it might be symptomatic of cardiovascular disease

12. During tinnitus retraining therapy, a patient:
    a. Receives biofeedback to minimize his anxiety relating to the tinnitus
    b. Receives counseling from a psychiatrist
    c. Wears an iPOD in order to listen to soothing music
    d. Receives counseling about how the brain learns to attenuate emotional and autonomic responses

13. One of the first steps in telephone training is:
    a. To ask the patient to call someone outside the clinic using a clinic phone
    b. To ask the patient to role-play with the clinician ways to instruct the telephone conversational partner
    c. To practice conversing with a familiar conversational partner via telephone
    d. To perform a task on the telephone such as making a dinner reservation at a restaurant or making an appointment for a haircut, while the clinician stands by as a "coach"

KEY RESOURCES

 ## THE NAL CLIENT ORIENTATED SCALE OF IMPROVEMENT (COSI)

(Used with permission from Oticon.)

COSI
The NAL Client Oriented Scale of Improvement

Name: _____
Audiologist: _____
Date: 1. Needs established _____
2. Outcome assessed _____

SPECIFIC NEEDS

Indicate Order of Significance

□	□	□	□	□

Degree of Change
"Because of the new hearing instrument, I now hear..."

					Worse
					No Difference
					Slightly Better
					Better
					Much Better

Final Ability (with hearing instrument)
"I can hear satisfactorily..."

					Hardly Ever 10%
					Occasionally 25%
					Half the Time 50%
					Most of Time 75%
					Almost Always 95%

469

ALERTING, ASSISTIVE, LISTENING AND VISUAL SUPPORT SYSTEMS CHECKLIST

Date: _____

Instructions to the clinician: Place an (X) in the column that best describes client's use of, interest in, or need for, each listed system.

SYSTEM	CURRENTLY USES	USED TO USE	IS INTERESTED IN	DOES NOT NEED
Assistive Listening Systems				
Closed-caption decoder for TV	☐	☐	☐	☐
Telecommunication for the Deaf (TDD)	☐	☐	☐	☐
Direct audio input (to speech processor from battery-operated radio, tape-player, or portable stereo)	☐	☐	☐	☐
Telephone adapter	☐	☐	☐	☐
Telephone amplifier	☐	☐	☐	☐
Telephone answering machine	☐	☐	☐	☐
TDD Relay message service	☐	☐	☐	☐
Group system (FM, loop, hardwire, infrared)	☐	☐	☐	☐
Fax machine	☐	☐	☐	☐
Oral interpreter	☐	☐	☐	☐
Alerting Systems				
Telephone signaler	☐	☐	☐	☐
Doorbell signaler	☐	☐	☐	☐
Door knock signaler	☐	☐	☐	☐
Smoke alarm signaler	☐	☐	☐	☐
Alarm clock signaler/vibrator	☐	☐	☐	☐
Baby cry signaler	☐	☐	☐	☐
Pet cat or pet dog	☐	☐	☐	☐
Trained hearing ear dog	☐	☐	☐	☐
Other (specify):	☐	☐	☐	☐
Comments: _____				

Note: From "Alerting and assistive systems: Counseling implications for cochlear implant users," by L. K. Schum and N. Tye-Murray, 1995. In R. S. Tyler and D. J. Schum (Eds.), *Assistive devices for persons with hearing impairment* (pp. 86–122). Needham Heights, MA: Allyn & Bacon. Adapted by permission.

THE SATISFACTION WITH AMPLIFICATION IN DAILY LIVE (SADL) SCALE

(adapted from Cox & Alexander, 1999, p. 320).

Instructions: Listed below are questions on your opinions about your hearing aids. For each question please circle the letter that is the best answer for you. The list of words below gives the meaning for each letter. Keep in mind that your answers should show your general opinions about the hearing aids that you are wearing now or have most recently worn.

A: Not at all

B: A little

C: Somewhat

D: Medium

E: Considerably

F: Greatly

G: Tremendously

1	Compared to using no hearing aid at all, does your hearing aid(s) help you understand the people you speak with most frequently?	A	B	C	D	E	F	G
2	Are you frustrated when your hearing aid(s) pick up sounds that keep you from hearing what you want to hear?	A	B	C	D	E	F	G
3	Are you convinced that obtaining your hearing aid(s) was in your best interest?	A	B	C	D	E	F	G
4	Do you think people notice your hearing loss more when you wear your hearing aid(s)?	A	B	C	D	E	F	G
5	Does your hearing aid(s) reduce the number of times you have to ask people to repeat?	A	B	C	D	E	F	G
6	Do you think your hearing aid(s) is worth the trouble?	A	B	C	D	E	F	G
7	Are you bothered by an inability to turn your hearing aid(s) up loud enough without getting feedback (whistling)?	A	B	C	D	E	F	G
8	How content are you with the appearance of your hearing aid(s)?	A	B	C	D	E	F	G
9	Does wearing your hearing aid(s) improve your self-confidence?	A	B	C	D	E	F	G
10	How natural is the sound from your hearing aid?	A	B	C	D	E	F	G
11	How helpful is your hearing aid(s) on MOST telephones with NO amplifier or loudspeaker?	A	B	C	D	E	F	G
12	How competent was the person who provided you with your hearing aid(s)?	A	B	C	D	E	F	G
13	Do you think wearing your hearing aid(s) makes you seem less capable?	A	B	C	D	E	F	G
14	Does the cost of your hearing aid(s) seem reasonable to you?	A	B	C	D	E	F	G
15	How pleased are you with the dependability (how often it needs repairs) of your hearing aid(s)?	A	B	C	D	E	F	G

THE INTERNATIONAL OUTCOME INVENTORY FOR HEARING AIDS (IOI-HA)

(adapted from Cox et al., 2000, p. 114S).

1. Think about how much you used your present hearing aid(s) over the past two weeks. On an average day, how many hours did you use the hearing aid(s)?

   ☐ none   ☐ less than 1 hour a day
   ☐ 1 to 4 hours a day   ☐ 4 to 8 hours a day
   ☐ more than 8 hours a day

2. Think about the situation where you most wanted to hear better, before you got your present hearing aid(s). Over the past two weeks, how much has the hearing aid helped in that situation?

   ☐ helped not al all   ☐ helped slightly
   ☐ helped moderately   ☐ helped quite a lot
   ☐ helped very much

3. Think again about the situation where you most wanted to hear better. When you use your present hearing aid(s), how much difficulty to you STILL have in that situation?

   ☐ very much difficulty   ☐ quite a lot of difficulty
   ☐ moderate difficulty   ☐ slight difficulty
   ☐ no difficulty

4. Considering everything, do you think your present hearing aid(s) is worth the trouble?

   ☐ not at all worth it   ☐ slightly worth it
   ☐ moderately worth it   ☐ quite a lot worth it
   ☐ very much worth it

5. Over the past two weeks, with your present hearing aid(s), how much have your hearing difficulties affected the things you can do?

   ☐ affected very much   ☐ affected quite a lot
   ☐ affected moderately   ☐ affected slightly
   ☐ affected not at all

6. Over the past two weeks, with your present hearing aid(s), how much do you think other people were bothered by your hearing difficulties?

      ☐ bothered very much   ☐ bothered quite a lot
      ☐ bothered moderately   ☐ bothered slightly
      ☐ bothered not at all

7. Considering everything, how much has your present hearing aid(s) changed your enjoyment of life?

      ☐ worse   ☐ no change
      ☐ slightly better   ☐ quite a lot better
      ☐ very much better

APPENDIX 12-1

Topics typically covered in a hearing aid orientation session. This list reflects the program offered at Veterans Administration hospitals (adapted from Reese & Hnath-Chisolm, 2005, p. 102).

Landmarks:

- Microphone position and function.
- Right hearing aid has red printing on it, left has blue.
- Manufacturer.
- Serial number is on hearing aids and written down in the information provided.

Batteries:

- Color and size.
- Remove tab before placing battery in hearing aid.
- Battery door won't close if battery is upside down.
- Opening the battery door when hearing aids are not in use helps batteries last longer.
- Brown box should be saved for hearing aid repairs.
- Batteries should last ____ days or longer.
- Batteries requested from the Denver Distribution Center.

Feedback:

- Normally occurs when hand held against the hearing aid.
- If feedback occurs when talking on phone, reposition phone OR use telecoil switch.
- If feedback occurs with jaw movement, hearing aid may not fit well.

Cleaning and care:

- Hearing aids should be cleaned every day.
- Greatest cause of hearing aid problems is ear wax accumulation in receiver tube.
- To clean hearing aids, use dry cloth/tissue or brush.
- Store hearing aids overnight in a dry, safe place.
- If hearing aid gets wet, don't dry it in an oven.
- If hearing aid isn't working, try replacing battery.
- If that doesn't help, call the clinic for an appointment.

During trial period:

- Read over the information provided by the audiologist.
- Pay close attention to what you do/do not like about the hearing aids so that the hearing aids may be adequately adjusted.
- Try to wear the hearing aids most of the day every day; it's OK to take the hearing aids out from time to time during the day or if otherwise instructed by audiologist.

Do expect:

- Listening to be easier.
- To hear better in many situations most of the time.
- Own voice may seem louder.
- May take several months to get used to.

Do not expect:

- Hearing aid to be painful.
- To hear better in noise.
- To hear better in all situations.

APPENDIX 12-2

Topics Covered in a Three-Class Group Follow-Up Program for New Hearing Aid Users (adapted from Northern & Beyer, 1999).

Class 1: Getting to Know Your Hearing Aids (pp. 260–261)
Objectives

1. To demonstrate an understanding of hearing loss and the goals of amplification.

2. To identify realistic expectations of using hearing aids.

3. To identify the limitations of using hearing aids.

4. To understand the importance of binaural amplification.

5. To initiate a comfortable and satisfying hearing aid orientation period.

6. To demonstrate an ability to insert the hearing aids, change batteries, clean the hearing aid, and utilize the telephone effectively.

Class 2: Overcoming Hearing Loss (pp. 261–262)
Objectives

1. To identify the psychological ramifications of hearing loss.

2. To promote the importance of accepting hearing loss as a (usually) permanent yet treatable condition.

3. To introduce positive and assertive coping behaviors that can assist the listener in overcoming communication hardships.

4. To provide tips and strategies for family members of the hearing aid user that will assist in overcoming communication hardships.

5. To identify listening strategies that can improve communication situations.

Class 3: Total Communication (p. 263)
Objectives

1. To identify conditions within a listening environment that can impact communication ability either positively or negatively.

2. To utilize positive and assertive listening strategies to overcome communication barriers.

3. To identify and utilize visual cues that will assist in communication settings.

4. To promote awareness of assistive listening devices and their applications.

5. To provide additional resources on hearing loss and hearing aids.

APPENDIX 12-3

Topics included in a one-session group follow-up session for experienced hearing aid users (adapted from Wayner, 2005, p. 35).

The overall goals are as follows:

- To offer patients who have used hearing instruments in the past and accompanying persons a review about insertion, care, operations, and a gradual schedule of adjustment for new hearing aid use.
- To review and practice the use of the telephone, assistive devices, visual clues, and supplementary listening strategies to facilitate effective communication.
- To review coping strategies.
- To provide troubleshooting methods for maintaining hearing aids.

The specific objectives are as follows:

- Provide description of session including goals and objectives.
- Complete *Hearing Aid Use and Satisfaction Measure* for experienced hearing aid user.
- Determine each participant's past experience with amplification to include: type/style, how long worn, how much worn, how amplification has helped, problems experienced, and special questions and concerns.
- Review hearing aid care, wearing schedule, maintenance, and troubleshooting.
- Provide overview of assistive listening devices and systems.
- Review communication strategies to include: listening strategies, visual strategies, and contextual and situational clues.
- Discuss factors that can control the communication environment to include: background noise, lighting, distance, preferential seating, restaurant/meeting place exercise, and implications for home.
- Telephone tips and practice.
- Distribute information about: equipment available for hearing aid maintenance, battery order form, Hearing Loss Association of America, warranty information, and insurance information.

APPENDIX 12-4

Self-Help and Professional Organizations That Serve Adults Who Have Hearing Loss in the United States and in the British Commonwealth and Other Related Web Sites

Alexander Graham Bell Association for the Deaf
www.agbell.org

American Athletic Association of the Deaf
www.usadsf.org

American Deafness and Rehabilitation Association
www.adara.org

American Hearing Research Foundation
www.american-hearing.org

American Tinnitus Association
www.ata.org

Americans with Disabilities Act (ADA) Home page
www.ada.gov

Association of Late Deafened Adults (ALDA)
www.alda.org

Australian Hearing
www.hearing.com.au

Better Hearing Australia
www.betterhearing.org.au

Better Hearing Institute
www,betterhearing.org

British Deaf Association
www.britishdeafassociation.org.uk

Canadian Association of the Deaf (CAD)
www.cad.ca

Canadian Hard of Hearing Association (CHHA)
www.chha.ca

Deaf Association of New Zealand
www.deaf.co.nz

The Ear Foundation (Australia)
www.earfoundation.org

Hearing Loss Association of America (Formerly Self-Help for Hard of Hearing People, SHHH)
www.shhh.org

Hearing Association Inc. of New Zealand
www.hearing.org.nz

Hearing Concern (United Kingdom)
www.hearingconcern.org.uk

National Association of the Deaf (NAD)
www.nad.org

National Captioning Institute (NCI)
www.ncicap.org

National Center on Employment of the Deaf National Technical Institute for the Deaf
www.ntid.rit.edu

National Foundation for the Deaf (New Zealand)
www.orl.org.nz

National Institute on Deafness and Other Communication Disorders
www.nidcd.nih.gov

APPENDIX 12-5

Example of a short-term communication strategies program (adapted from Abrahamson, 2000, p. 230).

Content area may include the following topics:

Environmental management

Factors influencing speech comprehension: environment, speaker, listener

Communication rules

Assistive devices

Coping strategies

Additional topics that may be included, especially if the program lasts more than one session: principles of behavior, stress management, including relaxation training and assertiveness training, and advocacy.

CHAPTER 13

Aural Rehabilitation Plans for Older Adults

OUTLINE

- Activity limitations and participation restrictions
- Audiological status and otologic health
- Life-situation factors
- Physical and cognitive variables
- Aural rehabilitation intervention
- Aural rehabilitation in the institutional setting
- Case study: Staying active
- Final remarks
- Key chapter points
- Terms and concepts to remember
- Multiple-choice questions
- Key Resources
- Appendix 13-1

This chapter is devoted to older adults, individuals who are 60 years of age and older. However, this age is an arbitrary benchmark, and people, agencies, and other concerns vary in how they define the term *older*. Theaters, shops, and national parks often confer the status of "senior citizen" to any individual over the age of 55 years. On the other hand, Congress has extended the mandatory age for retirement from 65 to 70 years. One reason for these ambiguous definitions relates to the heterogeneity of the population. One 65-year-old woman may be vibrant and healthy and be a "youthful old," whereas another woman who is 60 years old may be sedentary and afflicted with illness.

Most speech and hearing professionals will at some point in their careers likely work with older people (Figure 13-1). The elderly represent

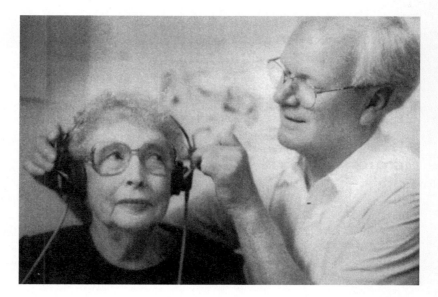

FIGURE 13-1. The expanding population of older persons. As the number of elderly persons in the U.S. population continues to increase, it is likely that they will comprise a significant segment of many speech and hearing professionals' case loads in the near future. *Photograph by Marcus Kosa, courtesy of the Central Institute for the Deaf.*

the fastest-growing segment in American society. More than 35.9 million people in the United States are over the age of 65 years, about 12% of the population. Within this population group, about 18 million persons are between the ages of 65 and 74 years, about 13 million are between 75 and 84 years, and about 5 million are 85 years or older. By 2030, the number of Americans over the age of 64 years will have ballooned to 72 million, or about 20% of Americans (He, Sengupta, Velkoff, & Debarros, 2006). Figure 13-2 shows the growth in this segment of the population in the

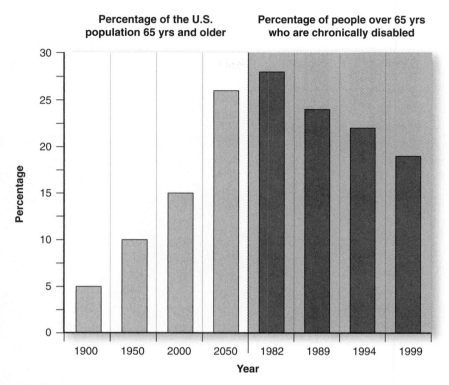

FIGURE 13-2. Better health. Not only is the older popluation growing, but elderly persons are becoming healthier. *Modeled after Lyman (2006).*

United States and its projected size in 2050. Figure 13-3 shows the projected growth rates by state for the years 2000–2030. The greatest growth will occur in the Sun Belt metropolitan areas, including cities such as Atlanta, Austin, and Las Vegas. Currently Florida has the greatest proportion of older residents of any state, but states like Pennsylvania and West Virginia also have a large proportion. As of 2000, nine states had more than 1 million people over the age of 65 years: California, Florida, New York, Texas, Pennsylvania, Ohio, Illinois, Michigan, and New Jersey (He et al., 2006).

Figure 13-2 also indicates that older individuals are healthier. In 1982, 25% of individuals over the age of 65 years had a chronic disability. In 1999, this proportion had dropped to less than 20% (Lyman, 2006). In addition to being healthier, today's older generation is more prosperous and better educated. In 1959, 35% of persons over the age of 65 years lived in poverty whereas in 2003, only 10% lived below the poverty line. In 1950, 17% of older persons had a high school diploma whereas in 2003, 72% held a diploma.

"Those first [baby] boomers were a year old when Howdy Doody first dangled on a TV screen the size of a dinner plate, 17 when John F. Kennedy was assassinated, 23 when they converged on Woodstock and 36 for the start of the great bull market of the 1980s."

Jerry Adler, reporter for *Newsweek.*

(Adler, 2005, p. 52).

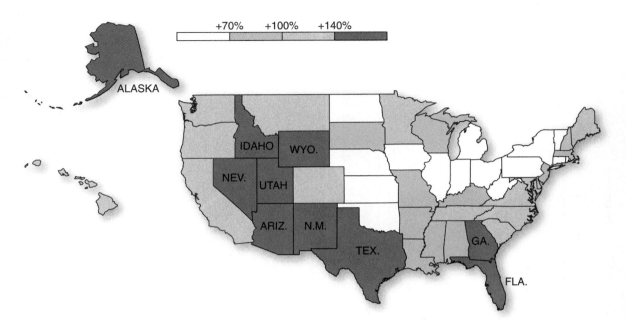

FIGURE 13-3. Projected growth of the U.S. population age 65 years and older for the years 2000–2030. *Modeled after Roberts (2007).*

"They [older persons] want the action, they don't want to be on the sidelines."

Ken Dychtwald, president of Age Wave

(Alder, 2005, p. 54)

Baby boomers are the generation born between the years 1946 and 1965.

The implication of these statistics for aural rehabilitation is that older persons will comprise the case loads of many speech and hearing professionals. These patients are relatively healthy, they are educated, and they have financial resources. Many will expect that hearing loss will not prevent them from living active and productive lives.

The older population is comprised of at least two groups, the more traditional seniors and the **baby boomers**. The estimated 78 million baby boomers include the generation born after World War II, between the years 1946 and 1965 (2005 U.S. Census Report). Many either have recently turned 60 years old or will turn 60 years in the near future. Researchers have suggested that traditional seniors and baby boomers differ in both their values and purchasing habits (Bloom, 1999; McGuire, 2002). Traditional seniors, sometimes known as the "Just Good Enough" generation, have experienced the deprivations of the Depression and World War II. They tend to save their money, and many dislike carrying debt. Traditional seniors value trust, service, and quality. Some are more resistant to technology, are price oriented, and have a tendency to follow medical advice (McGuire, 2002). By comparison, many baby boomers value active, youthful lifestyles. Convenience and cosmetics are likely to supersede price when they consider whether to use a hearing aid and whether to seek other aural rehabilitation services. Many are technologically savvy and many want control of their own decisions and health care (Goodale, 2003; McGuire, 2002; Threats, 2005). The traditional senior and the baby boomer may share many of the same listening difficulties, but they may pose different challenges in the design and implementation of an aural rehabilitation plan.

Figure 13-4 presents a design for providing aural rehabilitation to older persons. The model includes an evaluation and an intervention stage

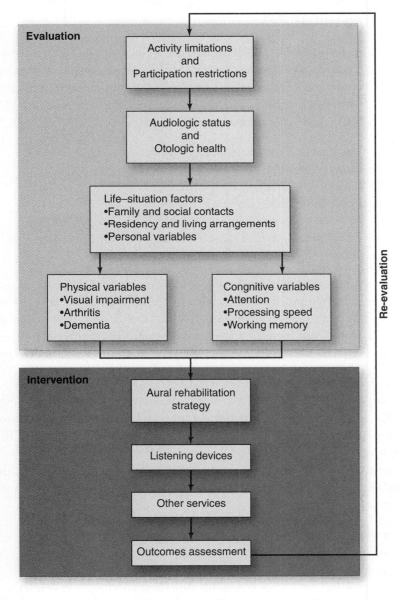

FIGURE 13-4. A model for providing aural rehabilitation services to older patients.

(see also Kiessling et al., 2003). Provision of reevaluation is also included, in recognition that as patients continue to age, their circumstances may alter and new interventions might become necessary. In the following sections, we will consider the separate components of the evaluation stage and the findings that might be obtained at each stage. We will then consider the intervention stage, including listening devices and other services.

ACTIVITY LIMITATIONS AND PARTICIPATION RESTRICTIONS

One of the first stages of evaluation is to determine a patient's activity limitations and participation restrictions. This evaluation will include collecting a case history and performing a structured inquiry, such as a checklist or inventory. As with younger adults, patients may be asked such questions as "Why are you here?" And "Tell me about . . ." (Kiessling et al., 2003, p. S297):

- The problems you are having with your hearing.
- The effects of hearing problems on your life.
- The kinds of activities you are involved in.
- The problems you have in these activities.
- The activities you would like to do that you have stopped doing.
- The activities that you find more difficult to do now than in the past.
- The new activities that you would like to undertake.

The responses to these questions will indicate a patient's listening goals and the priority that the patient places on each one. Some patients will identify a limited range of listening environments that are problematic whereas others will identify a large number and specify many priorities. Patients will also vary in their expectations of and in their attitudes toward aural rehabilitation (Gatehouse, 2003).

A case history will provide information about a patient's living arrangements, social interactions, vocational status, and hobbies. The case history also may include a conversation with a family member or caregiver, during which time the speech and hearing professional might ask about the patient's memory, emotional state, motivation to participate in an aural rehabilitation program, and the feasibility of doing so. It is important also to gather medical data about the following topics (Groher, 1989):

- Strokes, memory loss, vision problems, dizziness, and medications taken, because they may have an effect on the patient's ability to participate in testing and subsequent aural rehabilitation
- Arthritis and muscle weakness, because these conditions may interact with a patient's ability to handle a listening device

- Ambulation, behavioral changes, and other pertinent conditions, because they may affect the kinds of communication activities in which the patient may engage
- Dementia and Alzheimer's disease, because patients may require assistance from caregivers or family members to use hearing aids

During the case history, it is wise to be alert for symptoms of dementia. For example, if someone cannot remember his or her birth date or seems confused by simple tasks, such as completing a questionnaire, the audiologist may want to alter the test procedures. Otherwise, performance may not reflect true hearing ability.

Conversational fluency might be assessed informally. The speech and hearing professional might engage in conversation and note the frequency of communication breakdowns and the ways in which the patient attempts to repair them. Family members might be questioned about how well the individual can engage in conversation.

AUDIOLOGICAL STATUS AND OTOLOGIC HEALTH

In the evaluation stage, an older patient will likely undergo audiological testing that includes an audiogram and speech testing in both quiet and noise. Sometimes the evaluation will include measures of auditory processing, such as duration discrimination, **temporal-order discrimination**, and **dichotic-syllable identification** (e.g., Humes, 2005).

Other areas of evaluation may include otologic health, such as presence of cerumen and measures of middle ear pressure, and tinnitus. Age-related changes in the outer ear may include increased production of cerumen. Older adults have a greater likelihood of impacted cerumen and collapsed ear canals than younger adults, either of which might result in artificial air-bone gaps during audiological testing (see Chisolm, Willott, & Lister, 2003, for a review). Incidence of tinnitus in the older population has been estimated to be between about 25% and 30% (Nondahl et al., 2007; Sindhusake et al., 2003). There appears to be a clear association between the presence of tinnitus and reported quality of life in older persons (Nondahl et al., 2007).

Audiological Testing

Traditional audiological testing procedures may need to be adapted for the elderly. An audiologist will want to have ample time for patient instructions and may need to double-check to ensure that instructions are understood. If a patient is in the early stages of Alzheimer's disease, reinstruction may be necessary if the patient takes a short break because the person may have

---

Busy boomers are:
- Living active lifestyles
- Working longer
- Retiring later
- Interested in their health
- Willing to buy health products

(Engel, 2007)

Temporal-order discrimination requires a patient to attend to the order in which auditory stimuli are presented. For example, the patient may hear a series of three 2-element (or 4-element) tone bursts, with either burst having a different frequency. Two elements of the 3-element series will be identical, whereas one will have a reversed (or different) order of the bursts. The patient's task is to indicate which one is "different."

A **dichotic-syllable identification task** entails presenting two consonant-vowel syllables to a patient, one to each ear. The patient must identify the two syllables, sometimes from a closed set of alternatives.

forgotten the task. For someone in the later stages of dementia, testing may not be possible.

Other accommodations for the older patient that may be necessary include the following:

- During air or bone conduction testing, tone stimuli may need to be presented for a longer duration of time than for younger persons. Some older persons have difficulty in grasping the concept of listening for a soft, brief tone.
- Stimuli for speech recognition testing may need to be presented live voice rather than recorded voice, outside of the test booth, so that the patient and clinician can sit face-to-face (Hull, 1995). Some older persons are disconcerted by listening to a disembodied, impersonal voice over headphones.
- Time for rest periods may need to be allocated, or testing spread over more than one day, as some individuals may suffer from fatigue.
- Before testing begins, a visual examination should be made to ensure that there is not impacted cerumen in the outer ear. In some older persons, cerumen removal may be necessary.
- The use of insert earphones may be required to ensure that a correct audiogram is obtained. Softening of the cartilaginous tissue of the ear canal and pinna occurs with aging.

Presbycusis

Hearing loss is the third most common chronic condition afflicting the non-institutionalized elderly (Hazard, Andrews, Bierman, & Blass, 1990). Although estimates vary, about 30% of individuals over the age of 65 years who dwell in the community have some degree of hearing impairment. Fifty percent of those between the ages of 75 and 79 years have some degree of hearing loss (Willott, 1991). Up to 90% of seniors living in institutions have hearing loss (Hull & Griffin, 1992). Similarly, incidence of hearing loss is also high in the European elderly. For instance, 2.5 million people in the United Kingdom over the age of 70 years have enough hearing loss to benefit from using a hearing aid (although only one third of them own one, and 10% of these persons do not use them) (see Hanratty & Lawlor, 2000, for a review).

Presbycusis is a generic term used to refer to age-related hearing loss.

Presbycusis is the global term used to refer to hearing loss associated with the aging process. It does not refer to a single pathology but is typically diagnosed when an older person presents a high-frequency hearing loss. Physiologically, two major causes of age-related hearing loss are (a) neural, meaning a loss of sensory cells and supporting cells, nerve fibers, and neural tissue and (b) metabolic or strial, meaning a change in the blood supply to the cochlea. Neurologically, hair cells may die and/or the cell bodies of the auditory nerve that comprise the **spiral ganglion** may degenerate. Metabolically, the membranes of the cochlear tissues may begin to thicken, causing occlusion of the capillaries and a loss of blood supply. In addition to neural and metabolic causes, some evidence suggests that the central auditory system may also undergo age-related histopathology. For instance, the volume of the **cochlear nucleus** may shrink as the myelin surrounding the neural axons begins to thin (see Boettcher, 2002, for a review). A lifetime of noise exposure in both recreational and occupational settings, disease, and exposure to ototoxic agents can be contributing factors in some individuals. To date, no medical treatments exist to reverse age-related hearing loss, other than cochlear implants.

The **spiral ganglion** is comprised of the nuclei of the nerve fibers that connect to the hair cells and meet in the central core (which is called the modiolus) of the cochlea.

The **cochlear nucleus** is a cluster of cell bodies in the brain stem where the nerve fibers leading from the cochlea enter and synapse.

Audiological Findings Characteristic of Presbycusis

Figure 13-5 presents median thresholds for females and males for each half-decade of life between the ages of 60 and 84 years (Mills, Schmiedt, & Dubno, 2006). As can be seen, hearing loss increases with age and men experience a greater decline than do women. By the eighth decade, the display presents a falling slope, with the greatest loss occurring in the high frequencies. The decline in hearing thresholds accelerates over time, with the rate becoming more pronounced after individuals enter into their 70s.

A decline in speech recognition typically accompanies presbycusis. Beyond the age of 60 years, monosyllabic word recognition scores decline by 13% per decade in men and 6% per decade in women (Cheesman, 1997). Speech recognition difficulties are exacerbated when an older person attempts to listen in a noisy environment, more so than is the case for younger listeners (Pederson, Rosenthal, & Moller, 1991; Plath, 1991). As noted in Chapter 5, older persons also experience an age-related decline in their vision-only speech recognition skills (refer back to Figure 5-1).

"Age-related loss is generally gradual, starting at the higher frequencies. We might not notice it when we're in a quiet environment and looking at the speaker, but add a lot of background noise and dim lighting, and we lose the thread of conversation."

Jill Diesman, an audiologist with Hear USA

(Blackwood, 2005)

Auditory Processing

In addition to or in conjunction with sensorineural hearing loss and decreased word recognition, some older individuals may experience changes in their auditory processing abilities. These changes are indexed by performance on psychophysical tests and on tests of altered speech or demanding listening tasks. Two test batteries of auditory processing that are sometimes used with older adults are the *Test of Basic Auditory Capabilities* (*TBAC;* Chirstopherson & Humes, 1992) and the *Tonal and Speech Materials for Auditory Perceptual Assessment* (Humes, Coughlin, & Talley, 1996; Noffsinger, Wilson, & Musiek, 1994). The tasks in the TBAC require a patient to listen to a "standard" stimulus and then select which of two subsequent stimuli differs from the standard. An example of a task from the latter test battery is one that requires patients to recognize NU-6 monosyllabic words that have been time-compressed by 45%.

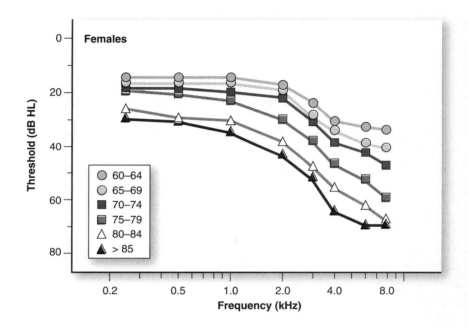

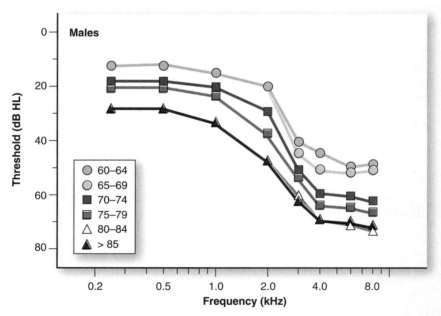

FIGURE 13-5. Average audiograms for groups of females (*n* = 1,358) and males (*n* = 935) at half-decade intervals between the ages of 60 and 84 years. *Modeled after Mills, Schmiedt, and Dubno (2006, p. 16).*

Some older persons have a reduced ability to discriminate two sounds that differ in pitch, intensity, or duration (Schneider, 1997), and these have been taken as indications of decreased auditory processing ability. For example, if an audiologist presents a 60-dB HL tone and a 65-dB HL tone to an older listener, the patient may say they are the same instead of different, whereas a younger person may clearly perceive them as different. Some persons have difficulty understanding time-compressed or frequency-filtered speech (Gordon-Salant & Fitzgibbons, 1999). Moreover, when a competing signal is presented to one ear, and the target speech signal to the other, as in a dichotic listening task, many elderly adults experience greater difficulty in understanding the target signal than do younger listeners (e.g., Roup, Wiley, & Wilson, 2006). Similarly, they will experience greater difficulty listening in environments that have severe reverberation and, as noted, background noise (Gordon-Salant & Fitzgibbons, 1999).

Much research has been conducted to determine the extent to which speech recognition difficulties result from peripheral cochlear pathology and the extent to which they result from changes in the central nervous system in general and/or to changes in modality-specific-age-related declines in the processing of auditory information (see Humes, 2005; Kricos, 2006, for reviews). This is a complex issue and has inspired varying opinions. The prevailing view is that hearing sensitivity for the higher frequencies in particular relates most strongly to speech recognition performance, at least in quiet listening conditions. For example, Humes (1996) concluded that an older person's average hearing loss at the frequencies 1,000, 2,000, and 4,000 Hz was the single best predictor of a variety of different speech recognition tests. However, other investigators have shown age-related differences in speech recognition performance, even after accounting for the presence of hearing loss (see Pichora-Fuller & Souza, 2003, and Pichora-Fuller & Singh, 2006, for overviews). What we do know is that the aging brain demonstrates a number of changes, which may have an impact on speech recognition performance, and they include the following (Willott, 1996):

- A loss of neurons
- A reduction in the number of synaptic connections between neurons
- Changes in the excitatory and inhibitory neurotransmitter systems
- Changes in neural transmission along the auditory pathway
- Possibly, changes in cognitive processing of the acoustic signal (e.g., information processing, labeling, retrieval, and storage)
- A decrement in long-term and short-term memory

These global changes in brain functioning might have some effect on an older individual's ability to process rapid streams of speech information. They also may affect how well the individual comprehends the gist of a message.

What Older Persons Have to Say About Hearing Loss

Sometimes an older person may make a comment that is consonant with hearing loss. Here are some remarks often made by older patients (Pichora-Fuller, 1997, p. 125):

- I hear, but I have trouble understanding.
- Sounds seem all jumbled up.
- It is difficult to tell where sounds are coming from.
- I understand when it is quiet, but I have trouble when it is noisy.
- I understand when I'm talking to one person, but I have trouble in a group.
- In a group, if I know who is talking then I can follow the conversation, but I have trouble when someone else starts talking.
- When someone else starts talking sometimes I have to look around to see who it is.
- If I know the topic of conversation then I do pretty well, but I often get lost when the topic changes.
- People seem to talk too fast; I need more time to make sense of what has been said.
- It is not so much that I can't understand what is said but that it is tiring to listen.
- I sometimes pretend to understand because it isn't worth it to ask the talker to repeat because I'm afraid that it would be an imposition and it could annoy or make the talker impatient.
- I don't know for sure when I hear correctly and when I don't.
- It's hard to get jokes; you have to get the punch line right away or it isn't funny.
- When I'm with two or more people, they start talking to each other and leave me out.
- I don't enjoy social events any more.

LIFE-SITUATION FACTORS

The next stage in the model presented in Figure 13-4 is the evaluation of life situation factors. These factors include family and social contacts, residency and living arrangements, and personal factors such as emotional health, mental health, temperament, sense of self-sufficiency and independence, and self-concept.

Family and Social Contacts

The number of people a patient interacts with and the frequency of interaction influence the person's morbidity, mortality, and physical functioning (Strawbridge, Cohen, Shema, & Kaplan, 1996). Older people who have five or more contacts are less likely to suffer from loneliness and depression and are more likely to have a higher quality of life than persons who have fewer social contacts. For example, a person who lives within a 30-mile radius of children and grandchildren and who works as a volunteer at the local zoo is more likely to have good mental health and be more interested in participating in an aural rehabilitation program than someone who has no family nearby and few interests outside of the home (Figure 13-6). Married people have lower mortality rates (He et al., 2005) and it is likely that marriage expands the social network of extended family members and friends who can provide social contact and support (House, Landis, & Umberson, 1988). As of 2003, about 40% of women 65 years or older lived alone whereas about 19% of men lived alone (U.S. Census Bureau, 2003).

The extent to which an older individual maintains frequent and significant contacts with family, friends, and community acquaintances can ameliorate or exacerbate the impact of hearing loss. Social contacts allow an individual to feel more a part of life and more involved in the community and provide motivation to address a hearing loss. Individuals who do not have communication partners available often do not seek aural rehabilitation services (Figure 13-7).

Just as social relationships influence the impact of hearing loss, hearing loss can affect social relationships. It is not uncommon for a hearing loss to trigger a negative feedback loop like that illustrated in Figure 13-8. Lindblade and McDonald (1995) suggested that older persons may withdraw from social interactions because conversation becomes too effortful. In turn, family and friends may begin to perceive them as unsociable, preoccupied with health matters, forgetful, or paranoid (Figure 13-9). These perceptions may lead to an older individual mistakenly being labeled as demented, confused, hostile, or senile. A son might find that his father frequently responds inappropriately to questions and suspect that he is experiencing cognitive decline. It may only be that the father has hearing loss, or has both hearing loss and mild confusion. As an older person withdraws, and appears to be less cooperative or less effective as a conversational partner, family and friends may begin to drift away and decrease contact. The older person may increasingly experience anger, frustration, apathy, and anxiety (Rousey, 1976). This situation may lead to more withdrawal and more negative reactions from communication partners.

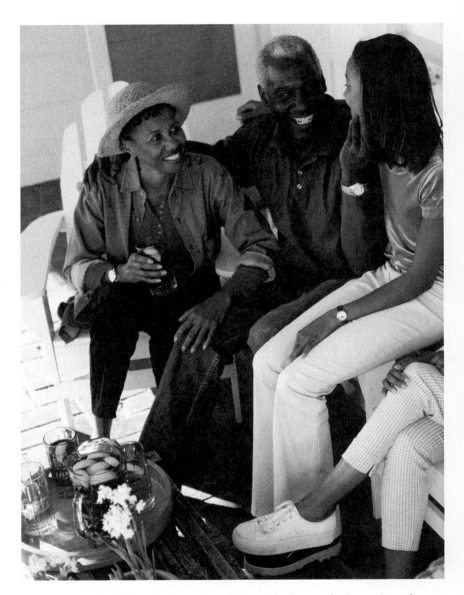

FIGURE 13-6. Proximity to family members. Persons who live near family members often are motivated to improve their communication effectiveness. *Copyright Photodisc/Getty Images.*

To the extent possible, when professionals working with an older individual recognize the potential exists for this circular chain of events, they might craft an aural rehabilitation plan that mitigates against undesirable outcomes. For example, it may be possible to encourage the patient to join small social activity groups that are not too demanding on his or her communication skills. If the patient enjoys playing cards or reading books, then the individual might be encouraged to join a bridge group or a book club. Provision of counseling for family and friends about the ramifications of hearing loss in general

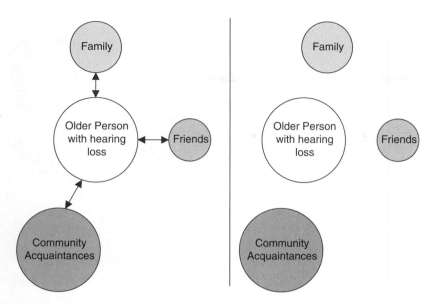

FIGURE 13-7. Social contacts. The number of social contacts and the frequency of contact can affect an older person's desire for aural rehabilitation.

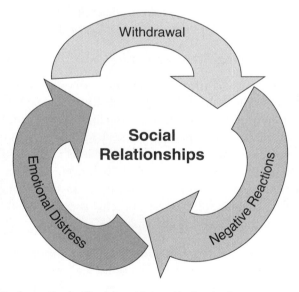

FIGURE 13-8. A negative feedback loop triggered by hearing loss.

and characteristics of the patient's particular loss may prevent the occurrence of the negative feedback loop depicted in Figure 13-8. Family, friends, and caretakers can learn how to counteract an older person's tendency to withdraw and avoid conversational interactions and encourage the individual to obtain aural rehabilitation services. In addition, they can actively participate in the aural rehabilitation program. They can learn how to use communication

"Yes, of course you feel stupid if you don't follow the way you used to. It can mean that you don't understand and you can't join in the discussion. Then you feel out of things. . . . You haven't really understood in some way and you might bring it up again later. Then they might say, 'Yeah, yeah, we've already talked about that.' Then I feel oh [groans] I'm so stupid! I should have kept my mouth shut."

An older patient speaking in an open-ended interview

(Espmark & Scherman, 2003, p. 109)

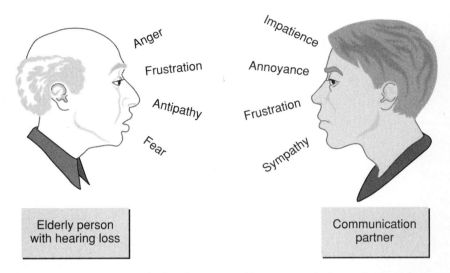

FIGURE 13-9. Miscommunications between an older person and a frequent communication partner. Miscommunications as a result of hearing loss sometimes result in an older person withdrawing from social interactions.

A **nursing home** is a residential, institutionalized facility that has three or more beds and provides nursing care.

strategies effectively or learn how to help the older person handle a hearing aid or assistive listening device, or to handle the device for the person if necessary.

Residency and Living Arrangements

Most older persons live in private residencies, with only about 5% residing in nursing homes (Nussbaum, Thompson, & Robinson, 1989). A **nursing home** is commonly defined as an institutionalized facility that has three or more beds and that provides nursing care. The majority of nursing home residents are women, and they may have previously resided in a private home, a hospital, or another nursing home before entering into their current residency (Gabrel, 2000). The majority of nursing home residents have hearing loss, and half of these have severe losses (Schow & Nerbonne, 1980; Voeks, Gallagher, Langer, & Drinka, 1990).

The residential-care population requires special attention, as patients are likely to have a multitude of health conditions, and their environments are likely to be noisier than private home environments (Figure 13-10). Noisy environments can magnify hearing-related communication difficulties, and may result in activity limitations and participation restrictions.

Most older persons desire to remain as independent as possible for as long as possible. One way to determine the level of supportive assistance required is to ask a patient to complete the *Activities of Daily Living* (*ADLs;* Katz, 1983) and *Instrumental Activities of Daily Living* (*IADLs;* 1969). For example, questions on the IADL include:

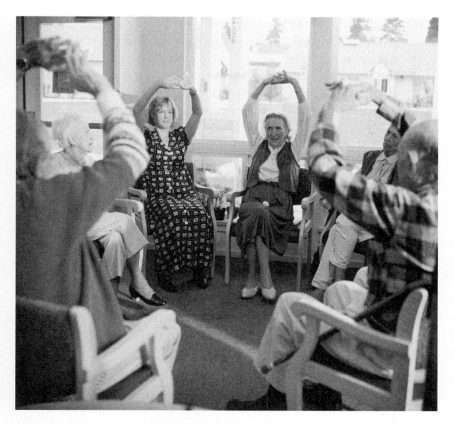

FIGURE 13-10. A patient's residency and the impact on an aural rehabilitation plan. A person in a health care facility or nursing home may have a particular need for assistive listening devices. In addition, health care workers may need special instruction.

- Can you use the telephone?
- Can you get to places that are out of walking distance?
- Can you prepare your own meals?

Response options are *Without help*, *With some help*, and *Completely unable to [do so]*."

Personal Variables

Many personal variables have the potential to influence the development of an aural rehabilitation intervention plan, and we considered several of these in Chapter 12 when we considered aural rehabilitation for adults under the age of 60 years. These variables include socioeconomic status, gender, and ethnicity and culture. For older patients, it will sometimes be appropriate to take stock of other personal variables in addition to those already reviewed.

It is not unusual for older people who have hearing loss to experience depression, isolation, anger, insecurity, and loneliness. Sometimes individuals feel shame, either from a sense of inadequacy or from a sense of being a burden on family, friends, and coworkers. They may be embarrassed that they must ask for message clarifications and that their ears may not be "what they used to be." Some may hesitate to ask their communication partners to exert the extra effort needed to communicate with them. Some older persons feel an overwhelming sense of wanting to "save face" and "save pride" and to hide from people that they need help in facilitating communication. These kinds of emotions and mindsets may lead older adults to undergo lifestyle changes and to experience a diminished quality of life.

Not only will the emotional state of an individual be influenced by the onset of hearing loss, but in turn, how the individual reacts to hearing loss will be influenced by the individual's psycho-emotional profile. A profile of a person's emotional state can be constructed by considering the following variables:

- Mental health
- Temperament
- Sense of self-sufficiency and independence
- Self-concept

Mental Health

A person is said to have a **mental health problem** if he or she has psychopathology or clusters of other acute or chronic symptoms. As with any age group, older individuals vary widely in their mental health. However, it is not uncommon for an older person to suffer from depression. The National Mental Health Association (2003) reports that about 15% of older community-dwelling adults and up to 25% of those who live in nursing homes and residential care experience depressive symptoms. The following situations may trigger depression (Kraaij, Arensman, & Spinhoven, 2002):

- Loss of or separation from friends and loved ones
- Change of residence
- Decreased ability to perform physical activities
- Retirement
- Empty-nest syndrome
- A decline in general health

A hearing loss can magnify feelings of hopelessness, loneliness, and help-lessness, and depression may decrease desire to seek hearing health care. Other mental conditions, such as anxiety, **obsessive-compulsiveness**, and **neuroticism**, also may increase the communication difficulties associated with a particular degree of hearing loss.

A **mental health problem** is defined as psychopathology or clusters of other acute or chronic symptoms; a psychological or physiological pattern that is not expected as a part of normal functioning, behavior, or culture.

Obsessive-compulsiveness is an anxiety disorder in which an afflicted person experiences unwanted and persistent thoughts. The person may seek to relieve anxiety by performing ritualized, seemingly purposeless acts, such as hand washing or checking.

Neuroticism is an enduring propensity to experience negative emotional states such as anxiety, anger, shyness, guilt, and/or self-consciousness.

One screening tool for depression often used with older patients is the *Geriatric Depression Scale* (Sheikh & Hesavage, 1986). The scale has 15 yes–no questions, including questions such as:

- Are you basically satisfied with your life?
- Do you feel that your life is empty?
- Do you often feel helpless?
- Do you prefer to stay at home, rather than going out and doing new things?

Responses on five or more questions that are consistent with depression may be reason for referral to a mental health expert.

Temperament

Some people are, by temperament, more or less able to cope with hearing loss. **Temperament** refers to stable personality traits. Such traits as introversion versus extroversion, assertiveness versus passiveness, and optimism versus pessimism will relate to the impact of hearing loss (e.g., Knutson & Lansing, 1990). For instance, an older person might routinely be frustrated by minor irritations, such as getting stuck in traffic, breaking a pencil lead, or forgetting to set an alarm clock. This person may be more affected by hearing loss than someone who has a more easygoing temperament. He or she may be intolerant of talkers who are difficult to understand and may overreact when a remark is missed or not recognized.

Temperament refers to stable personality traits.

Sense of Self-Sufficiency and Independence

Self-sufficiency and independence relate to whether an individual can conduct day-to-day activities without undue reliance on others. There appears to be a relationship between perceived control and adherence to an aural rehabilitation plan (Garstecki & Erler, 1998). In particular, older women who feel a sense of internal control over what happens in their lives tend to experience a greater sense of control over their hearing loss than do women who do not experience this feeling.

Self-sufficiency and independence relate to whether a person can conduct day-to-day activities without undue reliance on others.

Many older people feel increasingly dependent on others for daily activities. Some can no longer drive, some cannot do their own shopping, and some must have intermediaries accompany them to medical appointments. Hearing loss can be yet another signal of increased dependence, because an older person with hearing loss may have to rely on others to manage communication difficulties. One man complained, "My wife has to make all my telephone calls for me, and I hate it. It makes me feel like I'm 3 instead of 83!" One goal of the aural rehabilitation plan is to increase the older patient's sense of self-sufficiency and independence.

Self-Concept

As noted in Chapter 10, self-concept relates to how people view themselves; for example, does someone think of him or herself as having a hearing impairment? Does the person think that he or she is capable of coping with a disability? Often one's self-concept does not match other persons' perceptions, or an audiological report. One patient commented to her audiologist, "I don't feel old, and I certainly don't think of myself as a senior citizen. But the way people treat me reminds me I'm not young anymore. Someone will take my arm to help me up the stairs, or I go to buy a movie ticket, and they give me the senior citizen rate without even asking me if I'm eligible. It's weird." This woman was dismayed when her audiologist proceeded to describe the results of her hearing tests, and she learned she had a bilateral moderate hearing loss.

Persons' self-concepts interact with hearing loss. Some may experience difficulty in accepting aging altogether, and may refuse to wear a hearing aid. Conversely, another may accept hearing loss and will willingly engage in aural rehabilitation.

PHYSICAL AND COGNITIVE VARIABLES

Other health care professionals, such as a physician or psychologist, will be primarily responsible for assessing a patient's physical and cognitive status. Some of the possible conditions that they might identify may affect the aural rehabilitation plan and both the evaluation and intervention stages. Occasionally, a speech and hearing professional will administer a screening instrument, say for dementia. The results of a screening instrument might indicate that a patient should be referred to another specialist for further testing.

Physical Variables

Physical variables may influence the impact of hearing loss. Several physical changes occur as people age. Their skin wrinkles, age spots appear, hair may turn gray, joints stiffen, and muscles become weaker. Manual dexterity begins to decrease. The rate at which these changes occur varies among individuals, and some people are physically fit well into their 80s and even 90s. Physical fitness interacts with hearing loss to the extent that it may determine the kinds of communication interactions in which the individual engages (e.g., Does the person attend parties? Still work?) and the kinds of listening devices that can be used (e.g., Is manual dexterity a problem if the patient desires an in-the-canal hearing aid?).

In addition to changes in physical fitness, many older persons experience chronic ailments, and these may influence the impact of hearing loss. The most common chronic ailments include (in order of frequency of occurrence; National Center for Health Statistics, 1987):

- Arthritis
- Cardiac disease
- Hearing loss
- Hypertension
- Orthopedic problems
- Cataracts

Three common physical conditions are especially relevant when considering the impact of hearing loss for an older person: reduced vision, arthritis, and dementia.

Visual Impairment

The eyes undergo a number of physical changes with aging. The lens of the eye grows increasingly opaque, becoming more yellow, less elastic, and denser. The pupils shrink and admit less light. The muscles that control the eyes weaken. The number of optic nerve cells declines. As a result of these physical changes, the eyes are less able to shift focus from objects that are near to objects that are far. Vision may be reduced. Less light is able to pass through the lens, so paradoxically, older persons may require more illumination than younger persons for tasks such as reading, yet they may be more sensitive to glare. Some older adults experience a loss of contrast sensitivity, or an inability to discriminate dark from light (Marmor, 1998).

Even a slight or moderate vision impairment can create problems in everyday situations, interfering with the ability to read, to drive, or to watch television, and can restrict a patient's ability to live independently. Studies have suggested that anywhere between less than 5% and about 30% of individuals over the age of 70 years have impaired vision (Bergman & Rosenhall, 2001; Vinding, 1989), and that the prevalence of vision impairment increases as a function of age. **Visual impairment** is defined as a vision loss that cannot be corrected through the use of eyeglasses or contact lenses alone. Most persons over the age of 70 years use prescription lenses (Wun, Lam, & Shum, 1997). Of these, 18% must use a magnifying glass for reading and close work (Desai, Pratt, Lentzner, & K. Robinson, 2001). About 50% of persons over the age of 82 years have visual impairment and 78% over the age of 88 years (Bergman & Rosenhall, 2001). The frequency of blindness rises with age and peaks at 85 years of age

Visual impairment is a vision loss that cannot be compensated for through corrective lenses.

and older. The prevalence of blindness in both eyes is about 1% for individuals 74 years old and almost 3% for individuals 85 years and older (Centers for Disease Control and Prevention, 2001).

Many individuals who have severe visual impairments also have significant hearing loss (Bergman & Rosenhall, 2001; Kirchner & Peterson, 1980). It is a sad twist of fate that, in the face of hearing loss, when someone could utilize the visual signal probably more so than at any other time in life for the purpose of speech recognition, this sense also begins to decline. Visual difficulties may relate to **cataracts**, **glaucoma**, **diabetic retinopathy**, or **macular degeneration**, as well as other conditions (Nusbaum, 1999).

A **cataract** is a progressive retinal disorder that includes a clouding of the lens, causes blurred vision, and impairs contrast sensitivity. Lens-replacement surgery is available as a treatment.

Glaucoma is caused by high fluid pressure within the eye that may damage the optic nerve and result in reduced vision, especially in the peripheral visual field. Medication can often control the condition.

Diabetic retinopathy results from long-standing diabetes, causing blurred and distorted vision in the central visual field or patchy vision, and sometimes a detached retina. Management of the diabetic condition and laser surgery can limit damage to the eye.

Macular degeneration is a deterioration of sensory cells in the central region of the retina that may result in a progressive loss of both reading vision and distance vision.

Trends in Vision and Hearing

Older persons are more likely to seek intervention for impaired vision than impaired hearing. The Centers for Disease Control and Prevention (2001) report the following statistics:

- Percentage of people age 70 years and older with a visual problem who:
  Have seen a doctor: 99%
  Wear glasses: 93%
- Percentage of people 70 years and older with a hearing problem who:
  Have seen a doctor: 76%
  Use a hearing aid: 34%

Two of the more commonly used screening tests for reduced vision are the *Snellen Eye Chart* and the *Pelli–Robson Contrast Sensitivity Chart* (Pelli, Robson, & Wilkins, 1998). The *Snellen Eye Chart* presents alphabetic letters of diminishing height. Patients read the chart while sitting or standing at a distance of 20 feet. Acuity is expressed as a fraction, with the distance at which the patient is standing being the numerator, and the normal maximum legible viewing distance as the denominator. If at 20 feet, a patient can read the letters on the row marked "60," the patient has a visual acuity of 20/60 or better. The *Pelli–Robson Chart* requires patients to read large letters of a fixed size that vary in contrast. Figure 13-11 presents a sampling of letters from this kind of chart.

In addition to performance-based screening tests, vision screening questionnaires are available, including the *Functional Vision Screening Questionnaire for Older People* (Horowitz, Teresi, & Cassels, 1991) and the *National Eye Institute (NEI) Visual Functioning Questionnaire-25* (2000). The *Functional Vision Screening Questionnaire* consists of 15 yes–no questions, including:

- Do you ever feel that problems with your vision make it difficult for you to do the things you would like to do?
- When crossing the street, do cars seem to appear very suddenly?

A score of 9 or more suggests need for referral to an optometrist or ophthalmologist. The NEI questionnaire, which has an interviewer-administered format, has 25 items that have a graded scale of response options. For instance, to the question *Because of your eyesight, how much difficulty do you have finding something on a crowded shelf?*, the responses range from *No difficulty at all* to *Stopped doing this because of your eyesight.*

In some cases, visual skills cannot be enhanced through the use of corrective lenses or ophthalmologic intervention. Reduced visual acuity has the following implications for the impact of hearing loss and the design of an aural rehabilitation plan:

- Audiological testing: The test booth lighting may have to be adapted to ensure that it is neither darker nor brighter inside than the outside room, and the booth entry and any steps may need to be marked with bright contrasting tape. Furniture inside the booth should be high-contrast and glare should be minimized with evenly distributed incandescent light (Blumsak, 2003).
- Speechreading: Degraded visual acuity and decreased contrast sensitivity may mean that an individual will not be able to utilize the visual signal maximally so likely will experience more difficulty in day-to-day speech communication than a person who has similar hearing loss but normal vision.
- Speech perception training: Speechreading training may not be appropriate when vision is reduced, because the patient may not be able to adequately see lip movements and other facial gestures. Speech perception training might be aimed at helping the patient be alert to auditory stimuli and to utilize residual hearing to the fullest extent possible.
- Communication strategies training: The program may include instruction about ways to enhance the visual communication environment, such as a repair strategy of *Come closer.*
- Communication environment: A patient who is less visually able will need optimal lighting in his or her communication environment to maximize what clues are available from speechreading. Sometimes, the environment cannot be lit optimally for communication because

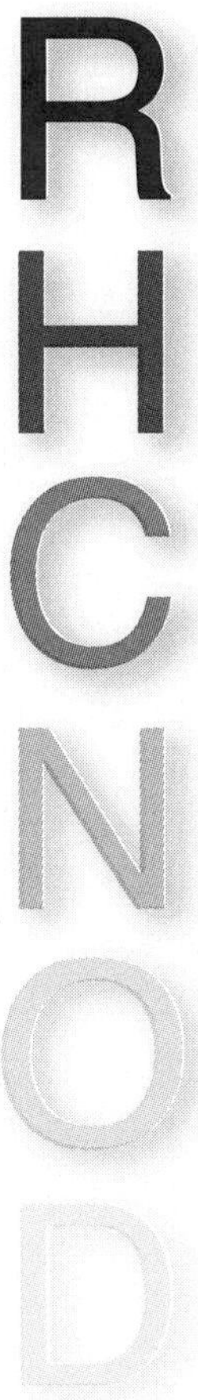

R
H
C
N
O
D

FIGURE 13-11. An example of a column of letters that appears on a contrast sensitivity chart.

bright lights cause the patient ocular discomfort. Harsh or "cold" fluorescent lighting is to be avoided when possible, whereas warm (incandescent) lighting is appropriate (Marmor, 1998).

• Hearing aids and assistive listening devices: Reduced vision may mean an individual is unable to manipulate the controls of a hearing aid, to see battery polarity, to recognize that cerumen has accumulated in the earmold, or to change the battery. These considerations may influence the kind of listening devices recommended. Family members or caregivers should receive instruction about how to check the batteries and handle the hearing aid. Any written materials should be in large print and reiterated with a different format. If a hearing aid is recommended, it is important to spend time with the patient so that he or she learns to feel the parts of the hearing aid and learns to adjust it by touch.

Arthritis

Arthritis encompasses more than 100 diseases and conditions and entails a painful inflammation of the joints, surrounding tissues, and other connective tissues. Arthritis decreases an individual's ability to perform fine motor activities. About 12% of persons between the ages of 65 and 74 years have activity limitations stemming from arthritis, and this percentage expands to about 19% for individuals 75 years and older (National Center for Health Statistics, 2002). Arthritis can decrease a patient's ability to use listening devices. For example, arthritis may pose the following difficulties for tasks related to using a hearing aid:

• Putting the hearing aid on and taking it off
• Opening the battery compartment and inserting batteries
• Removing ear wax and performing other cleaning tasks
• Operating the controls

Recommendations for listening devices will hinge upon a patient's ability to handle them. In some cases, it might be more appropriate to recommend an assistive listening device that has large controls and is easy to manipulate than to recommend a hearing aid. It also may be appropriate to instruct family members or caregivers on how to handle the listening devices.

Dementia

Dementia refers to a number of diseases that affect reasoning and intellectual faculties; symptoms may include memory loss, deterioration of thought processes, and orientation disorders.

Another common physical problem among older persons is dementia. **Dementia** is a generic term for a group of about 70 to 80 conditions that cause irreversible decline in cognitive functioning, and may relate to a variety of biological mechanisms that damage brain cells. The symptoms of dementia include gradual memory loss, disorientation, decline in the ability to perform everyday tasks, decline in the ability to process and interpret visual images, and loss of language skills.

Alzheimer's disease (AD) is a form of dementia. It is a progressive, degenerative, and irreversible disease. With AD, first memory, then reasoning, and finally language skills deteriorate. The time course between onset and death from AD is usually about 4 to 6 years, but may range from 3 to 20 years. An afflicted patient may become emotionally flat, confused, then incontinent, and eventually, mentally absent. In the final stages, patients lose their ability to use language and to recognize loved ones, and they become bed-bound. An estimated 5 million Americans suffer from AD. The prevalence could swell to 7.7 million by 2030. Normal aging does not necessarily cause AD, but the prevalence does increase with age. One out of eight people over the age of 65 years has AD, whereas nearly one in two over the age of 85 years has it. It is the seventh leading cause of death for people in the United States (Alzheimer's Association, 2007).

> **Alzheimer's disease (AD)** is a form of dementia that causes irreversible loss of brain cells.

Screening instruments for dementia include the *Mini-Mental State* (Folstein, Folstein, & McHugh, 1975), the *Clock Test* (Tuokko, Hadjistavropoulos, Miller, & Beattie, 1992), and the *Saint Louis University Mental Status Examination* (*SLUMS;* Banks & Morley, 2003). Sample items from the Mini-Mental State include:

- What is the year? Season? Date? Day?
- Spell the word *world* backwards.

The Clock Test includes three subtests: *Clock Drawing, Clock Setting,* and *Clock Reading.* Sample items of the SLUMS include questions about the week and year, as well as a simple math problem and a simple memory task. Other items in the SLUMS ask the patient to identify a triangle from three figure drawings and to name as many animals as possible in a 1-minute time interval.

Aural rehabilitation may be especially important for people who have dementia. There is some evidence that hearing loss can magnify cognitive dysfunction and accelerate dementia (Garahan, Waller, Houghton, Tisdale, & Runge, 1992), so it is important that hearing aid use be encouraged, when appropriate. Use of hearing aids appears to help maintain cognitive functioning (Mulrow, Aguilar, & Endicott, 1990) and reduce the consequences of dementia (Uhlmann, Larson, Rees, Koepsell, & Duckert, 1989). Instruction for family caregivers also may improve communication functioning.

Frank and Helen, a Happy Story with a Sad Ending

"A man is sitting next to her. She knows his name is Frank, but that is all she knows. She doesn't remember that when they met, she was head cheerleader and he was considered the best-looking guy in town. She doesn't remember that they've been married nearly 63 years and have raised two daughters. . . . She doesn't know that her daughters and Frank, 85, try to watch her constantly because they're terrified she will wander off. She doesn't even know her own name. It is Helen Erskine. She is 81 years old and she has Alzheimer's disease."

(Kantrowitz & Springen, 2007, p. 55)

Cognitive Abilities

Cognition refers to those mental processes involved in obtaining knowledge, in comprehending, and in thinking, including such mental acts as remembering, judging, and problem solving.

Attention is a selective narrowing of mental focus and receptivity.

Processing speed is the rate at which information is conducted and manipulated throughout the nervous system.

Working memory is the ability to store simultaneously and manipulate or transform items in memory.

Some older persons may display changes in cognitive functioning that occur as a natural process of aging, but usually not until after the age of 70 years. **Cognition** includes those mental processes that are used for perceiving, remembering, and thinking.

Some older persons may experience a change in **attention**, and slowed **processing speed** and reduced **working memory**. The extent to which these cognitive declines are present may affect how well the individual can comprehend speech. For example, if someone has a deficit in processing speed, that person may not understand connected discourse very well, especially if the talker speaks quickly. If the person has decreased working memory, the individual may forget the beginning of an utterance by the time the talker has reached the end of what he or she has to say, or the individual may not be able to process the meaning of the message because full attention has to be focused simply on remembering the words.

To the degree possible, it is worthwhile to examine the extent to which diminished speech recognition performance relates to a simple loss of audibility versus changes in cognitive processing. As Pichora-Fuller and Singh (2006) note,

> It is common for older adults to experience problems understanding spoken language in everyday life. Based on audiometric profile, some but not all of these older adults would be clear candidates for amplification. It is important to try to sort out how much of the effect of age on speech communication is actually due to simple loss of audibility and the associated

effects of cochlear pathology (e.g., loss of frequency selectivity) compared with how much is due to other changes in auditory or cognitive processing, or both, that are not predictable from the audiogram. (p. 34)

Other examples of how a patient's cognitive status may affect the aural rehabilitation plan include the complexity of instruction a clinician might provide to a patient and the controls or programs that might be included in a listening device.

Attention

Some older persons experience changes in their ability to focus on bits of information and to decide whether to process it further and if so, to what degree. This change in attention makes it difficult for some older individuals to distinguish relevant information from irrelevant information as when listening to a talker in the presence of background noise. It also may render some older individuals susceptible to distraction (McDowd & Shaw, 2000). Changes in attention may slow the speed at which they perform a mental task, may change their ability to attend to connected speech, and perhaps compromise their accuracy in task performance.

Processing Speed

Older adults, on average, are slower than younger adults when performing speeded cognitive tasks, and this slowness is often referred to as age-related general slowing. Evidence suggests that older adults are slower in processing both visuospatial and verbal information (e.g., Hale & Myerson, 1996). For example, older persons may have a harder time comprehending sentences that are spoken quickly than will younger persons, and they may have poorer recall for speeded speech (e.g., Stine, Wingfield, & Poon, 1986; Wingfield, Poon, Lombardi, & Lowe, 1985). If an older person is asked to decide, *as quickly as possible,* whether two words rhyme, that person will probably take longer to reach a decision than will a younger person.

Working Memory

One role of working memory for discourse comprehension is to hold in memory what has gone before and to integrate it with what is being heard at the present moment. Older adults tend not to perform as well as younger adults on tasks that require material to be held in memory for a short period and then recalled (Salthouse, 1994). Moreover, older adults often have greater difficulty in simultaneously holding onto and manipulating information (Wingfield, Stine, Lahar, & Aberdden, 1988).

"Functionally, attention is the means by which we actively limit the amount of information we process from the enormous amount of information available through our senses, memories, and cognitive processes. Attention serves to identify important features of one's environment."

Kathleen Pichora-Fuller and Gurjit Singh, researchers in the Department of Psychology, University of Toronto, Mississauga, Ontario, Canada

(Pichora-Fuller & Singh, 2006, p. 46)

Wingfield and Tu (2001) compiled data that suggests how verbal working memory might be affected by aging. Their analyses showed that young adults of about age 19 years and adults of about age 75 years were equally competent at repeating strings of digits after one hearing. When asked to listen to an increasingly long list of numbers, say "7, 3, 2, . . . ," both age groups were able to accurately repeat about seven digits on average. When the task became more difficult, the younger group outperformed the older group. In this more challenging task, participants were asked to listen to strings of sentences (e.g., *It snows when the weather gets cold.*) and determine whether or not each sentence in a string made sense. This type of task requires an individual to retain information and simultaneously perform a mental operation on the material. After hearing an increasingly long string of unrelated sentences, participants in the experiment were asked to recall the final word of each sentence in the particular string. Whereas the young adults were able to recall the final words from about three sentences, the older adults were able to recall only about two. In a similar vein, other studies have shown that older adults experience more difficulty in comprehending and recalling sentences that have complex syntax then do younger adults (Kynette & Kemper, 1988), sentences that are ambiguous, and sentences in which the pronoun is separated from the antecedent (Light & Capps, 1986; Zurif, Swinney, Prather, Wingfield, & Brownell, 1995). Another common difficulty is word retrieval, or recalling the name of a familiar person or object.

One screening measure that has been used to assess working memory is the backward digit section of the *Digit Span* subtest of the *Wechsler Scale of Adult Intelligence* (The Psychological Corporation, 1997). In this test, the examiner presents digits at the rate of one per second. The patient's task is to repeat the digits in reverse order. It has published norms based on age.

Cognitive Abilities Usually Unaffected by Aging

Despite the changes in attention, processing speed, and working memory that may occur with aging, it appears that older adults still can make good use of linguistic context. When listening to meaningful speech, they can often overcome some of the difficulties that they would otherwise experience when listening to rapid speech (Wingfield, Poon, Lombardi, & Lowe, 1985) or when listening to speech in the presence of background noise (Pichora-Fuller, Schneider, & Daneman, 1995). A simple experiment is illustrative. During a *word-onset gating* paradigm, a participant is presented with the first 50 msec of a word and then asked to guess its identity. If the guess is wrong, the participant hears the first 100 msec of the same word, and so forth, until the person guesses correctly. Studies have shown that older adults are often better at this task (i.e., they recognize words with less of the signal) than are younger adults (Wingfield, Alexander, & Cavigelli, 1994), suggesting that they have better facility with using linguistic context.

Vocabulary acquisition also appears to be age-resistant. Vocabulary usually continues to increase with age. In addition, knowledge that has been acquired over a lifetime, knowledge that has been accessed often and expanded, is typically retained (Nicholas, Barth, Obler, Au, & Albert, 1997).

AURAL REHABILITATION INTERVENTION

The evaluation stage of the plan presented in Figure 13-4 will provide information about a patient's activity limitations and participation restrictions, about a patient's priorities, about his or her audiological status and otologic health, and about life situation factors and physical and cognitive abilities. In designing an intervention strategy, goals can be developed to meet the patient's priorities and to alleviate activity limitations and participation restrictions. The intervention may include provision of listening devices and related instruction and training, and provision of other kinds of services.

Listening Devices

The National Council on Aging (1999) asked the question, "What happens to the quality of life if hearing loss goes untreated in an elderly person?" To answer it, they surveyed 2,304 seniors who have hearing loss. The survey centered only on the use of hearing aids. The findings illuminate what might happen if an older person fails to receive adequate aural rehabilitation intervention. A summary of the survey responses appears in Tables 13-1 and 13-2.

Table 13-1. Responses to a nationwide survey indicating the emotional status of older persons who have hearing loss. Those who responded affirmatively to the item pertaining to sadness and or depression had felt either emotion for 2 or more weeks during the previous year. Those who responded affirmatively to the item pertaining to worry, tension, and anxiety had felt these states for a month or more during the past year. All numbers represent percentages of persons with the indicated hearing loss who use hearing aids.

EMOTION	MILDER HEARING LOSS, USES HEARING AID	MILDER HEARING LOSS, DOES NOT USE HEARING AID	MORE SEVERE HEARING LOSS, USES HEARING AID	MORE SEVERE HEARING LOSS, DOES NOT USE HEARING AID
Sadness/Depression	14	23	22	30
Worry/Tension/Anxiety	7	12	12	17
Paranoia	13	24	14	36
Insecure/Irritable, Fearful/Tense	8	10	11	17

Source: From *The Consequences of Untreated Hearing Loss in Older Persons* by the National Council on the Aging, 1999, Washington, DC. Adapted by permission.

Table 13-2. Responses to a nationwide survey indicating the emotional status of older persons who have hearing loss. All numbers reflect percentages of hearing loss.

ACTIVITY	MILDER HEARING LOSS, USES HEARING AID	MILDER HEARING LOSS, DOES NOT USE HEARING AID	MORE SEVERE HEARING LOSS, USES HEARING AID	MORE SEVERE HEARING LOSS, DOES NOT USE HEARING AID
Participates Regularly in Social Activities	47	37	42	32
Participates in Senior Center Activities	24	15	21	16

Source: From *The Consequences of Untreated Hearing Loss in Older Persons* by the National Council on the Aging, 1999, Washington, DC. Adapted by permission.

As can be seen in Table 13-1, respondents who do not use hearing aids were more likely to report feeling sad or depressed for a period of 2 weeks or more during the previous year than respondents who used hearing aids, and they were more likely to report feeling worried, tense, or anxious for a month or more during the past year. They were also more likely to experience paranoia ("Other people get angry at me for no reason," when they misunderstand or ask people to repeat themselves). In fact, non–hearing aid users were almost twice as likely to report that "people get angry with me for no reason" than were hearing aid users. Finally, non–hearing aid users were more likely to describe themselves as feeling insecure, irritable, fearful, or tense than were hearing aid users. These differences between users and nonusers were robust, even when other variables such as income level and age were taken into account. The percentage of persons reporting negative emotions increased with the severity of the hearing loss.

Older persons who have hearing loss and who do not use hearing aids often suffer social consequences in addition to emotional consequences. As implied by Table 13-2, isolation becomes a real possibility. The survey showed that older persons who do not use hearing aids were more likely to avoid social activities, such as interacting with neighbors and participating in structured events, and were less likely to engage in activities sponsored by senior centers.

The results of this study demonstrate that older patients who have hearing loss, be it more mild or severe, experience both emotional and social consequences if the hearing loss goes untreated. Untreated individuals are more likely to experience depression, anxiety, worry, tension, paranoia, and emotional inner turmoil than are hearing aid users. In contrast, hearing aid users remain more active in their neighborhoods, in organized social activities, and in senior citizen centers.

Hearing Aids

The audiologist will want to assess carefully motivation to use amplification before the fitting and then ensure that support systems for hearing aid use are in place following fitting. Table 13-3 presents factors that affect a patient's motivation to use a hearing aid.

Table 13-3. Factors that may affect an older person's motivation to use a hearing aid.

- Degree of hearing loss
- Communication difficulties
- Self-concept
- Opinion of hearing aid users (e.g., "Only really old people use hearing aids, and I'm not there yet.")
- Number and quality of conversational interactions in which a patient engages
- The availability of communication partners
- Physical health (such as manual dexterity and visual acuity)

Many of the procedures that we reviewed for selecting hearing aids for adults (Chapter 12) are applicable for the elderly population. When selecting the hearing aid, the audiologist might select one that has easily manipulated battery compartments, especially if manual dexterity is problematic for the patient. A common trend has been self-adjusting aids that self-select the electroacoustic program according to the listening environment (Souza, 2004). Some hearing aids have automatic t-coils that detect the magnetic field of the telephone receiver. Remote controls are the answer to some dexterity problems. Other factors that will influence the recommendation include finances (Can the patient afford the device?), monaural versus binaural hearing aids, and whether assistive listening devices might be appropriate instead of, or as a supplement to, the hearing aid.

The importance of the hearing aid orientation cannot be overemphasized, and whether the older person becomes a successful hearing aid user may well hinge on the audiologist's willingness to take the time necessary to give a thorough orientation. There can be no shortcuts here. Ample time must be devoted to instructing the patient on how to insert and remove the earmold and how to handle the hearing aid. One patient, who stopped using his hearing aid shortly after purchasing it, was asked why he never developed a consistent use pattern. He responded that he did not know how to work the wax removal device, that the battery door was too difficult to operate, and that it hurt his ear to remove the aid at night. This man's audiologist may or may not have provided information about these topics during the hearing aid orientation. However, the audiologist obviously did not take enough time to ensure that the patient had an adequate understanding of how to handle the hearing aid and did not provide enough follow-up support to ensure successful use.

In addition to receiving a traditional hearing aid orientation, the audiologist might address specific difficulties that older persons often encounter with their hearing aids. These include changing batteries, inserting the aid into the ear (Figure 13-12), and adjusting the volume control. (Some hearing aid manufacturers accommodate the older patient by constructing aids that have a raised volume control and extraction handles.)

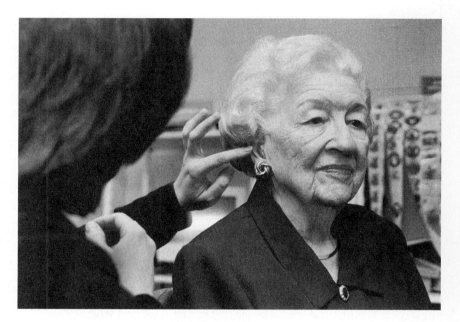

FIGURE 13-12. The hearing aid orientation. The older patient may require extra time to learn how to insert the earmold or ITE into the ear and to extract it. *Photograph by Kim Readmond, courtesy of the Central Institute for the Deaf.*

A component of a hearing aid orientation may be instruction for family members, caregivers, and others involved in the patient's health care. They may learn about caring for the hearing aid, and also develop realistic expectations about what the hearing aid can and cannot do for the patient.

A section of the survey conducted by the National Council on Aging (1999) focused on the benefits of hearing aid use. In addition to including responses from older persons who use hearing aids, this section also included responses from family members. Overall, both users and family members reported that following receipt of a hearing aid, improvements occurred in the patient's confidence, independence, relationships with family, and overall outlook on life. Interestingly, the families on average perceived greater improvements than even the users, suggesting that the patients' new ability to hear enhanced the family dynamics of communication. The findings are summarized in Table 13-4. Other studies suggest that hearing aid use by older persons improves their conversational fluency, helps maintain their psychosocial well-being, reduces hearing-related communication difficulties, and improves overall quality of life (Bess, 2000; Starck & Hickson, 2004; Vuorialho, Karinene, & Sorri, 2006).

Table 13-4. Percentage of hearing aid users who reported improvements as a result of hearing aid use.

IMPROVEMENT	% HEARING AID USERS	% FAMILY MEMBERS
Relationships at home	56	66
Feelings about myself	50	60
Life overall	48	62
Mental health	36	39
Self-confidence	39	46
Relationships with children and grandchildren	40	52
Willing to participate in group activities	34	44
Sense of independence	34	39
Sense of safety	34	37
Ability to play card/board games	31	47
Social life	34	41
Physical health	21	24
Dependence on others	22	31
Relationships at work	26	43
Ability to play sports	7	10

Adapted from The National Council on Aging (1999), *The consequences of untreated hearing loss in older persons*. Washington, DC:

Cochlear Implants

Somewhere between 250,000 and 400,000 adults 65 years and older have a severe to profound hearing loss and qualify, at least audiologically, for cochlear implantation (Blanchfield, Feldman, Dunbar, & Gardner, 2001). The procedure remains somewhat controversial for older persons because there has been, at least historically, the question of whether an older person has the potential to benefit from receiving a device due to reduced neural plasticity (i.e., an older brain may be less likely to learn to interpret the electrical signal than will a younger brain). Other concerns include (Leung et al., 2005; Pedley, Tari, & Drinkwater, 2003):

- Surgical risks, due to increased anesthetic risk, slow wound healing due to a thinning of the skin or reduced blood supply to the skin, or complications from preexisting illness
- General cognitive considerations, such as problems with memory, learning new tasks, and ability to manage the device
- Social considerations, such as a decreased motivation to use the device and participate in social interactions
- Cost–utility ratios in this day and age of health care rationing, where health care providers are increasingly asked to select the best candidates for expensive procedures

Most research suggests little reason why older persons who have profound hearing loss should not be considered for cochlear implantation. For instance, an investigation conducted by Leung and colleagues (2005) studied 258 patients over the age of 65 years and 491 patients under the age of 65 years. The investigators found no significant differences in the two groups' ability to recognize words in an auditory-only condition following cochlear implantation. Duration of deafness, and not age, appeared to be the best predictor of performance. Reports of medical complications for older patients are no greater than those for younger patients (Kelsall, Shallop, & Burmelli, 1995; Waltzman, Cohen, & Shapiro, 1993). Older cochlear implant recipients tend to use their devices. The cost-effectiveness of providing cochlear implants to older persons has been shown to parallel that achieved by providing cochlear implants to the general adult population, with improvements in hearing and emotional health being the chief contributors (Francis, Chee, Yeagle, Cheng, & Niparko, 2002).

Assistive Listening Devices (ALDs)

Sometimes the older patient will desire an ALD in addition to or in lieu of a hearing aid. For instance, an elderly person may be unable to handle a hearing aid or earmold because of arthritis and may need a simple FM system instead. Kaplan (1996) suggested that, when arthritis or reduced tactile sensation is present, a simple hardwired system with earphones or earbuds may be most appropriate. During conversation, a communication partner can talk into a microphone while the older person can wear earbuds. A microphone-earbuds system can be used for viewing television or listening to the radio. The patient can simply place the microphone by the system's speaker. Alternatively, an older person may be interested in obtaining a listening system that plugs directly into the earphone jack of the television set or radio. For watching television, there is also the option of closed captioning. When an elderly person lives alone, security is often an issue. It may be important to consider alerting devices to signal the doorbell and telephone ringing and the smoke alarm going off.

When the patient resides in a residential setting, maintenance and usage of an ALD might be simpler and less costly than use of a hearing aid (Lesner, 2003). Use of an ALD can simplify staff training because they are easy to use and troubleshoot compared to hearing aids, and ALDs are less likely to be lost.

Many older persons do not use ALDs, even though they may be prime candidates for doing so (see Southall, Gagné, & Leroux, 2006, for a review). Reasons why some patients choose not to use an ALD include: (a) fear of technology, (b) belief that their hearing loss is not problematic enough to warrant use, (c) lack of self-confidence or self-esteem, (d) fear of stigmatization because of hearing loss, (e) vanity, and (f) secondary health issues, such as reduced fine motor control and visual impairment. Many older patients are simply unaware of ALD options.

Southall et al. (2006) suggest that a series of landmark events occurs when an older person goes from not using to using an ALD (Figure 13-13). These landmark events include (pp. 257–258):

- Recognition that hearing difficulties compromise participation in valued activities. When patients realize that they cannot participate in social or leisure activities, they may reach a critical point where they decide to seek solutions. The opinions and encouragement of family and friends may factor into this recognition process.
- Awareness that technological solutions exist. Once recognition occurs, the patient may seek help, learning about ALDs through consultation with audiologists, hearing aid distributors, or other hearing and speech professionals.
- Consultation for and acquisition of the devices. The patient may receive professional recommendations for ALDs.
- Adaptation to use of device and modification of behavior. The final landmark entails patients adapting to using the ALD and modifying their behaviors accordingly. Patients learn how to use the ALD and begin to experience the benefits.

"Turn up that speaker phone, and boom. That's not bad. So, you know you hang on to some of the things that sound good."

An older person, commenting on how a telephone amplifier enhanced signal quality

(Southall et al., 2006, p. 256)

"My hearing aid dealer didn't mention anything like that to me. Which I am kind of ticked off about . . . But I wasn't aware of this. I was thinking to myself I have a stereo downstairs. And if I had a long cord . . . then I could listen to music . . . Didn't know at all!"

An older patient, commenting that he lacked knowledge about ALDs

(Southall et al., 2006, p. 255)

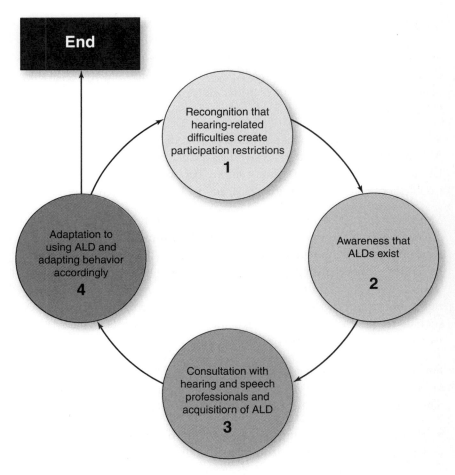

FIGURE 13-13. The four landmark events described by Southall et al. (2006) in acquiring an ALD.

Other Services

Some older people participate in group aural rehabilitation programs following receipt of a listening aid, or even without obtaining one. The program may include such topics as the following (Kricos & Lesner, 1995):

- Hearing aids (cochlear implants) and their functions
- Counseling about issues that are important to the participants
- Hearing and hearing loss
- Assistive listening device technology
- Auditory and visual nature of speech
- Communication strategies

Sometimes, family members will participate in the aural rehabilitation program with their older relatives (Figure 13-14). For instance, they may learn how to speak with clear speech. They may come to understand that conversation can be tiring for older persons who have hearing loss, and they may be encouraged to exercise patience and understanding in their interactions with them (e.g., Kramer, Allessie, Dondorp, Zekveld, & Kapteyn, 2005). The Appendix presents a list of resources for family members and caregivers to obtain information about legal, medical, and financial issues related to older persons and their health care needs.

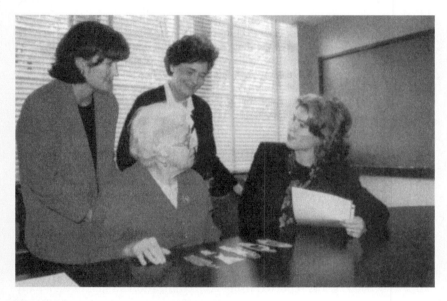

FIGURE 13-14. Participation of family members and other close acquaintances. Others might be encouraged to participate in the aural rehabilitation program for an older adult. *Photograph by Kim Readmond, courtesy of the Central Institute for the Deaf.*

Research suggests that some older patients benefit from participating in formal aural rehabilitation programs. Informational counseling and communication strategies may be especially helpful. For instance, many people may experience less perceived participation restrictions following a counseling-based aural rehabilitation program (Ventry & Weinstein, 1983) and quality of life may improve when both patients and frequent communication partners receive aural rehabilitation intervention (Kramer et al., 2005). Some patients benefit from participating in a program that provides analytic auditory training coupled with communication strategies training, but not a program that provides only analytic auditory training

(Kricos & Holmes, 1996). Perhaps the individuals who are most likely to benefit are those who have the greatest communication difficulties prior to the onset of training (Kricos & Holmes, 1996).

Hickson and her colleagues (Hickson, Worrall, & Scarinci, 2006) invited 96 people with hearing loss between the ages of 58 and 94 years, and their significant others when available, to participate in a 5-week interactive group education program called *Active Communication Education (ACE;* Hickson & Worrall, 2003). The groups met for 2 hours per week. The objectives of ACE were to improve the communication interactions of patients, to enhance quality of life, and to reduce participation restrictions. For individual groups, a speech and hearing professional helped participants to prioritize their communication needs during the first session. As such, program content for a particular group depended on the particular communication difficulties experienced by the participants. Typical needs included communicating more effectively around the house and listening with greater success to television. The Key Resources section presents an outline of the first session for an ACE program and an outline of how a particular communication difficulty might be addressed during a subsequent group session.

Participants completed a modified version of the *International Outcome Inventory-Hearing Aids (IOI-HA;* Cox et al., 2000), which appears in the Key Resources section in Chapter 12. Frequent communication partners completed a version of the IOI designed for significant others. At the end of the program, more than half of the participants with hearing loss and the significant other participants indicated that participating in the ACE meetings had been "very much worth the trouble." The majority of participants with hearing loss reported using communication strategies on a daily basis and about half of them reported that they had no remaining difficulties or only slight difficulty in the particular situations that they had identified as being problematic. The authors conclude that group interactions like ACE are beneficial for older patients and their frequent communication partners.

There are less tangible benefits for older persons who participate in group aural rehabilitation programs in addition to these just listed (see Taylor & Jurma, 1999). First, elderly patients benefit from affiliating with peers who are similar to themselves in a variety of ways, and the group experience permits them to expand the network of social contacts (see also Kricos, 2006). The social contacts not only alleviate age- and hearing-related loneliness, but they may also elevate their involvement and motivation for seeking help in managing their hearing difficulties. In the aural rehabilitation program, seniors can exchange stories and solutions, share frustrations, and talk about their hearing aids. Finally, the opportunity to interact with an audiologist or other speech and hearing professional can bolster their store of information and increase their number of opportunities to receive counseling.

AURAL REHABILITATION IN THE INSTITUTIONAL SETTING

If a patient resides in a nursing home or institutionalized setting, the aural rehabilitation program may have to be adjusted accordingly. Shultz and Mowry (1995) noted some of the problems associated with providing hearing health care to patients in a nursing home. These include:

- Managing the hearing loss when the patient may also have dementia or AD. Often patients with dementia also have depression, which can decrease motivation to participate in an aural rehabilitation plan.
- Preventing hearing aids from being lost. For instance, a patient may place the hearing aid in a bathrobe pocket, and the robe may end up in the laundry before the aid is removed.
- Maintaining the hearing aids. One study found that 45% of the hearing aids used by patients in four nursing homes and four retirement homes had at least one or more major problems (Ferguson & Nerbonne, 2003), suggesting a need for hearing aid monitoring programs.
- Involving the staff in the aural rehabilitation plan and providing in-service training. Personnel should be aware of the communication difficulties associated with hearing loss. They should be familiarized with communication strategies and learn how to optimize the listening environment. Staff need to know how to handle hearing aids; for example, how to change batteries, how to clean earmolds, and how to insert and remove the devices from an older person's ear, as many residents will not be able to manage them alone.
- Dealing with the high turnover of facility personnel. An audiologist may provide an in-service in August, only to discover that in December, half of the staff has been replaced.

An administrator of a nursing home may approach the speech and hearing professional to perform an **in-service** for the staff who work with the patients, or the clinician may approach the nursing home personnel. An in-service may be scheduled for a length of time ranging anywhere from a couple of hours (more common) to several half-day sessions (less common). Scheduling is often difficult because staff changes occur about three times during a 24-hour shift, so all workers may not be available at any given time. In addition, staff may not be financially compensated for the time they devote to receiving training, and some attendees may have

An **in-service** is continuing education provided to full-time employees.

just finished working an 8-hour shift and be eager to end their workday. Often the staff will have little knowledge about hearing loss, and some may not have received higher education so may lack appropriate background knowledge to understand some of the material you would like to present.

Material should be presented at level of difficulty that is appropriate for the audience and done in a way that maintains their interest and attention, as with the use of visual materials and hands-on teaching aids. In addition, the presentation of case studies, demonstrations (e.g., "Please try on the ear plugs in the package I gave you at the beginning of the class. Once you have them in place, I'll ask you to try to understand the sentences that I will read."), and group discussion ("Please help me generate a list of conditions that might make speechreading difficult.") serve to engage the staff in the learning process. The goal of an in-service is to provide basic information about hearing loss and hearing aids, to develop empathy for the person who has hearing loss, and to teach strategies for enhancing communication with patients. For example, a unit about speechreading may include the objectives:

- Participants will identify characteristics of a good speechreader.
- Participants will identify factors that influence the speechreading task.

Aural rehabilitation in an institutionalized setting can be effective. An investigation performed in Canada examined the benefits of providing an aural rehabilitation program to residents in a nursing home and the staff members with whom they most regularly communicated (Pichora-Fuller & Carson, 2001). The aural rehabilitation program focused on five areas: (a) providing hearing aids and assistive listening devices, (b) maximizing accessibility to communication opportunities, (c) educating nursing home staff, (d) promoting the use of communication strategies, and (e) providing a drop-in audiological clinic and residents' self-help group. As a result of participating in the program, the residents began to spend more time (hours/month) talking to acquaintances, attending religious services, and participating in meetings. The residents expressed increased satisfaction with their ability to talk on the telephone. Staff members became more familiar with assistive listening devices and improved their skills in handling hearing aids. They also changed their communication behaviors in ways that enhanced the residents' scope and quality of participation in nursing home activities.

CASE STUDY

Staying Active

A case study reported by Aarts (2006) illustrates the steps in planning an aural rehabilitation program for an older adult. The case study begins with an evaluation, then the development of an aural rehabilitation strategy, including prioritizing communication needs, and then the implementation of an intervention plan. Provision is made for follow-up and outcomes assessment.

At the time of his visit to an audiological clinic, "Mr. Whalen" was a 93-year-old widower in good health, other than poorly corrected vision and osteoporosis. He was concerned that poor hearing was hindering his ability to participate effectively in a variety of activities, including local service organizations, community boards, religious services, and out-of-town visits with his children and grandchildren. He came to the audiological clinic wearing two 4-year-old BTEs. During the case history, he reported that he used only one of the hearing aids' four programs and that he was unaware of whether they were equipped with t-coils (they were). He was frustrated by his communication difficulties and reluctant to use an FM system that had been recommended to him by another hearing-health care provider. Telephone communication was difficult. He reported that he was often unable to hear the telephone or the doorbell ring. When questioned, he admitted that he was unlikely to hear a smoke alarm while he was sleeping.

An audiological assessment revealed a sloping moderate-to-profound sensorineural bilateral hearing loss. Speech recognition testing showed that Mr. Whalen received limited benefit in quiet and no benefit in noise by wearing his hearing aids. Real-ear measures revealed that the hearing aids rendered only already loud sounds more audible.

The first step in developing an intervention plan was to prioritize Mr. Whalen's communication needs. His priorities were, in order of importance: (a) to improve functioning in quiet and in group meetings, (b) to improve telephone communication, and (c) to improve ability to hear environmental signals at home.

The next step was to create an intervention strategy that maximized his listening performance while maintaining cost-effectiveness. The audiologist reprogrammed the hearing aids, and suggested that if this did not resolve his listening problems, new aids might be purchased. The audiologist confirmed that the devices had telecoils and showed him how to work them. The audiologist also recommended a trial period with a midpriced FM system and a conference microphone. A lapel microphone was recommended, so Mr. Whalen could use the system in meetings as well as one-on-one settings such as in the car or sharing meals. Mr. Whalen also decided to participate in a trial period with a universal transmitter for smoke alarm, phone ringer, and dedicated doorbell, and a hearing aid–compatible device that would work with a cell phone.

In the first follow-up visit, which occurred immediately after the hearing aids were reprogrammed, real-ear measures showed that the hearing aids now somewhat improved the audibility of speech. The FM system's lapel microphone provided appropriate gain for normal conversational speech and the wireless phone devices appeared to provide benefit. Mr. Whalen received instruction about how to use the devices. He then spent the next period using the FM and telephone systems.

continues

CASE STUDY, *continued*

Staying Active, *continued*

About three weeks later, Mr. Whalen was seen for a second follow-up appointment. He had used the FM system on several occasions and had used the wireless phone devices, both at home and while traveling. About the FM system he said, "This system is going to be a wonderful gift. I can return to meetings and such, and be an active participant again" (Aarts, 2006, p. 64). During this follow-up visit, he received information about a universal ALD signaler, to be placed near his smoke alarm and landline home telephone.

On a subsequent visit, Mr. Whalen reported continued satisfaction with both the hearing aids and the FM system. He decided to forgo the hearing aid–compatible telephone device so he would not be tempted to talk on the cell phone and drive simultaneously. He also opted against purchasing the alerting devices due to financial concerns. The audiologist encouraged the patient to determine whether he could hear the smoke alarm when not wearing his hearing aids and to place an alerting device for a smoke alarm "at the top of his wish list" (Aart, 2006, p. 64).

 FINAL REMARKS

You may discover that working with older people provides some of your most rewarding professional experiences. One audiologist described how she tested an elderly woman who had terminal cancer. "Mrs. Kramer had a moderate, bilateral hearing loss," the audiologist related. "I knew by talking with her, and reviewing her medical records, that she only had a few months to live. I suggested that she might not be interested in purchasing a hearing aid." Much to the audiologist's surprise, Mrs. Kramer not only wanted to buy a hearing aid, she wanted to buy two. She also wanted to borrow a CD-ROM that provides speechreading training. Mrs. Kramer's rationale was simple: "There is so much going on in my body that I can't control. It feels good to be able to actually do something positive about my hearing problem."

 KEY CHAPTER POINTS

- The elderly represent the fastest growing segment of the U.S. population. By 2030, the number of citizens over the age of 64 years will be 72 million, or about 20% of the American population.
- The first stage of developing an aural rehabilitation plan is to determine a patient's activity limitations and participation restrictions.

- Degree of hearing loss increases with age. Age-related hearing loss is called presbycusis.

- Some older persons may experience a decline in auditory processing capabilities.

- The impact of hearing loss on the older individuals may vary as a result of the person's economic status, social circumstances, social contacts, and emotional and physical health. Two persons may be of the same chronological age, yet differ greatly on these variables.

- Three physical conditions that may influence dramatically the design and success of an aural rehabilitation plan include reduced vision, arthritis, and dementia.

- Many older persons experience changes in cognitive functioning, including decrements in attention, processing speed, and working memory. Vocabulary learning appears to remain intact.

- The use of hearing aids can prevent some of the negative consequences associated with presbycusis.

- Some changes may need to be made in the procedures for assessing hearing status, and for providing a hearing aid orientation. In particular, more time usually must be scheduled to provide aural rehabilitation services for an older adult than for a younger adult.

- Age should not be a determining factor in deciding whether an older person is a candidate for cochlear implantation.

- Some older persons desire assistive listening devices in addition to or in lieu of hearing aids.

- Group aural rehabilitation programs tend to work well with older patients, especially if they include their frequent communication partners.

- Staff at nursing homes and residential facilities need to learn about hearing loss, communication strategies, and listening aids.

TERMS AND CONCEPTS TO REMEMBER

Traditional seniors
Baby boomers
Patient priorities
Testing accommodations
Presbycusis
Auditory processing
Self-sufficiency
Self-concept
Vision screening
Arthritis
Dementia screening

Alzheimer's disease
Accommodations for visual impairment
Attention
Processing speed
Working memory
Cochlear implant candidacy
ALD landmark events
Group aural rehabilitation sessions
In-services

MULTIPLE-CHOICE QUESTIONS

1. An older adult is unable to understand a news broadcaster who speaks with a clipped and brisk speaking rate, even though she has normal audiometric thresholds bilaterally. This difficulty may be most indicative of:

    a. An activity limitation

    b. A participation restriction

    c. An auditory processing deficit

    d. A working memory deficit

2. An older person may present with a conductive hearing loss because:

    a. Softening of ear canal cartilage occurs with aging.

    b. Accumulation of ear fluid in the middle ear is commonplace among the elderly.

    c. Inattention affects bone conduction testing.

    d. Pure-tone stimuli are difficult for older persons to detect.

3. Hearing loss in the elderly is:

    a. Often best characterized as a flat audiogram configuration

    b. The number one chronic condition in this population

    c. Most commonly the result of a lifetime of noise exposure

    d. More common among men than women

4. Physiologically, the most common cause of presbycusis is:

    a. A loss of hair cells

    b. Cochlear conductive

    c. A combination of neural and metabolic factors

    d. A deterioration of the tectorial membrane

5. One older person is able to recite correctly 5 consecutive digits after hearing a talker speak 10 in a row whereas another person is able to recite 7. These two individuals differ in their:

   a. Attention

   b. Auditory processing capabilities

   c. Processing speed

   d. Working memory

6. Which of the following statements is true about cochlear implants and older persons?

   a. Older persons are at higher risk for surgical complications than are younger persons.

   b. Duration of deafness is a good predictor of benefit.

   c. Older cochlear implant recipients have been shown to have less motivation to engage in conversations than do younger cochlear implant recipients.

   d. Age is a good predictor of benefit.

7. Which is not a reason that an older person may opt not to use an ALD?

   a. That hearing aids are more user-friendly

   b. Vanity

   c. Belief that degree of hearing loss does not warrant use

   d. Secondary health issues

8. Contrast sensitivity refers to a patient's ability to:

   a. Determine whether two tones are the same or different in frequency

   b. Distinguish light from dark

   c. Determine whether a stimulus presented to one electrode in the cochlear implant electrode array is of equal amplitude to a stimulus presented to an adjacent electrode

   d. Adjust the volume control of an ALD so that speech recognition performance is maximized

9. An older person may have reduced processing speed. For example, this person:

   a. Might take longer than a younger person in deciding that the words *bat* and *bait* do not rhyme

   b. May become disoriented when taking a walk in his or her neighborhood

    c. May perform poorly on the *NU-6 Test* as a result

    d. May be unable to recognize speech in the presence of background noise

10. An older person who opts not to use a hearing aid, even if needed, is more likely than someone who does use a hearing aid to:

    a. Seek social support from a senior center

    b. Seek support from a network of family and friends

    c. Be fearful and tense

    d. Feel an internal locus of control

11. Mr. Freeman has arrived at your clinic for a hearing test. Mr. Freeman is 79 years old. During pure-tone testing, you might make the following adjustment in your test procedures:

    a. Forgo word recognition testing because Mr. Thomson likely will have poor speech discrimination

    b. Forgo bone-conduction testing because Mr. Thomson will likely tire before you are able to complete the procedure

    c. Use insert earphones to eliminate the possibility of collapsing ear canals

    d. Perform the testing as quickly as possibly to prevent fatigue

12. There are many difficulties inherent in preventing an in-service to personnel in a nursing home facility. One of the prime difficulties is that:

    a. Most nursing homes do not cater to the needs of persons who have hearing loss.

    b. In-services are difficult to schedule, because of work shifts.

    c. Most nursing home directors do not know about the importance of audiology and aural rehabilitation.

    d. There are no instructional designs available that maintain staff attention.

KEY RESOURCES

The *Active Communication Education (ACE)* program, developed in Australia, is designed for older people who have hearing loss. The program runs for 2 hours per week for 5 weeks. In the first session, a "Nominal Group Technique" is used to identify and prioritize the communication needs of the participants. In later sessions, a problem-solving approach is used to address those needs identified. Table 13-5 presents an outline of a typical first session in ACE whereas Table 13-6 presents a typical problem-solving session.

Table 13-5. Outline of the first session of ACE.

Objectives	• To welcome and introduce participants and to explain the aims of the program • To obtain measures of activity limitations, participation restrictions, quality of life, and communicative function • To explore the communication difficulties that participants experience in everyday life • To prioritize communication needs
Materials	• Folders with handouts • Whiteboard • Name tags, Post-it stickers
Introduction and welcome (15 minutes)	• Participants are invited to say who they are, what they have done about their hearing problems, and why they have come to the meeting
Communication needs analysis (20 minutes)	Participants brainstorm about such questions as (facilitator records answers on whiteboard): • What communication difficulties do you have in everyday life? • What activities do you have difficulty participating in because of your hearing loss? (ensure that every participant is allowed opportunity to speak, without going into too much detail at this stage)
Nominal group technique (15 minutes, followed by 15-minute coffee/tea break)	The group prioritizes communication difficulties: • Participants receive three Post-its, labeled 1, 2, and 3 • Each participant places the three Post-it stickers next to the most important (Label 1) and the least important (Label 3) difficulty listed on the whiteboard
Problem-solving process (40 minutes)	The group takes the top-priority item and considers these issues: • What is involved in the communication activity? Who, what, when, where, why? • What are the sources of difficulty in the activity? • What are some possible solutions? • What information is necessary to apply the solutions? • What practical skills are necessary to apply the solutions? • How can you test the solutions?
Conclusion (15 minutes)	Facilitator and group discuss next classes and facilitator assigns homework activity. Homework may include participants writing in a journal, addressing such issues as: "How do people describe you?"; "How well do you think you have coped with the changes associated with hearing loss?"; and "Describe a hearing-related difficulty when you used a strategy that worked, then describe a hearing-related difficulty where you used a strategy that did not work."

Adapted from Hickson and Worrall (2003, p. 2S88).

Table 13-6. Outline of a problem-solving session in the ACE program; in this session, the topic is conversation in noise.

Objectives	• To work through the problem-solving process as applied to an example situation in noise • To identify the component skills necessary for better communication in noise • To practice the component skills of requesting clarification • To work through the problem-solving process as applied to a situation that is unique to each participant
Materials	• Handouts • Whiteboard • Name tags and paper notebooks
Introduction (15 minutes)	• Discuss homework activity • Write session agenda on whiteboard
Example of a noisy situation (30 minutes)	• Ask each participant to look at the conversation described in a class handout and suggest ways to improve communication in that particular setting • List ideas on the whiteboard • Review a related handout
Identify necessary component skills (15 minutes, followed by a 15-minute coffee/tea break)	After making the modifications to the environment to optimize their chances of successful communication, facilitator suggests that communication breakdowns still occur. • Talk about repair strategies • Talk about the need to practice repair strategies • Review a related handout
Practice clarification skills (20 minutes)	Divide group into two and perform communication exercises. For example, a receptionist in a noisy medical waiting room tells you, "Your appointment will be next Thursday at . . ." You do not hear the time. What do you do?
Discussion of individual noisy situations (15 minutes)	• Have each participant identify a noisy situation that regularly presents communication difficulties • Work through the problem-solving process from Session 1 and ask group members to consider ways to repair likely communication breakdowns
Conclusion (10 minutes)	• Say good-byes and talk about what will happen next

Adapted from Hickson and Worrall (2003, p. 2S89).

APPENDIX 13-1

Resources for family members and caregivers of older patients who have hearing loss and other health-related issues (Adapted from Kantrowitz & Springen, 2007, p. 64).

- Administration on Aging (www.aoa.gov). Provides information on various services including elder rights.
- National Association of Area Agencies on Aging (www.n4a.org). Provides a national network of social services.
- Family Caregiver Alliance (www.caregiver.org). Offers programs at national, state, and local levels to support caregivers.
- AARP (www.aarp.org). Provides numerous benefits to members, who are age 50 and older.
- Eldercare Locator (www.eldercare.gov). Links caregivers with senior services; part of the U.S. Administration on Aging.
- National Academy of Elder Law Attorneys (www.naela.org). Provides searchable database to assist in finding an elder-law attorney.
- Medicare Rights (www.medicarerights.org). Provides health care information and assistance for people with Medicare.
- National Hospice and Palliative Care Organization (www.nhpco. org). Offers information on end-of-life issues and state-specific advance directives.
- Nursing Homes (www.medicare.gov/nihcompare). Provides detailed information on the past performance of every Medicare- and Medicaid-certified nursing home in the United States.

PART 4

Aural (Re)Habilitation for Children

CHAPTER 14

Infants and Toddlers Who Have Hearing Loss

OUTLINE

- Detection of hearing loss
- Identification and quantification of hearing loss
- Health care follow-up
- Parent counseling
- Early-intervention overview and development of an aural rehabilitation strategy
- Communication mode
- Listening device
- Early-intervention program
- Parental support and parent instruction

- Case study: A memorable journey
- Final remarks
- Key chapter points
- Terms and concepts to remember
- Multiple-choice questions
- Key resources
- Appendix 14-1
- Appendix 14-2
- Appendix 14-3
- Appendix 14-4

More than 1.4 million children in the United States have a significant hearing loss (Figure 14-1). Sensorineural hearing loss is the most common birth defect in the United States. About 3 babies born in this country out of every 1,000 have significant hearing loss and more lose their hearing during childhood (National Institutes of Health, 2006; White, 1996). Approximately 6 per 1,000 children in addition to the 3 per 1,000 will have permanent hearing loss by the time they begin school (American Speech-Language-Hearing Association, 1993).

In this chapter, the focus will be on infants and young children who have prelingual hearing loss. As noted in Chapter 1, children who have prelingual hearing loss had their hearing losses while learning language and speech. They may have been born with hearing loss or they may have lost their hearing early in life, perhaps as a result of meningitis, high fever, or head trauma. Figure 14-2 presents an overview of what happens when a baby is identified with hearing loss. The process begins with an evaluation, which entails detection and identification of the hearing loss and a consideration of etiology and other health concerns. This is followed by a preparatory process for the early-intervention program, which includes parent counseling and development of an aural rehabilitation strategy. It concludes with the implementation of the strategy and the program.

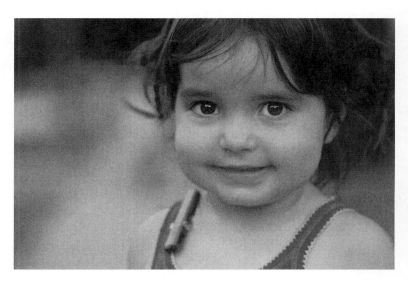

FIGURE 14-1. Incidence of hearing loss. More than 1.4 million children in the United States have a significant hearing loss. *Photograph courtesy of MED-EL Corp.*

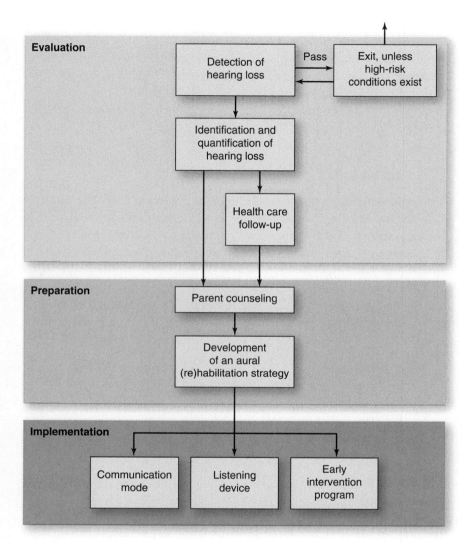

FIGURE 14-2. An overview of what happens when a baby is identified as having a hearing loss.

During the first 3 years of life, children experience their most intensive stage of speech and language development. If they are not exposed to language during this time because of hearing loss, they will likely experience difficulty in acquiring language and speech, and later, delays in developing literacy skills. During the early years, the brain develops the neural pathways and cognitive skills necessary for interpreting auditory information. If a child with significant hearing loss receives intervention early on, as opposed to later, he or she will have a much better chance of developing communication skills that are comparable to a child who has normal hearing (National Institutes of Health, 2006).

DETECTION OF HEARING LOSS

At least two events may trigger a parent or caregiver to bring a baby or young child to an audiologist for a hearing test. The first is that the child may have failed a screening test. The second is that a parent may have noticed the child is not responding to sound in the same way as children who have normal hearing.

Universal Newborn Hearing Screening

Universal newborn hearing screening (UNHS) results in the screening for hearing loss for all newborn infants.

The newborn nursery, also called the well-baby nursery, is a hospital unit designed to provide care for healthy newborn infants.

Universal newborn hearing screening (often referred to by the acronym UNHS) or Early Hearing Detection and Intervention (often referred to by the acronym EHDI), where every baby born is tested for hearing loss in the **newborn nursery**, has increasingly become the standard of care in the United States and in many places in Europe. Prior to the proliferation of UNHS, children who had hearing loss were often not identified until the age of 2 years or older. This reality was in contrast to goals established by national health organizations for persons with hearing loss. These organizations called for identification to occur in the first few months of life (Hergils & Hergils, 2000); for example:

- National Institutes of Health, United States (1993): 3 months
- Socialstyrelsen (The National Board of Health and Welfare), Sweden (1994): before 1 year
- National Deaf Children's Society, United Kingdom (1994): 80% by 12 months

In 1999, the federal Newborn Infant Hearing Screening and Intervention Act was signed into law in the United States, and was designed to provide up to 3 years of grant funding for states to develop screening and intervention services. The initiative grows increasingly successful. As of 2007, more than four out of five states and the District of Columbia had enacted legislation requiring newborn screening (Centers for Disease Control and Prevention, 2007) and several more states have voluntary compliance programs. About 90% of babies in the United States are screened before going home from the newborn nursery (White, 2004). In Europe, this percentage is as high as 98% (e.g., Poland, Sliwa, Kochanek, Durrant, & Smurzynski, 2008). Appendix 14-1 presents terminology that speech and hearing professionals might encounter if they work in a UNHS program.

Screening is a "pass/refer" procedure, meaning either that the baby is found to have normal hearing or that there is reason to suspect a hearing loss exists. If hearing loss is suspected (i.e., a "refer" result is obtained), the baby is referred for a complete audiological workup that will assess the child's hearing bilaterally and at all of the audiometric frequencies. Babies who fail the screening test but who turn out to have normal hearing are examples of **false-positive** results. In a typical newborn screening program, the false-positive rate may range from 2% of babies tested to 7%. Many programs rescreen babies who fail the screening the first time before they leave the newborn nursery. This practice pushes the false-positive rate toward the lower end of 2% (Gorga et al., 2001; Stewart et al., 2000). The use of rescreening can serve to minimize anxiety experienced by parents whose babies fail the screening the first time. In addition, because many babies who do not pass the hearing screening do not return for follow-up, more accurate screening means that fewer babies are lost to follow-up (Hall, Smith, & Popelka, 2004). Ideally the false-negative rate of UNHS programs is zero. The **false-negative** rate is the proportion of babies who have hearing loss who were missed during screening.

A **false-positive** occurs when a baby does not have a hearing loss but fails the screening test.

A **false-negative** occurs when a baby has hearing loss but passes the screening test.

Methods used for screening include otoacoustic emissions (OAEs) and automated auditory brain stem response testing (A-ABR), two procedures that will be described shortly. Screening is designed to detect hearing loss of 30 to 40 dB HL in the frequency region of about 500 to 4,000 Hz.

Support for UNHS stems from research showing that if hearing loss is identified before a child reaches the age of 6 months, and intervention is received, then that child will achieve language scores that compare favorably to children who have normal hearing, by the age of 3 years (Yoshinaga-Itano, Sedey, Coulter, & Mehl, 1998; Figure 14-3). This is not

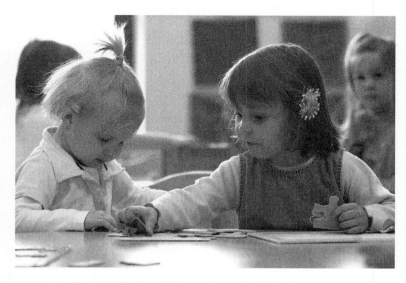

FIGURE 14-3. Early identification. Children who are identified as having hearing loss before the age of 6 months and who receive early intervention have a good chance of developing language skills that compare favorably with their peers who have normal hearing. *Photograph courtesy of MED-EL Corp.*

true of children who are not identified early and who do not receive intervention. Yoshinaga-Itano and Gravel (2001, pp. 63–64) summarize the importance of UNHS with the following checklist:

- Children with early-identified hearing loss who receive appropriate intervention services demonstrate significantly better language, speech, and social-emotional development than later-identified children.
- Early-identified children with intervention have language development similar to their nonverbal cognitive development.
- Early-identified children with intervention and normal cognitive development maintain language development in the low average range throughout the first 5 years of life.
- The better the language development, the less parental stress there is, and the better personal-social development of children.
- Four out of every five children born in hospitals with newborn hearing screening programs have language development in the low-average range between 1 and 5 years of age when they have hearing loss only and no secondary disabilities. These statistics compare to outcomes of later-identified children in which only one in every five children have language development commensurate with that of children who hear normally.

Some babies are particularly at risk for hearing loss. Risk factors associated with hearing loss include the following (Joint Committee on Infant Hearing, 1994):

- Low birth weight (less than 3.3 lbs)
- Family history of hearing loss
- In utero infections such as cytomegalovirus, rubella, or herpes
- Ototoxic medications
- Low **Apgar scores** (which reflect the normalcy of A = appearance, P = pulse, G = grimace, A = activity, and R = respiration at the time of birth)
- Need for use of a ventilator for 5 days or longer
- Craniofacial anomalies
- Physical manifestations consistent with a syndrome
- Bacterial meningitis
- Hyperbilirubinemia (severe jaundice) at levels that require an exchange transfusion

However, although these risk factors often trigger a suspicion of hearing loss, it is important to remember that almost 50 percent of children who have hearing loss do not have risk factors at birth.

An **Apgar score** is a numeric value between 1 and 10 assigned to newborns to describe their physical status at birth.

Once a baby has been identified in a screening program as potentially having a hearing loss, the results are communicated to the family in a "sensitive and timely manner" (Task Force on Newborn and Infant Hearing, 1999). A follow-up evaluation is scheduled as soon as possible. A baby who fails a newborn screening test should receive an appropriate audiologic and medical evaluation to confirm the presence of hearing loss, preferably by the age of 3 months. The baby with a confirmed hearing loss should begin to receive services before the age of 6 months (Joint Committee on Infant Hearing, 2000).

Even if a baby passes the newborn screening test, a speech and hearing professional might want to alert parents to watch for the tell-tale signs of hearing loss, especially if risk factors are present. Childhood hearing loss can occur after birth, so it is essential that some children undergo screening after leaving the hospital. At 6 months of age, babies with a risk factor for hearing loss should be retested, and then retested every 6 months thereafter until the age of 3 years (Joint Committee on Infant Hearing, 2000). A handout like that presented in the Key Resources section might be provided to parents when they leave the hospital with their new baby. Parents might be encouraged to monitor during the first year whether their babies react to loud noises, respond to their names, or localize to sound. At age 2 years, children should imitate simple words and play with their voices. At age 3 years, children usually begin to understand simple phrases, such as "all gone" and "time to go bye-bye."

Learning of the Hearing Loss Later On

Sometimes parents do not learn of their child's hearing loss until later on, perhaps because the loss occurred after the child left the newborn nursery or later in childhood. Parents may tell their speech and hearing professional how they suspected a hearing loss in their baby, and took the baby to the family doctor or pediatrician. The doctor may have dismissed the parents' concerns, and thereby have delayed diagnosis for several months or even years. As a result, the child was delayed in receiving amplification and intervention services. Some parents may express guilt because they did not follow their instincts and pursue second opinions. Other parents may express anger because they feel that the hearing loss could have been prevented. They may tell of taking their child to the hospital with a high fever and then being sent home with a diagnosis of a viral infection. Within hours, the child's condition worsened, with increased fever and seizures. Though the child will have survived a bout of what was ultimately diagnosed as meningitis, he or she will have been left with serious hearing loss that the parents believe might have been prevented (Kravitz & Selekman, 1992).

"People always seem surprised that I didn't discover my daughter's deafness until she was 19 months old. In fact, the possibility had crossed my mind when she didn't start talking. The pediatrician assured me that since she was babbling, she was also hearing. But I didn't do the one thing that would have told me for sure: I didn't make a loud noise when my baby was asleep to see if it would wake her up. Which is how I know that I had no intention of learning the truth just then."

Wendy Lichtman, mother of a college-age daughter with profound hearing loss
(Lichtman, 2005, p. 120)

IDENTIFICATION AND QUANTIFICATION OF HEARING LOSS

When a hearing loss is suspected, a child's hearing may be tested in a variety of ways. The selection of a measurement technique is dependent on the age of the child and his or her ability to participate in the test procedures. Once a hearing loss has been identified, hearing should be tested twice each year for young children, and four times or more annually if other problems are present or if there is concern about the accuracy of the test results. Older children usually need to be evaluated only once a year.

Objective Tests

Two objective tests are used to determine the presence of hearing loss: auditory brain stem response (ABR) and otoacoustic emissions (OAEs).

Auditory Brain Stem Response Test

Auditory brain stem response (ABR) testing often is used with babies between the ages of birth and 5 months. Surface electrodes are placed on the child's head, and neural activity elicited by the presentation of tone bursts or sound clicks is recorded. The auditory brain stem response is the electrophysiological response to an acoustic stimulus, and originates from the eighth cranial nerve and auditory brain stem. Potentials are categorized in terms of their latency, or the time at which they appear following acoustic stimulation. They usually occur between 1 and 15 msec following the presentation of a click. A standard ABR recording contains seven peaks. The "wave/peak V detection threshold" correlates well with hearing sensitivity in the 1,500–4,000 Hz region. For a comprehensive ABR test, the child usually must be sedated or at least asleep, as the patient must be very still in order to obtain accurate test results. ABRs can be used to determine the degree of hearing loss at the different audiometric frequencies. ABRs yield thresholds within 10 dB of behavioral thresholds (Stapells, 2002). However, ABRs cannot be used to determine how much residual hearing a child has beyond about 90 **dB nHL. Auditory steady state evoked potentials (ASSEP)**, a fairly new procedure that presents pure tones as stimuli, can be used to determine thresholds that are greater than 90 dB nHL.

For screening purposes, a variation of ABR, sometimes called an automated ABR (A-ABR), might be used. For example, ALGO is an automated ABR screening device, which compares the baby's ABR response to a stored template of expected brain waveforms (Herrman, Thornton, & Joseph, 1995). The response is scored as either a pass or a failure. It is effective in identifying infants with a moderate or greater degree of hearing loss (see Hayes, 2003, for a review of ABR as a screening instrument).

Otoacoustic Emissions Testing

Otoacoustic emissions (OAEs) are inaudible sounds that are the by-products of the mechanical actions of the outer hair cells in the cochlea. When sound stimulates the cochlea, the hair cells vibrate and initiate a signal in the eighth cranial nerve. Simultaneously, the vibration produces a sound that can be measured with a small probe inserted into the ear canal. Sound is presented, and the OAE is detected and traced. Persons who have normal hearing produce OAEs, whereas those who have hearing loss of 30–40 dB HL or greater do not. The procedure is widely used as a screening procedure. It is quick and painless to administer and does not require the cooperation of the patient, other than to remain relatively still.

When used for newborn screening, OAEs are often collected by a nurse, technician, or volunteer, although an audiologist may be on the hospital staff and will supervise the overall screening efforts. Only about 34% of the personnel who perform newborn screenings in the hospital are audiologists (Arehart, Yoshinaga-Itano, Thomson, Gabbard, & Brown, 1998). The screening professional often uses a hand-held otoacoustic emissions screener. It flashes a *pass* on the screening unit when an OAE is present, and a *refer* when it is not. Frequencies important for speech recognition are typically tested, such as 2,000, 3,000, 4,000, and 5,000 Hz (e.g., Hall et al., 2004). Children who do not pass are checked for middle ear effusion and then rescreened if necessary.

OAEs can also be used to assess hearing status of babies during more comprehensive diagnostic evaluations. **Distortion product otoacoustic emissions (DPOAE)**, or sometimes **transient evoked otoacoustic emissions (TEOAE)**, can be measured for frequency-select regions, which can help predict a baby's audiogram. DPOAEs entail the simultaneous presentation of two pure tones, and then the measurement of the resulting distortion product. Typically, an otoacoustic emission for a given frequency region may be recorded if the baby's hearing threshold for that region is better than 30 or 40 dB HL (Sininger, 2002).

Behavioral Tests

When a child is very young, it may not be possible to obtain an audiogram using traditional behavioral techniques. Thus, to obtain information about the child's ability to detect a range of frequencies, the audiologist may utilize behavioral/observational audiometry, visual reinforcement audiometry, or conditioned play audiometry.

Auditory brain stem response (ABR) is an auditory evoked potential that originates from the eighth cranial nerve and auditory brainstem structures. The electrophysiological record consists of five to seven peaks, which represent the neural functioning of the auditory pathway.

dB nHL (decibels normalized hearing level) is a decibel notation that is referenced to behavioral thresholds of a group of persons with normal hearing and is used to describe the intensity level of stimuli used in evoked potential audiometry.

Auditory steady state evoked potentials (ASSEP) are elicited by amplitude-modulated pure tones (or noise), and provide frequency-specific information; they may be used to determine thresholds that exceed 90 dB nHL.

Otoacoustic emissions (OAEs) are low-level sound emitted spontaneously by the cochlea on presentation of an auditory stimulus.

A **distortion product otoacoustic emission (DPOAE)** is the acoustic energy created by stimulating the ear with two simultaneous pure tones (f1 and f2), which results in energy created at several frequencies that are combinations of the two pure tones. DPOEs entail the measurement of 2f1-f2.

Transient evoked otoacoustic emission (TEOAE) is a means to access the integrity and function of the outer hair cells by presenting brief clicks. The low-level acoustic response emitted by the cochlea is measured.

Behavioral/Observational Audiometry

In **behavioral/observational audiometry (BOA)**, sometimes referred to as Auditory Behavior Index (ABI), the audiologist presents a sound stimulus and observes the child's behavior. Response to sound may be manifested by a change in sucking pattern, eye widening, cessation of activity, or a head turn.

One shortcoming of BOA is that babies vary in their responsiveness. Some 3-month-old babies will react to sound presented at 20 dB HL, whereas others will not react until the sound reaches 80 dB HL. For this reason, the procedure can reliably only eliminate the possibility of profound hearing loss. In addition, babies respond differently to sound, depending on their level of arousal, on how many times they have heard the sound (i.e., habituation occurs), and whether the sound is of interest to them (e.g., speech as opposed to tone pips). Finally, the observer's expectations can color the results: When someone wants to see a response from a baby, the person may see it, whether it really occurred or not.

Visual Reinforcement Audiometry

Visual reinforcement audiometry (VRA) is used with children between the ages of 6 months and $2\frac{1}{2}$ years. VRA takes advantage of a baby's natural inclination to turn toward sound. It is an example of an operant-**conditioned response**. The child is tested in a sound-treated room. Sound is presented through an audiometer. When sound is presented initially, a box in the room lights up. Inside of the box is a toy that moves. For example, a box may light up to reveal a toy monkey clashing cymbals or a video clip may play. The child learns to look at the box or video clip when the sound is presented, and then testing begins to determine the threshold for the frequencies of the audiogram. Ear-specific information may be obtained if the child is willing to tolerate insert earphones.

Conditioned Play Audiometry

Conditioned play audiometry (CPA) is used to assess children at about the age of 2 to $2\frac{1}{2}$ years. Children may place a peg into a pegboard each time a sound is presented (Figure 14-4). He or she may drop a block into a jar. The child is encouraged to wait and listen and then perform the response task when the sound is presented. The child's parent may sit in the sound-treated room with the child during testing, whereas the audiologist may be in the adjacent room with the audiometer, watching through the window. The parent must be coached to sit quietly and not provide cues about the presence or absence of sound to the child. When a child is capable of participating in CPA, it may also be possible to obtain

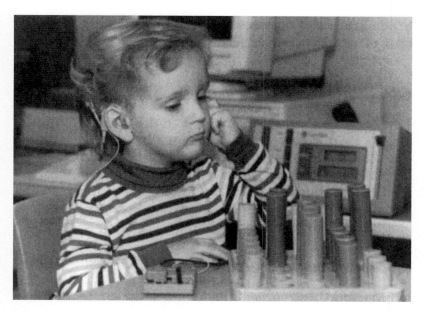

FIGURE 14-4. Conditioned play audiometry. A young child listens for a sound and places a peg into the pegboard every time he hears one. *Photograph by Patti Gabriel, courtesy of the Central Institute for the Deaf.*

speech detection thresholds (SDTs). The SDTs will provide a means to cross-check the audiometric thresholds obtained with CPA.

Speech detection threshold (SDT) is the level at which speech is just audible.

HEALTH CARE FOLLOW-UP

Many children who fail a hearing screening and most children who are identified as having hearing loss will be referred to other health care professionals and/or for additional audiological testing. The purpose is to determine etiology and to determine whether additional concerns are present besides hearing loss, including other disabilities and hearing-related conditions. Referrals may occur shortly after identification and/or several years following, when the child is a toddler or a preschooler.

Causes of Hearing Loss in Children

One of the first priorities of many aural rehabilitation plans for infants or toddlers is to determine etiology. Hearing loss can be sensorineural, conductive, or mixed. Sensorineural hearing loss may be **idiopathic**, meaning that the origin is unknown or uncertain, or may stem from nongenetic or genetic causes. Figure 14-5 presents causes of prelingual hearing loss in children.

An **idiopathic** hearing loss is a hearing loss with unknown origin.

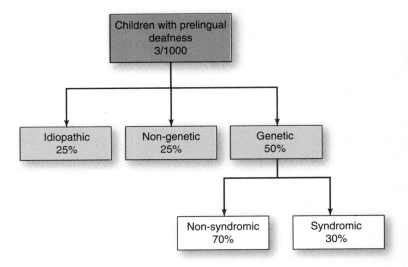

FIGURE 14-5. Causes of prelingual deafness in children. *Modeled after Smith and Camp (2007).*

Nongenetic Causes of Sensorineural Hearing Loss

Nongenetic causes may be **prenatal** (occurring before birth), **perinatal** (occurring at birth), or **postnatal** (occurring shortly after birth). Prenatal factors that may affect a child's hearing status include the following:

Prenatal means before birth.

Perinatal means during birth.

Postnatal means after birth.

Cytomegalovirus (CMV) is a member of the herpes virus.

- Intrauterine infections, including rubella, **cytomegalovirus**, and herpes simplex virus
- Complications associated with the Rh factor (wherein maternal antibodies affect the Rh-positive blood cells of the baby)
- Prematurity
- Maternal diabetes
- Parental radiation
- **Toxemia**
- **Anoxia**
- Syphilis

Toxemia is a condition during pregnancy that is characterized by hypertension, or a sharp spike in blood pressure, and edema, or a swelling of the hands and feet as a result of excessive body fluid.

Anoxia refers to a deficiency or absence of oxygen in the body tissues.

Hearing loss may be incurred during birth, in which case it stems from a perinatal cause. Perinatal causes of hearing loss include anoxia, which may be caused by a prolapse of the umbilical cord and a subsequent blockage of blood to the infant's brain. Although rare, the use of forceps during birth may cause damage to the cochlea, as might severe uterine contractions.

Cytomegalovirus: A Common Virus with a Potent Kick

Between 20% and 30% of childhood hearing loss may be caused by cytomegalovirus (CMV). CMV is a member of the herpes family that infects 50% to 80% of adults by age 40 years. Members of the herpes family cause chicken pox, infectious mononucleosis, and fever blisters. The herpes viruses are capable of remaining alive, if dormant, in the body for a lifetime. Typically, CMV causes no symptoms. It can be spread person to person, and is carried by body fluids, including blood, urine, breast milk, tears, and saliva. Usually, CMV is fairly harmless and many people will never know they have it. However, individuals who are at risk for active infection and serious complications are babies born to women who are infected with CMV for the first time during pregnancy and pregnant women who work with infants and children, as in a day-care facility.

In otherwise healthy children, symptoms of an active infection include prolonged high fever, chills, fatigue, headache, and general malaise. Most infected newborns are asymptomatic at birth, although some may present with **microcehpaly**, circulation problems, or abnormal tone. In some cases, infected babies will develop symptoms over the next few years. This means that they may not be identified as having hearing loss during a newborn screening procedure. Symptoms that may arise later, in addition to hearing loss, include mental retardation, developmental delays, coordination problems, and visual impairment. CMV is diagnosed with laboratory tests that detect antibodies within the body that have been developed in response to CMV or that detect the virus as an active infection (Directors of Health Promotion and Education, 2007; Rivera et al., 2002).

Microcephaly is an abnormally small head due to a failure of the brain to grow.

A postnatal loss may occur because of meningitis or other infection or use of ototoxic drugs. One report suggests that about 25% of bilateral childhood hearing loss is postnatal (Weichbold, Nekahm-Heis, & Weizl-Mueller, 2007), which is good motivation for continued surveillance of children after they leave the newborn nursery, particularly those at risk for hearing loss. A listing of ototoxic drugs appears in Table 14-1. Other postnatal factors include measles, encephalitis, chicken pox, influenza, and mumps.

Table 14-1. Medications that may be ototoxic.

• Aminoglycoside antibiotics, which are often used against gram-negative bacteria. Hearing loss is often bilateral and sensorineural. Some of the drugs may be more vestibulotoxic than cochleotoxic: **Amikacin** **Dihydrostreptomycin** **Garamycin** **Gentamicin** **Kanamycin** **Neomycin** **Netilmicin** **Streptomycin** **Tobramycin** **Viomycin**
• Salicylates, used in large quantities for the treatment of arthritis and other connective tissue disorders. Their use may result in sensorineural hearing loss and tinnitus: **Acetylsalicylic acid** **Aspirin**
• Loop diuretics, used to promote urine excretion. Their use may result in sensorineural hearing loss: **Ethacrynic acid** **Furosemide** **Lasix**
• Other drugs that may be ototoxic and that are used in chemotherapy regimens: **Cisplatin** **Carboplatin** **Nitrogen mustard**

Adapted from *Comprehensive Dictionary of Audiology* (2nd ed.) by B. A. Stach, 2003, Clifton Park, NY: Delmar Learning.

Genetic Causes of Sensorineural Hearing Loss

Genetic factors are thought to cause more than 50% of all incidents of congenital hearing loss in children. More than 400 kinds of genetic-based hearing losses have been described, and with increased activity in genetics research and the Human Genome Project, new types continually are being identified (Gorlin, Toriello, & Cohen, 1995).

Genetic hearing loss is distinguished from acquired (or nongenetic) hearing loss by physical examination, family history, ancillary medical testing such as a **computed tomography (CT) scan** of the skull, and molecular genetic testing (Smith & Van Camp, 2007). The physical examination may be performed by a physician specially trained to recognize genetic conditions, and may include a probing for subtle characteristics that relate to specific conditions (e.g., small pits in the front of the ears may implicate Branchio-oto-renal syndrome). In considering the family history, a genetic counselor may construct a **family tree**, covering about three generations. Special attention will be paid to family members who have/had hearing

A **computed tomography (CT) scan** creates a series of detailed pictures of areas inside of the body, taken from different angles or planes. The pictures are created by a computer that is linked to an x-ray machine.

A **family tree** is a genealogical diagram of a child's ancestry or kin.

loss, and other conditions that relatives may have manifested. Genetic testing may involve **chromosome** tests, where chromosomes are examined under the microscope to see if a part of a chromosome is missing or duplicated. Appendix 14-2 presents a list of terminology and corresponding definitions that might be encountered when discussing a diagnosis of genetic hearing loss.

A **chromosome** is a basic unit of genes; structures that carry the genes of a cell.

Hereditary hearing losses are often classified according to (a) the mode of inheritance (**autosomal dominant**, **autosomal recessive**, or **X-linked**), (b) whether they are syndromic or nonsyndromic, (c) the audiological configuration, (d) whether they are bilateral or unilateral, (e) the progression (e.g., sudden or gradual) and age of onset of the loss, and (f) whether or not the vestibular system is affected. Many people who have a hereditary hearing loss experience a delayed onset that is nonsyndromic (Tomaski & Grundfast, 1999). Patients who have a **delayed-onset hereditary** disorder may have normal hearing at birth and then begin to lose hearing later, sometimes not until they are in their 20s or 30s. A **nonsyndromic hearing loss** is one that has no other associated findings.

An **autosomal dominant** condition requires only one parent to have the affected gene in order to pass a trait onto an offspring.

An **autosomal recessive** condition requires both parents to have the affected gene in order to pass a trait onto an offspring; the parents may not exhibit the trait.

An **X-linked** condition involves genes carried on the X chromosome, or the sex chromosome.

Many hearing losses based in genetics are part of a **syndrome**, which refers to a number of conditions that occur together and characterize a common origin. For example, Waardenburg syndrome (WS) is the most common type of autosomal dominant syndromic hearing loss. It is characterized by a varying degree of sensorineural hearing loss, pigmentary discolorations of the skin, a white forelock in the hair, and the two irises of the eyes being of different color.

A **delayed-onset hereditary hearing loss** occurs when hearing is normal at birth, then declines later in life as a result of a hereditary disorder.

Nonsyndromic hearing loss is a hearing loss that has no other associated findings.

Usher syndrome is the most common type of autosomal recessive syndromic hearing loss. Affected individuals are born with a degree of sensorineural hearing loss and then develop **retinitis pigmentosa**, usually sometime after the first decade of life. Retinitis pigmentosa leads to night blindness and loss of peripheral vision and ultimately, possible blindness.

A **syndrome** is a collection of conditions that co-occur as a result of a single cause and constitute a distinct clinical entity.

Retinitis pigmentosa is any number of inherited, progressive conditions that cause abnormal pigmentation on the retina. Retinitis pigmentosa often impairs vision, with first a loss of night vision, then a loss of peripheral vision, and then the development of "tunnel vision." It finally causes blindness.

Alport syndrome is an example of X-linked syndromic hearing loss. It is characterized by progressive sensorineural hearing loss, renal disease, and ophthalmologic involvement. In Alport syndrome, the hearing loss usually does not manifest until the second decade of life (see Smith and van Camp, 2007, for a review of syndromes that involve hearing loss). Examples of other syndromes that may involve the auditory system appear in Table 14-2.

Mixed and Conductive Hearing Loss

Some children have mixed hearing loss, which is a combination of both conductive and sensorineural components, or a conductive hearing loss alone. The most common cause of a conductive component is otitis media,

Table 14-2. Examples of syndromes that may include hearing loss.

SYNDROME	CO-OCCURRING CONDITIONS
Alport	Nephritis and sensorineural hearing loss
Alstrom	Pigmentary retinopathy, diabetes mellitus, obesity, malformation of the brain, and progressive sensorineural hearing loss
Bjornstad syndrome	Congenital sensorineural hearing loss and pili torti
Branchio-otorenal syndrome	Branchial anomalies, including branchial clefts, fistulas and cysts; otologic anomalies including malformed pinna or preauricular pits; renal abnormalities; often, hearing loss, either conductive, sensorineural, or mixed
Crouzon	Premature closure of sutures, hypertension, downward displacement of eyeballs due to shallow orbits, mild to moderate conductive hearing loss, may entail mixed loss; closure of external auditory canal
Down	Mental retardation, characteristic facial features, often accompanied by chronic otitis media, and associated conductive, mixed, and sensorineural hearing loss
Edward	Microcephaly, agenesis of bones, congenital heart disease, craniofacial abnormalities, mental retardation, and outer, middle, and inner ear anomalies
Epstein	Macrothrombocytopathia, nephritis, and sensorineural hearing loss
Fetal alcohol syndrome	Low birth weight, failure to thrive, mental retardation, wide-set eyes, recurrent otitis media, sensorineural hearing loss
Formey	Joint fusion, mitral insufficiency, and conductive hearing loss
Harboyan	Characterized by progressive sensorineural hearing loss of delayed onset
Hunter	Sensorineural, conductive, or mixed hearing loss, growth deficiency, mental and neurological deterioration, coarse facial features
Jervell and Lange-Nielsen	Electrocardiographic abnormalities, fainting spells, and accompanied by congenital bilateral profound sensorineural hearing loss
Latham-Munro	Myoclonus epilepsy, ataxia, and sensorineural hearing loss
Lemieux-Neemeh	Nephritis, motor and neuropathy with sensorineural hearing loss
Mondini dysplasia	Congenital anomaly of the osseous and membranous labyrinths, severe loss of hearing and vestibular function
Pendred	Goiter and moderate-to-profound congenital sensorineural hearing loss
Pfeiffer	Premature closure of sutures, broad thumbs, broad great toes, short fingers and toes, hypertelorism, high arched palate, downward-sloping eyes, absent external auditory canals, conductive hearing loss
Richards-Rundle	Ataxia, muscle wasting, hypogonadism, mental retardation, and progressive sensorineural hearing loss
Robinson	Dominant onychodystrophy, coniform teeth, and sensorineural hearing loss
Stickler	Severe myopia, retinal detachment, flat facial profile, cleft palate, ocular anomalies, arthritis, sensorineural, conductive, or mixed hearing loss
Treacher Collins	Pinnae malformations, down-slanting eyes, small chin, depressed cheek bones, large mouth, eyelid colobomar, conductive hearing loss related to atresia and ossicular malformation
Usher	Congenital sensorineural hearing loss and progressive loss of vision
Waardenburg	Widely spaced eyes, joined eyebrows, a broad nasal root, and a minimal to severe unilateral or bilateral hearing loss (about 30% of patients have a white forelock)

which is the second most common childhood ailment, second only to the common cold. Other causes of conductive hearing loss include anomalies of the external ear canal, tympanic membrane, or ossicles and congenital **cholesteatoma**.

As noted in Chapter 1, otitis media is an inflammation of the middle ear, often associated with the buildup of fluid. The fluid may or may not be contaminated with infection. An estimated 35% of preschool children experience repeated episodes of otitis media (American Speech-Language-Hearing Association, 2007). Otitis media can result in a mild or moderate conductive hearing loss, particularly in the low frequencies, and can accentuate the amount of hearing loss in the presence of an existing sensorineural loss. The other symptoms of otitis media, besides hearing loss, and the severity, duration, and frequency of the inflammation vary between children. Some children will experience the condition one time and then never again and only experience slight pain and fever. Others will experience repeated bouts, with "glue-like" fluid, excruciating ear pain, and permanent hearing loss (due to damage to the ossicles and/or tympanic membrane).

A **cholesteatoma** is a tumorlike mass of epithelium cells and cholesterol in the middle ear that may invade the mastoid process and impinge upon the ossicular chain.

In the absence of pain and fever, the condition may go unnoticed by the child, and hence, untreated. As a result, the child may miss out on being exposed to some speech and language. Although the findings are inconsistent and the results somewhat contradictory, there is some evidence that academic performance may suffer in the early grades if children with otherwise normal hearing suffer from chronic otitis media (Golz, Netzer, & Westerman, 2005). Pediatricians report that otitis media between the ages of birth and 2 years can adversely affect speech and language development, although parents and day-care environments can mitigate against this outcome (Sonnenschein & Cascella, 2004). Otitis media in the early years puts children at risk for reduced consonant inventories, delayed babbling, and smaller expressive and receptive vocabularies, although these effects may disappear if the otitis media is resolved (see Shriberg et al., 2000, for a review). For instance, Keogh et al. (2005) reported that on average, children with a history of otitis media recognized connected discourse in noise as well as children without a history did, when they had reached the age of 9 or 10 years. The authors note that their participants who had a history of otitis media exhibited a wider range of performance, suggesting that a subset of children may indeed continue to be at risk for hearing-related difficulties. Some of the symptoms that might alert parents to the presence of otitis media in their young child include inattentiveness, reduced ability to discriminate speech, wanting the television turned up more loudly than usual, hands pulling the ear lobes, and undue fatigue.

Facts About Otitis Media

Here are some facts about children in the United States and otitis media (Janota, 1999, p. 48):

- About 50% of children have a bout of otitis media by their first birthday and 80% by their third.
- Otitis media is two to four times less prevalent in African American children than in White children.
- Otitis media is the most common reason a child under 15 years of age visits a physician.
- 30 million doctor visits a year are caused by otitis media.
- Otitis media is the most frequent reason why doctors prescribe antibiotic therapy for children.
- The surgical treatment of middle ear effusion is the most frequent reason for administering general anesthesia to children.

Other Disabilities

Cerebral palsy is a motor-control disorder caused by insult to the motor cortex of the brain.

Nearly 40% of children who have hearing loss have an additional disability (Gallaudet Research Institute, 2003). Co-occurring conditions include mental retardation, significant visual impairment, learning disabilities, and attention deficit disorder. Emotional or behavioral problems, **cerebral palsy**, and orthopedic problems also may co-occur with hearing loss. Sometimes, the multiple disabilities stem from similar causes, such as trauma at birth or prematurity. Causes may also relate to ethnic background and heredity. Table 14-3 presents conditions that commonly co-occur with hearing loss. The relatively high frequency of co-occurring conditions suggests that the speech and hearing professional will need to take these into account when developing a child's intervention plan and aural rehabilitation strategy and when working as a member of the child's multidisciplinary team.

Other Hearing-Related Conditions

Children may suffer from other hearing-related conditions besides sensorineural, conductive, and mixed hearing loss. Three such conditions are central auditory processing disorder (CAPD), auditory neuropathy (sometimes referred to as auditory dyssynchrony), and tinnitus.

Table 14-3. Conditions that may co-occur with hearing loss.

- Mental retardation
- Behavior or psychiatric disorders
- Learning disability, related to reading and/or writing
- Nervous system ailments, such as seizures, vestibular disturbances, or spina bifida
- Eye disease, including optic degeneration, ocular lens abnormalities, and retinitis pigmentosa
- Renal disease
- Musculoskeletal abnormalities in the skull, oral cavity, face, outer and/or middle ear, limbs, or joints
- Musculoskeletal disease, such as growth retardation or bone disease
- Growth retardation
- Cerebral palsy
- Skin disease, such as pigmentary disorder (e.g., albinism, white forelock, iris bicolor, or heterochromia), keratosis, sun sensitivity, thick, coarse hair, and malformed fingernails and toenails
- Metabolic disease such as diabetes, goiter, liver and spleen enlargement, or impaired metabolism or carbohydrates
- Cardiac and vascular disease

Central Auditory Processing Disorders (CAPDs)

Some hearing losses are due to central causes, which means that sound transmission between the brain stem and the cerebrum is disrupted, as a result of either damage or a malformation. Thus, the temporal cortex of the brain may receive incorrect information, or the information may not be processed correctly. These deficiencies in auditory processing skills sometimes are referred to as a **central auditory processing disorder (CAPD)**.

CAPD may result from head trauma, brain tumors, autism, or neurological vascular changes. Sometimes, a cause cannot be found. This is a difficult diagnosis to make. Many times, the problem is not implicit in the audiogram. A parent might comment, "He hears me, but many times I have to repeat myself several times before he gets what I'm saying." A day-care worker might note, "Whenever I talk to Mary, I find myself slowing down how fast I talk and accentuating my articulation. Otherwise, she gets this blank look on her face, as if her mind is somewhere else."

Children who have central hearing problems usually experience difficulty in one or more of the following:

- Localizing and lateralizing sound
- Auditory discrimination

Central auditory processing disorder (CAPD) is an inability to differentiate, recognize, and understand sounds. This inability is not due to either hearing loss or cognitive impairment.

- Auditory pattern recognition
- Associating meaning to sound
- Listening in noise
- Understanding degraded speech signals, fast speech, or speech with an unfamiliar accent
- Following rhythmic and melodic aspects of music
- Auditory memory

Although screening questionnaires, checklists, and related measures probe the kinds of difficulties included in this list, there is no universally accepted method of screening. There are, however, recognized CAPD diagnostic test batteries. The battery may include measures of auditory discrimination, auditory temporal processing and patterning, and dichotic speech tests. These diagnostic test batteries are typically inappropriate for children 3 years and younger, so diagnosis might have to wait until the child is older (American Speech-Language-Hearing Association, 2005b).

Auditory Neuropathy

Auditory neuropathy is a condition where the patient has a pure-tone audiogram that shows any degree of hearing loss, from mild to profound, and shows normal OAEs. ABRs are either absent or degraded, and word discrimination is reduced disproportionately to the pure tone loss.

Auditory neuropathy is thought to be related to CAPD, albeit different because it involves the peripheral auditory system. Children who receive a diagnosis of *auditory neuropathy* typically have a mild to moderate sensorineural hearing loss, and they exhibit OAEs. They have either absent or abnormal ABRs and poor word recognition, poorer than that which would be predicted by their audiological thresholds. Because OAEs are present, whereas ABRs are not, the disorder is believed to stem from problems with the auditory nerve or spiral ganglion, although the exact cause is unknown (see Rance, McKay, & Graden, 2004). Unfortunately, for many children who have auditory neuropathy, hearing aids are not very helpful.

Tinnitus

Not only do adults suffer from tinnitus (Chapter 11), children too may experience sound in their heads that has no external cause. In fact, tinnitus may be experienced by 25% to 55% of children who have hearing loss. Just like adults, tinnitus may inflict deleterious effects, including insomnia, emotional trauma (e.g., fear and worry), physical symptoms, attention difficulties, and listening challenges (Holgers & Juul, 2006; Kentish, Crocker, & McKenna, 2000). Tinnitus may be hard to detect in children because they may have always had it (so it seems like the normal state of affairs) or they may lack the words to describe the phenomenon.

PARENT COUNSELING

After their child's hearing loss has been identified, and before and/or during the time that they learn more about the nature of the hearing loss and related conditions, parents will receive counseling. Between 90 and 95% of children who have a severe or profound sensorineural hearing loss have parents who are normally hearing (Northern & Downs, 1991). This means that, prior to their child's birth, the parents may have been unfamiliar with the many ramifications of hearing loss. They also are unlikely to be members of the Deaf culture (Chapter 11). Thus, they will have much to learn about hearing loss and aural rehabilitation, and they will need to make a decision as to whether to try to learn how to sign. They may also need to consider issues concerning the Deaf culture. They may not (or may) be in agreement with the goal of enculturation of their child into a culture that is different from their own.

The advent of UNHS has in large measure changed the discovery mechanism of hearing loss. Whereas previously hearing loss was often suspected by parents through observation, now discovery is often "institution-initiated" (Luterman, 2001). There is an accelerated time scale between birth and identification, and identification occurs at a much earlier stage in the relationship formation between parent and baby. Sometimes, from very early on, the hearing loss is an integral part of the child's identity. Within weeks of giving birth, the parents may become involved in an intervention plan. Not surprisingly, many of them feel overwhelmed by the combination of new parenthood and their participation in the plan. Some speech and hearing professionals have suggested that parents may be unable to enjoy their baby before they have to deal with the consequences of the hearing loss. Others have argued that better bonding occurs because parents know from early on that their relationship is with a baby who has hearing loss (Figure 14-6). The parent–child relationship does not receive a jolt when later the hearing loss is discovered (See McCracken, Young, & Tattersall, 2008; Young & Tattersall, 2007).

Infancy is a time of great excitement and parent–baby bonding. When parents learn in the newborn nursery that their baby may not be who they had anticipated, the stages of grief that often accompany a child's diagnosis of hearing loss may be amplified compared with that experienced by parents who learn later of the hearing loss. This occurs because parents of older babies and children have lived with their child and may have gradually grown to suspect a problem. They have observed

"We just feel so lucky that she has been picked up and we know that she's going to have as much help as she needs and she's going to be able to do as much as she can with it being part of her life."

Mother of a 6-month-old baby who has a moderate hearing loss

(Young & Tattersall, 2007, p. 213)

"From our point of view it has been a nightmare really. I wish I hadn't been told, I wish I was just finding out now because I would have had nearly 8 months to just enjoy him. It has actually been 8 horrible months on and off. It hasn't affected me bonding with him or anything but I have not enjoyed him, like I did [my other child]. I wish I had never been told. I wish I was just finding out now."

Mother of an 8-month-old baby who has a moderate hearing loss

(Young & Tattersall, 2007, p. 215)

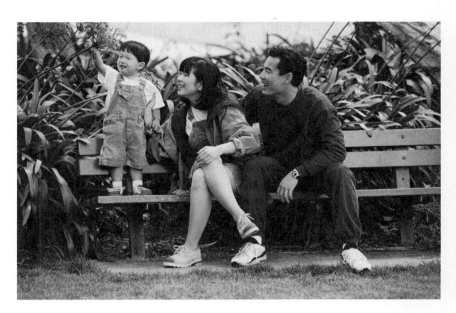

FIGURE 14-6. Reactions to early identification. Some speech and hearing professionals suggest that parents who learn of their baby's hearing loss early on are spared the surprise of learning about it later, and learn to accept the hearing loss as part of the baby's identity. *Copyright Photodisc/Getty Images. Reprinted by permission.*

their child not responding to sound, or have observed the child not developing vocal and listening behaviors that resemble those of his or her peers. Thus, they may not be totally caught off-guard at the diagnosis of hearing loss. In contrast, parents who learn that their baby might have a hearing loss while the baby is still in the hospital, and before they have had any chance to get to know and bond with the child, might be handed the news "cold turkey." Add the natural emotions of grief to the emotions associated with postpartum depression, the physical exhaustion of childbirth, and the stress of being a new parent, and the end result may be parents who feel fraught. It is critical that new parents receive counseling and support and that they have reason to believe there are mechanisms and support services that will steer them through this initial stage of coping with their baby's hearing loss.

Not every baby who fails a hearing screening test has a hearing loss. If a baby fails a screening test, then every attempt must be made to ensure that a comprehensive diagnostic evaluation is scheduled as soon as possible. Fast scheduling will minimize that period during which parents worry, not knowing one way or the other whether their baby has a hearing loss.

Luterman and Kurtzer-White (1999) surveyed a group of parents of babies who had been identified as having hearing loss as a result of neonatal hearing screening. They found (p. 16):

- The majority of parents supported early identification of hearing loss and would have wanted to know the diagnosis at birth.
- A minority of parents (17% of the respondents) would have preferred to wait to learn of their child's hearing loss.
- Parents would prefer to be informed of their child's hearing loss by an audiologist who is not only a skillful clinician but also an empathetic counselor.
- Parents wanted unbiased information, particularly concerning the issues of communication and education methodology.
- The parents' predominant need was to meet other parents of children with hearing loss.
- Parents wanted and needed time to process what they experience and the amount of information they receive at the time of diagnosis.

In Chapter 11, it was noted that adults often pass through a series of emotional stages, just as most people who experience grief. These stages of emotional adjustment may include shock, denial, guilt, anger, and acceptance. Parents and family members may also pass through these stages when they learn of their child's hearing loss. One goal of counseling may be to shepherd parents through these stages so they are best able to participate in their child's aural rehabilitation intervention plan.

Self-evaluation of counseling skills: *Do I . . . ?*

- Truly listen to [parents] without jumping ahead
- Demonstrate an ability to express own feelings
- Show sensitivity to [parents'] issues and timing
- Provide opportunities for [parents] to share feelings as well as content
- Support [parents'] feelings
- Offer experiences for [parents] to develop more skills in stating [their] own needs

(Edwards, 2003, p. 7)

Shock, Denial, and Grief

Shock and denial are ways of protecting oneself from a crisis and often result in parents focusing on minor details. Initially, parents may feel removed from a diagnosis, as if this were happing to some other family. Shock may be experienced as a feeling of numbness, confusion, and bewilderment.

Denial may quickly supersede shock. An individual may deny that the hearing loss exists or may deny the enormity of its consequences. Family members may need time and support to accept that their child has a hearing loss.

Grief may occur next, as parents realize that their ideal child has been lost. Grief is a normal and even healthy reaction, and is a means by which parents can deal with painful news and a disappointing reality. With time, the grieving process can bring the family back into balance and result in a resolve to move forward. Negative consequences of grief can be fatigue,

Table 14-4. Guidelines for working with families and caregivers.

AT DIAGNOSIS:	PARENTS SHOULD LEAVE WITH:
1. Allow families to "tell their story"	1. Written information (information packet)
2. Show kindness, empathy	2. A plan
3. Be honest	3. Phone number (to call whenever clarification is needed)
4. Express hope and confidence	4. Next appointment scheduled as soon as possible, in writing
WITHIN 4 TO 6 MONTHS OF DIAGNOSIS:	DURING THIS PERIOD, THE SPEECH AND HEARING PROFESSIONAL WILL:
1. Recognize/acknowledge the emotional responses	1. Ensure appropriate listening device is being used
2. Facilitate healthy attachment between child and caregivers	2. Model effective communication behaviors
3. Acknowledge imbalance and support work toward reestablishing a healthy family system	3. Provide parents with information about intervention services
4. Actively involve family in intervention choices—avoid "rescuing"—convey hope with all communication modes—convey that there are no failures	4. Refer to other professionals as necessary
5. Support involvement of extended family—siblings/grandparents	
6. Connect to other families with children of same age/similar hearing loss and to veteran families	

Adapted from Rall and Montoya (2005, p. 1).

stress, loss of sleep, headaches, and irritability. Montoya (2007) suggests that speech and hearing professionals can help parents resolve grief by:

- Actively listening
- Not judging the family
- Building parental self-esteem, self-confidence, and competence
- Providing immediate, resource-oriented support
- Having appropriate counseling skills
- Sharing expert knowledge and experience with living with hearing loss

Additional guidelines for working with families and caregivers during the first 6 months appear in Table 14-4.

Guilt and Anger

Guilt and anger may follow the denial stage, and often parents will become convinced that something they have done in the past may be responsible for the hearing loss. For example, one mother took anti-sea-sickness pills while on a cruise in the early weeks of her pregnancy. She experienced enormous guilt when her baby was diagnosed with profound hearing loss, because she was convinced the medication had resulted in abnormal fetal development. Guilt can cause a parent to overprotect a child ("I may have let this hearing loss happen, but I'm not going to let anything else bad happen to you") or to become superdedicated ("I'm going to make this up to you"). Luterman (2004) notes that overprotective parents may lead to a fearful child whereas superdedicated ones may result in siblings being neglected or a marriage being placed at risk.

Luterman (2004) considers the many sources that might provoke anger in parents. Most parents had the expectation that their child would have normal hearing and that their child would lead a "normal" life. The presence of hearing loss violated this expectation, and unmet expectations often incite anger. Anger may also arise from a sense of a loss of control. Most people like to think that they have limitless possibilities when it comes to operating in their child's best interests. The presence of hearing loss may restrict parents' options, and they may feel anger in response. Anger may also be a mask of fear, and may hide feelings of inadequacy.

Acceptance

Finally, acceptance may set in, as parents begin to accept that their child's hearing loss is a reality. Ideally, the parents and family are willing to take constructive steps to deal with their child's hearing condition.

Many parents feel confused and overwhelmed during the early stages following diagnosis, and these feelings may be magnified as they interact with a variety of different professionals who may provide abundant, and perhaps conflicting, advice about how to handle the child's loss. They may feel inadequate when they realize how much time and effort will be required on their part to maximize their child's potential. Sensitive counseling and empathetic listening on the part of the speech and hearing professional can help propel parents forward. As Luterman (2004) notes, "The hallmark of good counseling is careful listening and trusting that the parents will ultimately find the best solution for themselves and their child. Information should be given judiciously and parental confidence enhanced by emphasizing the skills and knowledge the parents already possess" (p. 220).

The stages just described are not necessarily like the rungs of a ladder, which parents climb up one step at a time and never climb back down. Rather, parents may pass from one stage to another, return to an earlier stage, and then advance again. For example, when a child enters kindergarten, the child's parents may look at his or her classmates who have normal hearing and realize more fully what a significant hearing loss may mean in terms of their child's academic achievement. This may trigger new feelings of grief, even if they have come to terms with the permanency of the hearing loss.

> "Angry people usually get things done and this can be a useful energy if directed appropriately. For parents of children with special needs, the anger often is displaced on to the professional. It behooves the professional to confront the parents' anger and unmask parental fears. This usually results in a fruitful encounter, which benefits the child."
>
> David Luterman, D.Ed., Professor Emeritus of Emerson College in Boston and expert in the psychological effects and emotions associated with hearing loss and parenting
>
> (Luterman, 2004, p. 217)

Dealing with Feelings and Moving Forward

Kozak and Brooks (2001) suggested ways for parents to deal with their feelings. These practical nuts-and-bolts recommendations are as follows.

- Accept your feelings: The situation is difficult and it is understandable and appropriate to be upset. Accept that it hurts and try to find something you can do to help your child. This will allow you to feel something more positive too.
- Talk to others: Find a spouse, parent, friend, or parent of another child with a challenge. Tell them what you are feeling and listen to them [talk about] their feelings. Get some support and see if you can give any . . .
- Write in a journal: If thinking and feeling are not enough to help but talking is too much for you right now or if you can't find the right listener, try writing some notes about your feelings in a journal, notebook or even a letter . . .
- Find a group to support you: You can find good listeners, help, support, and encouragement in a group of parents whose children have any special challenges . . . Your local children's hospital, clinics and schools may be resources for finding such a group . . . Most parents of children with challenges say that other parents of these children provided the most important help they received in the early years. This type of support can help you learn and move forward while you cope with all your feelings.
- Other ways: Some parents will look toward their ethical views or their religious values and comrades to help them find the way to feel better. Some people will delve into learning all they can about [hearing loss. Some may seek counseling] from a professional counselor or physician.
- Give yourself a break: Don't demand too much of yourself. Pat yourself on the back for doing what you've already done to help your child. Ask someone who cares about you for some words of encouragement. Get a hug from your child . . . Cry if it feels better to do so. Do something good for you, even if it's only taking time to watch the quiet beauty of a sunrise or sunset. Be thankful for your child. Don't expect yourself to do every job perfectly. No one is perfect in our imperfect world.

EARLY-INTERVENTION OVERVIEW AND DEVELOPMENT OF AN AURAL REHABILITATION STRATEGY

Once a child has been identified as having a hearing loss, an aural rehabilitation strategy will be developed, with the provision of early intervention. Early intervention starts as soon as the hearing loss has been identified. The goals of early intervention are (a) to enhance the infant's or toddler's development, (b) to minimize the possibility of developmental delay, and (c) to enhance the family's ability to accommodate the child's needs. Typically, the hospital staff will place the family in contact with personnel from the available early-intervention services in the child's region. A variety of early-intervention services have been established in states, with the help of federal grants, to provide children with appropriate services from birth until their third birthday.

Federal Law Concerning Early Intervention

In the United States, major legislation for children who have disabilities dates back to 1975, when Congress passed the *Education for All Handicapped Children Act of 1975*, known as PL 94-172 or the EHA law. This law guaranteed a free and appropriate education for all children with disabilities between the ages of 3 and 18 years of age, in the least restrictive environment possible. The disabilities covered included hearing loss, as well as specific learning disabilities, speech and language impairments, emotional disturbances, cognitive deficiencies, orthopedic impairments, visual impairments, and others. The term **free and appropriate public education (FAPE)** meant that children would receive special education

Free and appropriate public education (FAPE) refers to federal funding provided for the education of children with disabilities, and requires as a condition for receiving federal funds the provision of free and appropriate public education.

The Law That Started It All

Public Law 94-142 (November 29, 1975): It is the purpose of this Act to assure that all handicapped children have available to them, within the time periods specified in section 612(2) (B) a free appropriate public education which emphasizes special education and related services designed to meet their unique needs, to assure that the rights of handicapped children and their parents or guardians are protected, to assist States and localities to provide for the education of all handicapped children and to assess and assure the effectiveness of efforts to educate children.

A **least restrictive environment** is a basic principle of IDEA (*Individuals with Disabilities Education Act*) that requires public agencies to establish procedures to ensure that to the extent possible, children who have disabilities are educated with children who do not have disabilities, and that special classes, separate schooling, or removal from the regular educational environment occurs only when the severity of the disability is such that education in a regular class environment cannot be achieved satisfactorily.

and supporting services at public expense and under public supervision. These services were to comply with the standards of the state educational agency. A **least restrictive environment** was described as one in which a child who has a disability could be placed with the least limitations and still thrive when compared to peers who did not have a disability. The environment had to meet the child's unique needs and allow the child to be educated to the maximum extent appropriate with peers who have typical development.

Making Sense of the Numbers

Federal laws usually are designated with a tag number like PL 94-142. The *PL* is an acronym for *Public Law*. The first two numbers, in this case *94*, correspond to the number of the Congress that passed the law. The remaining three numbers indicate the piece of legislation. For instance, PL 94-142 was the 142nd piece of legislation passed by the 94th Congress of the United States. The congressional number advances once every 2 years (in even years).

The **Individuals with Disabilities Education Act (IDEA)** provides for specialized instruction for individuals who have disabilities and who meet eligibility requirements, typically that the disability causes adverse educational effects.

Part C of Public Law PL 108-446 refers to early-intervention services that are available to eligible children from birth through the age of 3 years and to their families.

The **No Child Left Behind Act of 2001 (NCLB)** (Public Law 107-110) reauthorized several federal programs aimed at improving the performance of U.S. primary and secondary schools by increasing the standards of accountability at the school, district, and state levels. NCLB enacts the theories of standards-based education (also known as outcome-based education) with the belief that high expectations and goals will result in success for all students.

PL 94-142 was amended in 1997 and reauthorized as PL 105-17, and became known as the **Individuals with Disabilities Education Act (IDEA)**. IDEA encompassed earlier amendments made to the original act, including PL 99-457 and PL 101-476, which mandated services for infants and toddlers and their families. IDEA changed the term *handicapped children* to *children with disabilities.* It expanded the age range of children covered by PL 94-142 to individuals from birth to the age of 21 (up to the 22nd birthday). The key additions afforded by IDEA are the provision of public services for infants and toddlers and their families (**Part C**), assistance to individuals making a transition from secondary school to postsecondary school settings, and the inclusion of assistive technology services in educational planning. The reauthorization underscored parent participation in decision making, made provisions for addressing the general education curriculum in education planning, and promoted high expectations for achievement.

In 2004, IDEA was revised and issued as Public Law No. 108-446, and was meant to align IDEA with the 2001 **No Child Left Behind Act**. In particular, the revised law revised performance goals and defined the term "highly qualified teacher." Provision of services under IDEA for infants might include any or all of the following:

- Family training, counseling, and home visits
- Special instruction
- Speech pathology and audiology
- Occupational therapy
- Psychological services
- Case management
- Medical services for diagnosis or evaluation
- Screening and assessment
- Transportation to and from services

Key provisions of the IDEA include the following (Messina & Messina, 2004):

1. *Identification*—the state and local education agencies must actively seek out and identify children who have special education needs (Child Find).

2. *Evaluation*—A child must be evaluated appropriately prior to placement. All methods used for testing and evaluation must be in the primary language or "mode of communication" of the child. No one test may be the determining factor for placement. [The Evaluation procedures cannot be racially or ethnically biased. Before a child is placed in an intervention program, a full and individualized evaluation will be conducted to determine the child's educational needs.]

3. **Individualized Education Plan (IEP)**—An IEP or an IFSP must be prepared for each child based on their individual educational needs.

4. *Parents* are equal participants in the decision-making process and students may be participants in their IEP development.

5. *Related Services*—Related servies shall be provided on an individualized basis to assist the child to benefit from special education.

6. *Least Restrictive Environment (LRE)*—Each child shall be educated to the maximum extent appropriate with children who do not have disabilities and children should be educated in more restrictive (different) settings only when less restrictive alternatives are not appropriate.

7. *Private School*—When children are placed in private schools by state or local education agencies in order to receive an appropriate education, this must be done at no cost to parents; private school programs must meet standards set by law.

An individualized education plan (IEP) is a team-developed, written plan that identifies goals and objectives that address the educational needs of a student aged 3–21 years who has a disability. The plan should take into account the family's preferred mode of communication, the child's linguistic needs, academic progress, social and emotional needs, and appropriate accommodations to ensure learning.

8. *Early Intervention and Preschools*—The IDEA makes early-intervention services available to children ages 0–5 years.

9. *Due Process*—Rights of parents and children must be guaranteed by states and localities; including notice, right to hearing, and appeal procedures. If parents have a complaint, they will have an opportunity for a due process hearing that is conducted by the state educational agency, the local educational agency, or intermediate educational unit. They have the right to be accompanied by counsel and other individuals with special knowledge with respect to their child's disability.

10. *Advisory Board*—Each state must set up an advisory board, including individuals who have disabilities, teachers, and parents of children who have disabilities.

11. *Funds*—IDEA provides flow-through funds per child per year to supplement state and local program efforts. Funds may be withheld for noncompliance. Payments by the state to local school districts may also be suspended for noncompliance.

12. *Records*—Parents have access to their child's educational records and can request that they be amended.

An **Individualized Family Service Plan** is a federally mandated plan for children age birth to 3 years that ensures appropriate early-intervention services for infants and toddlers and their families. The plan should take into account a child's current level of development, the family's resources and priorities, goals and services necessary for achieving the goals, and a time course.

An **individualized family service plan (IFSP)** is a federally mandated plan for the education of preschool children; it emphasizes family involvement and is updated annually. IDEA requires that states that receive funding for early-intervention provide services to a child who experiences developmental delays, as measured by appropriate test instruments. The IFSP must include a statement of the following (Johnson, 2006, p. 8):

- The child's present levels of physical, cognitive, communication, social, emotional, and adaptive development, based on objective criteria.
- The family's resources, priorities, and concerns related to enhancing the child's development.
- The major outcomes expected for the child and family, and the criteria, procedures, and timelines to be used in monitoring progress toward achieving the outcomes and whether modifications or revisions of the outcomes or services are necessary.
- Specific early-intervention services necessary to meet the needs of the child and family, including the frequency, intensity, and methods for delivering services.

- The environments in which early-intervention services shall be provided, including a justification of the extent, if any, to which services will not be provided in a natural environment.
- The projected dates for initiation of services and the anticipated duration of the services.
- An identification of a service coordinator.
- Steps to be taken to support the transition of the toddler to preschool or other appropriate services.

The Service Coordinator and the Medical Home

Once a child has been deemed eligible, a service coordinator is assigned to the family and child. The **service coordinator** coordinates the child's evaluations and assessments, facilitates and helps develop the IFSP, assists the family in receiving appropriate services, coordinates and monitors the delivery of services, and then helps develop a transition plan to preschool services if appropriate. Appropriate services might be provided by audiologists, family therapists, physical therapists, psychologists, social workers, speech and language pathologists, special educators, pediatricians and other medical specialists, and nutritionists.

The **service coordinator** is a designated person who helps the family during the development, implementation, and evaluation of the IFSP.

The pediatrician and any other primary care physician, working in partnership with the child's parents, and other health care professionals such as the audiologist, make up the infant's **medical home**. The medical home is not a hospital or a building, but rather "an approach to providing health care services where care is accessible, family-centered, continuous comprehensive, coordinated, compassionate, and culturally competent" (Joint Committee on Infant Hearing, 2000, p. 801). The professionals act in partnership with the family to develop a global plan of health and habilitative care, and advocate for the whole child within the context of the medical system. Often, the pediatrician helps parents to identify both medical and nonmedical services.

The **medical home** is the approach to providing health care services, and involves a partnership of health care personnel and family.

The Individualized Family Service Plan (IFSP)

The IFSP is a written document developed by a team, including the family. Appendix 14-3 presents some of the acronyms that might be encountered during the formulation of an IFSP. The IFSP describes the programs and services for a child, lists goals and objectives and procedures to be undertaken to ensure they are met, and identifies equipment that the public agency will provide the child and/or the child's family.

Implementation of the IFSP

During and/or after the IFSP has been developed, the aural rehabilitation plan can be fleshed out and implemented. This will entail initiating a communication mode that can be used between parent and child, providing appropriate amplification for the child, initiating early-intervention services, such as auditory training, and providing parent support, such as giving guidance about communication strategies and encouraging participation in parent support groups.

⬳ COMMUNICATION MODE

One of the first decisions to make about intervention concerns communication mode. Will the child use primarily speech to communicate? Manually coded English and speech? ASL? If a sign system is selected, the child as well as the family must learn the system.

The majority of persons with significant hearing loss who live in the United States use one of three modes to communicate: **American Sign Language (ASL)**, manually coded English, and spoken language. A relatively small minority use a system called Cued Speech.

American Sign Language (ASL) is a manual system of communication used by members of the Deaf Culture in the United States.

American Sign Language

ASL is a manual system of communication. A person does not use ASL and speak at the same time. ASL has a different grammar than spoken English. One ASL sign might represent a concept that would require many English words to express. Facial expressions and body language can impart a variety of meanings to the signs. In both ASL and manually coded English, fingerspelling may be used if there is no sign for a particular word or concept. In fingerspelling, one hand shape corresponds to each letter of the alphabet. The American manual alphabet appears in Figure 14-7.

In a bilingual/bicultural model, children with significant hearing loss learn ASL as their first language and then later learn English in school, as they develop reading and writing skills.

Some attention in recent years has been focused on the use of a **bilingual/bicultural model** for educating children with significant hearing loss. In this model, children use ASL as their first language for communication and then, later, learn English in school as they develop reading and writing skills. The premise is that, if children develop a language system for thought and expression first, basic skills will transfer to learning similar skills in a second language.

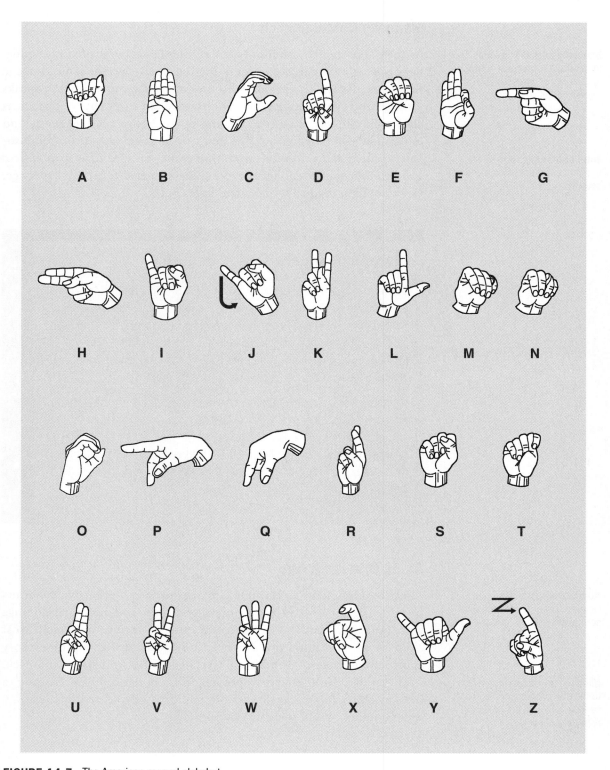

FIGURE 14-7. The American manual alphabet.

Manually Coded English

Manually coded English is a form of communication in which manual signs correspond to English words.

As the name implies, **manually coded English** is comprised of manual signs corresponding to the words of English. It also has the same syntactic structures. Typically, a person who uses manually coded English speaks simultaneously while signing. For instance, as a boy says, "The cat is inside," he will sign the article *the,* and then one sign each for *cat, is,* and *inside.* The combined use of sign and speech as an educational philosophy is called **total communication** (sometimes referred to as *simultaneous communication*). The child uses every available means to receive a message, including sign, residual hearing, and lipreading.

Total communication refers to a combined use of sign and speech.

More on Manually Coded English

There is no universally accepted English-based sign system. For example, under the rubric of manually coded English fall the systems of Signed English, Seeing Essential English (SEE 1), Signing Exact English (SEE 11), Linguistics of Visual English (L.O.V.E.), and the Rochester Method. People in one region of the country may sign a word one way, whereas those in another region sign it in a different way.

Many teachers and children who use manually coded English actually sign a Contact form of English, omitting function words such as *the* and morphemes, including those that mark past tense and plurality (Marmor & Pettito, 1979; Nix, 1983). Children who receive a Contact model of English may be at relatively high risk for developing deficits in language syntax.

Aural/Oral Language

Aural/oral language is the language used by persons with normal hearing.

Aural/oral language is the same language used by persons with normal hearing. The child with a hearing impairment who uses aural/oral language will speak messages and use speechreading to receive messages. Most children who use aural/oral language are educated with a multisensory approach, but a small number are educated with a unisensory approach. Children in a **multisensory approach** utilize both vision and hearing to recognize speech. In learning to talk, children rely on residual hearing, speechreading, and in some instances, touch.

Multisensory approach refers to the use of both vision and hearing, and sometimes touch, to recognize speech.

Children who have a communication mode based on a **unisensory approach** rely only on residual hearing to receive spoken messages. The preschool teacher may sometimes expect a child to recognize the signal auditorily, even if the youngster has minimal residual hearing. Several years ago, this approach was sometimes referred to as an **acoupedic approach**, and was defined by Pollack (1970) as follows: "The term *acoupedics* refers to a comprehensive habilitation program for the hearing impaired infant and his family, which includes an emphasis upon auditory training without formal lipreading instruction" (p. 13). In recent times, a unisensory approach is often referred to as an **auditory-verbal approach**. The auditory-verbal approach emphasizes the use of audition over vision for the learning of speech and language, and stipulates that a child makes habitual and optimal use of amplification or electrical stimulation (i.e., cochlear implant) in order to develop spoken communication. Auditory-verbal is considered to be a way of life. Children are expected ultimately to respond to sound and to use it in the same ways as do children who have normal hearing.

> **The unisensory approach** is one that advocates the use of only residual hearing to receive spoken messages.
>
> The **acoupedic approach** is a comprehensive habilitation program for infants and their families that emphasizes auditory training without formal lipreading instruction.
>
> The **auditory-verbal approach** encourages a child to develop listening behaviors and to develop spoken communication by relying on residual hearing rather than vision; the use of appropriate and habitual amplification or electrical stimulation (via cochlear implant) is strongly encouraged.

Cued Speech

Cued Speech is a communication system that uses phonemically based hand gestures to supplement speechreading (Cornett, 1967). Thus, the talker speaks while simultaneously cueing the message. By themselves, the hand signals are uninterpretable. When coupled with the audiovisual signal, speech recognition increases because viseme members are distinguished from one another. Although the system is not widely used, it has become an international phenomenon, having been adapted to more than 60 languages and dialects, including Spanish, Croatian-Serbian, Hindi, Swedish, and Telegu (Beck, 2006).

> **Cued Speech**, a system for enhancing speechreading, uses phonemically based gestures to distinguish between similar visual speech patterns.

In the Cued Speech system, eight different hand shapes are used to distinguish consonants, and six locations on the face and neck are used to distinguish vowels. For instance, the consonants /p/ and /b/ resemble one another on the mouth. The consonant /p/ is distinguished by a 1 hand shape and the consonant /b/ is shown by a 4 hand shape. If a talker said the word *pea,* he or she would hold a 1 hand shape to the corner of the mouth, because a 1 hand shape indicates the phoneme /p/, and a placement at the mouth corner indicates an /i/ vowel. If the talker instead said *bee,* he or she would hold a 4 hand shape at the mouth corner. The word *boo* would be signaled by a 4 hand shape at the throat. Figure 14-8 presents the Cued Speech system.

Cued Speech Configuration

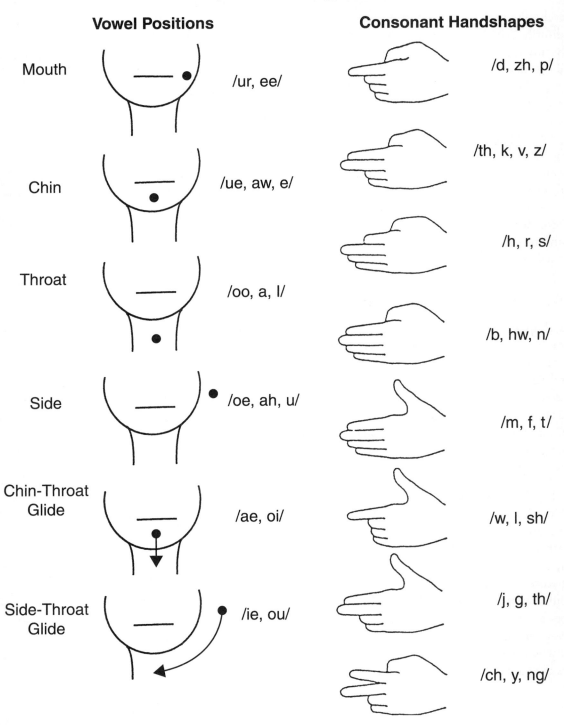

Vowel Positions

Mouth — /ur, ee/

Chin — /ue, aw, e/

Throat — /oo, a, I/

Side — /oe, ah, u/

Chin-Throat Glide — /ae, oi/

Side-Throat Glide — /ie, ou/

Consonant Handshapes

/d, zh, p/

/th, k, v, z/

/h, r, s/

/b, hw, n/

/m, f, t/

/w, l, sh/

/j, g, th/

/ch, y, ng/

FIGURE 14-8. Hand configurations and hand placement positions for Cued Speech.

Selection of a Communication Mode

Some debate and controversy surround the issue of communication mode, and many speech and hearing professionals take firm stands in favor of one mode versus another. Of all the decisions parents must make about their child's intervention plan, this decision can be the one they revisit most often.

Selection of communication mode is an area where there are no definitive answers as to the best way to go, and it is likely that the best route is different for different children. With this said, there is some evidence that children who utilize an aural/oral communication mode achieve better speech and language performance and literacy development than do children who rely on sign language. For instance, Markides (1988) found that children from an aural/oral-emphasis education program were more likely to achieve better speech intelligibility than children from total-communication programs, and their speech intelligibility was less likely to deteriorate over time. Dornan et al. (2008) found that a group of 29 children who have severe and profound hearing losses, and who were between the ages of 2 and 6 years at the time of their study, showed the same amount of progress in their speech and language skills over the course of 9 months as children who have normal hearing.

Although such studies suggest differences may exist between programs that implement different communication modes, most research investigations have provided relatively little control over other factors such as socioeconomic status or intellectual abilities. This is because there are many difficulties inherent in relating communication mode to outcome measures such as literacy or speech intelligibility. Complex interrelationships exist among demographic variables and the use of speech and sign. For example, children who use an aural/oral mode are more likely to have more hearing, to attend preschool, to come from higher-income families, and to use a hearing aid more often (Jensema & Trybus, 1978).

Perhaps where the issue of communication mode advantage is best resolved is in the population of cochlear implant users. Numerous studies have shown that children who use a cochlear implant and an aural/oral method of communication develop better speech and language skills than do children who use sign (e.g., Kirk et al., 2000) and better speech perception skills (Miyamoto, Kirk, Svirsky, & Sehgal, 1999). A group of researchers at Central Institute for the Deaf studied 181 children, 8 and 9 years of age, from across North America. They found that children who were in an aural/oral education program developed better speech (Tobey et al., 2003; see also Connor, Hieber, Arts, & Zwolan, 2000), language (Geers, Nicholas, & Sedey, 2003), conversational fluency (Tye-Murray, 2003), and reading (Geers, 2003) than did children who were enrolled in a total-communication environment. The aural/oral-communication advantage proved robust, even after they factored out child, family, and educational variables. The researchers also found that following cochlear implantation, more children switched from using a total-communication mode to an aural/oral mode than the converse (see also Watson, Archbold, & Nikolopoulos, 2006). Cochlear implantation was also associated with a shift from private school and special education settings to public school and mainstream programs.

LISTENING DEVICE

The goal of providing a listening device is to provide the infant or toddler with maximum access to the speech signal at a listening level that is safe and comfortable. For newborns and infants, estimated hearing sensitivity is supported by frequency-specific ABR threshold assessment. Behavioral measures may be available for older babies and toddlers to supplement the electrophysiological measures.

Amplification

Children usually receive hearing aids as soon as a hearing loss is identified, even if the child is only an infant. Even if the child is an excellent candidate for a cochlear implant, he or she must first go through a trial period with hearing aids to determine that it is not a viable option. The amplification fitting procedure typically employs prescriptive procedures that include individual real-ear measurements (see Chapter 3). The five steps of the amplification process are: (a) selection, (b) verification, (c) orientation, (d) validation, and (f) follow-up.

Selection

Selecting hearing aids for infants and young children differs in some ways from fitting hearing aids in adults (Hoover, 2001). First, there are physical differences. Children, especially infants, have smaller ears and ear canals, so hearing aid style options may be limited. Ear canal size might increase the occurrence of feedback and squeal, and the tiny pinna might not hold a hearing aid behind the ear. Second, because sound is funneled into a small space before the tympanic membrane, the sound pressure delivered to a child's ear might be greater than when the exact acoustic signal is delivered to an adult ear. Thus, it becomes important to ensure that sound is not too loud to cause damage. Finally, babies and young children often cannot participate in the fitting process. They cannot indicate when sound is too loud, and they cannot take a word recognition test.

Most young children receive BTEs. BTEs typically provide sufficient gain, even for profound hearing losses. Babies' ears are too tiny to accommodate an ITE, CIC, or ITC style of hearing aid. Moreover, these styles are impractical because the baby is growing quickly, and thus, a new aid would be required to accommodate the ongoing physical changes that occur. Even with a BTE style, parents have to monitor changes in the baby's ear size. New earmolds may have to be made every 6 to 8 weeks.

An advantage offered by BTEs is that they can be connected to many FM assistive listening devices. These systems include a wireless microphone worn by a talker and a receiver that the child uses, connected to the hearing aid.

Verification

The goal of verification is to determine whether speech is audible, and entails electroacoustic measures using a probe microphone and insertion gain protocol. Behavioral measures may be included in the verification procedure for older children. Verification provides frequency-specific information about speech audibility and estimates of real-ear aided responses.

Orientation

Once a hearing aid is fitted on a child, the audiologist provides instruction to the parents or caregivers about how to care for the device and how to perform a **listening check**, and provides the equipment to do so (Figure 14-9).

A **listening check** is an informal check of a hearing aid to ensure that it is functioning.

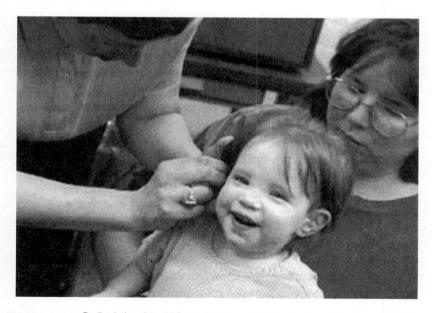

FIGURE 14-9. Pediatric hearing aid fitting. Parents receive instructions about how to handle, maintain, and troubleshoot the device. *From video footage by Rick Bernstein, courtesy of the Central Institute for the Deaf.*

Parent One: I'm not particularly good with equipment. I can just about work the video but you know it was like oh god I don't know what to do with [the hearing aid]. I suppose to start off I was frightened of it.

Parent Two: It just felt overwhelming 'cos [the audiologist] was talking how to look after them and do the thing, clean them, put them in . . . I was just thinking how am I going to manage this on a little baby . . . it was a nightmare really, it was all very well [to have the] hearing aids, but actually getting him to wear them and use them. . . .

Parent Three: It's a normal thing. They're just like putting on his clothes. They are just part of his clothing now and we can both . . . you know at first it was a bit distressing—but really it doesn't take very long to be able to fit them really quickly.

Three parents of babies identified with hearing loss, talking about becoming "hearing aid managers" while simultaneously trying to establish baby routines

(McCracken, Young, & Tattersall, 2008, p. 59)

The parent learns about device insertion, removal, overnight storage, and battery insertion and removal. Instruction will also include how to wash an earmold, how to monitor the child's ability to hear with the device, and how to troubleshoot the hearing aid (e.g., what to do if the hearing aid will not turn on, if the sound is weak or distorted, or if the hearing aid squeals). Written materials supplement the verbal instruction.

Validation

To validate the benefits of amplification, some toddlers of about age 3 years can take speech perception measures, such as the *Northwestern University Children's Perception of Speech Test* (*NU-CHIPS;* Elliot & Katz, 1980), a closed-set test of monosyllabic words (Chapter 2). Infants and most toddlers will require alternative means for validating benefit. Measures are typically subjective and depend on parent report or clinician observation. Examples of tests that can be used with infants and toddlers and that utilize parent report are the *Early Listening Function* (*ELF;* Anderson, 2002) and the *Infant-Toddler Meaningful Auditory Integration* (*IT-MAIS;* Zimmerman-Philips, 1997). These tests assess children's response to sound as well as their emerging speech and language skills, which are dependent on the child's hearing the spoken word. Such validation allows both the speech and hearing professional and the parents to realize the benefits and limitations of amplification.

The ELF takes several days to complete and is typically used with infants over the age of 6 months. It includes checklists and rating scales. For instance, a parent is asked to indicate whether the baby can detect the mother saying "sh, sh" or clicking her tongue loudly at a distance of 6 inches, 3 feet, 6 feet, 10 feet, and then from the next room. The mother must judge whether the baby is aware of her voice when the baby is wearing amplification.

The IT-MAIS is a structured interview conducted with the parent by the speech and hearing professional. It assesses a child's vocalization behaviors, alerting behaviors to sound, and ability to derive meaning from sound. One question on the IT-MAIS asks parents to, *Describe [child's] vocalizations when you first put his/her device on each day.* Points are awarded on a graduated scale, ranging from *no difference between when the device is turned on versus off* to *an increase of 100% when the child is wearing the device to when the child is not wearing it.* Parents are asked whether the child spontaneously responds to his or her name and whether the child is able to recognize auditory signals that are a part of the child's everyday routine.

Follow-Up

A typical follow-up schedule for children during the first year of using a hearing aid includes a recheck at 1 month following the initial fitting and then a visit at every 2 or 3 months. After the first year, visits to the audiologist may occur at 4- to 6-month intervals. At follow-up visits, hearing is assessed and the hearing aids are tested and adjusted as necessary. The follow-up includes a behavioral audiometric evaluation, current assessment of communication needs and abilities, adjustment of amplification system, periodic elecroacoustic evaluations, listening checks, earmold fit check, periodic probe-microphone measurements, and long-term follow-up including a check on ongoing auditory habilitation (American Academy of Audiology, 2004).

Some children reject their devices or want to control when they do and do not use it. Some children react negatively to amplified sound, and some may view the listening device as a means of asserting independence or gaining control over parents. A speech and hearing professional can encourage parents to take responsibility and foster full-time use. With a younger child, parents may provide reassurance and support to the child. Initially, the device can be worn for short periods and then gradually increased over time. Routines of use should be established. Putting the listening device on in the morning should be part of getting dressed, and removing it should be part of getting undressed in the evening.

Cochlear Implants

Multichannel cochlear implants were approved by the FDA in 1990 for the use in children who have profound hearing losses and who are between the ages of 2 and 17 years of age. Now, the FDA permits cochlear implantation for children as young as 12 months who have profound hearing loss and children 18 months and older who have severe to profound hearing loss. There is evidence that earlier implantation does not pose additional risks to babies and that it may lead to superior speech recognition skills (Lesinski-Schiedat, Illg, Heerman, Bertram, & Lenarz, 2004), so implantation before 12 months of age is becoming available in some countries and in some locales. Cochlear implant candidacy is determined by the degree of hearing loss, demonstration that the child receives minimal benefit from using hearing aids, enrollment in an early-intervention program that promotes auditory skill development, and the absence of medical contraindications (see Kirk, Firszt, Hood, & Holt, 2006, for a review).

Research suggests that children who use cochlear implants surpass hearing aid users who have similar degrees of hearing impairment in their speech recognition, speech production performance, and language and reading. Moreover, children who are younger when they receive a cochlear implant are more likely to perform better than children who are older on tests of speech perception, language, and speech production (e.g., Connor, Craig, Raudenbush, Heavner, & Zwolan, 2006; Fryauf-Bertschy, Tyler, Kelsay, Gantz, & Woodworth, 1997; Kileny, Zwolan, & Ashbaugh, 2001; O'Donoghue, Nikolopoulos, & Archbold, 2000; Robbins, Koch, Osberger, Zimmerman-Phillips, & Kishon-Rabin, 2004; Svirsky, Robbins, Kirk, Pisoni, & Miyamoto, 2000; Tye-Murray, Spencer, & Woodworth, 1995). In light of such experimental findings, it is likely that cochlear implant use will become more prevalent in the future. Indeed, there is potential for the cochlear implant to become the most commonly used listening device by young children who have significant hearing loss (Figure 14-10).

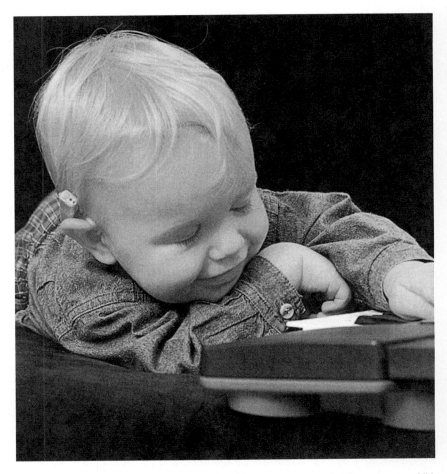

FIGURE 14-10. Benefits of early implantation. Research suggests that the younger a child is at the time of implantation, the greater the advantage afforded for speech, language, and auditory development. *Photograph courtesy of MED-EL Corp.*

The stages involved in a child's receiving a cochlear implant mirror those for the adult, and are summarized in Chapter 12, Table 12-1. These stages include initial contact, counseling, formal evaluation, surgery, fitting, follow-up, and aural rehabilitation.

Initial Contact

A parent might contact the clinical coordinator at the cochlear implant center and ask questions like those listed in Table 14-5.

Table 14-5. Questions parents may ask during the initial contact.

• Is my child an appropriate candidate?
• How does a cochlear implant work? How does it differ from a hearing aid?
• Will the cochlear implant help my child to talk and hear better?
• Can a cochlear implant electrocute my child? Is it dangerous to use?
• Can my child still play sports if he or she gets one?
• Will the cochlear implant last my child's entire lifetime? What happens if it "wears out"?
• Is the cochlear implant waterproof? Will my child be able to take a bath or shower?
• What happens if my child gets hit in the head?
• How often do the devices break?
• How much do they cost? Will my insurance pay for it?
• What's involved in obtaining a cochlear implant?
• Will my child have to use a particular communication mode?
• Are cochlear implants hard to take care of?

The clinical coordinator sends printed materials and schedules an appointment for a preliminary counseling session or formal evaluation. The printed materials may cover the following topics in a cursory fashion: the functions of a cochlear implant, how the cochlear implant differs from a hearing aid, who is a cochlear implant candidate, the reasons why some children may receive more benefit than others, the kinds of benefits that can be expected, insurance coverage, and the limitations of a cochlear implant.

Counseling

The pediatric audiologist typically conducts the counseling session. One goal of the preimplant counseling session is to establish realistic expectations about what the cochlear implant can do. The audiologist might explain that the child will always have a significant hearing loss, and that the cochlear implant is a communication aid and not a bionic ear. The audiologist will also explain in layperson's terms how other young users perform.

Ways to establish realistic expectations include the provision of opportunities for parents to talk with other parents of young cochlear implant users, some of whom receive more and some of whom receive less benefit from their devices. Scientific data about children's performance with a cochlear implant over time also might be shared with parents; data should indicate the best and poorest performance of groups of children and average performance. Data about listening, speech, and language might be discussed. When presenting research findings, it is important to do so in a way that is comprehensible and accessible to the parents.

Formal Evaluation

The goal of the formal evaluation is to establish candidacy. At the time of evaluation, children should show limited progress in the development of auditory skills and should have completed a trial period with appropriate amplification. The trial period usually lasts 10 weeks or longer to ensure that the cochlear implant is the optimal means of providing usable residual hearing. If the child appears to be acquiring speech and language skills with the use of a hearing aid, then candidacy is questionable. For young children, the evaluation of auditory skills and ability to benefit from the use of hearing aids might be performed through the use of parent questionnaires and informal measures of speech recognition.

Good general health, no chronic ear disease, and an unobstructed cochlea are typically prerequisites for most cochlear implant surgeries. A CT scan will provide a visual scan of the cochlea and reveal any cochlear anomalies or structural features that might preclude or complicate the implanting of an electrode into the spirals of the cochlea.

Surgery

Regardless of the counseling that has occurred beforehand, families often feel anxious before the surgery. Some worry about the anesthesia, potential surgical complications, the aftermath of surgery, and whether their child will receive benefit from the device. Some parents may experience guilt for inflicting a surgical procedure on their child. The speech and hearing professional will want to recognize and acknowledge these feelings and provide additional counseling when necessary.

The Cochlear Implant Fitting

The child returns to the cochlear implant center a few weeks following surgery for the cochlear implant fitting. The audiologist adjusts the stimulus parameters of the speech processor, which determine the signals delivered to the electrodes in the electrode array. The time necessary to fit and map a cochlear implant varies, depending on the maturity and cooperation of the child. Ideally a young child will learn to detect when sound is present and to indicate when it is soft and comfortably loud. Initial thresholds may be high, and maximum current levels may be low; these may change as the child becomes accustomed to hearing. In addition, due to a limited attention span, only a few electrodes may be programmed during the initial fitting session. Although most children can use their cochlear implant after one or two fittings, an optimum fitting may require several months.

When the device is activated, the prelingually deaf child may show no response to sound. Other responses include fright, surprise, rejection, distress, or wonderment. Children with verbal skills might report a sensation in the neck or head.

Before leaving the cochlear implant center, parents receive instruction about how to handle the device. Topics will include how to turn the device on and off, battery information, troubleshooting, warranty, and general care and maintenance.

Follow-Up Visits

After the first year of cochlear implant use, the child returns to the cochlear implant center at regular intervals, anywhere from every 3 months to annually. Audiological evaluation indicates whether the cochlear implant is functioning properly and whether performance has changed. Decreased performance is cause for concern because it may signal problems with the device or physiological changes in the auditory system. The audiologist may adjust the speech processor to enhance performance. During the annual visit, the family is advised whether the manufacturer has made new software or other options available for the cochlear implant and the child may be provided with an opportunity to try them.

Aural Rehabilitation

Listening and speech skills do not emerge spontaneously as a result of children receiving cochlear implants and then being exposed to conversation in their everyday environments. A concerted, deliberate aural rehabilitation effort is required before they learn to utilize the electrical signal for the purpose of speech recognition and speech and language acquisition. The aural rehabilitation plan must include participation by the parents, speech and hearing professionals, and educators. The child will continue participation in an early-intervention program, one that emphasizes spoken language and includes auditory training.

◉ EARLY-INTERVENTION PROGRAMS

Early intervention ideally begins as soon at the permanent hearing loss is confirmed, and it includes the receipt of a listening aid. Families may be given a list of all of the available programs in the geographic area and/or referred to a statewide early-intervention system. Some families will have many options whereas others will have only a few. The service coordinator assigned to the family typically is responsible for ensuring that the IFSP is developed and that the appropriate services are identified (Sass-Lehrer, 2004).

The Joint Committee on Infant Hearing (2000) presents guidelines for early-intervention programs. The goals are to support families in developing a child's communication skills, to help the family understand an infant's strengths and needs, and to promote the family's ability to advocate for the child. Early intervention builds upon family support and bolsters the family's confidence in their ability to parent a child who has hearing loss.

Early-intervention programs provide families with general information about language development and specific information about how hearing loss might affect development. Families are encouraged to engage in home-based activities that facilitate language acquisition. Programs usually ensure access to peer and language models. Peer models include other families who have children with hearing loss, as well as adults who have hearing loss. Language models may include individuals who use an aural/oral mode of communication or a mode that includes the use of sign. Overall, services should address a child's communicative competence, social skills, emotional well-being, and self-esteem.

Types of Programs

In a **center-based** program, children attend therapy for a designated number of hours per week.

In a **home-based** program, an early interventionist visits the infant's home and provides instruction for the child and parents.

Parents might consider a center-based program or a home-based program, or a combination of the two. In a **center-based program**, children attend therapy for a designated number of hours each week. Their parents may participate too. In **home-based programs**, an early-intervention specialist visits the infant's home and provides instruction to the parents and child (Figure 14-11). Home-based programs occur in the home and emphasize one-on-one rather than group instruction.

Examples of early-intervention programs are the SKI-HI curriculum (www.skiho.org) and the John Tracy Clinic home study programs (www.jtc.org). The SKI-HI curriculum is a family-oriented program for children who are between the ages of infancy and 5 years, and has been implemented

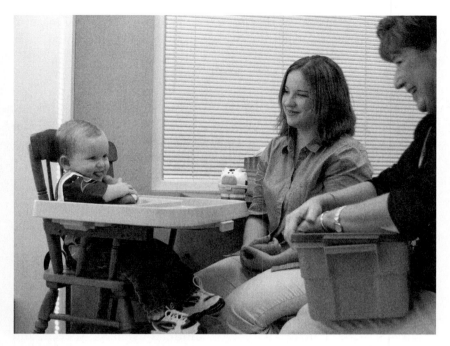

FIGURE 14-11. Home-based programs, in which a professional provides one-on-one services for the baby in the home environment and works with the baby's family. *Photograph by Kim Readmond, courtesy of the Central Institute for the Deaf.*

throughout the United States and Canada. National and local trainers provide training to service providers in participating states, and some training occurs at the SKI-HI Institute in Logan, Utah. The program includes early amplification, a focus on early communication approaches, language programs, and early literacy. Portions of the curriculum are devoted to natural environments and everyday routines, parent support, and conversation training.

The John Tracy program offers both an on-site early-intervention program for families who reside in Southern California and a correspondence course. Programs are available for infants, toddlers, and preschoolers, and aural/oral communication is promoted. For example, topics included in the infant program are family relationships, deafness, child development, and communication. Videotapes are available to demonstrate techniques, such as those associated with auditory training.

Once a child enrolls in an early-intervention program, ongoing assessment is critical to determine its effectiveness. The family and service coordinator usually review the IFSP at 6-month intervals to determine whether progress has been achieved and whether outcomes should be revised or modified. The IFSP must be updated on an annual basis, taking into consideration the results of formal evaluation, progress made, and other pertinent information.

Lesson Plans for Infants and Toddlers

Implementing an aural rehabilitation lesson typically entails involving parents, providing auditory training, and stimulating speech and language development. Parents can learn to provide speech and language models to their children and to use communication strategies like those reviewed in Chapter 9. Parents can be encouraged to respond to their child's communication attempts. Formal and informal auditory training can maximize the child's use of residual hearing. Programs such as CAST and DASL, which were described briefly in Chapter 4, can serve as a template for providing auditory training to very young children, although they likely will need to be modified to accommodate a child's language skills and maturity. In addition, cochlear implant manufacturers such as Advanced Bionics and Cochlear Corporation have programs that stimulate very young children's listening, speech, and language skills and these programs are described on their Web sites (see Chapter 3, Appendix). Programs aimed at speech and language development are considered in Chapter 15.

Warren Estabrooks (2006) presents examples of lesson plans for babies through the age of 3 years. These examples represent the kinds of activities that are appropriate for very young children and how important goals such as mastering the concept of turn taking can be accomplished through simple play routines. One lesson plan is reviewed in detail in this section in order to illustrate how a lesson may be implemented.

In the illustrative lesson plan, a sample of goals, which was designed for a 6-month-old baby named Arthur who has a bilateral severe to profound hearing loss, included the following (Estabrooks, 2006, pp. 91–93):

- Audition: To detect environmental and speech sounds, as indicated when Arthur stops the activity, smiles, and widens his eyes; to recognize friendly and angry voices by responding appropriately.
- Speech: To experiment and explore his own vocalizations by encouraging cooing and vocal play; to produce varied suprasegmentals.
- Language: To listen to the narration of life provided by the caregivers; to encourage vocalization for wants and needs; [to develop the vocabulary words of *round, up,* and *down*]

- Cognition: To imitate facial expressions; to understand cause and effect.
- Communication: To develop joint attention; to develop early turn-taking skills.

In this lesson plan, the clinician first addressed the goals by engaging Arthur and his mother in a game with a jack-in-the-box toy. The clinician began by turning the crank on the box toy (with its lid closed) and singing the child's song, "Round and round." When the toy clown popped out of the box, the clinician said, "Oh look! It's a clown. The clown says, *ha ha ha.*" Arthur was encouraged to touch the clown and to "push it down—push the clown dowwwn." The game was repeated, with the mother turning the crank and engaging in similar repartee. Tips for Arthur's mother, to be pursued later in the home environment, included the following (p. 93):

- Point out wheels, tops, fans, or mobiles that turn or spin around, and say, "Round and round."
- Think about all the natural ways in which you [the parent] might incorporate the word *round* and its concept throughout the day.
- When you're going down the stairs, or when you are putting Arthur down onto a blanket, use the word *dowwwn.* Contrast "dowwwn" with "up, up, up."

This lesson plan also included activities with a toy airplane, a squeaky toy duck, a ball, a fish, a musical clock, and a toy train. With the musical clock activity, the clinician and mother indicated when the music was playing and when it was not. They provided positive feedback to Arthur when he cooed in response to the music's onset. "Do you want more?" the clinician asked. He waited for a few seconds before answering, "Yes!"

At the end of the lesson, the clinician and parent collaborated in compiling diagnostic information based on their observation of Arthur during the lesson. This information was recorded in Arthur's file and used to tailor his next intervention session. Their observations included the following (Estabrooks, 2006, pp. 98–99):

- Audition: Alerts to low- and mid-frequency [sounds] by widening eyes and smiling, and searching for toys; does not detect whispered speech.
- Speech: Uses a variety of vocalizations (*uh, nn*); quality of vocalizations sounds natural.
- Language: Engages in and enjoys vocal play; vocalizes more frequently with intent to make things happen.

- Cognition: Demonstrated understanding of "cause and effect" with musical clock; did not demonstrate anticipation in games or routines.
- Communication: Laughs, smiles, and coos while socializing; maintains appropriate eye contact.

PARENTAL SUPPORT AND PARENT INSTRUCTION

The intervention team will provide parental support throughout early intervention. Members of the team may include the pediatric audiologist, the pediatrician and/or family practitioner, the otolaryngologist, the service provider, a speech-language pathologist, and an early-childhood educator. Appendix 14-4 presents a list of agencies and Web sites that parents and caregivers may contact for additional support.

Other parents of children who have hearing loss may share their experiences with families and provide empathetic listening by means of **parent support groups**. Opportunities to interact with other parents may lessen the stress associated with having a child with a hearing loss. Parent support groups provide a community wherein parents can express and explore their emotions. They can talk about their anxiety or anger or confusion with others who not only empathize with their situation but who have experienced it first hand.

Parent support may include the provision of communication training by the speech and hearing professional. An extensive body of literature suggests that parents can positively affect their child's communication abilities. Moreover, parent-implemented interventions, where parents are taught ways to enhance their child's communication skills in the context of everyday life, can be effective (Kashinath, Woods, & Goldstein, 2006). For instance, many parents demonstrate the use of multiple communication strategies following intervention. Kaiser, Hancock, and Nietfeld (2000) effectively taught parents to use such strategies as language expansions and following of the child's lead. Subsequent to their parents' experience with an intervention program, children who have disabilities tend to show an increased frequency of verbalizations and spontaneous speech (Laski, Charlop, & Schreibman, 1988) and an increased amount of engagement and responsiveness during interactions (Krantz, McDuff, & McClannahan, 1993; Moran & Whitman, 1991).

One approach to early language intervention is known as *milieu* teaching. The emphasis is on the function of communication and on embedding learning within ongoing routine interactions. Daily life routines offer families a naturally occurring and supportive framework

Parent support groups provide opportunities for parents to share their feelings and issues related to having a child with hearing loss with others who have experienced them firsthand.

"... just by talking in group sessions we realized there are common interests, common concerns, 'I'm not the only one.' In most cases you think, 'I'm the only one that's feeling this way,' and you start discussing and you're going, 'Oh, everybody is in the same boat.'"

Dave, parent of a child with hearing loss, who joined a parent support group

(Ericks-Brophy et al., 2007, p. 14)

"Sharing our story became useful to others."

Jackie Busa, mother of two young children who have significant hearing loss

(Busa, 2005, p. 9)

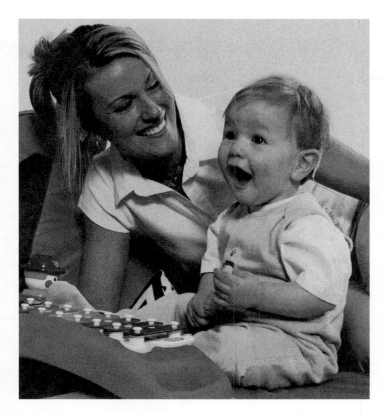

FIGURE 14-12. Language stimulation techniques, in which parents learn to use facilitative language techniques in the context of everyday routines and play periods. *Photograph courtesy of MED-EL Corp.*

in which they can use specific strategies to promote their child's language and conversational abilities (Figure 14-12). By embedding conversational strategies into play and caregiving routines, the intervention becomes individualized to the family and becomes part of their unique combination of personal and cultural values, ecological constraints, and resources (Kashinath et al., 2006). Parents learn to attend to their child's attentional lead and to stimulate conversation based on the child's focus. They learn to expect participation. Everyday events, such as getting dressed in the morning, playing with toys, or fixing dinner, become opportunities for language development (Kashinath et al., 2006; Warren & Yoder, 1996).

Speech and hearing professionals may encourage parents to use facilitative language techniques. **Facilitative language techniques** are communication acts that facilitate language development in young children. Table 14-6 presents a list of facilitative strategies and examples of each one.

Facilitative language techniques stimulate language growth in young children through the course of conversational interactions.

Table 14-6. Facilitative language techniques and examples of each one.

COMMUNICATIVE TECHNIQUE	DEFINITION	EXAMPLE
Signaling Expectations and Time Delay	Adult waits for the child's response and signals expectations by tilting the head or raising the eyebrows.	Parent: "Hmmm, you have a block. I wonder what you'll do with it." (Looks expectantly at the child)
Self-Talk	Adults speak aloud what they are doing and what they are thinking, thereby illustrating that language can be used to organize, analyze, and direct actions.	Parent: "I'm unpacking the groceries. I'll take out the apples. Maybe we'll make a pie. . . ."
Expansion and Modeling	Adult copies the meaning of a child's utterance and adds one or more morphemes or words. When new information is included, this technique is sometimes referred to as *expatiation*.	Child: "Baby cry." Parent: "The baby is crying." Child: "Baby sad." Parent: "The baby is sad because she's hungry."
Parallel Talk	Adult matches language to an activity a child is performing or an object that the child is looking at.	Parent: "You're holding a teddy. Now you're feeding the teddy. Oh, hug the bear."
Recast	Adult "recasts" a child's utterance into a question.	Child: "Daddy go." Parent: "Did Daddy go into the store?"
Comment	Adult makes a comment to keep the conversation going or to positively reinforce the child.	Parent: "Yes, that's right. Good job!"
Linguistic Mapping (Labeling)	Adult expresses in words or interprets the child's intended message using context as a clue.	(Child hands parent a toy car and vocalizes) Parent: "That's a car."

Adapted from Spencer (1994) and DesJardin and Eisenberg (2007, p. 462).

Informal Instruction

A speech and hearing professional might shape parents' communication behaviors in an informal manner. For example, the clinician might observe parent and child as they engage in a conversation during a play session in the home or clinical setting. Afterward, the clinician might say to the mother, "You seemed very attentive to Teri's focus of attention as you played with the *Lego* pieces. It was very effective the way you named the colors of each piece he picked up." With this remark, the clinician has given the mother positive reinforcement and provided instruction about how to increase vocabulary through the use of labeling. Such a remark might also serve to bolster the mother's self-confidence and sense of satisfaction about the play session.

When providing informal instruction, clinicians should exercise tact and respect for the parent and avoid being critical or negative. The goal is to empower and enable parents to use their own talents, knowledge, and experiences to foster language growth and conversational skills; criticism or an undue display of professional expertise will only diminish well-intentioned efforts. When providing instruction to parents or guardians, it is important to remember that they know their child better than anyone, including all speech and hearing professionals.

Formal Instruction

Instruction for parents or primary caregivers might also be more structured and systematic (e.g., Kashinath et al., 2006; Tye-Murray, 1994a), and might follow a similar model that we consider for communication strategies training in Chapter 9, with the stages of didactic instruction, guided learning, and real-world practice.

Didactic Instruction

During didactic instruction, a clinician might begin by discussing selected language-stimulation strategies and reviewing related examples. Parent and clinician might jointly "problem solve," brainstorm about intervention strategies, and discuss the pros and cons. The selection of strategies to be taught will depend on the age and language sophistication of the child and the parent's current behaviors. For example, if a clinician observes that a mother routinely uses expansion when interacting with her child, then there is no need to provide further instruction about the technique. If the child never uses language to communicate, then there is no language upon which to expand.

The clinician might ask a parent to describe family routines and to identify one or two that happen regularly. Initially, these routines might be selected for practicing the selected strategies. Later, use of the strategies might generalize to other situations.

Instruction may begin with a parent-friendly written handout explaining particular language stimulation and conversational strategies. The strategies can be discussed and parents might be asked to explain the strategies in their own words and to provide examples of when they might use them.

The clinician might provide audio- or videotaped examples of other parents using the strategies in order to demonstrate how they work. Two film clips might be shown to a parent (or to a parent group). For example, a first video clip might show an adult who signals low expectations that her

---

Ways for a Parent to Signal Expectation

- After asking a question, wait for an answer. Cock your head and look expectantly at your child.
- Raise your eyebrows and look inquisitive.
- Shrug your shoulders, holding your palms up.
- Maintain visual contact as you wait for your child to respond.
- Lean forward and look interested.

child will communicate, as in the following interchange taken from a film transcript (from Spencer, 1994):

Child:	(Points toward crayons)
Mother:	What are you pointing at?
Child:	(Grabs a color)
Mother:	You wanted the color. Here's some paper, too.
Mother:	What are you drawing? It looks like a cat.
Child:	(Continues drawing)
Mother:	Here is the black. You can color the tail black. (p. 52)

In this clip, the mother asks questions, but does not expect her child to answer them. She does not pause and allow the child to initiate a remark. By providing the paper and crayon to her child, she has eliminated the need for him to ask for them. A second film clip demonstrates how an adult can signal higher expectations for communication, and thereby elicit more language from her child (Spencer, 1994):

Child:	(Points toward crayons)
Mother:	What? (looks around expectantly)
Child:	Ka.
Mother:	Color?
Child:	Cala.
Mother:	Color. Green or black? (waits)
Child:	Bak.
Mother:	(Gives the child the black crayon . . . waits)
Child:	Papa.
Mother:	Paper—here's a big piece. (Holds paper up)
Child:	Mine.
Mother:	Draw me a picture. (pp. 52–53)

After a parent views this second clip, the parent and clinician can talk about how the mother frequently paused and allowed time for her child to talk. She used facial expressions that signal expectation for more information and established a turn-taking pattern. Actually seeing meaningful, concrete examples of strategies in action demonstrates their potency. A clinician can say that a technique works, but observing someone not use a strategy and then comparing the outcome to when someone uses a strategy affords an explicit contrast. In the event that no film clips are available, printed transcripts like the ones presented here can be discussed.

The clinician might then model the target strategy(ies) with the child, and when possible, do so in a simulation of a family routine or even in the home environment. The parent can observe the clinician and child and then the two of them might discuss the effectiveness of a strategy after the demonstration.

Guided Practice

The parent might then practice the strategy with the child, using the same routine that the clinician engaged in. When appropriate, the clinician might join in, while still maintaining the integrity of the parent's sequence and interaction style. This can continue until the parent feels comfortable in implementing the strategy. After practicing, the parent and clinician might identify other situations in which the practiced strategy might be implemented and/or useful. They might complete workbook activities like the one presented in Table 14-7. If groups of parents are involved, parents might share ideas about how they interest their children in using language in the home environment.

Real-World Practice

Parents might tape-record themselves while playing with their child at home and then review the tapes, checking to see whether they have implemented language-expansion and conversation-stimulating techniques. This practice will help them be more mindful of their efforts and also will provide an opportunity to appreciate the success of their efforts.

Real-world practice might be monitored by asking parents to keep a journal about their communication interactions with their child on a daily basis for a week or two. They might also complete daily checklists, indicating whether they consciously performed any of the techniques that day.

Table 14-7. Workbook exercise that an adult might complete to practice expansion.

On the lines below are some typical utterances a child might say during dinnertime. The meal consists of hamburgers and french fries. Beside each utterance, write ways that you might expand on what the child has said by modeling good grammar and/or adding a little more information.

CHILD'S UTTERANCE	YOUR EXPANDED MODEL
1. "More."	
2. "Give me."	
3. "Cup fall."	
4. "Down chair."	

Possible expatiations: (a) "I want more french fries, please"; (b) "Give me the ketchup, please"; (c) "The cup fell over"; (d) "You want to get down from your chair."

CASE STUDY

A Memorable Journey

Luanna Shibuya relates "one's family's journey into the hearing world" (Shibuya, 2006). The journey began with her son Parker, who was born in November of 1998 in Maryland, before the state had implemented newborn screening. During early infancy, Parker did not babble as much as his older sister Sydney had at the same age. His parents wrote this off to gender differences between boys and girls. They became suspicious of a hearing loss only later, when Parker continued not to respond to his name or other auditory stimuli. Shortly before his first birthday, an audiologist confirmed that he had a severe-to-profound hearing loss.

Initially, the parents "mourned the loss of their perfect son" (p. 20). Shibuya writes of unanswerable questions and a sense of unknown fear: What caused the deafness? How should the family change their goals, expectations, and desires for him? How would Parker's life differ from Sydney's? How does a family raise a child who has hearing loss? The parents' one certainty was that they wanted Parker to be a part of the hearing world, and to learn to talk and listen.

Shibuya and her husband received advice from a family friend who was an audiologist about cochlear implants and they conducted their own research as well. The parents contacted a cochlear implant center and learned about the different brands of cochlear implants available for children. They talked to as many parents of children who use implants as they could. They made a "comparison chart" that helped them to visualize the characteristics of the various cochlear implant models. They selected a particular cochlear implant brand because it had a simple head piece, a body-worn processor, and company commitment to the product. Parker underwent successful surgery, and once having received a cochlear implant, began to progress with his speech and language skills.

In October 2001, the Shibuya family welcomed a third child into the home, Sebastian. The youngest child failed his newborn hearing screening and was later diagnosed as having hearing loss. Although the mother reports of having the same sense of loss at Sebastian's diagnosis, she and her husband were more comfortable navigating the road toward cochlear implantation than they had been 3 years earlier.

Through the years, the parents have attended numerous audiological appointments and have experienced many challenges in the IFSP and IEP processes. On the whole, however, they are pleased with how well their boys are doing with their cochlear implants. The parents sometimes have to remind teachers and adults that the two boys have hearing loss, and that they cannot hear in the swimming pool or at a distance. As of 2006, Parker and Sebastian are "boys who are deaf [but] functioning in the hearing world" (p. 21). A few months before her article was published, Shibuya overheard Parker, then a student in a mainstream kindergarten class, introduce himself to an adult, "Hi, I'm Parker, I'm deaf." He said this in a matter-of-fact way, and it was the first time that his mother had heard him include hearing loss as a part of his identity.

FINAL REMARKS

In this chapter, we have focused on children who have severe and profound hearing losses. Children with lesser degrees of hearing loss also may experience listening difficulties. For instance, a child with a mild, high-frequency hearing loss may appear to have no problem in recognizing speech or responding to environmental sounds. However, the child may not be performing optimally in everyday listening settings, because he or she may have degraded listening performance in the presence of background noise. A child with a mild-to-moderate hearing loss may have decreased speech recognition and may be delayed in both speech and language development if appropriate amplification is not provided.

Children who have a lesser degree of hearing loss represent a fairly significant segment of children in the United States. Ross (1990) suggested that 16 of every 1,000 school-age children have pure-tone-averages (PTAs, Chapter 6) between 26 and 70 dB HL. These children may need special accommodations in the classroom, as we discuss at the end of Chapter 15, and may benefit from the use of special assistive listening devices, such as FM trainers (Chapter 3).

"We understand the need for speech and language services and work closely with the school, but we know that we cannot depend on the schools to manage all the boys' needs. We must be responsible and ensure services are provided adequately, and we are active participants in this process."

Luanna Shibuya, mother of two young cochlear implant users

(Shibuya, 2006, p. 21)

KEY CHAPTER POINTS

- If children are not exposed to spoken language during the first 3 years of life, they will likely experience delays in acquiring language, speech, and literacy skills.

- Most states have implemented universal newborn hearing screening (UNHS), which requires that every baby born is tested for hearing loss in the newborn nursery.

- Methods used for screening are otoacoustic emissions (OAEs) and automated brain stem response testing (A-ABR).

- If hearing loss is identified before a child reaches the age of 6 months, and intervention is begun, the child may develop language skills comparable to those of peers who have normal hearing.

- Behavioral tests for identifying hearing loss in young children include behavioral/observational audiometry (BOA), visual reinforcement audiometry (VRA), and conditioned play audiometry (CPA).

- About 40% of children who have significant hearing loss also have another disability.

- Hearing loss may arise from a variety of causes that may be prenatal, perinatal, or postnatal. The hearing loss may be due to environmental factors or genetic factors.

- Some hereditary hearing losses have a delayed onset, and some are nonsyndromic.

- Otitis media overlaid on a sensorineural hearing loss results in a mixed hearing loss. Some evidence suggests that if untreated, the child may experience related speech and language delays.

- Parents often have difficulty in accepting their children's hearing loss and may pass through a series of psychological stages before acceptance occurs. A primary role of the speech and hearing professional is to empower parents to interact effectively with their child and to make important decisions about their child's aural rehabilitation plan.

- Public Law 94-142, passed in 1975, was a landmark event in the history of children who have disabilities. It guaranteed a free and appropriate education for all children between the ages of 3 and 18 years, in the least restrictive environment.

- The acronym IDEA stands for the Individuals with Disabilities Education Act and was passed by Congress in 1990. Stemming from Public Law 94-142, it expanded the range of children covered to individuals from birth to the age of 21. It was amended in 1997 and again in 2004.

- Early and appropriate amplification is critical for normal speech and language development. Children often receive behind-the-ear hearing aids. In-the-ear aids usually are not prescribed, for a variety of reasons, including the fact that children's ears may still be growing, so aids must be frequently recast. Cochlear implants may be received after an appropriate hearing aid trial.

- Goals of the early-intervention program are to support families in developing a child's communication skills, to help the family understand the child's strengths and needs, and to promote the family's ability to advocate for the child.

TERMS AND CONCEPTS TO REMEMBER

Universal newborn hearing screening (UNHS)
Support for UNHS
Risk factors
Objective hearing tests
Behavioral hearing tests
Etiologies
Cytomegalovirus
Syndrome
Ototoxicity
Otitis media
Other disabilities
Auditory neuropathy
Stages of acceptance
Goals of early intervention
Individuals with Disabilities Education Act (IDEA)
Individualized Family Service Plan (IFSP)

Service coordinator
Medical home
American Sign Language (ASL)
Bilingual/bicultural
Total communication
Auditory-verbal approach
Validation of hearing aid fitting
Cochlear implant fitting
Family support
Facilitative language techniques

MULTIPLE-CHOICE QUESTIONS

1. The percentage of children who have hearing loss and who also have another disability is:

    a. 50%

    b. 80%

    c. 15%

    d. 40%

2. The percentage of children who have hearing loss and who are born to parents who have normal hearing is:

    a. 55%

    b. 75–80%

    c. 90–95%

    d. 40%

3. Parental radiation that results in hearing loss is an example of what kind of cause for hearing loss?

    a. Nonsyndromic

    b. Environmental

    c. Genetic

    d. Autosomal dominant

4. A child may experience a delayed-onset hearing loss most likely as a result of:

    a. Complications associated with the Rh factor

    b. Toxemia during pregnancy

    c. Hereditary condition

    d. Perinatal anoxia

5. Otitis media can result in what kind of hearing loss?

   a. Mild to moderate conductive

   b. Moderate to severe conductive

   c. Moderate sensorineural

   d. A high-frequency loss audiometric configuration

6. Alport is an example of:

   a. A syndrome

   b. A screening device

   c. A measuring unit for indexing a newborn baby's hearing thresholds

   d. A kind of inherited hearing loss that is related to an autosomal recessive genetic condition

7. The goal of the National Institutes of Health in the United States is that all children who have hearing loss are identified by:

   a. The first week of life

   b. The third month of life

   c. The first birthday

   d. The age of 2 years

8. Which of the following statements is false?

   a. Children who have hearing loss and who are identified early may have language development similar to their nonverbal cognitive development.

   b. Children who have hearing loss and who are identified early and who receive intervention maintain language development in the low-average range throughout the first 5 years of life.

   c. Before children can receive a cochlear implant, they must undergo a trial period with a hearing aid.

   d. Children who fail a screening test in the newborn nursery have a hearing loss.

9. OAEs occur because of:

   a. Electrical activity generated by synapses in the auditory nerve

   b. The elasticity of the tympanic membrane

   c. Vibration of the outer hair cells

   d. Movement by the inner hair cells

10. A medical home is:

    a. The location of the early-intervention program

    b. An approach to providing health care to infants and their families

    c. The location of the service coordinator and the IFSP

    d. The location where screening occurs

11. In audiology, the acronym BOA stands for:

    a. Benign OAE-ABR results

    b. Baby otologic awareness campaign

    c. Brain stem overview assessment

    d. Behavioral observational audiometry

12. Auditory neuropathy is characterized by:

    a. Normal ABRs and absent OAEs

    b. Present OAEs and abnormal ABRs

    c. Normal bone conduction thresholds and normal ABRs

    d. Hearing loss that is centered at the level of the cortex

13. Mary Jones has pure-tone averages of 10 dB HL in each ear. She has a hard time distinguishing between a series of three tone pips and a series of four tone pips. Mary most likely has:

    a. CAPD

    b. Auditory neuropathy

    c. Severe tinnitus

    d. Syndromic hearing loss

14. Which statement is true?

    a. Parents often go through a stage of grieving when they learn their child has hearing loss. Once this stage passes, these emotions related to the hearing loss will likely not resurface.

    b. Guilt often precedes denial during parents' adjustment period to their child's hearing loss.

    c. Shock and grief often co-occur.

    d. Good support from professionals typically allows parents to bypass the anger and guilt stages of adjustment to a child's hearing loss.

15. A service coordinator is a person who:

    a. Facilitates and helps develop the IFSP

    b. Arranges for the screening test

    c. Is involved in the first stage of receiving a cochlear implant, and provides the family with general information

    d. Arranges for the objective and/or behavioral audiological tests after a baby has failed a newborn hearing screening test

16. Babies who have hearing loss:

    a. Typically are fitted with body aids because they can be strapped to the body, so the baby won't lose it.

    b. Typically are fitted with BTE.

    c. Typically are fitted with ITE, because the pinna will not support a BTE.

    d. Typically are fitted with CIC, so they will appear like any other infant.

17. What is meant by the term *least restrictive environment?*

    a. A child is placed in the home community.

    b. A child is placed in an environment that does not impede his or her academic development.

    c. A child is placed in an environment that imposes the least limitations while still allowing the child to thrive when compared to peers who do not have a disability.

    d. A child is placed in an environment that allows him or her to be included in all aspects of the general classroom's daily routines and activities.

18. What is due process with respect to the IDEA?

    a. All children will receive a comprehensive evaluation of hearing, speech, language, cognition, and academic performance before goals and objectives are formulated for the IEP.

    b. Parents will have an opportunity to question the IEP, and if necessary, have a due process hearing. They have the option to be accompanied by counsel and other individuals with specialized knowledge about their child.

    c. Each state must set up an advisory board, including individuals with disabilities, teachers, and parents of children who have disabilities. This board will ensure that due process is followed in providing education to children who have disabilities.

    d. For parents who opt to send their children to private schools, the state government will provide them the same funds toward tuition that would have been expended had their children received due process services in the home community via public education mechanisms.

19. What best describes the IFSP?

   a. A federally mandated plan for providing elementary education to children with disabilities, which is updated annually

   b. Individualized Federal Service Plan

   c. An amendment made to IDEA in 1997

   d. A federally mandated plan for the education of preschool children, which emphasizes family involvement

20. Which of the following statements is false?

   a. Cued Speech supplements lipreading.

   b. Cued Speech is equivalent to the manual alphabet.

   c. Cued Speech is used by a minority of children who are deaf or hard of hearing.

   d. In Cued Speech, the position of the hand on the face and neck conveys vowel information.

21. For cochlear implant users, which mode of communication results in the development of optimal speech and language skills?

   a. Cued Speech

   b. Aural/oral

   c. Total communication

   d. ASL

KEY RESOURCES

 A PARENT'S GUIDE TO HEARING AND LANGUAGE MILESTONES HANDOUT

Your baby will reach a series of milestones as he or she grows. If you suspect that your baby is not reaching these milestones, talk to your doctor or speech and hearing professional, because your baby may have a hearing loss or some other condition that is delaying development.

Newborn

• Cries
• Startles to loud and/or sudden sound

2 to 3 Months

• Laughs
• Forms sounds in the back of the mouth ("gah")

- Responds to your (parent's) voice
- Distinguishes changes in the tone of voice (happy vs. sad)

4 to 6 Months

- Turns head toward sound
- Begins to put sounds together, typically a consonant and a vowel ("bah")
- Makes nonspeech sounds playfully (squeals, yells, makes "raspberries")

6 to 12 Months

- Babbles strings of syllables ("bah-bah-bah")
- Attempts nonverbal communication through facial expression, eye gaze, vocalization, and gestures such as pointing, reaching, and head shaking
- By 12 months, responds to name; understands the word *no* and simple instructions; gives a toy in response to a request

12 to 18 Months

- Strings sounds together that have an adultlike speech rhythm
- Speaks first words
- By 18 months, understands about 50 words and speaks up to 20 words, usually in isolation and not sentences or phrases

18 to 36 Months

- Demonstrates rapid speech development: learns new words rapidly and puts them together in strings of two or more
- By 36 months, can understand up to 3,600 words; constructs sentences with an average of 3 to 4 words; can tell a simple story; can sing songs; can provide simple information verbally, such as the name of the family's street or his or her age

APPENDIX 14-1

A speech and hearing professional might encounter these abbreviations and acronyms when reading the medical or audiological records for an infant or very young child (adapted from Mize & Wigley, 2002).

- BMT: Bilateral myringotomy and tubes
- Chemotx: Chemotherapy
- CHL: Conductive hearing loss
- CNT: Could not test
- DNT: Did not test

- ENT: Ear-nose-throat
- F/u: Follow-up
- H/o: History of
- M/o: Month old
- NBHS: Newborn hearing screening
- PCHI: Permanent childhood hearing impairment
- Pt: Patient
- R/o: Rule-out
- SF: Soundfield
- SLP: Speech-language pathologist
- SNHL: Sensorineural hearing loss
- S/p: Status post
- TEOAE: Transient evoked otoacoustic emissions
- TM: Tympanic membrane
- Tymps: Ympanogram
- UNHS: Universal newborn hearing screening
- WNL: Within normal limits
- Y/o: Year old

APPENDIX 14-2

Important Terms to Know When Discussing Genetics (adapted from Clark & Russell, 1997, pp. 13–26)

Allele: One particular version of a gene.

Chromosome: Structures bearing the genes of a cell and made of a single strand of DNA.

DNA: (deoxyribonucleic acid) Nucleic acid polymer of which the genes are made.

Dominant allele: The allele whose properties are expressed as the phenotype.

Gene: A unit of genetic information contained within the chromosome that can be inherited.

Genotype: The total genetic makeup of an organism.

Heterozygous: Having two different alleles of the same gene.

Homozygous: Having two identical alleles of the same gene.

Mutation: An alteration in the genetic information carried by a gene.

Phenotype: The visible effect of the genotype.

Recessive allele: The allele for which properties are not observed because they are masked by the dominant allele.

Sex-linked: A gene is sex-linked when it is carried on one of the sex chromosomes.

APPENDIX 14-3

Some of the acronyms used when talking about children and their educational needs include the following:

- FAPE: Free appropriate public education
- IDEA: Individuals with Disabilities Education Act
- IEP: Individualized Education Plan
- IFSP: Individualized Family Service Plan
- IAT: Intervention assistance team, a multidisciplinary group of professionals who work together to provide intervention for a child
- LRE: Least restrictive environment
- SST: Supplemental services teacher, who interacts with a child's regular teacher to help the child

APPENDIX 14-4

Family Support Services (adapted from the Centers for Disease Control and Prevention, www.cdc.gov/ncbddd/ehdi/links.htm, retrieved July 16, 2007, and Florida Resource Guide, 2005)

Agencies:

1. The Alexander Graham Bell Association for the Deaf and Hard of Hearing (www.agbell.org) helps families understand childhood hearing loss and the importance of early diagnosis and intervention. Through advocacy, education, research, and financial aid, the society ensures that children with hearing loss have the opportunity to listen and talk. There are chapters throughout the United States and a network of international affiliates.

2. American Society for Deaf Children (ASDC; www.deafchildren .org) is an organization of parents and families that advocates for children's total quality participation in education, the family, and the community.

3. Auditory-Verbal International (www.auditory-verbal.org) provides resources and information to parents and speech and hearing professionals on teaching children who have hearing loss to speak with residual hearing and amplification.

4. Babyhearing (www.babyhearing.org), created by Boys Town National Research Hospital, has centers for research and clinical

services for hearing loss in children. Parents are invited to ask questions about infant hearing screening and follow-up testing, steps to take following diagnosis, hearing aids, language and speech, and parenting issues.

5. Family Voices (www.familyvoices.org) is a national organization that is a clearinghouse for information and education concerning the health care of children with special needs.

6. Hands & Voices National (www.handsandvoices.org) is a parent-driven, nonprofit organization supporting families with children who have hearing loss, regardless of communication method or mode. Membership includes families, professionals, and individuals who are deaf or hard of hearing who collaborate to empower families with newly identified babies with hearing loss, to advocate for better educational outcomes, and to provide information and technical support on related subjects without a bias toward one form of communication over another.

7. John Tracy Clinic (www.jtc.org) is a nonprofit organization that provides, worldwide and without charge, parent-centered services to young children with hearing loss. Services include audiological testing, parent/infant programs, parent classes, a preschool, and a correspondence course.

8. Laurent Clerc National Deaf Education Center (www.clerccenter .gallaudet.edu), part of Gallaudet University, provides information on various topics related to deafness.

9. Marion Downs National Center for Infant Hearing (www.colorado .edu/slhs/mdnc/links.html) provides information on newborn hearing screening, assessment, diagnosis, and early intervention.

10. National Association of the Deaf (NAD; www.nad.org) is the oldest and largest organization representing people with disabilities in the United States. They provide information about grassroots advocacy and empowerment, captioned media, legal assistance, policy development and research, public awareness, and youth leadership.

11. National Cued Speech Association (www.cuedspeech.org) promotes and supports the use of Cued Speech for communication, education, language acquisition, and literacy.

12. National Policy Center for Children With Special Health Care Needs is concerned with the promotion of complete, family-centered systems of health care for children with special needs. The Center is dedicated to producing information that is relevant to benefit managed care organizations, state agencies, families, and program administrators.

13. The SKI-HI Institute (www.skihi.org) is devoted to providing information for assisting infants, toddlers, and young children and their families through research, development, promising practices, training, technical assistance, and information sharing.

Additional Web Sites

1. Animated American Sign Language Dictionary, www.bconnex.net. Provides animated demonstrations of signs and fingerspelling.

2. Center for Disease Control, www.cdc.gov/ncbdd/ehdi. Provides information about hearing detection and intervention.

3. Children's Medical Services, www.cms-kids.org. Provides children with special health care needs a family-centered, managed system of care.

4. National Center for Hearing Assessment and Management, www.infanthearing.org. Assists families with managing hearing loss.

5. Oral Deaf Education/Oberkotter Foundation, www.oraldeafed.org. Provides support to parents of children with hearing loss.

6. Sign with Your Baby, www.sign2me.net. Promotes benefits of teaching sign language to babies.

CHAPTER 15

School-Age Children Who Have Hearing Loss

OUTLINE

- Creation of an Individualized Education Plan (IEP)
- The multidisciplinary team
- School and classroom placement
- Amplification and assistive listening devices
- Classroom acoustics
- Speech, language, and literacy
- Other services
- Children who have mild or moderate hearing losses
- Case studies: IDEA(s) for all
- Final remarks
- Key chapter points
- Terms and concepts to remember
- Multiple-choice questions
- Key resources

A t about the age of 3 or 4 years, a child who has hearing loss is ready to enroll in preschool. The next decade and a half of formal education will present rewarding and challenging years, as the child continues to develop communication skills, learns to read, studies academics, and engages in social activities with classmates. In this chapter, we consider children who are of school age, and the aural rehabilitation services that will enhance and promote their educational experiences. The bulk of the chapter concerns children who have severe and profound hearing losses. At the end of the chapter, we consider children with mild and moderate hearing losses.

Figure 15-1 presents a schematic of a child entering the school system. At the point of entry, the child likely is using a listening device and has begun to use a communication mode, such as spoken language or total communication. Changes in either listening device or communication mode might be made once the child enters into a preschool or kindergarten, depending on how well he or she is progressing. He or she may have received early intervention services, such as center-based or home-based aural rehabilitation, which will have equipped him or her with school-readiness skills. Examples of school-readiness skills are knowing how to sit quietly at a table or desk and knowing how to change in an orderly fashion from one structured activity to the next. The formation of a multidisciplinary team, the creation of an Individualized Education Plan, and the selection of school and classroom placement are illustrated as sections of a pie chart because these events do not necessarily happen sequentially. Sometimes they happen almost simultaneously and sometimes the determination of one, say selection of a school, will have an impact on the determination of another, say the selection of members for the multidisciplinary team. From this triad, the child emerges into a school setting. An aural rehabilitation intervention strategy will ensure that his or her listening device is maintained and that he or she has access to appropriate assistive listening devices. Special steps will be taken to promote development of speech, language, and literacy skills and to facilitate social adjustment.

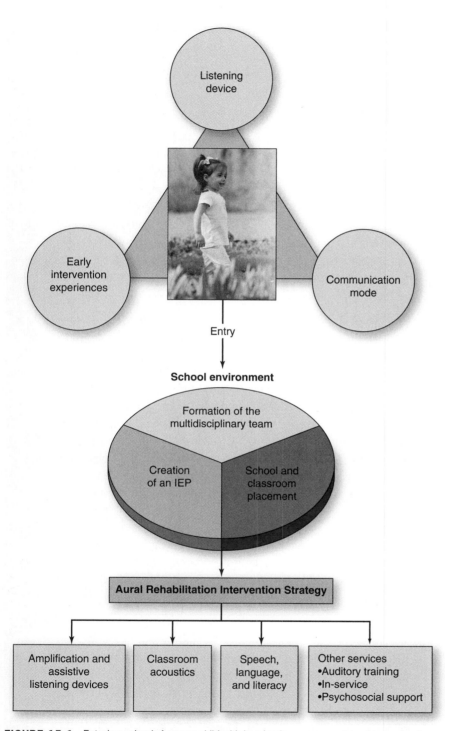

FIGURE 15-1. Entering school. A young child with hearing loss prepares to enter a school setting. She brings with her experience with a listening device, a communication mode, and experiences from an early intervention program. *Photograph courtesy of MED-EL Corp.*

The Beginnings of Education for Children Who Are Deaf and Hard of Hearing in the United States

The beginnings of education for children who are deaf and hard of hearing in the New World follow two threads, manual communication and aural/oral communication (or oralism). Although there were sporadic attempts to educate children with significant hearing loss in the United States before Alice Cogswell, many historians date the dawn of deaf education in this country to her birth in 1805. Alice was born into a well-to-do family in New England. At the age of 2 years, she contracted "spotted fever" and lost her hearing. Treatments of salt water poured into her ears, leeches, and special creams could not return what was lost. An ear trumpet bought by her distraught parents allowed her to hear a church bell, but not much more.

Alice's father, Dr. Mason Fitch Cogswell, a physician who performed some of the first cataract surgeries in the United States, commissioned his young neighbor, Thomas Hopkins Gallaudet, to travel to Europe and learn instructional methods for the deaf. Gallaudet originally planned to visit the Braidwood family in England and Abbé Sicard in France, to gather instructional techniques in aural/oral communication and manual communication in the two countries, respectively. The Braidwood family proved to be secretive and unwilling to share their oral teaching methods. Thus, in 1816 Gallaudet left London for Paris, where he learned a manual communication system from Abbé Sicard and Laurent Clerc (himself deaf). Gallaudet returned to the United States, along with Clerc, and provided instruction to Alice. The two men went on to establish the American Asylum for the Education of the Deaf and Dumb (now the American School for the Deaf) in 1817, a school with a manual orientation. During the next 40 years, Clerc became one of the most influential educators of children who were deaf and the first (and one of the few) deaf teachers in the 19th century. Gallaudet's son, Edward Miner Gallaudet (1837–1917), became the president of the first college for students who are deaf in the new world, now named Gallaudet University.

The thread of oralism in the United States can be picked up several years later. This moment in time, too, was triggered when a young girl of a prominent family lost her hearing. Mabel Hubbard suffered scarlet fever in 1863 and, as a result, incurred an irreversible hearing loss. Her father, Gardiner Greene Hubbard, a lawyer in Massachusetts, helped to establish the Clarke School in Northampton, Massachusetts, in 1867,

The Beginnings of Education for Children Who Are Deaf and Hard of Hearing in the United States, *continued*

with the assistance of Samuel Howe, who also was the principal of the first school for the blind in the United States.

When Mabel Hubbard grew up, she married Alexander Graham Bell (Figure 15-2). In the latter half of the 19th century, Bell became an articulate and passionate advocate for oralism in the United States. In fact, an impetus for developing the telephone was a desire to develop an amplification device for his wife-to-be and for his mother, who also had a hearing loss. His counterpart, who advocated an orientation that incorporated manual communication, was Edward Gallaudet. In the late 1800s, these two men often were engaged in debate as to the merits of one method versus the other.

Throughout the 20th century, debates and controversies flared on and off as to which of the two basic educational approaches, manual or aural/oral, is most appropriate for educating children who are deaf. The debate continues into the 21st century.

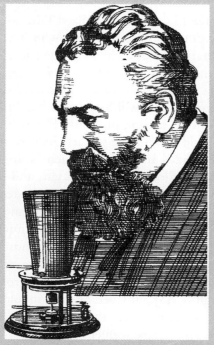

FIGURE 15-2. Alexander Graham Bell, advocate for an aural/oral mode of communication.

CREATION OF AN INDIVIDUALIZED EDUCATION PLAN (IEP)

IDEA and the Child Who Has Hearing Loss

Section 300.346 of the IDEA (1997) states:

The IEP team shall also:

(iv) Consider the communication needs of the child, and in the case of the child who is deaf or hard of hearing, consider the child's language and communication needs, opportunities for direct communications with peers and professional personnel in the child's language and communication mode, academic level, and full range of needs, including opportunities for direct instruction in the child's language and communication mode; and

(v) Consider whether the child requires assistive technology devices and services.

As noted in Chapter 14, an Individualized Education Plan (IEP) is a written statement developed for children who have a disability. The plan includes a description of a child's present levels of performance, a statement of annual goals (e.g., a listing of language structures that will be mastered), a recommendation for special education support with an indication of how support will be provided and to what extent, and objective criteria for evaluating progress. The IEP also indicates the extent to which a child will be able to participate in regular educational programs. Specific details are included, such as the location and plan for service delivery, how long services will last, and how and when the child will be promoted within the public school system. The IDEA stipulates that in the development, review, and revision of an IEP, the plan takes into account the language and communication needs of the child and the opportunities available for direct communication with peers and professionals in the child's language and communication mode. Interpreting services, such as an educational interpreter who is proficient in signed English, ASL, or Cued Speech, should be made available as needed. Table 15-1 summarizes the components of an IEP whereas Table 15-2 presents an example segment.

Table 15-1. Components of the Individualized Education Plan.

1. A statement of the present level of performance
2. A statement of annual goals
3. Short-term instructional objectives
4. Special education and related services to be provided
5. Extent of participation in the regular educational program
6. Projected date for services to begin
7. Anticipated duration of services
8. Appropriate criteria to determine if objectives are achieved
9. Evaluation procedures to determine if objectives are achieved
10. Schedules for review
11. Assessment information
12. Placement justification statement
13. A statement of how special education services are tied to the regular education program

Adapted from Haynes, Moran, and Pindzola (2006, p. 9).

Table 15-2. Example segment of an Individual Education Plan.

DOMAIN	STATUS	ANNUAL GOAL	SHORT-TERM OBJECTIVE
Audiologic	Can discriminate two utterances that differ in syllable length and intonation, such as *hello* from *how are you?*	To achieve closed-set identification of monosyllabic everyday words	Will correctly identify a spoken word when presented in the context of four then six alternatives with 80% accuracy
Language	Does not use bound morphemes, such as *-ed* or *-ing*	To establish consistent use of word endings in expressive and written communication	Will demonstrate use of past tense endings in 80% of written samples and in 70% of spontaneous and spoken language samples
Speech	Neutralizes vowels and omits final word consonants	To improve speech intelligibility	Will distinguish between /i/, /a/, and /u/ in imitated speech tasks with 80% accuracy, and produce final consonants in at least 50% of words spoken during a spontaneous speech task
Psychosocial	Does not follow classroom rules	To demonstrate grade-appropriate classroom behavior	Will receive positive reinforcements for adhering to classroom regulations, and accumulate 100 points during a 3-month period
Educational	Reading is delayed by one grade level; can read aloud but has reduced comprehension	To improve reading comprehension	Will demonstrate comprehension on 85% of grade-appropriate reading samples

Table 15-3 presents an example segment describing a child's present level of performance. This segment describes academic/educational achievement and learning characteristics. The IEP may also include a description of a child's present level of performance in the domains of social development, physical development, and needs within a classroom setting.

Table 15-3. An example segment from an IEP describing "Andrew Johnson" and his present level of academic performance. Andrew is an 8-year-old boy with profound hearing loss. Similar descriptions to this one are included in Andrew's IEP that describe his social development, physical development, and classroom needs.

> *Andrew is a curious boy who enjoys variety. His grades range from Bs to Cs. He responds well to visual aids, hands-on activities, and novelty. Andrew experiences moderate difficulty in working independently, and often requires teacher encouragement to complete an assignment. Andrew recognizes common words during reading class and is performing just below grade level on reading comprehension tests. He enjoys listening to stories and appears to have good auditory comprehension with the use of his cochlear implant. Mathematics may be a strength. He is able to add and subtract three- and four-digit numbers.*

The IEP is developed in a meeting attended by representative(s) of the local educational agency, the teacher, the parents or guardians, and sometimes, the child and/or other individuals at the discretion of the parents. When the child has a communication disorder, a speech-language pathologist and/or an audiologist likely attends. These meetings are usually held annually.

THE MULTIDISCIPLINARY TEAM

A **multidisciplinary team** is a group of professionals with different expertise who contribute to the assessment, intervention, and management of a particular individual.

The members of the **multidisciplinary team** implement the IEP. This team may include an audiologist, a speech-language pathologist, an educator, and a psychologist (and/or a counselor). Depending on the situation, the team also may include an interpreter and an itinerant teacher (and/or a resource teacher). Each professional provides a different perspective of the child's abilities and needs and provides different services.

The Role of the Audiologist

An audiologist may perform any of the following duties:

- Evaluate hearing and speech recognition skills
- Assess central auditory function
- Select, fit, and help maintain appropriate listening devices, including hearing aids and FM systems

- Analyze classroom environment and make recommendations about improving classroom acoustics and reducing classroom noise
- Provide speech perception training
- Provide consultation to parents and other professionals on the multidisciplinary team

Audiologists identify and evaluate children's hearing capabilities and speech recognition skills. Although very young children may not be able to participate in word recognition testing, assessment of hearing thresholds can be performed with almost all age groups. Following identification, the audiologist may make any necessary referrals, such as to a physician or other health care professional. The audiologist also may initiate the formation of the multidisciplinary team and the case-management process.

Audiologists also select and ensure proper use of listening devices. They may select and fit a new hearing aid or make a recommendation for the child to receive a cochlear implant. They likely will explore the child's home and school environments, either through parent and teacher questionnaires or through site visits to the home and school. For instance, the audiologist may see that the child is in a noisy classroom and often misses much of the teacher's speech. The audiologist then may recommend that the child and teacher use an FM system to reduce the effects of background noise. Follow-up maintenance and repair also will be provided.

Sometimes audiologists provide formal speechreading and auditory training rather than, or in addition to, the speech-language pathologist or classroom teacher. In some cases, they may make recommendations to the person who provides training. Finally, audiologists consult with parents and teachers about the child's listening potential and difficulties and ways to encourage the development of listening skills.

Educational Audiologists: Here, There, and Where?

Educational audiologists are audiologists who work in the school systems. Although there are no hard and firm figures about how many audiologists serve U.S. schools, the American Speech-Language Association (ASHA) estimates the number to be about 1,200. The number working within states varies. Whereas a state like Iowa employs about 55 full-time educational audiologists working in 12 area education agencies (AEAs),

continues

Part B is the section of Public Law PL 105-17 (IDEA) that refers to intervention services for eligible children between the ages of 3 and 21 years in the public school system.

Educational Audiologists: Here, There, and Where?, *continued*

a state like Oklahoma employs only 1 to serve its largest school district of 42,000 students. Audiological services for children between the ages of 3 and 21 years are authorized by **Part B** of IDEA. Services include hearing screening, provision of aural rehabilitation services, creation and administration of prevention programs, provision of counseling and guidance, and selection, fitting, and evaluation of listening devices. School districts are not required to employ an educational audiologist, but they are required to ensure that children who require audiological services receive them (Pallarito, 2006).

The U.S. Department of Education allocates funding for IDEA, but for many years, appropriations have fallen short of authorized funding. In the fiscal year 2002, for example, states and localities had to absorb about $10.5 billion in shortfalls. States vary in how they divvy up their funds, and it is not uncommon for audiologists to have to compete on behalf of school-based hearing programs against others seeking funding for other services. Ensuring that children are supplied with appropriate and functioning listening aids and assistive listening technology is very difficult for many school districts.

The Role of the Speech-Language Pathologist

An ASHA Omnibus Survey (2003) suggests that about 46% of school-based speech-language pathologists serve children who have hearing loss and on average, they have about three children with hearing loss in their caseloads. A speech-language pathologist may perform any of the following functions (see also American Speech-Language-Hearing Association, 2004c):

- Evaluate speech and language performance
- Evaluate preliteracy and literacy skills, including phonological awareness
- May evaluate speechreading skills
- May select assistive listening devices and perform visual inspection and listening check of amplification devices
- Collaborate in the assessment of central auditory processing disorders
- Provide speech and language therapy
- Consult with parents and classroom teachers

- Provide instruction in sign language to child, classroom teacher, and parents, if appropriate
- Maintain bridges of communication between clinical setting, classroom, and home, and ensure that therapy objectives are reinforced informally throughout a child's day
- Advise audiologists about appropriate language levels for audiological tests
- Provide speech perception training

A speech-language pathologist evaluates speech and language performance and provides speech and language therapy. Test results are used to identify initial therapy objectives, and a hierarchy of steps to be followed over time is developed. Often, the objectives coincide with a curriculum that has been developed specifically for children who have hearing loss.

The speech-language pathologist also provides consultation to parents, teachers, audiologists, and other members of the multidisciplinary team. For instance, they may familiarize parents and teachers with their child's speech and language skills and how the child's skills compare to those of other children. They also can describe both how speech and language skills progress in children with normal hearing and children with hearing loss, and factors that may accelerate or impede progress. Such information helps those who know the child to develop appropriate expectations and provides them with ideas about how best to nurture the child's development.

For families who use total communication or ASL, speech-language pathologists may help parents and teachers learn sign language. They may recommend printed or video resources that include sign dictionaries, and may even provide direct instruction and practice.

Speech-language pathologists also can suggest ways for helping children generalize what they learned in therapy to more real-world settings by informing parents and teachers about their child's current therapy objectives and by suggesting practice materials. For example, a speech-language pathologist might observe a child in the classroom and then suggest ways the classroom teacher can integrate speech and language practice into the daily routine.

Speech-language pathologists may provide information about the child's language skills to audiologists and help them select appropriate audiological tests. For instance, if the speech-language evaluation reveals that a child has an extremely limited vocabulary, the audiologist may opt not to evaluate the child's speech recognition skills with recorded sentence lists.

In some cases, the speech-language pathologist provides formal speechreading and auditory training and may even perform hearing screenings. Again, the speech-language pathologist interacts with teachers and parents so they can reinforce auditory and speechreading training in everyday communication situations.

The Role of the Educator

The teacher provides academic instruction in the classroom setting. Sometimes the teacher is a regular classroom teacher and will have had little experience in working with children who have hearing loss, and sometimes the teacher has a degree in deaf education. A regular education teacher knows the general curriculum and knows strategies that might help a child learn appropriate behavior, if behavior is at issue. A teacher of children who are deaf and hard of hearing has expertise in modifying the curriculum for a child who has hearing loss so that the child has an optimal opportunity to learn. The teacher of children who are deaf and hard of hearing has completed a planned curriculum of educational coursework and practicums that include observation, student teaching, planning, implementing, and evaluation of educational outcomes with respect to children who have hearing loss. This teacher can individualize instruction and can advise other adults about modifications in either the physical classroom or classroom procedures that may facilitate learning. The roles of the classroom teacher may include (American Speech-Language-Hearing Association, 2004c, p. 3):

- Assessment, diagnosis, and evaluation
- Planning instructional content and practice
- Planning and managing the learning environment
- Managing student behavior and social interactions skills

Ideally the classroom teacher will understand a child's specific needs, and will help to ensure that a child with hearing loss receives additional support in relation to his or her listening, speaking, language, and reading comprehension abilities. The teacher may perform a listening check on a child's hearing aid on a daily basis and troubleshoot problems. The teacher may also act as a liaison between the child and the family and the school district.

The Role of the Psychologist

The psychologist often performs a psychoeducational assessment. The psychoeducational assessment may include an evaluation of the following child variables (Heller, 1990, p. 62):

- Intelligence, both *verbal* (cognitive abilities demonstrated via language-based performance) and *nonverbal* (cognitive abilities demonstrated by performance that is not language based)

- Verbal function, written language, and reading
- Arithmetic skills
- Visual-motor skills
- Visual and auditory memory and multimodal integration
- Social and emotional function and problem solving
- Attention
- Behavior

The results of this assessment may be used to design a child's intervention plan and to assess whether the child is progressing within his or her current program. The psychologist can also provide support to a student. This professional can talk with a child and provide the youth with the language necessary to express feelings about having a hearing loss, and can help facilitate interactions with fellow classmates (e.g., Dworkin, 2004).

Sometimes the psychologist is also the school counselor. In this role, the professional can provide structured programs that promote coping skills, psychosocial adjustment, a positive self-concept, and problem-solving abilities. For the older student, the professional may provide information about postsecondary programs that cater to students who have hearing loss.

The Role of the Interpreter

The interpreter presents the ongoing classroom dialogue to the child using the child's preferred mode of communication. Most often, an interpreter is part of the multidisciplinary team when the child uses sign language and the classroom teacher does not sign. The interpreter may provide in-class support as well, especially in elementary schools when a child stays in the same classroom for most of the day. The interpreter also promotes communication and interactions between the student and classmates by conveying spoken and signed information back and forth.

The Role of the Itinerant Teacher

A general education teacher may receive the assistance of an **itinerant teacher** for children who are deaf and hard of hearing. The itinerant teacher works with the student with hearing loss on a one-on-one basis, with the objective of reinforcing classroom instruction. Concepts, vocabulary, and literature that have been covered in the regular classroom may be reviewed. The itinerant teacher will receive copies of classroom materials, such as handouts and visual aids, and may go through these with the student. The itinerant teacher may also prepare a student for new material, teaching key concepts, words, and phrases before the student encounters them in the

Itinerant teachers work in several schools, providing support services to children who are deaf and hard of hearing and to their teachers.

"Itinerant teachers. These people are lifelines or whatever, I mean you can't sing their praises enough."

Liz, parent of a child with hearing loss who attends a public school, commenting on what makes inclusion possible

(Eriks-Borphy et al., 2006, p. 64)

"Families want flexibility in methodology and placement decisions. What may be the 'right decision' at a given point in time may change later on. Families want to be supported in the options they choose, and not made to feel 'locked in' to these important decisions."

Jackson Roush, professor, University of North Carolina at Chapel Hill

(Roush, 1994, p. 349).

regular classroom. Sometimes the itinerant teacher will provide auditory and speechreading training and sign language instruction, and will sometimes develop individualized programs that promote a student's language, social, and academic skills. The itinerant teacher also might educate classroom teachers and peers about issues related to hearing loss and might help the teacher learn how to handle assistive technology.

SCHOOL AND CLASSROOM PLACEMENT

Because urban and rural areas of the United States afford different educational opportunities, decisions about school and classroom placement are to some extent dependent on geographic location. In large cities, parents often have several choices whereas in rural areas, familial choice may be limited.

School Placement

Options for school placement include public or private institutions and day or residential programs. Public placements are funded by government sources whereas private placements are funded by tuition and charitable donations.

A residential school provides comprehensive academic, health, and socialization programs. Students live in dormitories with other children who are deaf and hard of hearing. The staff at the school are expected to communicate with the students fluently, using the students' mode of communication.

A day school for children who are deaf and hard of hearing employs teachers of children who are deaf and hard of hearing to teach all academic subjects. These schools have support personnel readily available, such as an audiologist and speech-language pathologist. Children commute to a day school for children who are deaf and hard of hearing from their homes on a daily basis, and the school is usually located in a central location so it serves children from all over the geographic region. Another version of a day-school placement is enrollment within a general education school, where students receive instruction either in a self-contained classroom or in a regular classroom.

Since the passage of U.S. Public Law (PL) 94-142 (the Education for All Handicapped Children Act) in 1975, there has been a substantial increase in the number of children who remain in their home communities and receive a public education. Concomitantly, there has been a decrease in the number of children who attend residential and day schools for children who are deaf and hard of hearing. Less than 10% of children between the ages of 6 and 21 years attend a residential facility and less than 10% attend a day school for children who are deaf and hard of hearing (U.S. Department of Education, 1998).

Classroom Placement

Two distinct classroom placement options, self-contained and mainstream, are available in many public school districts and a third, resource rooms, may also be available. **Self-contained classrooms** are contained within neighborhood or community schools and include only students with hearing loss (Figure 15-3) or may also include children who have other disabilities, in which case it is classified as a *multicategorical self-contained* classroom. In **mainstream classrooms**, children with hearing loss attend classes together with children who have normal hearing. Some children attend a self-contained classroom for part of the school day and a mainstream classroom for some subjects, such as art and physical education (Figure 15-4). When in a mainstream classroom, children often utilize support services, such as the use of a sign or oral interpreter and/or an FM system. Some children attend a mainstream classroom and also receive individualized instruction in a resource room. Children who attend **resource rooms** spend some part of their school day in a regular classroom, and receive instruction from a speech and hearing specialist or a special education teacher for certain topics, such as language.

In some mainstream scenarios, children are treated more like "visitors" to the regular classroom than active members (Antia, Stinson, & Gaustad, 2002). Because of academic or behavioral considerations, the classroom teacher might believe a child is best served in the special classrooms. The upside of this model is that in some ways the child might get the best of both worlds. He or she receives needed support and still has an opportunity to interact with a peer group. The downside of this model is that a student's "visits" to the classroom might be disruptive to the classroom routine, and the child may not be able to slip into the flow of what is happening at the moment (e.g., the child might not have performed an assignment that is under current discussion).

An alternative or a supplement to a resource room is an itinerant teacher. The child attends school in a regular classroom, but receives support services from an itinerant teacher, who works in several schools and has expertise in issues related to hearing loss.

Two derivatives of mainstreaming are inclusion and coenrollment. Like mainstreaming, **inclusion** entails placing children who have hearing

"When I attended the school for the deaf, I took deafness for granted, I did not understand then, that if you are deaf, you do not hear. Then you are not like the others. Then you are different. I did not understand it. I took being deaf for granted. . . . but when I got my own [hearing] friends and I wanted to talk with them, instead of my family, then I met with obstacles. That was a great barrier. Bang."

Gro, a high school student living in Norway

(Ohna, 2003, p. 7)

Self-contained classrooms include only children who are deaf and hard of hearing.

In **mainstream classrooms**, children who are deaf and hard of hearing attend classes with their normally hearing peers.

Resource rooms provide instruction in particular areas for children who spend part of their day in regular classrooms.

Inclusion integrates all students and activities into the daily routine of the general education classroom.

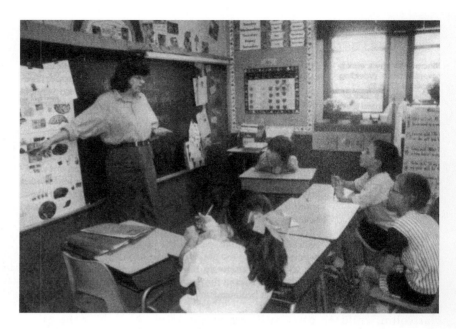

FIGURE 15-3. Self-contained classroom placement. Class sizes are usually small, and children sit in a circle around the teacher. *Photograph by Kim Readmond, courtesy of the Central Institute for the Deaf.*

loss in classrooms with children who have normal hearing. A child in an inclusion classroom is included in all aspects of the class life and the school (Figure 15-5) (Antia et al., 2002; Marschark, Young, & Lukomski, 2002). The classroom teacher has the primary job of educating every child in the classroom, but may also have a partnership with a special education teacher in making adjustments to the curriculum and structuring the classroom environment to meet the learning needs of the child with hearing loss. The philosophical difference between mainstreaming and inclusion is that, in the former, the child must adapt to the classroom, whereas in the latter, the classroom must adapt to the child (Stinson & Antia, 1999). Children in an inclusion setting usually communicate with spoken language, total communication, or Cued Speech. Children who use ASL typically are not placed in this setting. Inclusion is not without its challenges. Many classroom teachers feel unprepared to handle the multifaceted needs of both children who have normal hearing and children who have hearing loss, and sometimes the child with hearing loss has problems integrating socially with his or her peers who have normal hearing (e.g., Israelite, Ower, & Goldstein, 2002) and feels "different" from classmates (Leigh, 1999). The advantages of

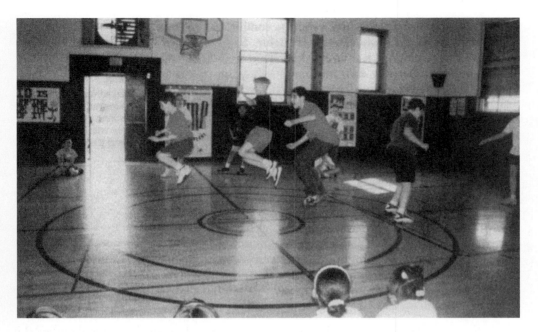

FIGURE 15-4. Partial mainstream classroom placement. Children may be mainstreamed for nonacademic subjects during the school day, such as physical education class. *Photograph by Kim Readmond, courtesy of the Central Institute for the Deaf.*

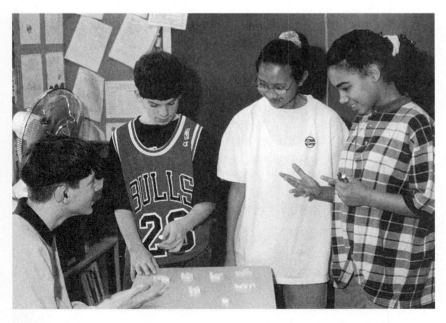

FIGURE 15-5. Inclusion classroom placement. The child with hearing loss is an active member of the classroom, participating in all academic and social interactions. *Photograph by Marcus Kosa, courtesy of the Central Institute for the Deaf.*

"Deaf kids do have deficits in just general knowledge and background knowledge of things that hearing kids understand because they have experience with something similar . . . so you have to be watching all the time for what they don't get because they don't have experience with it before . . . I think a lot of times regular teachers assume a depth of knowledge that deaf kids really don't have and they sit a lot of times without having a clue what you're talking about."

Helen, a regular classroom teacher who taught in a coenrollment class with children with hearing loss

(Jiménez-Sánchez & Antia, 1999, p. 221)

Coenrollment refers to a model of educating children who have hearing loss that entails a team of teachers, one a regular classroom teacher and the other, a trained teacher for children who have hearing loss.

inclusion include opportunities for children with hearing loss to participate more readily in extracurricular activities with their neighborhood peers and to learn from speech and language modeling afforded by children with normal hearing. For children with normal hearing, advantages include being exposed from an early age to students with disabilities, which may lead to better acceptance and understanding of differences (Eriks-Brophy et al., 2006).

In a **coenrollment model**, the classroom is conducted by two teachers, a regular classroom teacher and a teacher of children who are deaf and hard of hearing (Antia & Levine, 2001; Jimenez-Sanchez & Antia, 1999). The class may include students who have normal hearing and students who have hearing loss and who may use sign. The ratio of children who are deaf and hard of hearing to children with normal hearing is about 1:4 (e.g., Mellon, 2005). When there is a balanced mix of students, the model may be referred to as *reverse mainstream.* All students have access to the school district's adopted grade-level curriculum, and teachers hold the same expectations for students with normal and impaired hearing. This model aspires to place children who have hearing loss on the same playing field as children who have normal hearing. This kind of team-teaching gives all students exposure to their own culture and that of others, and helps students establish a self-identity and self-esteem. The students with normal hearing may be expected to learn sign and to learn about the Deaf culture.

School Days

High school students who had hearing losses ranging from moderate to profound were queried about their school experiences and interactions with their peers. These students live in Toronto, Canada. They attended special classes for hard-of-hearing students for their elementary schooling and now attend a regular public high school with children who have normal hearing. Here are some of their comments about fitting in to the mainstream (Israelite et al., 2002, pp. 141–142):

About fitting in, a student named Sam said: "My biggest challenge was grade 9. Trying to fit in a school where I had never been, where people from my neighborhood attended too. . . . When I was there, people would put me down because I was different from them. But my challenge was to fit with them, to tell them that I could do the same thing as [them] or possibly better."

School Days, *continued*

About revealing her hearing loss to peers, a student named Kate said: "I realized when I first entered my mainstream English class they don't know I'm hard of hearing so they treat me like everyone else. If I say I'm hard of hearing, then they will treat me differently. . . . So I don't say anything so they treat me the same as everyone else."

About interactions with the classroom teacher, a student named Jade said: "One thing I hate is when I was in grade 9, one of my English teachers told a teacher I was going into her grade 10 class, and my teacher told her that I was hard of hearing. My teacher was making sure [my grade 10 teacher knew] I was hard of hearing. Every need of mine would be granted. I hated that [grade 10] class so much. The teacher was so nervous around me. I don't need special treatment. I don't like it when I come to a classroom and the teacher knows me because I'm hard of hearing."

Appropriate format accommodations allow children with hearing loss to participate with children who have normal hearing on a "fair playing ground."

The full-time inclusion classroom option may offer various levels of support. Direct services may be provided by an itinerant teacher who works with the child in the regular classroom, either by helping the student to engage in regular classroom learning or by providing direct instruction with a specialized curriculum. Alternatively, an itinerant teacher might provide indirect services by helping the classroom teacher implement **appropriate format accommodations** or by providing training and in-services about how to teach a child with hearing loss. Full-time inclusion with accommodations may mean that the student has access to assistive technology devices, captioning, acoustical improvements to the classroom, and/or a sign interpreter (Burns, 2004).

Figure 15-6 illustrates one model for determining classroom placement. The goal is to move the child toward a regular mainstream classroom placement as expediently as appropriate. Only when necessary is a child placed outside of the mainstream classroom or taken out of the classroom to receive special support services.

Not all speech and hearing professionals adhere to such a model. Sometimes a child is placed in a regular classroom at the onset of his or her educational program, so that the youth has normal classroom experiences from the outset and learns to identify with the hearing world. Alternatively, some children are educated in a self-contained classroom throughout their

Examples of appropriate format accommodations:

- Abbreviated assignments
- Alternative test format
- Content enhancement
- Content reduction
- Copies of class notes
- Extra credit
- Flexible scheduling
- Interpreter
- Language simplification
- Modified grading
- Paraphrasing
- Study guides

(Burns, 2004, p. 109)

Self-contained Classroom	Part-time Self-contained Classroom;	Part-time Mainstream Classroom;	Full-time Mainstream Classroom
	Part-time Mainstream Classroom	Part-time Resource Classroom	– Direct Services – Indirect Services – Accomodations – No Services

FIGURE 15-6. One model for determining classroom placement. The goal is to move a child from a placement on the left to one towards the right. Once a child enrolls in a full-time mainstream classroom (far right), the child may receive direct services, as when an itinerant teacher provides ancillary instruction, indirect services, as when the itinerant teacher provides guidance to the classroom teacher, accomodations (e.g., an FM system), or no services.

Recommended Equipment to Have in the Classroom:

- Hearing aid **stetoclip** for listening check
- Battery tester
- Air blower to remove moisture and wax from earmold and tubing
- Extra supplies (batteries, and for the FM system, cords, receiver buttons, teacher microphones)

(Oticon, 2006)

A **stetoclip** is a nonelectric device that resembles a stethoscope, which enables someone to perform a listening check on a hearing instrument.

school years, with special emphasis on becoming enculturated into the Deaf community.

AMPLIFICATION AND ASSISTIVE LISTENING DEVICES

Part B of the IDEA states that "each public agency must ensure that hearing aids worn in school by children with hearing impairments, including deafness, are functioning properly" (300.113). Ensuring appropriate amplification requires that good communication occurs between the school staff, the family, and the members of the child's medical home or audiologic care system. Assistive listening devices may be required to optimize a child's ability to function in the classroom.

Amplification

An audiologic assessment will determine the range, nature, and degree of hearing loss and determine whether a child needs amplification and/or whether the child receives adequate benefit from a current listening device. The assessment usually includes a case history, an otoscopic examination, acoustic immittance audiometry, pure-tone audiometry, speech testing, and tests to determine the benefits afforded by the child's current hearing aid or cochlear implant.

Once a student is fitted with an appropriate listening device, then a procedure for ensuring that the device is working properly must be implemented. This may entail periodic checks by an educational audiologist. School staff may learn how to conduct daily visual and listening checks and learn how to troubleshoot the device for common causes of malfunction. The Key Resources section includes a handout about checking hearing instruments. It is important that school staff, such as the classroom teacher, understand the limitations of amplification. Most students will still experience difficulties in hearing, especially in a noisy classroom.

Assistive Technology

The IDEA defines assistive technology as any equipment or system that will increase, maintain, or improve the functional capabilities of children who have a disability. If the IEP stipulates that assistive technology is needed in order for a child to have access to the regular classroom curriculum, then the school district will provide it at no extra cost to the child's family. The school system may purchase, borrow, or lease the device.

In Chapter 3, FM systems were described. In this system, the speech signal is transmitted via radio signal from a microphone worn by the teacher to an FM receiver worn by the student. The teacher talks into a microphone placed near his or her mouth and the signal passes through to an FM personal receiver, which either stands alone or is incorporated into the child's hearing aid or cochlear implant. Because the signal is conveyed directly to the child's ear, the impact of a noisy classroom environment is minimized. The disadvantage of an FM system is that a child can listen to the speech signal of only one person, the person who is wearing the microphone. The child may not have good access to the speech of others in the classroom, such as classmates, particularly if there is only one microphone.

One of the more widely used options is an FM sound field amplification system, which provides an optimal signal-to-noise ratio (SNR) for both children who have hearing loss and children who have normal hearing. Recall that an SNR is the relative difference in dB between the sound source of interest (e.g., the teacher's voice) and the background noise. The FM sound field amplification system is like a public address system, comprised of an FM receiver and a microphone for the teacher. Speakers are placed along the periphery of the classroom or on individual students' desks. FM sound field systems have been shown to lead to improvements in academic achievement, speech recognition skills, and student's attending and learning behaviors, for both students with hearing loss and students with normal hearing. Teachers are less likely to suffer laryngitis when using sound field amplification (see ASHA, 2002, Appendix F, for a review).

The educational audiologist often has the responsibility of ensuring that the classroom teacher is comfortable using the FM system. The audiologist may perform a demonstration and show the teacher how to perform a listening check to make sure that the system is functioning properly and how to troubleshoot it and make minor repairs.

CLASSROOM ACOUSTICS

Classrooms are noisy environments. Shoes scuffling, children whispering, papers crackling, books slamming, chairs scraping, a student laughing, footsteps falling in the hallway, doors closing, air-handling systems humming—these are just some of the sources blasting sound into the classroom. These **background noises** can cover up, mask, and even distort speech. Sounds also bounce from wall to wall, and from floor to ceiling, **reverberating** from one hard surface to another. An extensive body of literature documents the deleterious effects of excessive classroom noise and reverberation levels on speech recognition performance and educational/social development (see ASHA, 2005c, for a review). Classroom noise can also have a negative impact on students' ability to pay attention, their task persistence, and their overall levels of reading achievement (see Anderson, 2004).

Noise may average 50 to 60 dBA SPL in a regular classroom (Crandell & Smaldino, 1995). Children who have hearing loss will be at a double disadvantage in trying to attend to the teacher's speech and to hear other children in a noisy classroom (Crandell & Smaldino, 2000). They experience difficulty even in quiet, and background noise and reverberation exacerbate already degraded word recognition and speech comprehension abilities. For example, if a teacher's voice arrives at a child's desk at a level of 65 dBA SPL (which is about a normal conversational level) and the classroom background noise is 60 dBA SPL, the SNR is only +5. Students with normal hearing require an SNR of about +6 dB for optimal auditory comprehension (Crandell, 1992). Children with even a mild hearing loss perform 13% worse in their speech recognition at the relatively good SNR of +6 and perform 33% worse when the SNR falls to –6 (Crandell, 1993). Reverberation magnifies the effects of noise, and many classrooms have reverberation levels long enough to degrade speech recognition for most listeners, even those with normal hearing (Crandell & Bess, 1986).

Some simple steps can be taken to minimize the level of noise in a classroom and the amount of reverberation. These include any or all of the following (ASHA, 2002; Johnson, 2000, p. 269):

- Installing carpeting or cork on the floor
- Applying rubber tips on chair and desk legs
- Hanging acoustical panels, cork, felt, or flannel bulletin boards on walls
- Placing bookshelves or wall dividers to create quiet areas within the classroom

Background noise is any undesirable auditory stimuli that interferes with someone's ability to attend to a target signal or to concentrate.

Reverberation is the persistence of a sound due to the signal being reflected from the surfaces of walls, ceiling, and floor. Long reverberation times (more than 500 msec) cause a speech signal, such as a teacher's words, to merge with other signals and to lose clarity.

- Angling mobile whiteboards to reduce the amount of reverberation
- Applying window treatments such as draperies or shades to reduce the amount of reverberation
- Covering ceiling with suspended acoustic tile
- Using cushions in place of chairs
- Obtaining a solid-core, well-fitted door with a noise lock or door-way treatment
- Arranging desks and tables in a staggered formation, so sound will not travel directly to reflective surfaces
- Arranging the classroom so instruction occurs away from sound sources, such as an air vent

Other strategies include encouraging children to wear soft-sole shoes, such as tennis shoes, and keeping the door and windows closed during academic instruction.

More invasive and global initiatives can be taken to minimize noise and reverberation. The air-handling system can be adjusted to minimize noise generation. Siebein, Gold, Siebin, and Ermann (2000) found that the primary noise source in classrooms came from heating, ventilating, and air-conditioning (HVAC) systems. The following air-conditioning systems were found to be especially noisy: (a) self-contained, wall-mounted units, (b) decentralized fan coil units, (c) central rooftop units that serve multiple rooms, and (d) central systems with variable air volume systems (p. 380). They suggested possible solutions to HVAC-related noise, including the use of silencers, adequate duct length, and vibration isolators.

Selection of a classroom might be an option. Classrooms that are smaller, with lower ceilings, and classrooms that are not perfect squares or rectangles will minimize reverberation. If the school administration has not selected a classroom for a self-contained or inclusion class, a teacher might encourage them to allocate this kind of room. Moreover, an instructor might select a room away from special-purpose rooms (such as the gym or the band room) and away from environmental noise (e.g., a classroom facing a back alley would be preferable to a classroom facing a busy urban street).

Teachers in noisy classrooms can learn strategies to accommodate students with hearing loss. These strategies include the following:

- Using visual aids for instruction
- Gaining students' attention before speaking so to optimize their chances for successful speechreading
- Encouraging all students to help minimize the noise level in the classroom

- Facing the students when talking and avoiding covering one's mouths
- Becoming aware that most children with hearing loss cannot simultaneously speechread or read sign and perform another task that requires them to look away (such as using a computer or taking notes)
- Providing handouts to provide context cues for speechreading
- Ensuring that the child with hearing loss has favorable seating, typically at the front of the classroom, where the teacher's face will be most visible

SPEECH, LANGUAGE, AND LITERACY

A formal evaluation of a child's speech, language, and literacy will probably be performed in order to develop an IEP and then at regular intervals to assess progress. Test results will help shape and modify the objectives that are included in the plan. In the following sections, we review speech, language, and literacy difficulties that are likely to occur in the presence of hearing loss and procedures for evaluating current levels of performance, and then consider intervention strategies for speech and language.

Speech Characteristics

Segmental errors are errors in speech sounds.

Suprasegmental errors are errors in speech rhythm and prosody, the pitch, rate, intensity, and duration imposed on phonemes and words.

Overall intelligibility, **segmental errors** (errors in the sounds of speech), and **suprasegmental errors** (errors in speech rhythm and prosody) are often considered when compiling a description of children's speech (Figure 15-7). As a general rule, children with more residual hearing and/or better benefit from a listening device speak better and produce fewer segmental and suprasegmental errors than children with less residual hearing or children who receive less benefit from amplification (e.g., Tye-Murray, Spencer, &

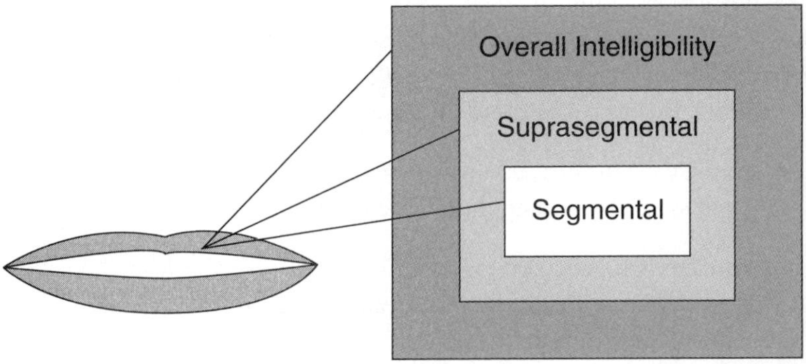

FIGURE 15-7. Assessment of speech production. Speech proficiency is determined with a consideration of overall intelligibility, segmental errors, and suprasegmental errors.

Woodworth, 1995; Yoshinaga-Itano, 2006). The effects of hearing loss are most pronounced with children who have a congenital loss or who lose their hearing in early childhood. In the presence of adventitious hearing loss, even when the loss is profound, speech usually remains intact (e.g., Kishon-Rabin, Taitelbaum, Tobin, & Hildesheimer, 1999).

What a child speaks relates to what a child hears. For instance, young co-chlear implant users who can hear the place of articulation, nasality, and voicing features, as determined by an information transmission analysis (see Chapter 2), are more likely to speak these features correctly than are children who do not hear them very well (Tye-Murray, Spencer, & Gilbert-Bedia, 1995). Figure 15-8 illustrates the relationship between speech recognition scores on the *Word Intelligibility Picture Index* (*WIPI*; Ross & Lerman, 1971) and speech production scores on an imitative sentence test. These data were collected from young cochlear implant users who had at least 5 years of device experience (Tye-Murray, Tomblin, & Spencer, 1997). There is a strong relationship between children's abilities to produce phonemes and their abilities to recognize them. A **Pearson correlation**, which tests how well one set of data predicts another, was $r = .88$, which is a significantly strong correlation (see also Levitt, McGarr, & Geffner, 1987; Smith, 1975). In addition, there is a moderately positive relationship between the severity of hearing loss and the severity of concomitant speech difficulties (e.g., Wake et al., 2004).

A **Pearson correlation** indicates the strength and the direction of a linear relationship between two variables.

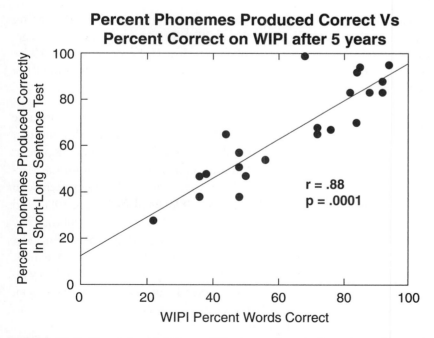

FIGURE 15-8. The relationship between children's speech production and speech recognition skills after 5 years of cochlear implant experience.

A child's intelligibility also depends on numerous other factors, including age at identification, the speech therapy received, motivation to speak, the consistency of appropriate amplification use, the age of first receiving a hearing aid and/or a cochlear implant, and the child's speech environment. For example, does the child hear speech often? Do those around the youngster provide good speech models? Is reinforcement provided when the child tries to speak?

> ## Some Hearing Can Make a Big Difference
>
> Children who have mild-to-moderate hearing loss, especially if they wear appropriate amplification, tend to develop near-normal speech production and good intelligibility (Elfenbein, Hardin-Jones, & Davis, 1994). Their speech errors tend to resemble those of children who have normal hearing and developmental articulation disorders. For instance, children with a less than severe hearing loss may misprounouce such fricatives as /s/ or /ʃ/ but may pronounce most other sounds with good accuracy (see Eisenberg, 2007, for a review).

Overall Intelligibility

Historically, most children with profound and prelingual hearing impairments who use hearing aids are difficult to understand. On average, listeners identify less than 20% of their words (John & Howarth, 1976; Markides, 1970; Monsen, 1978). Very few studies have examined the intelligibility of children who use modern-day hearing aids.

Research suggests that children with significant hearing loss demonstrate different developmental patterns than children with normal hearing and that they reach a plateau in their speech skills relatively early in their development. For example, the phonetic repertoires of infants who have profound hearing loss have been found to be restricted when compared to their peers with normal hearing (Lach, Ling, Ling, & Ship, 1970; Stoel-Gammon, 1988) and their babbling patterns aberrant (e.g., Von Hapsburg & Davis, 2006). They demonstrate fewer instances of **canonical babbling** and their babble includes a more limited range of consonants (Stoel-Gammon, 1988; Wallace, Menn, & Yoshinaga-Itano, 1998). Although children with profound hearing loss who use hearing aids may be idiosyncratic in several aspects of speech production, many demonstrate similar error patterns when speaking and they demonstrate universally poor intelligibility.

Canonical babbling is an advanced form of babbling that consists of well-formed consonant-vowel combinations; in children with normal hearing, this kind of babbling begins to occur around the 10th month of life.

Children who use cochlear implants speak better than children who use hearing aids. For example, in a study of 181 children, 8 and 9 years of age, who had used cochlear implants since before the age of 5 years, Tobey et al. (2003) found that listeners understood on average more than 60% of the children's words. More than half of the children produced words that were 80% intelligible or better. Similarly, Peng, Spencer, and Tomblin (2004) found that 24 children with prelingual hearing loss achieved an average intelligibility level of about 72% words repeated correctly on a sentence imitation task, after about 7 years of device experience. Half of the children achieved a score of 85% or better whereas 6 out of the 24 scored below 50%. Peng et al. also presented evidence that speech intelligibility scores continue to show steady improvement beyond even 5 or 6 years of device use.

Segmental Errors

Children with significant prelingual hearing loss produce many segmental errors, both when speaking vowels and diphthongs and when speaking consonants. In one group of hearing aid users who had a mean hearing level of 95 dB HL, 56% of all vowels and diphthongs and 72% of all consonants were rated by a group of listeners as deviant (Markides, 1970). Not surprisingly, there exists an inverse relationship between the number of vowel and consonant errors and overall intelligibility: As the number of errors in a child's speech increases, intelligibility decreases (Smith, 1975).

Children who have significant hearing losses and who use hearing aids most commonly neutralize vowels. Some physiological studies have focused on how the tongue moves during vowel production. These studies suggest that talkers with profound hearing loss may not move their tongue bodies in the anterior–posterior (front–back) dimension as much as talkers with normal hearing and may rely primarily on jaw displacement for distinguishing vowel height (e.g., the low vowel /a/ vs. the high vowel /I/) (Dagenais & Critz-Crosby, 1992; Tye-Murray, 1987, 1991). This restricted tongue movement is likely a primary component underlying the perceptual phenomenon of neutralized vowels. Children who have been studied longitudinally between the ages of 11 and 14 years demonstrate little change in the average number and types of vowel and diphthong errors they make over time (McGarr, 1987).

A list of vowel error types includes the following:

- Neutralizations
- Substitutions

- Dipthongizations
- Prolongations
- Nasalizations

Children who have severe and profound hearing losses and who use hearing aids tend to produce characteristic consonantal errors (e.g., Smith, 1975). These errors include voiced/voiceless confusions, substitutions, omissions, distortions, and errors in consonant clusters. Many children produce consonants that are visible on the face more accurately than consonants that are not visible. For instance, a child is more likely to produce the word *pat* correctly than the word *cat*. Manner of production errors are also common. Affricates, fricatives, glides, and laterals are especially difficult for many children to produce.

Children who use cochlear implants acquire speech sounds in about the same order as do children who have normal hearing, and at a much faster rate and with better proficiency than children with comparable hearing loss who use hearing aids (e.g., Blamey, Barry, & Jacq, 2001; Paatsch, Blamey, & Sarant, 2001; Tobey, Geers, & Brenner, 1994; Tye-Murray & Kirk, 1993). Use of a cochlear implant can result in greater accuracy in vowel production and a more complete repertoire (e.g., Blamey et al., 2001; Tye-Murray & Kirk, 1993; Warner-Czyz, Davis, & Morrison, 2005). For instance, in one study, 12 children acquired good production of vowels by the time they had achieved 4 years of cochlear implant experience (Blamey et al., 2001). Tye-Murray, Tomblin, and Spencer (1997) found that the errors made by cochlear implant users resembled those made by hearing aid users, with central vowels produced with greatest accuracy and front vowels produced with least accuracy.

Consonantal inventories also approach those of children who have normal hearing after children receive prolonged cochlear implant experience (e.g., Chin, 2003; Serry & Blamey, 1999). Though experience with a cochlear implant leads to good consonant acquisition, fricatives and affricates remain slow to emerge, perhaps because they are high-frequency sounds and difficult to hear (Blamey et al., 2001; Tye-Murray et al., 1997). Interestingly, just like children who have similar hearing losses but who use hearing aids, young cochlear implant users tend to produce the more visible bilabial consonants correctly more often than the less visible palatals, velars, and glottals (Tye-Murray et al., 1997). Such findings suggest that young cochlear implant users rely on both auditory and visual signals for acquiring consonant sounds.

Suprasegmental Errors

Children with significant hearing loss and who use hearing aids tend to have a distinctive speech quality. Their speech often sounds breathy, labored, staccato, and arrhythmic. Errors in suprasegmental patterns

The Roles of Auditory Information in Speech Acquisition

To understand the difficulties children with minimal hearing capability have in developing intelligible speech, it is helpful to think about the ways in which auditory information helps us learn to talk. Auditory information plays at least five important roles during a child's acquisition of speech:

1. Auditory information potentiates the development of specific principles of articulatory organization. By listening to the speech of others in their community, children learn how to regulate their speech breathing, learn how to flex and extend their tongue bodies, and learn how to alternate rhythmically between vowels and consonants. Children who cannot hear often do not learn to (a) manage their breath streams for speech, (b) rotate their tongue forward and backward in the mouth to establish vowel postures, and (c) move the articulators smoothly and continuously from one articulatory posture to the next.
2. By listening to others, children learn how to produce specific speech events. For instance, they learn to distinguish /p/ with a relatively rapid-velocity opening gesture and /w/ with a slow velocity gesture.
3. Children develop a system of phonological performance (i.e., they learn the phonemes of their language community) through listening. Often children who cannot hear do not acquire some sounds in their language, especially those associated with high-frequency auditory information, such as /s/ and /ʃ/.
4. Auditory feedback informs children about the consequences of their articulatory gestures and how these consequences compare to sounds produced by other talkers. For example, if a talker explodes air through his or her lips, he or she learns that this will produce a plosive sound. If the talker does it with too much vigor, he or she will hear a sound that may be inappropriately loud, when compared to other talkers of his or her language. It is not uncommon for a talker who is deaf to produce a slight popping sound when producing plosives.
5. Auditory feedback may provide information for monitoring ongoing speech production and for detecting errors. For instance, you might hear yourself say "See went," and then quickly correct yourself and say "She went." Talkers who are deaf are unable to monitor themselves in this way.

(Tye-Murray, Spencer, & Woodworth, 1995).

"The choice and use of the most appropriate teaching strategies for a given child require sound knowledge of the potential of the senses in speech reception and the sensory-motor mechanisms underlying feedforward and feedback control of speech production."

Daniel Ling, an influential speech teacher for children who are deaf and hard of hearing

(Ling, 1975, p. 3)

"The intelligibility of a deaf child's speech is frequently lowered by permitting him to produce each element in a word exactly as it would be produced if it stood by itself."

S. Sibley Haycock, Superintendent of the Langside School for the Deaf, Glasgow, Scotland, 1901–1923

(Haycock, 1933, p. 29)

contribute to this aberrant speech quality. These include errors in stress, speaking rate, coarticulation, breath control, pitch, and intensity. Many children place equal stress on all syllables or stress words inappropriately. For instance, the word *baby* may be produced with the stress on the second syllable instead of the first, as in "bah-BEE" (e.g., Robb & Pang-Ching, 1992; Tye-Murray & Folkins, 1990).

Typically, children with severe and profound losses speak very slowly, pausing often, both within words and between words. They may insert extraneous sounds and prolong words. Voelker (1938) found that children with profound hearing loss spoke 70 words per minute as compared to 164 words per minute spoken by children with normal hearing.

Many children do not coarticulate sounds in the same way as normally hearing talkers. For instance, a child might say the word *basket* as "ba-a-sa-kat." In this production, the child has articulated sounds as if they were isolated units (e.g., Monsen, 1976; Rothman, 1976; Tye-Murray, Zimmermann, & Folkins, 1987). Whereas talkers with normal hearing begin to move their tongue body and jaw towards the vowel posture during a preceding consonantal closure, talkers with profound hearing loss may not.

Adult talkers who have profound and prelingual hearing loss demonstrate normal respiratory and aerodynamic behaviors for nonspeech tasks and aberrant behaviors for speech (Forner & Hixon, 1977; Itoh, Horii, Daniloff, & Binnie, 1982). Poor breathing behavior correlates highly with poor speech intelligibility. Adults often inefficiently manage the speech airstream, as characterized by higher air volume expenditure during connected speech (Forner & Hixon, 1977; Metz, Whitehead, & Whitehead, 1984). They tend to initiate speech at low lung volumes and to speak fewer syllables per breath cycle (Whitehead, 1982).

Children's voice quality may be unpleasant, and may be described as breathy, hoarse, or strained (Hudgins & Numbers, 1942; Markides, 1970). Their pitch may sound excessively high or variable (Horii, 1982). Some children speak with a monotone. Pitch breaks, with pitch abruptly changing from high to low, are common.

There is at best only limited information about how receipt of a cochlear implant affects children's suprasegmental production performance. At least two studies suggest that use of a cochlear implant may affect nasalization of speech (e.g., Svirsky, Jones, Osberger, & Miyamoto, 1998; Tye-Murray, Spencer, Bedia, & Woodworth, 1996). One study demonstrated that use of a cochlear implant may enhance management of intraoral air pressure (Jones, Gao, & Svirsky, 2003). In contrast, McCleary, Carnye, and Schulte (2003) found that seven children who used early versions of cochlear implant speech processors (they were implanted in the 1990s) and who were educated in a total-communication environment continued to demonstrate deviant aero-dynamic speech behaviors, even after 5 or 6 years of cochlear implant use.

Language

As noted earlier in this chapter, 90% of children with significant hearing loss are born to parents who have normal hearing. As a result, many children are not exposed to language early on because they do not have access to the auditory speech signal and their parents do not sign. One consequence is that many children have delays in their **expressive** and **receptive** language. One way to appreciate how hearing loss affects language development is to compare normally hearing and hard-of-hearing groups. Eight-year-old children with normal hearing have a better knowledge of grammar than do adults with prelingual profound hearing loss. Moreover, most adults with significant hearing loss never acquire a vocabulary better than that of a fourth grader with normal hearing (Bamford & Saunders, 1985; DiFrancesca, 1972). Language difficulties are often categorized as problems of either form (syntax and morphology), content (semantics and vocabulary), or pragmatics (use).

Expressive language refers to the language we speak (or sign).

Receptive language refers to the language that we either hear (or receive via sign).

Form

The list comprising problems of **form** is extensive (for reviews, see Rose, McAnally, & Quigley, 2004; Seyfried & Kricos, 1996;). Children with significant hearing loss may overuse nouns and verbs and rarely use adverbs, prepositions, or pronouns. They may omit function words. Many of their sentences have a simple subject-verb-object structure, and their sentences have fewer words compared to those produced by children who have normal hearing. Compound or complex sentences are rare, as are morphemes that mark plurality, possession, the third singular "s" (e.g., *she walks*), or past tense. In telling a story about her cat, one child said, "Socks jump. Cup fall over. Mess big. Mom mad about Socks." In this narrative, the child omitted function words such as *was,* articles such as *the,* and tense markers such as *-ed.* (See Griswold & Cummings, 1974, who report a paucity of connectives, articles, and auxiliary modal verbs in the language of children with profound hearing loss.) Her syntactic structures were simple. Although a listener might follow her story, her sentences sound telegraphic.

Form refers to the proper use of the elements of language, such as nouns and verbs, prepositions, and so on.

Even a moderate hearing loss may impair morphological development. For instance, McGuckian and Henry (2007) compared the production accuracy of grammatical morphemes between 10 children with moderate hearing loss and a mean age of 7 years, 4 months and 10 children with normal hearing and a mean age of 3 years, 2 months. The children with hearing loss displayed a different pattern of morphologogical development than the children with normal hearing, a pattern that was more like that demonstrated in second language learners. For instance, whereas the children with normal hearing tended to produce the possessive "s" and the plural "s" with a high level of accuracy, the children with moderate hearing loss rarely produced the possessive "s" and were somewhat inconsistent in their production of plural "s."

Sometimes children order their words incorrectly. A child may say, "Saw cat big," meaning she saw a big cat.

Not only do they rarely produce compound or complex sentences, children with significant hearing loss often cannot interpret them when they speechread or read. For example, someone might say to a child, "The cat was chased by the dog." The child may interpret this sentence in the active tense: *The cat chased the dog.* A talker might speak a nominal sentence, such as, "The ending of the school year saddened the teacher." The child might interpret it in an objective sense: *The school year saddened the teacher* (Russell, Quigley, & Power, 1976).

Children who receive cochlear implants may have accelerated and enhanced language acquisition. Tomblin, Spencer, Flock, Tyler, and Gantz (1999) looked at the syntax of a group of 29 young cochlear implant users and a comparable group of 29 young hearing aid users with a measure called the *Index of Productive Syntax* (IPSyn; Scarborough, 1990). The cochlear implant users demonstrated greater rates of growth in English grammar over time than did the hearing aid users. Geers, Nicholas, and Sedey (2003), in a study 181 8- and 9-year-old implant users (the same group of children studied by Tobey et al., 2003), found that about half of the children demonstrated English syntax at a level comparable to their peers who have normal hearing. It also appears that postimplant language acquisition rate parallels that of normal development (Svirsky, Chute, Green, Bollard, & Miyamoto, 2002). There is a wide range shown within this population, and not all children receive as much benefit as do others (Kirk, Miyamoto, Ying, Perdew, & Suganelis, 2002).

Content

Content refers to the extent of vocabulary and use of words.

Content refers to the words and meanings used during communication. A pervasive language problem among children with hearing loss is a restricted vocabulary, and the greater the hearing loss, the greater will be the effects on vocabulary acquisition (e.g., Kiese-Himmel & Reeh, 2006). Their performance on standard achievement tests such as the *Standard Achievement Test* (Gardner, Rudman, Karlsen, & Merwin, 1982) shows that their vocabulary growth lags behind that of children with normal hearing during the school years (Spencer & Lederberg, 1997). Many children learn only common everyday words. They may have gaps in their vocabularies, wherein they do not know words relating to an entire concept, such as outer space. Hence, words such as *planet, Martian, star, spacemen,* and *rocket* may be unfamiliar. They often use words in limited ways. For instance, a child may use a word such as *happy* as a predicate (e.g., *The boy is happy*) but not as a modifier (e.g., *The happy boy is here*). Many children cannot identify synonyms and antonyms or understand idioms such as, *She was mad as a hornet*. Similarly, many experience difficulty handling words with multiple meanings. For example, children may understand the word *stand* in the context of, *Please stand by the piano*, but not in the context of, *Please move the music stand*.

In general, children who have significant hearing loss will learn words that are concrete more readily than they will learn words that are abstract (Green & Shephard, 1975). They may associate meanings to words like *bird, chair, sit, telephone,* and *ball*, but words that do not pair up with a physical object or an overtly observable behavior will be more difficult to learn, words such as *rephrase, sentimental, admirable,* and *wise*. There is some evidence that children with profound hearing loss and who use hearing aids, and who are exposed to sign early in the home, as with ASL or total communication, develop larger vocabularies than children who are not exposed to sign (Connor, Hieber, Arts, & Zwolan, 2000; Griswold & Cummings, 1974; Schafer & Lynch, 1980).

Vocabulary acquisition is enhanced by the use of a cochlear implant. Waltzman et al. (1997), who obtained language data from 38 children who received their cochlear implants before the age of 5 years, reported they demonstrated 4 years of vocabulary growth during a 3-year period.

Pragmatics

Children with hearing loss sometimes demonstrate **pragmatic** errors, using language in inappropriate ways (Kretschmer & Kretschmer, 1994). For instance, some may use questions inappropriately. One child's first question to a new acquaintance was to ask how much money the girl's father made. A child may not know how to initiate or maintain a conversation or know how to repair breakdowns in communication. In some circumstances, the child may nod and bluff, pretending to understand.

Pragmatics refers to the study of how language is used.

A child also may not know some of the social graces of conversation. For example, he or she may not know how to take turns while conversing, how to acknowledge that the message has been heard, and how to change the topic of conversation. In the following conversation, a child with hearing loss introduced a topic abruptly and did not respond to the adult's request for clarification:

Adult: Do you want to come with me?

Child: Car fell off table, boom!

Adult: What did you say?

Child: Mine.

These inappropriate responses may relate to both the child's hearing loss (the child may not have recognized the adult's utterances) and an unfamiliarity with conversational rules.

In general, there at least three reasons why some children do not learn conversational pragmatics well. These are (e.g., see Gfeller & Schum, 1994; Schum & Gfeller, 1994):

- First, they do not receive extensive practice in using language. Their unfamiliarity with many language structures and reduced vocabulary limit their ability to converse. Moreover, if they do not use an aural/oral communication mode, they have fewer conversational partners to interact with because few normally hearing persons know manually coded English or ASL.
- Second, they cannot overhear their parents or other people talking. Thus, they do not receive the everyday, incidental models of how to use language.
- Third, they may not receive the same formal instruction as children who have normal hearing. For instance, a parent may carefully explain the rules of politeness to a child with normal hearing (do not interrupt; say "thank you"; let someone else say something). The parent may not explain the rules to his or her child with a hearing loss, either because of the child's limited language or because of the parent's limited skill in using sign. A child using manually coded English or ASL may not receive the same language experiences as a normally hearing child, because few people in the child's environment will be familiar with these means of communication.

Literacy

Literacy is an issue closely related to language development. Literacy is indexed by performance on reading and writing measures. Given many children's difficulties using English language, it is not surprising that many also have difficulty learning to read and comprehend and to compose written text. Literacy skills are the foundation for mastering academic material, and poor skills may hinder academic progress.

Reading

Children who are deaf and hard of hearing and who use hearing aids often show delays or differences when compared to children who have normal hearing (see King & Quigley, 1985, for a review). The average reading and writing levels of high school students with profound hearing loss are at a third- or fourth-grade level (Allen, 1986). This level is barely adequate to allow them to read a newspaper. Rarely does a student with significant hearing loss exceed a 7.5-grade reading level (DiFrancesca, 1972; Trybus & Krachmer, 1977).

There are at least two major reasons for reading deficits and several other contributing factors. First, reading problems may relate to an inadequate language system. Deficits in vocabulary, unfamiliarity with groups of related words, and unfamiliarity with complex syntactic structures appear to interfere with children's ability to understand printed text (Connor & Zwolan, 2004).

In addition, some children who have profound hearing loss do not develop an auditory basis for mapping sound to print (Golding-Meadow & Mayberry, 2001). Typically, when children crack the code of deciphering the written word, they grasp the principle of associating sound to words. They learn **word decoding**, which allows them to associate the orthographic form of a word to its phonological properties and hence, its meaning. Access to a phonological code allows them to "sound out words" for sound–print mapping. Many children who have never heard sound, or who have had access to degraded speech signals, do not develop the phonological awareness of their counterparts with normal hearing. Other factors that compound the reading task include deficits in experience and world knowledge (see Marshark, 2003).

Word decoding is the ability to apply one's knowledge of letter-sound relationships, including a knowledge of letter patterns, to the task of recognizing and interpreting written words.

Use of cochlear implants appears to mitigate the deleterious effect of hearing loss on reading achievement but not eliminate it (Figure 15-9). Spencer, Tomblin, and Gantz (1997; see also Geers, 2003; Spencer, Barker, & Tomblin, 2003) studied groups of young cochlear implant users and hearing aid users. Children completed the *Woodcock Reading Mastery Test*, which assesses children's ability to comprehend short two- to three-sentence paragraphs. Fifty percent of the children who used cochlear implants were reading at grade level. They achieved higher reading levels than the hearing aid users and exhibited faster performance growth rates over time. Vermeulen, Van Bon, Schreuder, Knoors, and Snik (2007) found that Dutch children who had used a cochlear implant for at least 3 years achieved better reading performance levels than children who used hearing aids, but that both groups still performed poorly compared to children with normal hearing.

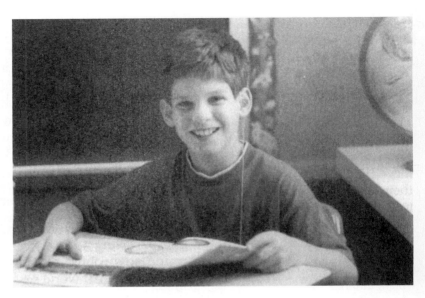

FIGURE 15-9. Literacy and cochlear implant use. Use of a cochlear implant appears to lead to better reading skills than use of conventional amplification. One reason may be that enhanced listening skills allow children to acquire English language more readily, which in turn may promote literacy. *Photograph by Patti Gabriel, courtesy of the Central Institute for the Deaf.*

Writing

The writing samples of children with hearing loss often contain syntactic errors, such as omission of articles, inappropriate use of pronouns, and omission of bound morphemes (e.g., *'s* and *-ed*). There is a tendency to use a preponderance of subject-verb-object sentences, and rarely construct complex syntactic structures. Use of synonyms, antonyms, metaphors, or cohesive forms of substitution or ellipsis is rare (Yoshinaga-Itano, Snyder, & Mayberry, 1996).

Some children have difficulty writing narratives, in which there is a clear beginning, middle, and end to their story. Sometimes, they have difficulty focusing on the important parameters of a story (Pakkulski & Kaderavek, 2001). For example, a third-grade boy, when asked to write a story about a girl holding a scorched dress and an iron, wrote the following sample: *Girl have red sweater. Hair yellow. Girl work hard!*

In this example, the child appears to have focused on surface details of the picture rather than the underlying story. The child also used inappropriate verb tense (e.g., *have* instead of *has*) and omitted function words. Most children progress beyond this level of expression and often demonstrate gains in their narrative skills between the ages of 7 and 18 years of age, although they rarely achieve the competency of age-matched peers with normal hearing (Yoshinaga-Itano & Downey, 1996). Even if they receive a cochlear implant, children with significant hearing loss appear to experience difficulties in using grammatical structures such as conjunctions and correct verb forms in writing sentences (Spencer, Barker, & Tomblin, 2003).

Writing Samples from 10- and 11-Year-Old Children with Hearing Loss

Three children who attend a private school for the deaf on a full-time basis wrote the stories that follow: Michelle, Jelyyn, and Allison. The samples are characteristic of the writing skills demonstrated by a group of children of this age and with significant hearing loss, both in terms of variability in their length and in their types of errors. The class assignment was to describe the scene depicted in Figure 15-10. The children were shown this picture after their teacher read them a story about a girl and her purchase of a magic sled.

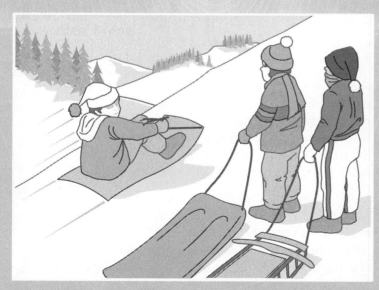

FIGURE 15-10. The picture that was used to elicit the written language samples presented in this chapter. The picture illustrates a story about a magic sled that can glide uphill. Students were asked to look at the picture and then write a story about the magic sled.

Michelle wrote only two sentences:

> *The gril going up the hill.*
>
> *The boys look the gril going up the hill.*

continues

Writing Samples from 10- and 11-Year-Old Children with Hearing Loss, *continued*

Michelle described the key element of the picture: The girl was sledding upward and the boys were impressed enough by the action that they stopped and watched. Some of the errors include omission of the function word *is* in the first sentence, and the word *at* in the second sentence. She also misspelled the word *girl*. She used the commonplace word *going* in lieu of the more descriptive word *sledding*.

Although Jelyyn's writing sample also included many errors characteristic of children who have significant hearing loss (including spelling errors, tense disagreement, omission of morphemes, omission of function words, run-on sentences, verb disagreement, and inappropriate change in verb tense), her narration of the story and of the accompanying picture was more complex and more informative than that of her classmate, Michelle. She also used more appropriate punctuation. However, notice how she missed writing about the key element of the story: The sled was magic, and hence able to glide uphill.

> *A girl name Tiffany. She walking by the stroe and she saw a macigi sleding and she went into the store and buy the macigi sleding and she can't wait to go sled down the hill. When she finish buy the sled. She was in a hurry. When she got home she put her snowpant on, hat, boots, mittens, scarft. And ran up the hill and she try to sleding down.*

The final sample presents the most narratively sound and grammatically correct paragraph of the three. In writing it, Allison described the key elements of the story. Also, in the final sentence, she inserted dialogue, which is an advanced component in narrative writing. Grammatically, even though Allison did not use quotation marks and did not use a question mark where appropriate, she preceded the dialogue with a comma and capitalized the first word. Other grammatical errors included the omission of function words and inappropriate changes in verb tense. Allison wrote:

> *It was winter time, and it was snowy in the picture. Dave, Kathy and Dan went sleding on big hill. They are tired to walk up on big hill but Kathy and her sled went up! Fanilly they get on top of hill. They ask her, How your sled went up*

Speech and Language Evaluation

The purposes for conducting a speech and language assessment include (a) determining the need for intervention, (b) developing intervention goals, and (c) evaluating progress and effectiveness of intervention.

There are several general principles to remember when testing the speech and language abilities of children who have hearing loss. The principles pertain to the following topics:

- Task type
- Mode of communication
- Rapport
- Test procedures
- Test norms

Children often use speech and language differently in one setting than in another, and they perform differently on varying tasks. For example, children are more likely to produce a sound correctly when they imitate their speech-language pathologist than when they tell a story to their classmates. By using a variety of speech tasks, a clinician can determine how robust certain skills are and whether they have generalized to real-world settings.

Evaluation should be performed with a child's preferred mode of communication (Figure 15-11). For example, the child may use total communication. If the clinician does not know the child's sign system, then a sign language interpreter should be secured. The child must understand the tasks and the test items to provide a true reflection of speech and language skills.

Before formally evaluating a child, a rapport must be established between tester and child. Some children with hearing losses are shy about using their voices, especially among strangers. If children do not feel comfortable in the tester's presence, they will not provide speech or language samples that represent their true skills.

It is important to select specific test procedures appropriate for the child's age and language. For example, if an articulation test has picture cards, the child must have the vocabulary necessary to name the pictures.

For children who have mild or moderate hearing loss, it is usually standard practice to use assessement instruments that have been developed for use with children who have normal hearing. For children who have significant hearing loss, the clinician might try to use at least some tests that have been developed for children with hearing loss, although this

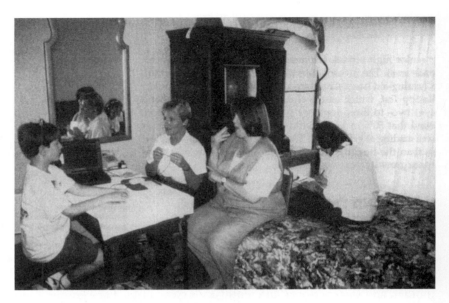

FIGURE 15-11. Mode of communication and assessment. A speech and language evaluation usually is performed with a child's preferred mode of communication. Here, an interpreter cues the messages of a speech-language pathologist who does not know Cued Speech. *Photograph by Kim Readmond, courtesy of the Central Institute for the Deaf.*

may not always be possible, because few tests are available. For children who use total communication, not many tests have been designed to be administered with sign.

Assessing Speech Skills

To assess speech intelligibility, a speech sample first must be collected and then evaluated. To obtain a speech sample, the clinician might ask a child to perform any or all of the following tasks:

- Imitate a series of isolated words or sentences. For example, a speech-language pathologist might say, "The boy saw the cat," and the child then repeats the sentence. This procedure typically elicits a child's best performance (Figure 15-12).
- Create a citation speech sample. A speech-language pathologist might instruct a child, "Tell me the name of the picture," or, "Tell me what is happening here." The child then speaks the name or describes what is occurring in the picture. This task is highly structured like an imitated-sentence task, but the child does not receive a speech or vocabulary model to imitate.

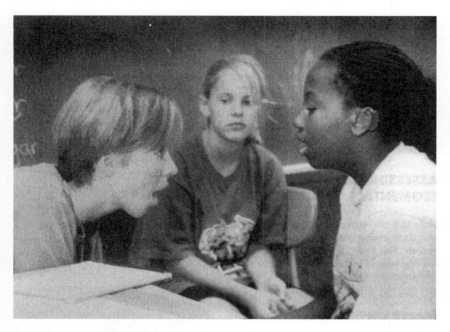

FIGURE 15-12. Imitation task. One way to collect a speech sample from a child is to use an imitation task. The clinician speaks an utterance and the child imitates it. *Photograph by Marcus Kosa, courtesy of the Central Institute for the Deaf.*

- Retell a story. A speech-language pathologist may show the pictures in Figure 15-13 to a child one at a time and tell a corresponding story, picture by picture. The child then retells the story. This procedure constrains the language that children use in the sample, but still allows for the evaluation of spontaneous speech and language production.
- Speak spontaneously, using continuous speech. A speech-language pathologist might observe informally a child in therapy, in the classroom, or on the playground while he or she speaks to other children. In the therapy session, they may engage in casual conversation, and the speech-language pathologist pays close attention to the child's articulation proficiency and language structures.

Once a speech sample has been collected, overall intelligibility can be evaluated in at least three different ways. First, the recordings can be played to a group of listeners who can assign each sample a value from a rating scale (Johnson, 1975). For example, 1 on a 5-point scale might correspond to *I understood none of the child's message,* and 5 correspond to *I understood all of the child's message.* There are some disadvantages to using rating scales. A group of listeners must be assembled, which is not always easy to do in settings such as a public

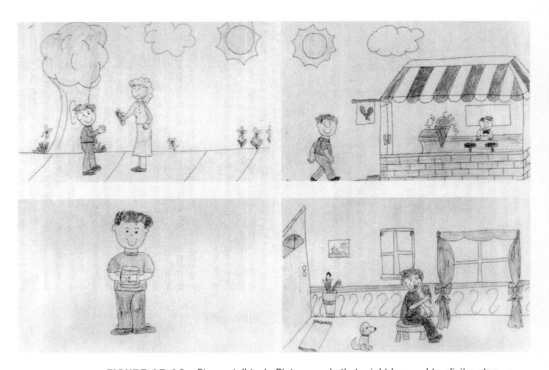

FIGURE 15-13. Story-retell task. Picture cards that might be used to elicit a story-retell speech and language sample. A clinician first tells a story, using a prepared text that corresponds to each picture in the picture series (here, organized clockwise, beginning with the top left-hand corner). Then the child tells the story back.

school. Moreover, some have questioned whether rating scales present an accurate portrait of children who vary from one another in their intelligibility (Samar & Metz, 1988; but see Wilkinson & Brinton, 2003). It may be that judges have a tendency to cluster scores at one end of the continuum or the other. A second way to evaluate intelligibility is to play the speech samples to a group of listeners, and ask them to write down what they hear. The number of words correctly identified constitutes a percentage words correct intelligibility score. The listeners might estimate how much of the child's speech they understood, such as 10% of the words, 20%, and so forth. Although the transcription procedure also requires a panel of listeners to be assembled, it has high face validity because it shows how many of their words can be identified by listeners. A third way to quantify speech intelligibility is for a speech-language pathologist to transcribe phonetically the spoken message and reference the spoken transcription to the printed text. The speech-language pathologist then can determine what percentage of the words or sounds were spoken correctly. This way is probably the most commonly used procedure for assessing intelligibility in clinical and educational settings.

Speech intelligibility scores vary as a function of several different variables (Figure 15-14). For instance:

- A child will be more intelligible when reading a paragraph than speaking a list of unrelated sentences.
- Listeners will understand more of a child's speech if they have heard the speech of other children with hearing loss before, than if they are naive listeners.
- Listeners will recognize more speech if they can hear and see children rather than only hear them.

When recording intelligibility scores it is wise to comment on these variables, especially if the child's progress is to be monitored over time. If this is not done, the child's intelligibility score might improve because of a change in an extraneous variable. This may be misinterpreted as an improvement in the child's speaking proficiency.

Segmental speech testing determines which sounds children can articulate and which sounds they cannot. Variables to consider when selecting test procedures include context, methodology, and whether to use conventional tests of articulation.

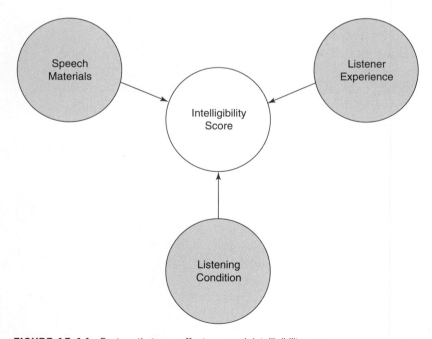

FIGURE 15-14. Factors that may affect a speech intelligibility score.

Segmental speech production can be evaluated with a variety of contexts, including nonsense syllables, isolated words, sentences, and spontaneous speech. It is common to evaluate how well children produce various features of articulation, such as place and manner.

Methodologically, a child may imitate a clinician or might produce the sounds by naming picture cards or reading printed words aloud. The child also may speak spontaneously, and then the clinician can determine what sounds were produced in a set number of words (say, the first 200 words spoken by the child).

Often, conventional articulation tests are used to assess segmental speech skills, such as the *Goldman–Fristoe Test of Articulation* (Goldman & Fristoe, 1969) and the *Test of Minimal Articulation Competence* (*T-MAC;* Secord, 1981). Some clinicians modify the tests by eliminating test words that are not in the child's vocabulary. If modifications are made, they should be recorded alongside the child's scores. Tests designed specifically for children with significant hearing loss include:

- The *Phonetic Level and the Phonologic Level Speech Evaluation* (Ling, 1976): In the phonetic level segment, children's imitative vocal characteristics are judged on the basis of pitch, duration, and intensity. Children are asked to produce vowels and diphthongs as single syllables, repeated syllables (e.g., *ba ba ba*), alternated syllables (e.g., *ba bee ba bee*), and as syllables with varying pitch and loudness. The phonologic level segment of the test focuses on the quality and complexity of the child's speech at a discourse level. The clinician completes a checklist that concerns the child's vocal control, linguistic structure, phonemic inventory, and intelligibility.
- The *CID Phonetic Inventory* (Moog, 1988): Very similar to Ling's (1976) phonetic level test in structure, this inventory also bases the evaluation of a child's speech production primarily on the syllable unit. Children are shown printed cards and then asked to imitate the clinician's spoken model. Vowels, diphthongs, and consonants in a variety of syllable configurations are tested.
- The *Speech Intelligibility Evaluation* (*SPINE;* Monsen, 1981): The SPINE documents overall intelligibility at the single-word level. It consists of 40 cards with a single word printed on each (the cards must be constructed by the clinician as they are not commercially available). The cards are sorted into contrastive sets of four, each set designed to contrast vowel characteristics and voicing. The child sees a set of four cards at a time and speaks the name of

one of the depicted images. The clinician records what he or she hears. The percentage of words correctly recognized constitutes the child's intelligibility score. Monsen, Moog, and Geers (1988) developed a similar test, *The CID Picture SPINE*, for children who cannot read.

Suprasegmental speech skills can be evaluated by rating children's spontaneous speech as described by Subtelny, Orlando, and Whitehead (1981) or by asking them to perform specific speech tasks. For instance, a speech-language pathologist might determine whether a child can sustain the vowel /a/ for 5 seconds (to assess breath management) or whether the child can speak two-syllable phrases with correct stress and pitch variation (to assess his or her ability to imitate stress patterns) (Levitt, 1987).

Assessing Language Skills

Table 15-4 presents examples of language tests sometimes used with children who are hearing impaired. They are organized according to whether they primarily assess form, content, or pragmatics.

Table 15-4. Language tests that are sometimes used to test children who have hearing loss. Assessment instruments designed specifically for children and teenagers who are deaf and hard of hearing are denoted with an asterisk (*).

Form
Rhode Island Test of Language Structure (RITLS) (Engen & Engen, 1983)*
Grammatical Analysis of Elicited Language (GAEL) (Moog & Geers, 1979)*
Grammatical Analysis of Elicited Language, presentence level (GAEL-p) (Moog, Kozak, & Geers, 1983)*
Test of Syntactic Ability (TSA) (Quigley, Monranelli, & Wilbur, 1976)*
Written Language Syntax Test (WLST) (Berry, 1981)
Berko Morphology Test (Berko, 1984)
Test for Auditory Comprehension of Language–Third Edition (TACL–III) (Carrow-Woolfolk, 1999)
Oral and Written Language Skills (OWLS) (Carrow-Woolfolk, 1996)
Developmental Sentence Analysis (DSA) (Lee, 1974)
Index of Productive Syntax (IPSyn) (Scarborough, 1990)
Content
Semantic Content Analysis (Kretschmer & Kretschmer, 1978)
Peabody Picture Vocabulary Test–Revised (PPVT–R) (Dunn & Dunn, 1981)
Reynell Developmental Language Scales (Reynell, 1977)
Function
Pragmatic Content Analysis (Kretschmer & Kretschmer, 1978)
Performative Content Analysis (Hasenstab & Tobey, 1991)

Assessment procedures generally can be classified as checklists (e.g., Moog & Geers, 1975), tests (e.g., Quigley, Monranelli, & Wilbur, 1976), or language sample analyses (e.g., Kretschmer & Kretschmer, 1978). In compiling a checklist, a clinician checks whether a particular behavior is present. For example, a clinician might check *yes* or *no* for the statement, *The child recognizes the meaning of subject-verb-object sentences.*

Many tests contain items that assess formally a child's ability to use language structures. For example, if negation is assessed, the child might be asked to change the sentence, *He will go* to *He will not go.*

Language sample analyses usually are performed on samples of both the child's receptive and expressive language. A clinician might describe the semantic classes children use and recognize, their complex sentence productions, and their communication proficiency. For example, a child produced the following language sample:

The boy watched the boy eat. The boy eat again. The boy smiles.

Quantitative measures for a sample like this would usually include (see Rose, McAnally, & Quigley, 2004, p. 201):

- Type-Token Ratio (TTR). A ratio of the number of different words compared to the total number of words used. In the sample above, the TTR is 6:12.
- Mean Sentence Length (MSL). The mean number of words per sentence. In the sample above, the MSL is four.

Assessing Reading Skills

With the reauthorization of IDEA and passage of the No Child Left Behind Act (Chapter 14), one purpose of assessing reading skills is to determine whether children are meeting the goals and standards established by each state. The results can also guide the formulation of instructional objectives and indicate whether a student has progressed in learning how to read and in reading comprehension.

Although a few assessment tools have been designed specifically for children who have hearing loss (the *Test of Early Reading Ability-Deaf or Hard of Hearing [TERA-D/HH]* is an example), instruments developed for children with normal hearing are often utilized to evaluate a child's reading readiness and reading skills. The disadvantages of using assessment instruments designed for children with normal hearing include: (a) The items of the test may be too difficult for the children with hearing loss to complete and (b) it is difficult to assess how well a child is doing compared to the peer group comprised of children with hearing loss. On the other hand, if a child is in a mainstream or an inclusion classroom, test scores may indicate how well he or she may be expected to perform in that setting and how well the child performs with respect to classmates who have normal hearing. Table 15-5 presents a sample of instruments used for assessing reading, as well as the grades (for children who have normal hearing) appropriate for testing and the areas of skill evaluated. These areas of skill include reading and language comprehension, phonology, syntax and semantics, decoding, phoneme awareness, alphabetic principles, letter knowledge, and concepts about print.

Table 15–5. A sample of assessments used to assess reading performance.

ASSESSMENT	GRADE	AREAS ASSESSED
Analytical Reading Inventory (6th ed.) (Woods & Moe, 1999)	K, 1, 2, 3, and higher	Reading comprehension, language comprehension, decoding
Bader Reading and Language Inventory (3rd ed.) (Bader, 1998)	Pre-K, K, 1, 2, 3, and higher	Reading comprehension, language comprehension, phonology, syntax, semantics, decoding, phoneme awareness, letter knowledge, concepts about print
Brigance Comprehensive Inventory of Basic Skills-Revised (CIBS-R) (Brigance, 1999)	Pre-K, K, 1, 2, 3, and higher	Reading comprehension, phonology, semantics, decoding, letter knowledge
Durrell Analysis of Reading Difficulty (3rd ed.) (DAR) (Durrell & Catterson, 1980)	Pre-K, K, 1, 2, 3, and higher	Reading comprehension, language comprehension, semantics, decoding, phoneme awareness
GOALS: A Performance Based Measure of Achievement (Psychological Corp., 1994)	1, 2, 3, and higher	Reading comprehension, language comprehension
Gray Oral Reading Test-Diagnostic (GORT-D) (Bryant & Wiederholt, 1991)	K, 1, 2, 3, and higher	Reading comprehension, syntax, decoding
Kaufman Assessment Battery for Children (K-ABC) (Kaufman & Kaufman, 1983)	Pre-K, K, 1, 2, 3, and higher	Reading comprehension, semantics, decoding
Reading and Oral Language Assessment (ROLA) (Littcon Inc., 2000)	K, 1, 2, 3, and higher	Reading comprehension, language comprehension, decoding, lexical knowledge, phoneme awareness, letter knowledge, concepts about print
Signposts Early Literacy Battery and Pre-DRP Test (Touchstone Applied Science Associates, Inc., 2001)	K, 1, 2, and 3	Reading comprehension, language comprehension, syntax, semantics, decoding, phoneme awareness, letter knowledge
Test of Early Reading Ability-Deaf or Hard of Hearing (TERA-D/HH) (Reid, Hresko, Hammill, & Wiltshire, 1991)	Pre-K, K, 1, and 2	Letter knowledge, concepts about reading
Woodcock Diagnostic Reading Battery (WDRB) (Woodcock, 1997)	K, 1, 2, 3, and higher	Reading comprehension, semantics, decoding, letter knowledge
Woodcock-Johnson Psycho-Educational Battery (WJ-R) (Woodcock & Johnson, 1989)	K, 1, 2, 3, and higher	Reading comprehension, lexical knowledge

For children who are on the cusp of reading readiness, sometimes a teacher completes a simple checklist to assess preliteracy performance. For example, the teacher might indicate whether a child *never, sometimes,* or *always* demonstrates some of the following developmental benchmarks (adapted from Bodrova, Leong, Paynter, & Semenov, 2000):

- Holds a book upright and turns the pages of the book from front to back
- Pretends to read familiar books; joins in with predictable phrases (e.g., "I will huff and puff and blow your house down.")
- Reads environmental print (such as a McDonald's sign or a stop sign)
- Identifies letters in his or her name
- Tells a story when stimulated with a sequence of pictures
- Pretends or creates using language
- Listens responsively to narratives and books
- Tells stories

Speech and Language Therapy

Most children with significant hearing loss benefit from receiving speech and language therapy. Speech and language skills often do not emerge spontaneously. Concerted attention over many years must be placed on developing skills if a child is to learn to speak and use English.

Speech Therapy

Goals for a comprehensive speech development program may include the following (Carney & Moeller, 1998, p. S62):

- Increase vocalizations that have appropriate timing characteristics and that require numerous vocal tract movements
- Expand phonetic and phonemic repertoires
- Establish link between audition and speech production
- Improve suprasegmental aspects of speech
- Increase speech intelligibility

Results from the speech evaluation are used to select therapy goals. The phonetic transcriptions of elicited and spontaneous speech may be used for phoneme and phonological error pattern analysis. Phonetic error analysis yields an inventory of sounds a child can produce, as well as a catalog of the child's deletions, substitutions, and distortions. Phonological error analysis reveals phonological process errors. These may include final-consonant deletions, cluster reductions, and frontings. Therapy goals may focus on increasing a child's phonetic repertoire and on reducing phonological process errors. Auditory modeling is used extensively, sometimes in conjunction with a visual and tactile supplement.

Therapy curricula often differ according to the way speech is presented to the child and how feedback is provided (see Kosky & Boothroyd, 2001). In an auditory approach, children may receive instructions and correction about their speech via the auditory modality primarily, although often, no attempt is made to limit children's use of nonauditory cues, such as natural facial cues. In a more visual approach, visual stimuli are presented purposefully to supplement the auditory signal. A visual program may entail the use of mirrors, Cued Speech, or graphic symbols that are paired with specific speech sounds or prosodic features. Multisensory approaches, which may be somewhat eclectic, usually will present instruction through more than one sensory modality.

A widely implemented speech therapy program based on an auditory approach was developed by Daniel Ling (1976). This program rests on the premise that there is a hierarchy of speech skills. The most effective and efficient way to learn how to talk is to learn skills in an appropriate sequence and to build on an existing skill to develop a new one. For instance, before a child can learn specific speech sounds, he or she must first learn to regulate voice level and pitch. A child should be able to speak homophenous syllable strings, such as *bee-bee-bee*, before being asked to speak heterogeneous strings, such as *bee-boo-bee-boo*.

Visual methods include the *Northampton Charts*, developed at Clark School for the Deaf in 1885 and updated in 1925. Sounds are associated with a letter, and the sounds are represented on charts, which are on display during the therapy session, and even in the classroom throughout the day. Visual methods also include the use of computer-based visual feedback systems, such as the *IBM Speech Viewer* (no longer commercially available). Computer-based visual aids may present a visual response to a child's production, indicating the "goodness" of production or overall accuracy (e.g., Pratt, 2003). For instance, a child may sustain phonation into a microphone connected to the computer, and a balloon shown on the computer monitor is shown growing in size throughout the duration of phonation (Figure 15-15).

Carhart (1947; 1963) was an advocate of a multisensory approach in the last century. He proposed that children should receive auditory and speechreading training to learn the sounds of the language, and that speech instruction should be analytic and should incorporate auditory, visual, vibrotactile, and kinesthetic cues. The Lexington School for the Deaf advocated a more synthetic multisensory approach (Vorce, 1971; 1974).

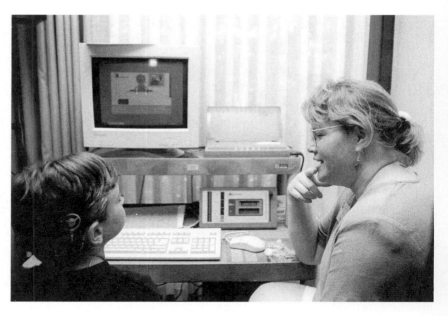

FIGURE 15-15. Computer-based visual aids during speech and language therapy. *Photograph by Kim Readmond, courtesy of the Central Institute for the Deaf.*

The guiding premise was that speech training should be stimulated in naturally occurring contexts, with emphasis placed on the whole utterance rather than individual sounds and syllables.

Language Therapy

Therapy goals in language development may include the following (Carney & Moeller, 1998):

- Increase communication between parent and child
- Promote an understanding of complex concepts and discourse units
- Enhance vocabulary growth
- Increase world knowledge
- Enhance self-expression
- Enhance growth in use of language syntax and pragmatics
- Develop narrative skills

A number of curricula have been developed for promoting language growth. Language curricula vary from highly structured to naturalistic. Content, form, and pragmatics are addressed in the development of a language intervention plan. Special emphasis may be placed on vocabulary development if the child is younger, and children might be encouraged to use conjunctions, pronouns, and modals.

Structured models usually exploit teacher modeling, student imitations, and sometimes, metalinguistic symbols. By being focused on structured stimuli, children may learn to perceive language patterns, practice them, and eventually, produce them spontaneously.

An example of a structured language curriculum is *A Patterned Program for Linguistic Expansion Through Reinforced Experiences and Evaluation* (*APPLE TREE;* Anderson, Boren, Kilgore, Howard, & Krohn, 1999). Designed for children in the primary and intermediate grades, the program consists of a sequence of procedures for developing children's ability to construct and comprehend 10 basic sentence patterns. Structures taught early in the curriculum include NOUN + VERB (BE) + ADJECTIVE (e.g., *The ball is red*) and NOUN + VERB (e.g., *The boy walks*). A structure taught later is NOUN1 + VERB + NOUN2 + VERB (e.g., *The boy sees the bird sit in the tree*). The program is designed so that each sentence pattern builds upon the previous pattern, and students advance to increasingly difficult levels of syntactic and semantic complexity. The curriculum also includes vocabulary building, spontaneous sentence production prompted with visual aids such as a picture story, and construction of transformations, such as asking a child to convert one of the sentence patterns into a question format. A sample activity is illustrated in Figure 15-16. Here, a child has been asked to arrange a set of word cards into patterns corresponding to the NOUN + VERB (BE) + ADJECTIVE sentence structure.

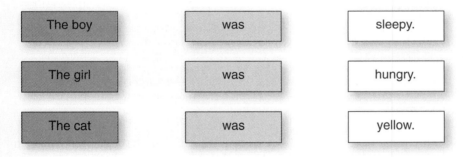

FIGURE 15-16. Structured language activities. During a structured language activity, a student might be asked to arrange word cards into a NOUN + VERB (BE) + ADJECTIVE pattern.

Many modern curricula advocate more naturalistic methods, where language is learned in the context of everyday, meaningful communication. Teachers and clinicians use conversation to expand vocabulary and to model syntax and pragmatics. The underlying premise is that children learn language when they are surrounded by language that describes what is relevant, meaningful, and/or of interest to them at the moment.

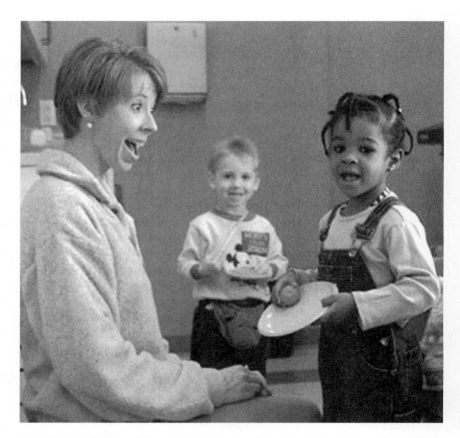

FIGURE 15-17. Naturalistic methods of language instruction. Naturalistic methods include optimizing everyday events (and structuring the environment so that events occur) to promote the growth of form, content, and pragmatics. In this encounter, a student is showing her teacher an apple on a plate. The teacher repeats the child's production of the word *apple* and expands on it by saying, "The apple is on the plate." Her goal is to fine-tune the child's understanding of the preposition *on*. The teacher also expands the child's pragmatic skills by asking, "Please, may I have the apple?" This utterance demonstrates the use of the word *please*. *Photograph by Kim Readmond, courtesy of the Central Institute for the Deaf.*

In a naturalistic approach, therapy goals often are based on information about the language development of children with normal hearing, and goals are reinforced throughout the day, whether at school or at home (Figure 15-17). If a child is school-age, concerted attention may be placed on the development of syntax and semantics. The speech and hearing professional may spend time observing the child in the classroom. The clinician then makes specific recommendations about how the classroom teacher might reinforce language therapy goals in a naturalistic setting and incorporate goals into the academic curriculum. The classroom observation also may reveal specific language error patterns that the child is producing.

OTHER SERVICES

The aural rehabilitation intervention plan might include other components, including those we have considered in preceding chapters, such as auditory training, communication strategies training, and assertiveness training and counseling. A speech and hearing professional might provide an in-service to classroom teachers and other staff about hearing loss and accommodations in the classroom. Classmates might be sensitized to the communication difficulties associated with hearing loss.

Services may include psychosocial support (Chapter 10). There is evidence that children and adolescents with significant hearing loss have a greater likelihood of experiencing psychosocial problems than children who have normal hearing (see Wallis, Musselman, & MacKay, 2004, for a review). Social problems may include:

- Social isolation (e.g., Antia, 1982; Suarez & Torres, 1996; Kluwin, 1999)
- Naiveté about peer interests and customs
- Difficulty in empathizing (e.g., Bachara, Raphael, & Phelan, 1980)
- Limited understanding about internal states such as feelings
- Feelings of frustration or intimidation during social interactions

Although children with hearing loss vary from one another as in any group of children, and some children will experience few difficulties in psychosocial adjustment, increasing magnitudes of hearing loss can cause increasing difficulties. Table 15-6 describes how varying degrees of long-term hearing loss may affect psychosocial well-being and associated educational needs.

An example of an assessment instrument for psychosocial adjustment for school-age children is the *Meadow-Kendall Social Emotional Assessment Inventories for Deaf and Hearing-Impaired Students* (*SEAI;* Meadow, 1983), one of the few instruments developed specifically for children with hearing loss. This inventory includes 59 items divided into three subscales: social adjustment, self-image, and emotional adjustment. Norms are established for ages 7 to 21 years and are based on inventories collected from more than 2,400 students. A classroom teacher or other educational professional who is in close contact with the student rates behaviors on a 5-point scale, ranging from *Very true* (description of an observed behavior) to *Does not apply.*

Several discussions about the development of social skills are available in the literature, as are ways to alleviate such social difficulties as those just listed (Gfeller & Schum, 1994; Paul & Jackson, 1993; Schum, 1991; Schum & Gfeller, 1994; Schloss & Smith, 1990). Some research suggests that children with severe and profound hearing loss can learn to enhance

Enhancing Children's Self-Image and Social Adjustment: Suggestions for the Classroom Teacher in a Mainstream Setting:

- Develop a program that includes coping strategies
- Enable the student to accept how hearing loss makes him or her different, while still enabling him or her to realize that hearing loss is not the student's primary descriptive characteristic
- Identify attributes that describe the student as a valued individual
- Help the student and classmates to understand the nature of hearing loss
- Develop activities to foster inclusion
- Create situations that encourage a student to take chances

(Oticon, 2006, pp. 6–7)

Table 15-6. Relationship between the degree of hearing-loss and psychosocial impact (adapted and updated from Anderson & Matkin, 1991, pp. 17–18).

DEGREE OF HEARING LOSS	POSSIBLE PSYCHOSOCIAL IMPACT	POTENTIAL EDUCATIONAL NEEDS AND PROGRAMS
Minimal or Borderline 16–25 dB HL	May be unaware of subtle conversational cues that could cause child to be viewed as inappropriate or awkward. May miss portions of fast-paced peer interactions that could begin to have an impact on socialization and self-concept. May have immature behavior. Child may be more fatigued than classmates due to listening effort needed.	May benefit from mild gain hearing aid or personal FM system depending on hearing loss configuration. Would benefit from sound field amplification if classroom is noisy and/or reverberant. Favorable seating. May need attention to vocabulary or speech, especially with recurrent otitis media history. Appropriate medical management necessary for conductive losses. Teacher requires in-service on impact of hearing loss on language development and learning.
Mild 26–40 dB HL	Barriers beginning to build with negative impact on self-esteem as child is accused of "hearing when he or she wants to," "daydreaming," or "not paying attention." Child begins to lose ability for selective hearing, and has increasing difficulty suppressing background noise, which makes the learning environment stressful. Child is more fatigued than classmates due to listening effort needed.	Will benefit from a hearing aid and use of a personal FM or sound field FM system in the classroom. Needs favorable seating and lighting. Refer to special education for language evaluation and educational follow-up. Needs auditory-skill building. May need attention to vocabulary and language development, articulation or speechreading, and/or special support in reading. May need help with self-esteem. Teacher in-service required.
Moderate (41–55 dB HL)	Often with this degree of hearing loss, communication is significantly affected, and socialization with peers with normal hearing becomes increasingly difficult. With full-time use of hearing aids/FM systems, child may be judged as a less competent learner. There is an increasing impact in self-esteem.	Refer to special education for language evaluation and for educational follow-up. Amplification is essential (hearing aids and FM system). Special education support may be needed, especially for primary children. Attention to oral language development, reading, and written language. Auditory-skill development and speech therapy usually needed. Teacher in-service required.
Moderate-to-Severe (56–70 dB HL)	Full-time use of hearing aids/FM systems may result in child being judged by both peers and adults as a less competent learner, resulting in poorer self-concept and social maturity, and contributing to a sense of rejection. In-service may foster improved self-concept and a sense of cultural identity.	Full-time use of amplification is essential. Will need resource teacher or special class depending on magnitude of language delay. May require special help in all language skills, language-based academic subjects, vocabulary, grammar, pragmatics, as well as reading and writing. Probably needs assistance to expand experiential language base. In-service of mainstream teachers required.
Severe (71–90 dB HL)	Child may prefer other children with hearing impairments as friends and playmates. This may further isolate the child from the mainstream; however, these peer relationships may foster improved self-concept and a sense of cultural identity.	May need full-time special aural/oral program with emphasis on all auditory language skills, speechreading, concept development, and speech. As loss approaches 80–90 dB HL, may benefit from a total-communication approach, especially in the early language-learning years. Individual hearing aid/personal FM system essential. Need to monitor effectiveness of communication modality. Participation in regular classes as much as is beneficial to student. In-service of mainstream teachers essential. May be a candidate for a cochlear implant.

continues

Table 15-6. *continued*

DEGREE OF HEARING LOSS	POSSIBLE PSYCHOSOCIAL IMPACT	POTENTIAL EDUCATIONAL NEEDS AND PROGRAMS
Profound (91 dB HL or more)	Depending on auditory/oral competence, peer use of sign language, parental attitude, etc., child may or may not increasingly prefer association with the Deaf culture.	May need special program for children who are deaf and hard of hearing with emphasis on all language skills and academic areas. Program needs specialized supervision and comprehensive support services. Early use of amplification likely to help if part of an intensive training program. May be a cochlear implant candidate. Requires continual appraisal of needs in regard to communication and learning mode. Part-time in regular classes as much as is beneficial to student.
Unilateral (one normal-hearing ear and one ear with at least a permanent mild hearing loss)	Child may be accused of selective hearing due to discrepancies in speech understanding in quiet versus noise. Child will be more fatigued in classroom setting due to greater effort needed to listen. May appear inattentive or frustrated. Behavior problems sometimes evident.	May benefit from personal FM or sound field FM system in classroom. May benefit from **CROS** hearing aid. Needs favorable seating and lighting. Student is at risk for educational difficulties. Educational monitoring warranted with support services provided as soon as difficulties appear. Teacher in-service is beneficial.

their social competency (Figure 15-18). Suárez (2000) developed a program consisting of two parts—(a) an interpersonal problem-solving training program with 15 lessons of a cognitive approach to social competence and (b) six lessons of social skills—and then conducted an experiment to test its efficacy. During the first part, participants developed the interior language

A **CROS** (contralateral routing of signals) hearing aid is designed for unilateral hearing losses. A microphone is placed on the poor ear and the signal is routed to a hearing aid worn on the better ear.

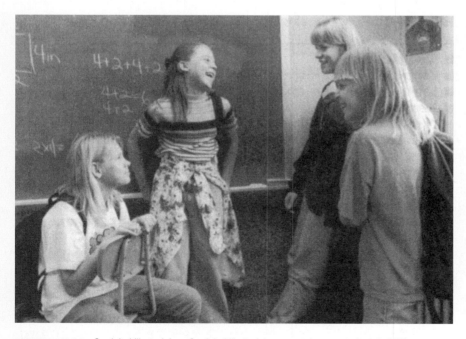

FIGURE 15-18. Social skills training. Social skills training can enhance students' abilities to function in groups and to solve interpersonal problems. *Photograph by Patti Gabriel, courtesy of the Central Institute for the Deaf.*

for cognitive problem solving (e.g., *What do I have to do? Which way is best? How well did I do?*). Participants learned to identify emotions, with the use of drawings and photographs, and to explore the causes of their emotions. They learned to evaluate solutions to interpersonal problems. In the second part, they learned specific social abilities, including how to apologize, how to negotiate with peers, how to avoid problems with others, how to withstand group influence, and how to cooperate and share in group interactions. Training activities included modeling, role-playing, feedback and reinforcement, and homework. Results showed that the 18 participants improved their social problem-solving skills and increased their assertive behavior, as determined by both teacher- and self-report.

CHILDREN WHO HAVE MILD OR MODERATE HEARING LOSSES

Heretofore, we have focused primarily on children who have severe and profound hearing loss. However, there is a huge population of children who have mild and moderate hearing losses who may require services from a speech and hearing professional at some point. It has been estimated that about 15% of children in the United States (more than 7 million) have a low-frequency or high-frequency hearing loss in at least one ear (Niskar et al., 1998). Two factors thought to contribute to the high prevalence of hearing loss in children are otitis media and noise exposure.

Many of these children experience particular difficulty while listening in noisy and reverberant classrooms. As a result, they experience deficits in speech recognition, academic learning, social skills, and self-image. They may have difficulty recognizing speech that is spoken quietly or at a distance. For these reasons, children who have mild and moderate hearing losses also may need aural rehabilitation, although usually not to the same extent as children who have severe and profound hearing losses. Children with a mild hearing loss (hearing thresholds between 20 and 40 dB HL) are often diagnosed later in childhood, perhaps during an elementary school screening program, because they rarely seem to have significant problems in hearing or in developing speech and language.

Children with a moderate loss (thresholds between 40 and 70 dB HL) have difficulty understanding speech presented at a conversational level and may have difficulty comprehending speech in a group setting. However, children with either a mild or moderate loss tend to receive a great deal of benefit from the use of hearing aids.

Children with mild or moderate hearing losses usually have an IEP developed. In particular, they should receive a speech-language evaluation to determine whether their speech and language acquisition is progressing according to age-level normally hearing peers. Sometimes, children will have mild misarticulation errors, such as errors in the production of fricatives and affricates (Elfenbein, Hardin-Jones, & Davis, 1994). Children with moderate hearing losses may also have some delays in vocabulary development (Davis, Elfenbein, Schum, & Bentler, 1986; Pittman, Lewis, Hoover, & Stelmachowicz, 2005; Stelmachowicz, Pittman, Hoover, & Lewis, 2004). Children with mild or moderate hearing losses may or may not need speech-language therapy, and they may need to use a free-field FM assistive listening device system. Often a child's classroom teacher will consult with a speech and hearing professional about how to adjust the classroom environment to accommodate the child with hearing loss. A handout like that presented in the Key Resources might be provided to the classroom teacher.

CASE STUDIES: IDEA(s) for ALL

IDEA(s) for All

Seaver and DesGeorges (2004) present a number of case studies to illustrate the nuances of the IDEA, and how its reauthorization in 1997 specifically addressed the needs of children who have hearing loss. Three of the case studies are summarized in this section.

V.S., Assistive Listening Technology (p. 22)

V.S. has a mild-to-moderate hearing loss and attends a public school. Her classroom faces a busy highway and is heated by a noisy air-handling system. Audiological tests have shown that her speech recognition scores decrease by 50% in the classroom environment as compared to a sound-treated booth. An audiologist measured the SNR and the reverberation times of the classroom and found them to be unacceptable. V.S.'s IEP team determines that accommodations are necessary so she can continue to function in her neighborhood school. She is supplied with an FM system, which boosts her speech recognition scores to 84% correct. The classroom receives carpeting and is treated with acoustic ceiling tiles.

L.R., Least Restrictive Environment (p. 21)

L.R. lives in the suburbs outside of a city. She received a cochlear implant 3 years previously, at the age of 4 years. She attends a centrally located day school for children who are deaf and hard of hearing, and one that has a total-communication educational philosophy. Until recently, L.R.'s parents used sign with her in the home but have noticed that her spoken-language skills have progressed to such a level that signing is no longer necessary. Her current teachers are strong advocates of sign language and they have no prior experience with children who use cochlear implants. The speech-language pathologist at

continues

IDEA(s) for All, *continued*

her day school has also never worked with a child who has a cochlear implant, but has opted to treat her like other children who use hearing aids. L.R. has friends at school but has not made friends in her own neighborhood. Her parents decide that she could benefit by being exposed to strong spoken-language models during her school day.

Although L.R.'s original placement in a total-communication program was appropriate, her needs have changed following the receipt of a cochlear implant. Her school district is not large enough to offer an aural/oral option and there are few children in the mainstream in her district. Her parents would like her to enroll in the neighborhood school and be fully integrated with children who have normal hearing, and receive services from an itinerant teacher. The members of her IEP team agree that L.R. should return to her local school so as to have more spoken-language models, but they also believe that the professionals who work with L.R. should have special expertise with children who have cochlear implants. The special education director from L.R.'s school district performs some field research and learns that a neighboring school district has a cochlear implant staff, assembled to serve a group of four children. The special education director solicits support from this district. Their cochlear implant staff agrees to provide ongoing mentorship to the itinerant teacher who will serve L.R. Their staff also agrees to provide in-services to L.R.'s classroom teacher and help the teacher to understand and implement the accommodations that are appropriate for a cochlear implant user.

J.M., Direct Instruction (p. 19)

J.M. is 4 years old and the daughter of Deaf parents who use ASL. She has a severe-to-profound hearing loss. Currently she is in a center-based preschool for children who have disabilities. Three of her classmates have hearing loss, two have autism, and the other children have other "special needs." The program uses total communication. Her parents want J.M. to have the opportunity to use her native language and to maintain the family's values of culture and community.

The IEP team considers ways to provide direct instruction in J.M.'s primary mode of communication. Because the school uses the SEE sign system, they must accommodate her language through other means. A neighborhood school district has a charter school with teachers who provide instruction using ASL. The IEP team decides that this would be the optimal placement for J.M.. This alternative placement will also permit J.M. to interact with other children who use her communication mode. The home school district funds transportation to the ASL charter school. Her parents become a resource for the charter school about Deaf culture and community.

FINAL REMARKS

This chapter presented an overview of school-age children's intervention programs. Federal law mandates that children receive a "free and appropriate public education" in the least restrictive environment, ideally at whatever public school children would have attended on the basis of where they live. However, given the relatively low incidence of hearing loss and deafness, not every school district has the critical mass to justify the expense of creating a program for children with hearing loss nor for hiring the appropriate staff. In many cases, creative solutions must be sought, with the overt goal of meeting children's unique communication requirements and related needs. IEP teams have the charge of helping to ensure that children receive the services that they need. Special provisions of the IDEA stipulate accommodations for a child's language and communication needs, for opportunities to interact with peers and teachers, for assistive technology, and for other academic needs. Integral to developing an IEP and ensuring that children receive appropriate services is the child's family (Figure 15-19). Parents many times must become advocates for their children, participating in the IEP process and ensuring that their children receive the optimal services available (e.g., Flanders, 2006; Underwood, 2006).

> "We knew our daughter, we knew hearing loss, we knew her goals, we attended every meeting with the school and we knew IDEA as it related to hearing loss."
>
> Nicole Underwood, who filed for due process so that her daughter would receive the family's preferred school placement and services related to her use of a cochlear implant
>
> *(Underwood, 2006, p. 42)*

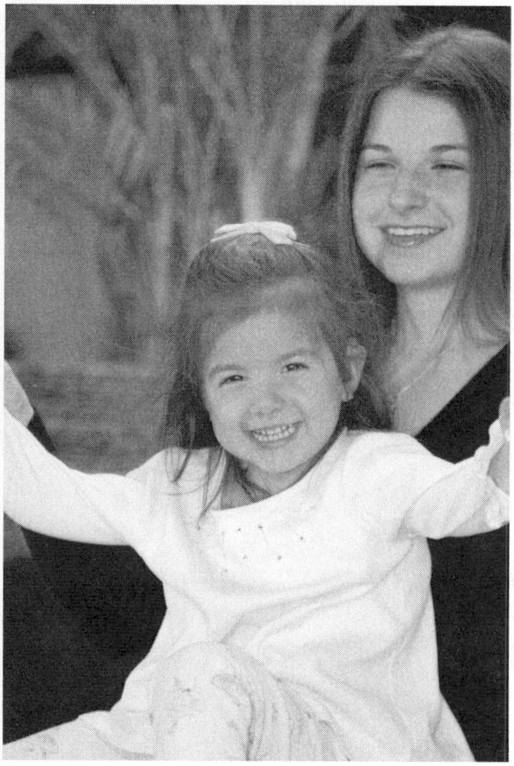

FIGURE 15-19. Parent advocacy. Parents many times must be advocates for their children, participating in the IEP process and soliciting appropriate services. *Courtesy of MED-EL Corp.*

KEY CHAPTER POINTS

- An Individualized Education Plan (IEP) is a written document that describes the child's current levels of performance, a statement of annual goals, a recommendation for special education support with an indication of how support will be provided, and objective criteria for evaluating progress.

- A multidisciplinary team is assembled to provide support and services to the child and his or her family. The team may include an audiologist, speech-language pathologist, classroom teacher, psychologist, interpreter, itinerant teacher, and/or resource room teacher.

- School placement may be public or private, residential or day. Classroom placement may be self-contained or mainstream. Variations of a mainstream placement include partial mainstreaming, inclusion, and coenrollment.

- Most children in the United States who have severe and profound hearing loss live at home and attend school in their home community. The majority of children use total communication.

- Use of assistive devices and favorable classroom acoustics can enhance a student's academic performance.

- Children with significant hearing loss may make characteristic speech errors, such as neutralizing vowels and omitting final consonants. These errors underlie generally low intelligibility levels.

- Children with significant hearing loss often have problems in content, form, and pragmatics of language. For instance, many have reduced vocabulary and have mastered fewer syntactic structures than children with normal hearing.

- Children with significant hearing loss often experience difficulty in learning to read. Many adults never attain better than a fourth-grade reading level.

- Evidence suggests that receipt of a cochlear implant may enhance and accelerate speech, language, and literacy growth.

- A speech and language evaluation is performed in order to develop a hierarchy of speech-language therapy objectives.

- Some children with hearing loss can benefit from psychosocial support and social skills training.

- Most children with mild and moderate hearing losses can attend classrooms with children who have normal hearing. Usually, they will receive an IEP, although they may or may not require specialized speech and hearing services.

TERMS AND CONCEPTS TO REMEMBER

Individualized Educational Program (IEP)
Multidisciplinary team
Itinerant teacher
Classroom placement

Self-contained classroom
Mainstream classroom
Resource room
Coenrollment
Appropriate format accommodations
Segmental speech errors
Suprasegmental speech errors
Roles of auditory feedback
Form
Content
Pragmatics
Literacy
Impact of cochlear implants
Rating scales
Transcription procedures
Checklists
Language sample analysis
Preliteracy skills
Structured language curriculum
Naturalistic language instruction
Social skills training

MULTIPLE-CHOICE QUESTIONS

1. The IDEA stipulates that the IEP team will do all but the following for the child who has a profound and congenital hearing loss:

    a. Provide opportunity for direct communication with classmates

    b. Provide access to assistive listening devices, as needed

    c. Ensure that the child learns the native language of the Deaf culture

    d. Provide access to a sign interpreter, as needed

2. Which professional is most likely to prepare a student for new material before the student encounters it in the regular classroom?

    a. The speech-language pathologist

    b. The classroom teacher

    c. The itinerant teacher

    d. The interpreter

3. School districts that have a self-contained classroom for students who are deaf and hard of hearing are required to do which of the following:

    a. Ensure that children who require audiological services receive them

    b. Follow a coenrollment model

    c. Employ an educational audiologist

    d. Purchase an assistive listening device for students who would benefit by using one

4. Which of the following is an example of an appropriate format accommodation:

    a. Open-book tests

    b. Study guides

    c. Resource room

    d. Inclusion

5. Reverberation refers to:

    a. A SNR of greater than −5 dB

    b. The effects of PL 94-142 since 1975

    c. The sound absorption potency, or grade, of acoustic ceiling tile

    d. Presence of sound due to signals being reflected from room surfaces

6. A coenrollment classroom is an example of:

    a. An educational placement where the child receives services from a resource room for part of the school day

    b. Mainstreaming

    c. Self-containment

    d. Educational models that entail a team of teachers, one a regular classroom teacher and the other, a teacher with specialized training

7. Typical segmental errors made by children who have profound deafness include:

    a. Breathiness

    b. Arrhythmic speech patterns, characterized by abnormal syllable stress patterns

    c. Substitution of high vowels for low vowels

    d. Voicing confusions

8. On average, children who have profound hearing loss achieve about what level of intelligibility?

    a. 5%

    b. 40%

    c. 20%

    d. 60%

9. Which of the following is not a common error associated with vowel production by children who have significant hearing loss?

    a. Neutralization

    b. Diphthongization

    c. Shortening

    d. Nasalization

10. Of the following sounds, which one is most likely to be produced correctly by a talker who has a profound hearing loss?

    a. /b/

    b. /t/

    c. /g/

    d. /n/

11. Which is an example of a problem related to form?

    a. The child has a restricted vocabulary, where words related to an entire concept may be unknown.

    b. A child asks a brand new acquaintance to lend her $20.

    c. A child sees a car driving by and says, "Car go fast."

    d. A child can understand the word *bank* when talking about a receptacle for money, but not when the word is used in reference to the ground flanking a river.

12. When writing an essay, a fourth grader who has significant hearing loss is likely:

    a. To omit function words such as *of* and *to*

    b. Underuse subject-verb-object sentence structures

    c. Follow too rigidly the narrative template of beginning, middle, and ending

    d. Overuse adverbs

13. Reading levels of high school graduates who have significant hearing loss and who use hearing aids:

    a. Hover around the 9th-grade level

    b. Permit them to understand articles in *Time,* a periodical geared toward the general U.S. readership

    c. Barely allow them to read a local newspaper with understanding

    d. Have improved gradually during the past half century

14. Janice is a 5-year-old girl. She lost her hearing at the age of 2 months, following a severe viral infection. Eleven months ago, Janice received a cochlear implant. She is beginning to articulate the following sounds accurately:

    a. Central vowels

    b. Front vowels

    c. Alveolars

    d. Palatals

15. When collecting a speech or language sample, it is important to:

    a. Make sure the child practices the sample several times before it is collected for assessment purposes

    b. Collect a variety of measures, as children's performance may vary as a function of task type

    c. Use an aural/oral communication mode

    d. Remain unfamiliar to the child until you actually begin testing, as talker familiarity may cause the child to speak with conversational speech

16. Which of the following factors probably has the least effect on a child's speech intelligibility score?

    a. Listener experience

    b. Listening condition

    c. Speech materials

    d. A guardian present in the room when the sample is collected

17. The speech therapy program developed by Daniel Ling is based on:

    a. The premise that formal instruction precedes informal instruction

    b. A hierarchy of speech skills

    c. The *Northampton Chart*

    d. Computer games, such as a balloon growing in size as the child phonates into a microphone

18. Sometimes children who have significant hearing loss experience socialization issues. For example, they:

    a. May experience social isolation

    b. Prefer to avoid interacting with other children who have significant hearing loss, so as not to appear a part of a minority

    c. Prefer the company of adults

    d. Experience excessive degrees of sympathy, as they can empathize with persons who face difficult situations

KEY RESOURCES

 ## CHECKING HEARING INSTRUMENTS

(adapted from Oticon, 2006, pp. 8–9)

Hearing aids

- Visual inspection: Look for dents, cracks in the hearing aid case, cracks in the tubing, wax in the earmold, moisture in the tubing, corrosion in the battery compartment.
- Listening check: Insert tip of the hearing aid's sound hook tightly into the end of the stetoclip, which you wear in the same way that a physician wears a stethoscope. Turn the instrument on and, while speaking into the hearing aid's microphone, rotate its volume control (if the device has one) while listening.
- Battery check: Check and replace the batteries if necessary.

FM systems

- Visual inspection: Check cords and hearing instrument. Turn the power on and be sure the LOW battery and NO FM indicators are not lit. If the NO FM indicator is lit, check that the batteries in the transmitter are in place and the unit is switched ON.
- Listening check: Listen to the system and ensure normal function.

 ## GUIDELINES FOR THE CLASSROOM TEACHER

The following suggestions should help _____'s teacher understand although he/she receives benefits from his/her hearing aid, it does not make speech clearer, only louder. What he hears might be called indistinct speech since there are individual sounds that are distorted or that she may not hear at all. Therefore anything that can be done to improve the listening conditions would be helpful.

1. Let _____ sit as close to the teacher as possible. In this way he/she will be able to benefit from both the auditory and visual cues. This seat should be far away from noisy distractions of hallways, radiators, or windows. Expect _____ to have more trouble listening and paying attention when the room is noisy than when it is quiet.

2. Speak naturally to _____ in a good clear voice. The hearing aid is an amplifier therefore it is unnecessary to shout.

3. If _____ does not understand something that was said, the teacher can:

   a. repeat—perhaps a little slower.
   b. rephrase.
   c. write the word or sentence on the board.

4. In order to follow a group discussion, it would be helpful if _____ could sit where she could see most of the faces, and if the teacher or children could try to let her know who is talking and let her look before the speaker begins to talk. It is also ideal if the teacher can repeat the most important things said.

5. In order to understand what is said, it is usually helpful for _____ to see the speaker's face and lips. This is called speechreading. For speechreading it is helpful if

   a. _____'s back is to the major light source.
   b. The speaker does not move around too much.
   c. The speaker speaks clearly and distinctly and faces _____ when talking.

6. Sometimes a child with hearing loss may miss the small words and misunderstand a sentence, especially if it is a long sentence and the room is noisy. If _____ seems confused or gives a silly answer, repeat what was said and if he/she said something inappropriate let her in on the joke. _____ may not always tell the teacher if he/she has not understood, but she should be encouraged to do so. Children who are hearing impaired are sometimes embarrassed to keep asking for repetitions.

7. New vocabulary words may be difficult for _____, and he/she may require a little extra help in vocabulary development.

8. In some cases a notetaker can be a help to the student with hearing loss. Sometimes a "buddy" in the class can be assigned to repeat directions to the child with hearing loss without disrupting the classroom routine.

Source: A handout from Central Institute for the Deaf Hearing, Language, and Speech Clinics. Reprinted with permission.

APPENDIX

Answers to Multiple-Choice Questions

Chapter 1: Introduction

1. c
2. d
3. a
4. b
5. d
6. c

Chapter 2: Assessing Hearing Acuity and Speech Recognition

1. c
2. b
3. a
4. b
5. a
6. d
7. a
8. b
9. c
10. d
11. a

Chapter 3: Listening Devices and Related Technology

1. b
2. d
3. b
4. a
5. c
6. b
7. d
8. c
9. a
10. c
11. a
12. c
13. d
14. c
15. a
16. b

Chapter 4: Auditory Training

1. c
2. a

3. a
4. b
5. d
6. d
7. b
8. a
9. b
10. c
11. a
12. c

Chapter 5: Speechreading

1. c
2. c
3. a
4. b
5. d
6. a
7. c
8. b
9. a

10. a
11. b

Chapter 6: Speechreading Training

1. a
2. b
3. c
4. a
5. c
6. a
7. d
8. d

Chapter 7: Communication Strategies and Conversational Styles

1. a
2. a
3. d
4. d
5. c
6. b
7. a
8. b
9. d
10. c

Chapter 8: Assessment of Conversational Fluency and Communication Difficulties

1. a
2. b
3. d
4. d
5. b
6. b
7. c

8. a
9. d

Chapter 9: Communication Strategies Training

1. c
2. a
3. d
4. b
5. c
6. b
7. d
8. a
9. c
10. b
11. d

Chapter 10: Counseling, Psychosocial Support, and Assertiveness Training

1. a
2. c
3. a
4. c
5. b
6. c
7. c
8. d
9. d
10. c

Chapter 11: Adults Who Have Hearing Loss

1. a
2. b
3. d
4. a

5. b
6. d
7. b
8. c
9. d
10. a

Chapter 12: Aural Rehabilitation Plans for Adults

1. a
2. b
3. d
4. c
5. c
6. c
7. a
8. b
9. c
10. a
11. b
12. d
13. b

Chapter 13: Aural Rehabilitation Plans for Older Adults

1. c
2. a
3. d
4. c
5. d
6. b
7. a
8. b
9. a
10. c

11. c

12. b

Chapter 14: Infants and Toddlers Who Have Hearing Loss

1. d
2. c
3. b
4. c
5. a
6. a
7. b
8. d
9. c
10. b
11. d

12. b
13. a
14. c
15. a
16. b
17. c
18. b
19. d
20. b
21. b

Chapter 15: School-Age Children Who Have Hearing Loss

1. c
2. c
3. a

4. b
5. d
6. d
7. d
8. c
9. c
10. a
11. c
12. a
13. c
14. a
15. b
16. d
17. b
18. a

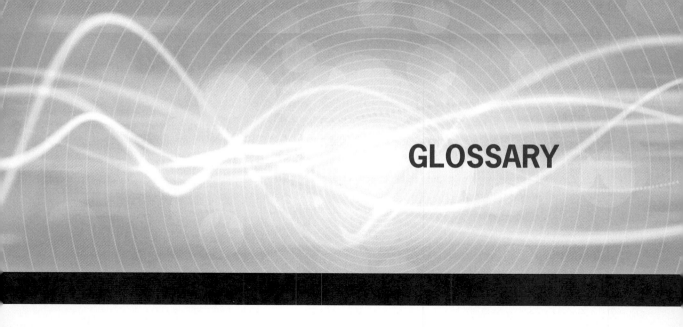

GLOSSARY

Terms and acronyms used in this text and other terms related to aural rehabilitation.

AAA: American Academy of Audiology.

AARP: American Association of Retired Persons.

ABR: Auditory brain stem response.

Academy of Doctors of Audiology: ADA; a national organization that fosters and supports qualified audiologists in their efforts to dispense hearing aids and to provide related aural rehabilitation services; formerly known as the Academy of Dispensing Audiologists.

Acknowledgment gesture: A head nod or a head shake made in response to a remark from a frequent communication partner.

Acoupedic approach: A comprehensive habilitation program for infants and their families that emphasizes auditory training and listening for communication, without formal lipreading or speechreading instruction.

Acoustic cue: Acoustic information in a segment of speech that conveys phonetic information.

Acoustic feedback: Sound produced when the amplified sound from a device

receiver is picked up again by the microphone and reamplified; a high-pitched squeal.

Acoustic feedback cancellation: A feature that avoids the annoying squeal produced by hearing aids when the microphone picks up the amplified sound from the hearing aid and reamplifies it.

Acoustic lexical neighborhood: A set of words that are acoustically similar and have approximately the same frequency of occurrence.

Acoustic neuroma: A tumor of the auditory or eighth nerve, usually benign, which may cause gradual hearing loss, tinnitus, and dizziness.

Acquired hearing loss: Hearing loss that is acquired after birth.

Activity limitation: A change at the level of the person brought about by an impairment at the levels of body structure and function.

Acute otitis media: Inflammation of the middle ear that lasts for 3 weeks or less.

AD: Alzheimer's disease.

ADA: Americans with Disabilities Act; Academy of Doctors of Audiology.

Adaptive strategies: Methods of counteracting maladaptive behaviors that stem from hearing loss.

ADD: Attention deficit disorder.

Adjacency pairs: Linked speaking turns.

ADM: Automatic directional microphone.

Adventitious hearing loss: Hearing loss occurring after birth.

Affricate: Consonants that include a vocal tract obstruction (or a stop consonant) and a prolonged frication; for example, /tʃ/.

AGC: Automatic gain control.

Aggressive conversational style: Conversational style characteristic of some persons who have hearing loss, characterized by hostility, belligerence, and a bad attitude.

Aided thresholds: Hearing thresholds obtained from a patient using hearing aids, indicated by an "A" on the audiogram.

Air–bone gap: The difference between air and bone conduction thresholds; a difference may indicate a conductive component in the hearing loss.

Air conduction: Sound travels through the air, enters the external auditory canal, and progresses through the middle ear, inner ear, and then to the brain; air conduction thresholds are represented by "O" (right ear) and "X" (left ear) on the audiogram.

ALD: Assistive listening device.

ALGO: An automated ABR screening device used for screening newborns.

Allele: One of two or more alternative forms of a gene, occupying the same position on paired chromosomes, which are responsible for alternative traits or for controlling the same inherited characteristic.

Altered speech: Human speech that is recorded and then altered in some manner.

Alzheimer's disease: AD; refers to a disease that affect reasoning and intellectual faculties; symptoms may include memory loss, deterioration of thought processes, and orientation disorders.

Ambient noise: Surrounding noise in a listening environment.

American Academy of Audiology: AAA; professional society for audiologists, founded in 1988.

American Association of Retired Persons: AARP; consumer group for persons over the age of 50 years.

American National Standards Institute: ANSI; group that determines standards for measuring instruments, including audiometers.

American Sign Language: ASL; a manual system of communication used by members of the Deaf culture in the United States; sometimes referred to as Ameslan.

American Speech-Language-Hearing Association: ASHA; professional organization of speech and hearing professionals, including speech-language pathologists, audiologists, and speech and hearing scientists.

American Tinnitus Association: ATA; consumer organization for persons who have tinnitus.

Americans with Disabilities Act: ADA; U.S. law enacted in 1990 to provide equal access to persons with disabilities.

Amplification: Provision of increased intensity of sound.

Amplifier: A transducer that converts an audio signal into an electronic signal and usually increases the intensity of sound.

Analytic training: Speechreading or auditory training that focuses the student's attention on individual speech units.

Anomaly: A structure that is irregular or deviates from the norm, such as a cochlear anomaly.

Anoxia: Deficiency or absence of oxygen in the bodily tissues.

ANSI: American National Standards Institute.

Anticipatory strategies: Methods of preparing for a communication interaction.

Aperiodic: Not occurring at regular intervals; not periodic.

Apgar score: A numeric value between 1 and 10 assigned to a newborn to describe physical status at birth; determined by the baby's color, heart rate, respiration, muscle tone, and responsiveness.

Appropriate format accommodations: Accommodations that allow children with hearing loss to participate with children who have normal hearing on a "fair playing ground."

Articulation: Movement and positioning of the oral-cavity structures, including tongue tip, tongue body, jaw, and lips, during speech production.

ASHA: American Speech-Language-Hearing Association.

ASL: American Sign Language.

ASSEP: Auditory steady state evoked potential.

Assertive conversational style: Conversational style used by some persons with hearing loss, characterized by a respect for the rights of others and assuming responsibility for the success of the conversational interaction.

Assertiveness training: Training that is aimed at teaching patients to express themselves assertively in their interpersonal communication interactions and to state both negative and positive feelings directly.

Assistive listening device: ALD; instrument designed to provide awareness or identification of environmental signals and speech and to improve signal-to-noise ratios.

Asymmetrical hearing loss: Hearing loss in which the degree and/or configuration of loss in one ear differs from that in the other ear.

ATA: American Tinnitus Association.

Atresia: A congenital closure of the external auditory canal.

Attack time: The time between when a signal begins and the onset of its steady-state amplified value.

Attention: A selective narrowing of mental focus and receptivity.

Attention deficit disorder: ADD; cognitive deficit that limits an individual's ability to pay attention and stay focused on a task; may involve restlessness, distractibility, and hyperactivity.

Audible: Loud enough to be heard.

Audio boot: A device that is used with a behind-the-ear hearing aid for coupling to a direct audio input cord; sometimes called a *shoe.*

Audiogram: A graphic representation of hearing thresholds as a function of stimulus frequency.

Audiologic rehabilitation: Term often used synonymously with aural rehabilitation or aural habilitation; sometimes may entail greater emphasis on the provision and follow-up of listening devices and less emphasis on communication strategies training and speechreading and auditory training.

Audiologist: Allied health care professional who has academic accreditation in the practice of audiology; professional who provides an array of services related to hearing evaluation and rehabilitation.

Audiometer: An instrument for testing the ability of the human ear to detect sound over a range of frequencies and intensities; may also be used to determine most comfortable listening levels and uncomfortable listening levels.

Audiometric zero: Lowest sound pressure level that can just be detected by an average adult ear at any particular frequency; designated as 0 dB Hearing Level (HL) on an audiogram.

Audiovisual: Situation wherein speech is presented to both the auditory and visual modalities.

Audiovisual integration: The cognitive process whereby information from the auditory and the visual signal are combined to form a unified percept.

Audition: Hearing.

Audition-only: Presentation of only an auditory signal in testing or training.

Audition-plus-vision: Presentation of both auditory and visual signals simultaneously in testing or training.

Auditorily: With audition.

Auditory: Pertaining to hearing.

Auditory brain stem implant: Implant that has an electrode that implants to the juncture of the eighth cranial nerve and the cochlear nucleus in the brain stem; provides crude sound awareness.

Auditory brain stem response: ABR; auditory evoked potential that originates from the eighth cranial nerve and auditory brainstem structures; the electrophysiological record consists of five to seven peaks, which represent the neural functioning of the auditory pathway.

Auditory canal: External auditory meatus.

Auditory cortex: The region of the brain that is responsible for processing auditory information and is located in the temporal lobe of the cerebral hemisphere, just forward of the occipital lobe.

Auditory feedback: One's own speech signal that is heard while speaking.

Auditory memory: Acquisition, storage, and retrieval of previously experienced auditory sound patterns.

Auditory neuropathy: Condition where the patient has a pure-tone audiogram that shows any degree of hearing loss, from mild to profound, and shows normal OAEs and either absent or degraded ABRs. Also called auditory dyssynchrony.

Auditory training: Instruction designed to maximize an individual's use of residual hearing by means of both formal and informal listening practice.

Auditory steady state evoked potentials: ASSEP; auditory evoked potentials elicited by amplitude-modulated pure tones (or noise), and provide frequency-specific information that can be used to estimate hearing sensitivity; they may be used to determine thresholds that exceed 90 dB nHL.

Auditory-verbal approach: A communication and educational approach that encourages a child to develop listening behaviors and to develop spoken communication by relying on residual hearing rather than vision; the use of appropriate and habitual amplification or electrical stimulation (via cochlear implant) is strongly encouraged.

Auditory-verbal therapy: An intervention in which technology, techniques, and strategies are used to enable children to listen and understand spoken language, with a primary emphasis on the auditory modality for learning.

Aural habilitation: Sometimes used synonymously with aural rehabilitation; intervention for persons who have not developed listening, speech, and language skills; may include diagnosis of communication and hearing-related difficulties, speechreading and auditory training, counseling, speech and language therapy, communication strategies training, manual communication, and educational management.

Aural/oral communication: The communication mode used by persons with normal hearing, which entails listening and speaking.

Aural/oral method: An instructional method used to teach children with significant hearing loss using hearing, speechreading, and spoken language, but not manual communication.

Aural rehabilitation: Intervention aimed at minimizing and alleviating the communication difficulties associated with hearing loss; may include diagnosis of hearing loss and participation restrictions, amplification, counseling, psychosocial support, assertiveness training, communication strategies training, speechreading and auditory training, family instruction, speech-language therapy, and educational management.

Auricle: Pinna; external or outer ear.

Automatic directional microphone: ADM; a microphone that automatically switches between an omnidirectional and directional mode according to environmental conditions.

Automatic gain control: AGC; nonlinear hearing aid compression circuitry that changes gain as signal level changes or limits the output of the hearing aid when the level reaches a specified value.

Autosomal dominant: One parent passes a dominant allele to the child; the probability of the trait being expressed in the child is 50%.

Autosomal recessive: Transmission of genetic characteristics in which both parents must pass on matching alleles to the child in order for the characteristic to be expressed.

Autosome: Any of the 22 pairs of 23 chromosome pairs not related to determination of gender.

Baby boomers: The generation born between the years 1946 and 1965.

Background noise: Extraneous noise that masks the acoustic signal of interest.

BAHA: Bone-anchored hearing aid.

Barotrauma: A condition caused by a drastic change in air pressure, as when flying; often occurs in divers and snorkelers and then relates to water pressure.

Battery: A cell that provides electrical power.

Behavioral audiometry: Pure-tone and speech audiometry that requires a behavioral response from the patient.

Behavioral/observational audiometry: BOA; method of testing a child's hearing in which the tester presents a sound stimulus and observes the child's behavior for change.

Behind-the-ear hearing aid: BTE; a hearing aid worn over the pinna and coupled to the ear canal by means of an earmold.

Bilateral: On both sides; involving both ears.

Bilingual: A term that describes a person who speaks two languages.

Bilingual/bicultural model: In aural rehabilitation and in the United States, teaching children with significant hearing loss ASL as their first language and then later English in school as they develop reading and writing skills.

Binaural: For both ears.

Binaural advantage: The advantage of using both ears instead of one, such as better hearing thresholds and enhanced listening in the presence of background noise.

Binaural amplification: Use of a hearing aid in each ear.

Binaural squelch: Improvement in listening in noise when hearing with two ears instead of one, resulting in a 2- to 3-dB improvement in signal-to-noise ratio.

BOA: Behavioral/observational audiometry.

Body hearing aid: A hearing aid worn on the body; includes a box worn on the torso and a cord connecting to an ear-level receiver.

Bone-anchored hearing aid: BAHA; A bone-conduction hearing aid anchored to the mastoid via a titanium screw and attached percutaneously to an external processor; primarily used for conductive hearing loss and when there is an intractable middle ear disorder or significant atresia.

Bone conduction: Transmission of sound through the bones in the body, particularly the skull.

Bone conduction hearing aid: A hearing aid that delivers the amplified signal via a bone vibrator placed over the mastoid directly to the cochlea, bypassing the middle ear.

Bone conductor: Vibrator or oscillator that is used to transmit sound to the cochlea by means of vibration of the bones of the skull.

BTE: Behind-the-ear hearing aid.

Calibration: Checking of a measuring instrument, such as an audiometer, against an accurate standard to determine whether deviations or errors exist.

Canonical babbling: An advanced form of infant babbling that consists of well-formed consonant-vowel combinations.

CAPD: Central auditory processing disorder.

Carrier phrase: In speech audiometry, a phrase that precedes the target word, such as, "Say the word _____."

Cataract: Progressive retinal disorder that entails a clouding of the lens; causes blurred vision and impairs contrast sensitivity.

CAT scan: Computerized axial tomography scan.

CDT: Continuous discourse tracking.

Center-based program: Program wherein children attend therapy outside the home environment for a designated number of hours per week.

Central auditory processing disorder: CAPD; an inability to differentiate, recognize, and understand sounds that is not due to either hearing loss or cognitive impairment.

Cerebral palsy: A motor-control disorder caused by insult to the motor cortex of the brain, characterized by a lack of muscle control, especially in the limbs.

Cerumen: Ear wax.

Cholesteatoma: A tumorlike mass of epithelium cells and cholesterol in the middle ear that may invade the mastoid process and impinge upon the ossicular chain.

Chromosome pair: The basic unit of genes; structures carrying the genes of a cell and made up of a single strand of DNA.

Chronic: Of long-standing duration.

Chronological age: Age of an individual referenced to birth.

CIC: Completely-in-the-canal hearing aid.

CICI: Completely implantable cochlear implant.

Circuit: A combination of electronic components that conveys electronic current.

Circuitry: The parts of an electric circuit.

Classroom acoustics: The background noise and reverberation properties characteristic of a classroom, determined by the size and surfaces of the room, the sound sources inside and outside, furnishings, people, and other factors.

Clarification: A counseling technique whereby clinicians abstract the essence of a patient's remarks and summarize them back to their patient.

Clear speech: Speech that is spoken at a moderately loud conversational level, and is characterized by precise but not exaggerated articulation, pauses at appropriate linguistic boundaries, and somewhat slowed speaking rate; often used to increase the message recognition of listeners with hearing loss.

Clinical significance: Whether an experimental result has practical meaning to either patient or the clinician.

Clock-time orientation: An orientation driven by the clock and characterized by an adherence to time as a factor in determining the length of an interaction or the time course of an intervention.

Closed captioning: Printed text or printed dialogue that corresponds to the auditory speech signal from a television program or movie.

Closed-ended questions: Questions with a constrained number of response options, often used to gather quantitative information.

Closed set: A stimulus or response set that contains a fixed number of items, known to the patient.

Cluster analysis: A statistical approach to information in a database that aims to determine which data points fall into groups or clusters on the basis of similarity.

CMV: Cytomegalovirus.

CNT: Could not test.

Coarticulation: The influence of one phoneme on either a preceding or succeeding phoneme.

Cochlear implant: Device implanted in the skull that permits persons with significant hearing loss to receive stimulation of the auditory mechanism; typically comprised of a microphone, a speech processor, and an electrode array inserted into the cochlea; directly stimulates the auditory nerve by means of electrical current.

Cochlear implant mapping: Process of programming the cochlear implant's speech processor.

Cochlear implant team: Group of professionals who are part of the cochlear implant process; usually includes an otolaryngologist, audiologist, and clinical coordinator and may include an educator, aural rehabilitation specialist, speech-language pathologist, psychologist, and/or social worker.

Cochlear nucleus: Cluster of cell bodies in the brain stem where the nerve fibers leading from the cochlea enter and synapse.

Coenrollment: A model of educating children who have hearing loss that entails a team of teachers, one a regular classroom teacher and the other, a trained teacher for children who are deaf and hard of hearing.

Cognition: Those mental processes involved in obtaining knowledge, in

comprehending, and in thinking, including such mental acts as remembering, judging, and problem solving.

Comfortable loudness level: Intensity level at which it is comfortable to listen to sound; sometimes referred to as the most comfortable listening level.

Completely implantable cochlear implant: CICI; a cochlear implant comprised of only internal components.

Communication: The act of exchanging messages; may entail the use of speech, sign, writing, or hand gestures.

Communication breakdown: Instance in the course of a conversation when one participant does not recognize the message presented by another.

Communication disorder: An impairment in one's ability to communicate.

Communication mode: The means used to share information between a sender and a receiver and may include speech, sign, writing, hand gestures, or any other system of shared symbols.

Communication partner: Person with whom one engages in conversation.

Communication strategies training: Instruction provided to a person with hearing loss or the person's frequent communication partner that pertains to communication strategies and the management of communication difficulties.

Communication strategy: A course of action taken to enhance communication.

Completely-in-the-canal hearing aid: CIC; a hearing aid that fits entirely within the external ear canal.

Comprehension: In auditory training, a higher level of auditory skill development characterized by an ability to understand spoken messages.

Compressed speech: Speech that has had segments removed and then has been compressed in such a way that the frequency composition remains intact.

Compression: In hearing aid circuitry, nonlinear amplifier gain used to determine and limit output gain as a function of input gain.

Compression ratio: The ratio in decibels between the acoustic input to a hearing aid amplifier and its auditory output.

Computerized axial tomography: CAT; a computer-generated picture of a section of the brain compiled from sectional radiographs obtained from the same plane; also know as CT scan.

Concha: The bowl-like depression of the outer ear that forms the mouth of the external ear canal.

Conditioned play audiometry: Method of testing young children in which the child is trained to perform a task in response to presentation of a sound.

Conditioned response: A new or modified response to a previously neutral stimulus.

Conductive hearing loss: Hearing loss that stems from an impairment in the outer or middle ear and that does not involve the inner ear.

Configuration: Refers to the shape of the audiogram and gives an overall description to the hearing loss.

Congenital: Present at birth.

Congenital hearing loss: Hearing loss that exists at or dates from birth; reduced hearing sensitivity related to pre- or perinatal causes.

Congruence with self: A tenet of person-centered counseling in which clinicians act as themselves in interactions with patients and do not assume a facade of professionalism.

Consonant-vowel-consonant: CVC; a monosyllabic word structure; CVCs often are used as stimuli in isolated-word speech recognition tests.

Construct: An abstract or general idea that is inferred or derived from a constellation of measures or from a group of specific instances.

Construct validity: Statistical term meaning the extent to which a test measures what it is supposed to measure, usually a trait or skill; for example, speech perception.

Constructive strategy: Tactic designed to optimize the listening environment for communication; a kind of facilitative strategy.

Content: In language, a child's extent of vocabulary and use of words.

Content validity: Statistical term meaning the extent to which a test adequately samples what it is supposed to measure.

Contextual information: Linguistic support available for identifying a target word, phrase, or sentence.

Continuous discourse tracking: CDT; aural rehabilitation technique in which the receiver (listener) attempts to repeat verbatim text that is presented by a sender (speaker); performance is summarized as the number of words repeated per minute.

Conversational fluency: Relates to how smoothly conversation unfolds and is reflected by the time spent in repairing communication breakdowns, the exchange of information and ideas, and the sharing of speaking time.

Conversational rules: Implicit rules that guide the conduct of participants engaged in conversation.

Conversational turn: During the course of a conversation, the period during which a participant delivers a contribution to the conversation.

Corner audiogram: An audiogram that displays a profound hearing loss, with thresholds measurable only in the low frequencies.

Cost-effectiveness: The relationship between the money spent and the benefits accrued.

Critical period: The early years of a child's life in which the language and vocal patterns of the individual's language community are acquired most easily.

CROS (contralateral routing of signals) hearing aid: Hearing aid that is designed for unilateral hearing losses, where a microphone is placed on the poor ear and the signal is routed to a hearing aid worn on the better ear.

Counseling: When provided for persons who have hearing loss (or their family members), a professional service designed to help patients better understand and solve their hearing-related problems.

Cued Speech: A system for enhancing speechreading; hand configurations are placed at different mouth and throat positions to distinguish between similar visual speech patterns.

Cultural and linguistic competence: A set of congruent behaviors, attitudes, and policies that come together in a system, in an agency, or among professionals that enables effective work in cross-cultural situations.

CVC: Consonant-Vowel-Consonant.

Cycling: In speechreading or auditory training, coming back to a training objective that has been achieved with some success in order to provide reinforcement and additional learning.

Cytomegalovirus: CMV; a member of the herpes virus that may cause hearing loss and other disorders in newborn babies.

DAI: Direct audio input.

Daily log: A procedure for assessing conversational fluency and communication difficulties, in which respondents perform a self-monitoring procedure about behaviors of interest and provide self-reports; usually completed more than once, over a set period of time.

dB: Decibel.

dB nHL: Decibels normalized hearing level; a decibel notation that is referenced to behavioral thresholds of a group of persons with normal hearing and is used to describe the intensity level of stimuli used in evoked potential audiometry.

Dead-air spaces: Unventilated air spaces, as exists between the inner and outer walls of some sound-treated booths.

Deaf: Having minimal or no hearing.

Deaf culture: A subculture in society that shares a common language (American Sign Language), beliefs, customs, arts, history, and folklore; primarily comprised of individuals who have prelingual deafness.

Decibel: dB; logarithmic unit of sound pressure; one tenth of a Bel; unit for expressing sound intensity.

Delayed-onset hereditary hearing loss: Hearing is normal at birth, then declines later in life as a result of a hereditary disorder.

Dementia: Term that refers to a number of diseases that affect reasoning and intellectual faculties; symptoms may include memory loss, deterioration of thought processes, and orientation disorders.

Deoxyribonucleic acid: DNA; molecules that carry genetic instructions.

Dependent variable: The factor or item measured in an experiment.

Describing: A language stimulation technique wherein an adult uses an event a child is interested in to talk about various aspects of the event.

Desensitization: A way to reduce a patient's negative reactions in specific situations by means of repeatedly exposing the person to them in mild form, either in reality or in role-playing or imagination.

Detection: The ability to recognize when a sound is present and when it is absent.

Developmental delay: Lagging behind in development relative to age-matched peers.

Diabetic retinopathy: A condition resulting from long-standing diabetes, which causes blurred and distorted vision in the central visual field and sometimes a detached retina.

Digital hearing aid: Hearing aid that utilizes digital technology to process the signal.

Digital signal processing: DSP; performed by a hearing aid, a procedure that converts the signal from analog to digital form, processes the signal to achieve a target, then converts the signal back to analog form.

Direct audio input: DAI; hardwired connection that leads directly from the sound source to the hearing aid or other listening device.

Directional microphone: Microphone that is more sensitive to sound originating from in front of the hearing aid user than from behind.

Disability: A physical or mental impairment that substantially limits one or more life activities in the individual.

Discourse: Communication of thoughts by use of language.

Discrimination: In speechreading or auditory training, the ability to distinguish whether stimuli are the same or different.

Disorder: An abnormality in functioning.

Dissonance theory: Theory concerning situations in which one's self-perceptions do not coincide with reality.

Distortion: Undesirable change in the audio signal.

Distortion product otoacoustic emission: DPOAE; the acoustic energy created by stimulating the ear with two simultaneous pure tones (f_1 and f_2), which results in energy created at several frequencies along the outer hair cells that are combinations of the two pure tones; DPOAEs typically entail the measurement of energy produced at $2f_1-f_2$.

DNA: Deoxyribonucleic acid.

DNT: Did not test.

Dominant hereditary hearing loss: Hearing loss that stems from a genetic characteristic on at least one gene of a pair.

Dominating conversational behaviors: Characteristic of an aggressive conversational style; includes taking extended speaking turns, frequent interruptions, and abrupt topic changes.

DPOAE: Distortion product otoacoustic emission.

Dri-aid kit: A small package used to keep moisture out of the internal components of listening devices.

Drill activity: Repeated exercises and rote activities.

DSP: Digital signal processing.

Dynamic range: The difference in decibels between an individual's threshold of sensitivity for a sound and the level at which the sound becomes uncomfortably loud.

Dysfunction: Abnormal function.

Ear protection: Term used to refer to hearing protectors such as ear plugs and ear muffs.

Earache: Pain in the ear.

Earhook: The curved apparatus of a behind-the-ear hearing aid and some other types of listening devices that connects the device case to the earmold, and hooks over the pinna.

Earmold: A device that fits into the concha and directs sound from the earhook of a listening device to the ear canal.

Earmold acoustics: The influence of the earmold's configuration and structure, such as bore length and venting, on the acoustic properties of the sound delivered to the tympanic membrane by a listening device.

Earmold bore: A hole in the earmold through which an amplified audio signal travels.

Earmold impression: Cast made of the concha and ear canal.

Earmold vent: A canal drilled in the earmold for the purpose of aeration or alteration of the audio signal.

Earplug: A kind of ear protection, consisting of a material that is inserted into the ear canal for the purpose of sound attenuation.

EBP: Evidence-based practice.

Effective gain: Difference in decibels between a patient's aided and unaided thresholds.

Effusion: In the middle ear, exudation of body fluid from the middle ear membranous walls as a result of inflammation.

Eighth cranial nerve: The cranial nerve consisting of an auditory and vestibular branch.

Electrical threshold: The amount of current that must be passed through an electrode so that the cochlear implant user is just aware of sound sensation.

Electroacoustic: Related to the conversion of an acoustic signal to an electrical signal or an electrical signal to an acoustic signal.

Electrode: Metal ball or plate through which electrical stimulation is applied to the body or electrical energy is measured.

Electrode array: Electrodes placed in pairs on a carrier wire and inserted into the cochlea; component of a cochlear implant.

Elicitation techniques: A technique that a clinician might use to ensure that a communication breakdown or other desired event or behavior occurs.

Emotional acceptance and adjustment counseling: Explores individuals' reactions to loss of hearing.

Empathetic understanding: A tenet of person-centered counseling; the counselor listens to the patient's concerns and feelings about a hearing problem, reflects them back to the patient, and helps the patient identify solutions.

Encephalitis: An inflammation of the brain, often caused by a viral infection.

ENT: Ear, nose, and throat.

Equivalent lists: In speech recognition testing, test lists that contain items that are presumed to be equally difficult to recognize.

Event-time orientation: An orientation that is process-driven wherein issues are pursued to their natural conclusions no matter how long that might take.

Explicit categorization: A way to ensure retention; an informational counseling technique wherein a clinician enumerates the topics that will be covered and then announces each one before talking about it.

External components: In cochlear implants, the external components are worn on the outside of the body.

Evidence-based practice: EBP; clinical decision making that is based on a review of the scientific evidence of benefits and costs of alternative forms of diagnosis or treatment, and a critical examination of current and past practices.

Evoked potential: Electrical activity generated in the brain in response to a sensory stimulus.

Expanded speech: Recorded speech that is altered by duplicating small segments of the signal so that the speech sounds as if it were produced with a slow speaking rate; no additional spectral information is introduced.

Expansion: Language stimulation technique in which an adult copies the meaning of a child's utterance but modifies or expands the grammar of the message.

Expectation: The patient's attitude about the benefit that will be provided, such as with a hearing aid.

Expressive language: The language we speak or sign.

Expressive repair strategy: Tactic taken by an individual when a communication partner has not understood one of his or her messages.

Extended repair: Repair of a communication breakdown that requires many repair strategies and many exchanges between the communication partners involved.

External auditory meatus: External ear canal.

External ear canal: The canal of the outer ear leading from the concha to the tympanic membrane.

Eyeglass hearing aid: Style of hearing aid rarely used in which the hearing aid is housed in the temple piece of a pair of eyeglasses.

f_0: Fundamental frequency.

f_1: First formant.

f_2: Second formant.

Facilitative language techniques: Techniques used to stimulate language growth in young children through the course of conversational interactions.

Facilitative strategy: A strategy used to facilitate communication; includes means taken to instruct the talker, structure the listening environment, enhance the structure of the received message, and affect the speech recognition performance of the individual using the strategy.

False-negative response: In reference to newborn hearing screening, occasions when a baby has hearing loss but passes the screening test.

False-positive response: In reference to newborn hearing screening, occasions when a baby has normal hearing but fails the screening test.

Familial deafness: Deafness reoccurring in members of the same family.

Family tree: A genealogical diagram of a child's ancestry or kin.

FAPE: Free and appropriate public education.

Favorable seating: Includes being close enough to see the talker's lip movements, being able to see the talker full-face rather than in profile, and having the talker's face well lit; may also include selecting seating in a quiet area of a room, as in a restaurant.

FDA: Food and Drug Administration.

Fetal alcohol syndrome: Syndrome found in children whose mothers abused alcohol while the child was in utero; children who have the syndrome may have mental retardation, low birth weight,

unusual eye spacing, chronic otitis media, and sensorineural hearing loss.

Filter: In listening devices, a component that differentially amplifies and attenuates certain bands of frequencies in the incoming signal.

Filtered speech: Speech that has been passed through filter banks for the purpose of removing or amplifying frequency bands in the signal.

Fingerspelling: A kind of manual communication in which words are spelled letter-by-letter using standard hand configurations.

Flat audiogram: Audiogram configuration in which the thresholds across frequencies are similar.

Fluctuating hearing loss: Hearing loss that varies in magnitude over time.

FM: Frequency modulation.

FM trainer: Classroom assistive listening device in which the teacher wears a microphone and the signal is transmitted to the student(s) by means of frequency modulated radio waves.

FM boot: A small bootlike device worn on the bottom of a user's hearing aid that attaches to or contains an FM receiver; used as part of an FM assistive listening device system.

Food and Drug Administration: FDA; U.S. government agency that oversees the regulation of medical devices such as hearing aids and cochlear implants.

Form: In language, refers to the proper use of the elements, such as nouns, verbs, prepositions, and so forth.

Formal instruction: The first stage in a communication-strategies training program in which individuals receive information about various types of communication strategies and other appropriate listening and speaking behaviors.

Formal training: In reference to speechreading or auditory training, highly structured activities that may involve drill, usually scheduled to occur during designated times of the day, either in a one-on-one lesson format or in a small group.

Formant: A resonance in the vocal tract that results in some frequencies in the speech signal having more energy than other frequencies.

Formant 1: f_1; the first frequency band above the fundamental frequency that demonstrates high energy in the speech signal.

Formant 2: f_2; the second frequency band above the fundamental frequency that demonstrates high energy in the speech signal.

Formant transition: Segment in the speech signal that displays rapid change in the frequency or spectral composition of the formants.

Free and appropriate public education: FAPE; refers to federal funding provided for the education of children with disabilities, and requires as a condition for receiving federal funds the provision of free and appropriate public education.

Frequency: The number of regularly repeated events in a given unit of time; usually measured in cycles per second and expressed in Hertz (Hz).

Frequency modulation: FM; the process of creating a complex signal by means of sinusoidally varying a carrier wave frequency.

Frequency of usage: A measure indicating how often a particular word occurs during everyday conversation; sometimes referred to as frequency of occurrence.

Frequency response: Output characteristics of a listening device; denoted as gain as a function of frequency.

Frequent communication partner: A particular person with whom another often converses; often a family member.

Fricative: Speech sound generated by creating turbulent airflow through a constriction in the oral cavity; for example, /f, s/.

Full-on gain: Hearing aid setting that results in the maximum acoustic output.

Functional gain: Difference in decibels between unaided and aided thresholds.

Fundamental frequency: f_0; in speech, the lowest frequency in the speech output; voice pitch.

Gain: In hearing aids, the difference in decibels between the input level of an acoustic signal and the output level.

Gain/frequency response: The difference between the amplitude of the input signal and the amplitude of the output signal across frequencies.

Gene: A basic unit of heredity that is responsible for transmitting characteristics from one generation to the next; a sequence of DNA that occupies a specific place on a chromosome.

Genetic: Concerning heredity.

Genetic counseling: Provision of information to prospective parents about the likelihood of an inherited condition or disorder in their children.

Genotype: The genetic makeup of an individual.

Geriatric: Concerning the aging process.

Glide consonant: A consonant sound that is characterized by gradual change in the acoustic signal; for example, /w, l, r/.

Glaucoma: An eye condition characterized by unusually high pressure within the eyeball, which may lead to damage to the optic disc and irreversible loss of vision.

Goal: The result toward which training or instruction is directed; it is the desired aim or outcome.

Grounding: A conversational occurrence in which communication partners establish a body of information as shared common ground for an ongoing conversational interchange.

Group discussion: A meeting that provides a forum for class members to discuss communication issues.

Guided learning: The second stage in a communication strategies training program, in which individuals use conversational strategies in a structured setting.

Habilitation: Program or intervention aimed at the initial development of skills and abilities.

HAE: Hearing aid evaluation.

HAO: Hearing aid orientation.

HAT: Hearing assistive technology.

Hair cells: Sensory cells in the cochlea that attach to the nerve endings of the eighth cranial nerve.

Handicap: Consists of the psychosocial disadvantages that result from a functional impairment; use of this term is discouraged by the World Health Organization.

Hard-of-hearing: HOH; having a hearing loss; usually not used to refer to a profound hearing loss.

Hardwired: Directly connected by wires.

Head shadow: Attenuation of sound to one ear because of the presence of the head between the ear and the sound source.

Headphone: Earphone.

Health maintenance organization: HMO; managed care organization that offers prepaid, comprehensive health coverage for both hospital and physician services; a type of insurance that stipulates which doctors and medical facilities can by used by a patient, and which medical tests and procedures will be covered.

Health-related quality of life: HRQoL; the impact of a health condition on the well-being experienced by an individual or a group of people; includes such dimensions as physiology, function, social activity, cognition, emotions, energy, vitality, health perception, and general life satisfaction.

Hearing aid: An electronic listening device designed to amplify and deliver sound from the environment to the listener; includes a microphone, amplifier, and receiver.

Hearing aid evaluation: HAE; procedure wherein an appropriate hearing aid is selected for an individual.

Hearing aid orientation: HAO; process of instructing a patient (and a patient's family member) to handle, use, and maintain a new hearing aid.

Hearing aid use pattern: The times, situations, and locations in which a hearing aid user wears the hearing aid(s).

Hearing assistive technology: HAT; technology that facilitates access to auditory information.

Hearing conservation: Prevention or reduction of hearing loss through a program of identifying and minimizing risk, monitoring hearing sensitivity, education, and providing protection from noise exposure.

Hearing culture: The mainstream culture in the United States; includes auditory experiences in addition to or in lieu of visual experiences.

Hearing impairment: Abnormal or reduced hearing sensitivity; hearing loss.

Hearing level: HL; decibel level referenced to audiometric zero.

Hearing loss: Abnormal or reduced hearing sensitivity; hearing impairment.

Hearing Loss Association of America: HLAA; an organization for people who have hearing loss, which exists for the purpose of enhancing members' communication success through information, education, advocacy, and support.

Hearing protection: Devices designed to minimize the risk of noise-induced hearing loss.

Hearing-related disability: A loss of function imposed by hearing loss; the term denotes a multidimensional phenomenon.

Hearing-related stress: Stress that includes the stress of adjusting to a new self-concept, the stress of living with an impaired sensory system, and the stress of living with the reactions of society to people who have a disability and who experience communication difficulties.

Hearing threshold: Level of intensity at which a sound is just audible to an individual.

Hertz: Hz; a unit of frequency that is equal to one cycle per second.

Heterozygous: Having genetic variants; having dissimilar alleles at corresponding loci of a chromosome pair, which may result in offspring differing in a trait, depending upon which version of the gene they inherit.

High-pass filtered speech: Speech that has been passed through filter banks, leaving the higher but not the lower frequencies.

HL: Hearing level.

Holistic: An approach to speechreading that incorporates several methods and includes the child in setting goals.

HMO: Health maintenance organization.

Home-based program: An early interventionist visits the infant's home and provides instruction for the child and parents.

Homophenes: Words that look identical on the mouth.

Homozygous: Having two identical alleles of the same gene.

HRQoL: Health-related quality of life.

Hz: Hertz.

IDEA: Individuals with Disabilities Education Act.

Identification: In reference to auditory or speechreading training, the ability to label auditory or audiovisual stimuli.

Idiopathic: In reference to hearing loss, a loss with unknown origin.

IEP: Individualized educational plan.

IFSP: Individualized family service plan.

Immitance: The energy flow through the middle ear, and includes admittance, compliance, conductance, impedance, reactance, resistance, and susceptance.

Impairment: Reduced or abnormal function.

Impedance audiometry: Battery of measures designed to assess middle ear functioning, including tympanometry and acoustic reflex threshold determination; immitance audiometry.

Incidence: Frequency of occurrence.

Inclusion: Integrates all students and activities into the daily routine of the general education classroom.

Independent variable: The experimental factor that is manipulated or influential.

Individualized education plan: IEP; federally mandated plan for providing education to children with disabilities, updated once a year.

Individualized family service plan: IFSP; federally mandated plan for the education of preschool children with disabilities, with an emphasis on family involvement, updated annually.

Individuals with Disabilities Education Act: IDEA; provides for specialized instruction for individuals who have disabilities and who meet eligibility requirements, typically that the disability causes adverse educational effects.

Induction loop system: A length of wire surrounding the circumference of a room or table that conducts electrical energy from an amplifier, and thus creates a magnetic field; the current flow from an induction loop can induce the telecoil in a hearing aid to providing amplified sound to the user.

Informal training: In reference to speechreading or auditory training, activities that occur during the daily routine, often incorporated into other activities, such as conversation or academic learning.

Information transmission analysis: A statistical procedure that analyzes the transmission of speech features by scoring confusions between test stimuli that are grouped based on the presence or absence of those features.

Informational counseling: Includes imparting information about the hearing loss and the benefits and limitations of amplification.

Infrared system: Assistive listening device that broadcasts from the sound source to a receiver/amplifier by means of infrared light waves.

Inner ear: Part of the hearing mechanism that houses the structures for hearing and balance and includes the cochlea, vestibules, and semicircular canals.

Input signal: Acoustic signal that enters a listening device.

Insert earphone: An earphone whose receiver is attached to a tube that leads to an expandable cuff and that can be inserted into the ear canal.

Insertion gain: Hearing aid gain.

In-service: Continuing education provided to full-time employees.

Instructional strategy: Instruction provided to a communication partner so that the person converses in a way that maximizes the patient's recognition of messages and minimizes the possibility of communication breakdown; a kind of facilitative communication strategy.

Intelligibility: The degree to which speech can be recognized.

Interactive communication behaviors: Consistent with an assertive conversational style; includes a sharing of responsibility for advancing a topic of conversation, choosing what to talk about, showing interest, and responding to remarks appropriately.

Interdisciplinary team: A group of professionals with different expertise working together for the purpose of providing assessment and intervention in a coordinated and cooperative fashion.

Interleave pulsatile stimulation: A cochlear implant processing strategy whereby trains of pulses are delivered across electrodes in the electrode array in a nonsimultaneous fashion.

Internal components: Components of a cochlear implant that are implanted within the skull.

Interpreter: A person specially trained to translate oral or signed communications from one language to another.

Interview: An assessment procedure to assess conversational fluency and communication difficulties, in which

individuals talk about their conversational problems and consider possible reasons as to why communication breakdowns happen.

In-the-canal hearing aid: ITC; hearing aid that fits in the external ear canal, with only a partial filling of the concha.

In-the-ear hearing aid: ITE; hearing aid that fits into the concha of the ear.

Ipsilateral: Pertaining to the same side.

ITC hearing aid: In-the-canal hearing aid.

ITE hearing aid: In-the-ear hearing aid.

Itinerant teachers: Teachers who work in several schools, providing support services to children who are deaf and hard of hearing and their teachers.

JND: Just noticeable difference.

Just noticeable difference: JND; the smallest increment of stimulus change in which the stimulus can be perceived as different; difference limen.

K-AMP circuit: Hearing aid circuit designed to provide more gain for moderate-level sound, no gain for high-intensity sound, and compression limiting for the highest level sound; also often provides more amplification for high frequencies.

Keying: Occurs when a talker's tone of voice, cadence, lexical emphasis, prosody, and other speaking characteristics imbue an emotional stance to an utterance.

Kinesthetic: Relating to the perception of movement, position, and tension of body parts.

Kneepoint: Point on an input–output function of a hearing aid where compression is activated.

Labeling: A language stimulation technique in which an adult provides names for objects, actions, and events.

Language: Complex system of symbols that are used in a rule-governed fashion for the purpose of communication.

LD: Learning disability.

LDL: Loudness discomfort level.

Learning disability: LD; a lack of ability in an area of learning that is inconsistent with an individual's cognitive capacity and is not a result of a deficit in sensory, motor, or emotional functioning.

Learning effect: Performance on a test improves as a function of familiarity with the test procedures and test items and not because of a change in ability.

Least restrictive environment: LRE; a basic principle of IDEA that requires public agencies to establish procedures to ensure that to the extent possible, children who have disabilities are educated with children who do not have disabilities, and that special classes, separate schooling, or removal from the regular educational environment occurs only when the severity of the disability is such that education in a regular class environment cannot be achieved satisfactorily.

LEP: Limited English proficiency.

Level: Intensity of sound.

Lexical: Concerning the lexicon; relating to the vocabulary of a language.

Lexicon: The total stock of morphemes in a language.

Life factors: Conditions that help define one's life, such as relationships, family, and vocation.

Life stages: Stages in the life span in which a hearing loss may have a differing impact.

Limited English proficiency: LEP; used in reference to persons who are limited in their English proficiency.

Limited set: When the response items in a stimulus or response set are limited by situational or contextual cues; for example, words related to summer.

Linear amplification: Hearing aid amplification system in which there is a one-to-one correspondence between the input and output until the maximum output level is reached.

Linked adjacency pairs: Two remarks that often are linked in conversation, as when one communication partner asks, "How are you?" and another responds, "Fine, thank you."

Lipreading: The process of recognizing speech using only the visual speech signal and other visual cues, such as facial expression.

Listening check: Informal assessment of whether a listening device is functioning appropriately.

Live-voice testing: Stimuli in a test of speech recognition are presented by a talker in real time.

Localization: The ability to locate the source of a sound in space due to the normal ear's sensitivity to interaural differences in phase and intensity.

Loudness: Perception of the intensity of a sound.

Loudness balancing: Matching the loudness of two sounds, as between the two ears, when taking an alternating binaural loudness balance test or as when mapping a cochlear implant, so stimulation follows the loudness contour of the speech signal.

Loudness comfort level: Level at which sound is perceived to be comfortably loud.

Loudness discomfort level: LDL; level at which sound is perceived to be uncomfortably loud.

Loudness summation: A summing of the signals received by each ear, resulting in a 3-dB advantage for binaural over monaural hearing.

Loudspeaker: Device that converts electrical energy into sound.

Loudspeaker azimuth: The position of the loudspeaker relative to the listener, measured in angular degrees in the horizontal plane.

Low-pass filtered speech: Speech that has been passed through filter banks, leaving the lower but not the higher frequencies.

LRE: Least restrictive environment.

Luminance: The intensity of light per unit area of the source.

Macula: A small area at the back of the eye where vision on the retina is keenest.

Macular degeneration: Progressive loss of both reading vision and distance vision due to damage or breakdown of the macula.

Mainstream classrooms: Classrooms in which children who have a hearing loss attend classes with their peers who have normal hearing.

Mainstreaming: Reassignment of children with disabilities from a special education classroom to a classroom in the regular school environment.

Maladaptive strategies: Inappropriate behavioral mechanisms for coping with the difficulties caused in conversation by hearing loss, such as avoidance behavior; they often yield short-term benefit in exchange for long-term negative consequences.

Managed care: A health care reimbursement plan in which an organization intercedes between patient and provider and determines the kind and extent of services that will be provided.

Manner of articulation: Classification of a speech sound as a function of how it is produced in the oral cavity; for example, glide.

Manual alphabet: Series of hand configurations that correspond to each letter in the alphabet; used to fingerspell words in manual communication.

Manual communication: Communication modes that entail the use of fingerspelling, signs, and gestures.

Manually coded English: A form of communication in which manual signs correspond to English words.

Map: Specifications of threshold, suprathreshold, and frequency by which the speech processor of a cochlear implant processes the speech signal and delivers it in electrical form to the electrodes in the electrode array.

Masker: For tinnitus, an electronic listening device that delivers low-level noise to the ear for the purpose of masking the presence of tinnitus.

Masking: Noise that interferes with the perception of another sound.

Maximum comfort level: MCL; highest intensity level at which sound is considered to be comfortable.

Maximum power output: MPO; the maximum level intensity that a hearing aid can produce; SSPL.

MCL: Most comfortable loudness; maximum comfort level.

Mean length speaking turn: MLT; used in the assessment of conversational interactions, computed by determining the average number of words a person speaks during a set number of conversational turns.

Mean length turn ratio (MLT ratio): The ratio of the MLTs of two participants in a conversation.

Medicaid: A program in the United States authorized by Title XIX of the Social Security Act that is jointly funded by the federal government and state governments, which reimburses hospitals and physicians for providing health care to qualified people who cannot otherwise afford services.

Medical home: An approach to providing health care services, and involves a partnership of health care personnel and family.

Medicare: A program under the U.S. Social Security Administration that reimburses hospitals and physicians for medical care they provide to qualified people who are 65 years or older.

Ménière's disease: An inner ear disorder that is related to idiopathic endolymphatic hydrops and may cause vertigo, hearing loss, tinnitus, and the sensation of fullness in the ear.

Meninges: The membranes that cover the brain and spinal cord.

Meningitis: A common cause of childhood sensorineural hearing loss caused by bacterial or viral inflammation of the meninges.

Mental health problem: A psychological or physiological pattern that is associated with distress or disability, and that is not expected as part of normal development or functioning.

Mental retardation: Intellectual function is below normal range.

Message-tailoring strategy: Phrasing one's remarks in a way that constrains the responses of a communication partner; a kind of facilitative communication strategy.

Metacommunication: Communication about communication.

Metalinguistic: To think about and attend to the use of language.

Microcephaly: An abnormally small head due to a failure of the brain to grow.

Microphone: Transducer that converts an audio signal into an electronic signal.

Microtia: A congenitally small external ear.

Middle ear: Portion of the hearing mechanism extending from the tympanic membrane to the oval window of the cochlea; includes the ossicles and middle ear cavity.

Mimetic: Imitating or copying the movements.

Mixed hearing loss: A hearing loss that has a conductive and sensorineural component.

Mobile unit: A mobile van that is equipped to screen hearing; used for educational and on-site industrial hearing screening programs.

Modality: Any of the five senses, including audition and vision.

Modeling: An instructor demonstrates a desired behavior and a student attempts to imitate it.

Monaural: Concerning one ear.

Monolingual: Term that describes a person who speaks only one language.

Monosyllabic word: A word comprised of one syllable.

Morpheme: Smallest unit of language that conveys meaning.

Most comfortable loudness: MCL; level at which sound is most comfortable for a listener, usually measured in dB HL.

Multiband compression: A method of shaping the loudness growth of a signal to maximize speech for the listener using different degrees of compression and output limiting for different frequencies.

Multichannel: More than one channel of information; often used to describe cochlear implants that present different channels of information to different regions of the cochlea.

Multidimensional scaling: A statistical procedure whereby data points are represented in a geometric space; for example, two phonemes that sound similar to a patient will be plotted near to each other; two phonemes that sound dissimilar will be plotted far from each other.

Multidisciplinary team: A group of professionals with different expertise contributing to the assessment, intervention, and management program for a particular individual.

Multiple channels: A listening aid that filters the signal into frequency bands so that some bands (usually the high-frequency bands) can receive more gain than others.

Multiple-memory hearing aid: A hearing aid that can be programmed to process the speech signal in more than one way, so that the user can adjust the processing strategy for different listening environments.

Multisensory approach: Educational approach for children with significant hearing loss that emphasizes the use of vision, residual hearing, and sometimes touch to enhance communication.

Myringitis: Inflammation of the tympanic membrane.

NAD: National Association of the Deaf.

Nasal consonant: Consonant that entails resonance in the nasal cavities and a lowered velum; for example, /m, n/.

National Association of the Deaf: NAD; advocacy group for members of the Deaf culture.

NCLB: No Child Left Behind Act.

NECCI: Network of Educators of Children with Cochlear Implants.

Neckloop: A transducer worn around the neck as part of an FM assistive device system, consisting of a cord from a receiver; transmits signals via magnetic induction to the telecoil of the user's hearing aid.

Neonatal: Concerning the first 4 weeks of life.

Network of Educators of Children with Cochlear Implants: NECCI; professional organization of speech and hearing professionals and educators who are involved with children who receive and use cochlear implants.

Newborn nursery: Well-baby nursery; a hospital unit designed to provide care for healthy newborn infants.

NIHL: Noise-induced hearing loss.

NIPTS: Noise-induced permanent threshold shift.

NITTS: Noise-induced temporary threshold shift.

No Child Left Behind Act of 2001: NCLB; reauthorized several federal programs aimed at improving the performance of U.S. primary and secondary schools by increasing the standards of accountability at the school, district, and state levels.

Noise: Unwanted sound.

Noise exposure: Level of noise and duration of exposure.

Noise-induced hearing loss: NIHL; sensorineural hearing loss that is the result of exposure to excessive levels of sound; auditory trauma caused by loud sound and resulting in permanent hearing loss.

Noise-induced permanent threshold shift: NIPTS; permanent decrease in an individual's hearing thresholds as a result of exposure to excessive sound levels.

Noise-induced temporary threshold shift: NITTS; transient shift in an individual's hearing thresholds as a result of exposure to excessive sound levels; temporary threshold shift.

Noise notch: A pattern of audiometric thresholds characterized by a dip in hearing sensitivity at 4,000 Hz and is often found in someone who has a history of noise exposure.

Noise reduction: The difference in sound pressure level (SPL) of a noise, measured at two different locations.

Noninteractive communication behaviors: Characteristic of a passive conversational style; includes failure to contribute to the development of a conversational topic, minimal response to turn-taking signals, and a proclivity to bluff.

Nonlinear amplification: Amplification system that does not provide a one-to-one correspondence between input and output at all input levels.

Nonsense syllable: Single syllable of speech that has no meaning.

Nonspecific repair strategy: A repair strategy used to repair a communication breakdown that does not provide specific instruction to the communication partner about what to do next.

Nonsyndromic hearing loss: A hearing loss that has no other associated findings.

Norm: Standards derived from a sample of the population of interest, thought to represent typical values of the characteristic under study or test.

NR: No response.

Nursing home: A residential, institutionalized facility that has three or more beds and provides nursing care.

OAE: Otoacoustic emission.

Objective: Physically measurable; in speechreading or auditory training, leads to a measurable result, expected within a particular time period and/or after a particular lesson, the accomplishment of which represents

a milestone toward achieving the corresponding goal.

Occlusion effect: Enhancement of the level of low-frequency sound in bone-conducted signals as a result of occlusion of the ear canal.

Occupational hearing loss: Noise-induced hearing loss incurred on the job.

Occupational Safety and Health Administration: OSHA; federal agency that regulates occupational health and safety hazards and establishes and enforces minimum standards for industrial hearing conservation programs.

Omnidirectional microphone: Microphone that is sensitive to sound coming from all directions.

On–off control: A small switch that moves back and forth to turn the hearing aid off when not in use and on when needed; may be incorporated into the volume wheel or the battery door.

Open-canal fitting: A hearing aid fitting that has an open earmold or a tubing-only to the ear canal, with no earmold.

Open-ended questions: Questions that elicit qualitative information.

Open-set: Testing or training task that does not provide a set of choices to the patient.

Oral interpreter: A professional who silently repeats a talker's message as it is spoken, so that a person with hearing loss may lipread the message.

Oralism: Method of instruction for children who have significant hearing loss that emphasizes spoken-language skills to the exclusion of manual communication.

Oral transliteration: The act of lagging a talker by a few words, mouthing or speaking the words with a normal speaking rate and good enunciation for the purpose of conveying a spoken message by another to a person who has hearing loss.

Organized messages: Communications that are not wordy and do not use complex verbiage; terminology is precise.

OSHA: Occupational Safety and Health Administration.

OSPL90 curve: An electroacoustic assessment of a hearing aid's maximum level of output signal, expressed as a frequency response curve to a 90-dB signal, with the hearing aid volume control set to full on.

Ossification: A conversion of tissue into bone.

Otitis media: Inflammation of the middle ear often accompanied by the accumulation of fluid in the middle ear cavity.

Otoacoustic emission: OAE; low-level sound emitted by the cochlear spontaneously or following the presentation of an auditory stimulus.

Otolaryngologist: Physician who specializes in the diagnosis and treatment of diseases and conditions of the ear, nose, and throat.

Otologist: Physician who specializes in the diagnosis and treatment of diseases and conditions of the ear.

Otoscope: Instrument for visual examination of the external ear and tympanic membrane.

Ototoxic: Having a poisonous effect on the structures of the ear, particularly the hair cells in the cochlea and vestibular organs.

Outcome measure: Indicates the amount or type of benefit experienced by either an individual or a group of individuals to a treatment or series of treatments, and/or indicates a response.

Outer ear: Peripheral part of the auditory mechanism that includes the

pinna, the concha, the external auditory canal, and lateral wall of the tympanic membrane.

Output: Energy or information exiting from a listening device.

Output limiting: Limiting the output of a listening device by means of peak-clipping or compression.

Output sound pressure level: An electroacoustic assessment of a hearing aid's maximum level of output signal, expressed as a frequency response curve to a 90-dB signal, with the hearing aid volume control set to full on.

Ownership: The feeling of responsibility and need to manage or oversee.

Parallel talk: A language stimulation technique, wherein an adult matches language to an activity a child is performing.

Parent-support group: A group that provides opportunities for parents to share their feelings and issues related to having a child with hearing loss with others who have experienced them firsthand.

Part B: The section of Public Law PL 105-17 that refers to intervention services for eligible children between the ages of 3 and 21 years in the public school system.

Part C: The section of Public Law PL 108-446 that refers to early-intervention services that are available to eligible children from birth through the age of 3 years and to their families.

Participation restriction: An effect of an activity limitation that results in a change in the broader scope of a patient's life.

Passive-aggressive conversational style: Conversational style in which aggression is expressed in indirect ways.

Passive conversational style: Conversational style of some persons who have hearing loss, characterized by withdrawal from conversation, frequent bluffing, and avoidance of social interactions.

Patient orientation: An orientation centered on the patient's background, current status, needs, and wants, on which the design and delivery of rehabilitative services are based.

Pattern perception: A kind of discrimination that requires a listener to distinguish between words or phrases that differ in the number of syllables.

PB: Phonetically balanced.

Peak-clipping: A method of limiting hearing aid output in which a constant or linear amount of gain is provided across a range of input levels until it reaches a saturation level at which the amplifier begins to "clip" off the peaks of the signal.

Pearson correlation: A statistical analysis that indicates the strength and the direction of a linear relationship between two variables.

Perilingual: Hearing loss acquired during the stage of spoken language acquisition.

Perinatal: During birth.

Personal adjustment counseling: Counseling that focuses on the permanency of the hearing loss and on psychological, social, and emotional acceptance.

Personal FM trainer: A listening device in which the speaker wears a wireless microphone and the speech is frequency modulated on radio waves transmitted through the room to the listener, who wears a receiver.

Phenotype: Visible expression of a genotype of an individual.

Phoneme: Speech sound.

Phonetic alphabet: Symbols that represent the sounds of a spoken language.

Phonetically balanced word lists: PB word lists; sets of words that contain speech sounds with the same frequency of occurrence as in everyday conversation.

Pinna: Auricle; the cartilaginous structures of the outer ear.

Pitch ranking: Determines the ability to discriminate pitch from stimulation of the basal to apical electrodes of a cochlear implant.

Place of articulation: Classification of a speech sound according to where in the vocal tract it is produced; for example, bilabial.

Plasticity: Term used to refer to the physiological changes in the central nervous system that occur as a result of sensory experiences.

Play audiometry: Behavioral method for testing the hearing thresholds of young children, in which correct identification of a stimulus presentation is rewarded by allowing the child to perform a play-oriented activity.

Plosive: Stop consonant that is produced by creating an oral-cavity closure, building air pressure behind the closure, and then releasing it; for example, /p, t, k/.

Postlingual: Hearing loss incurred after the acquisition of spoken language.

Postnatal: After birth.

Pragmatics: The study of how language is used in a social context, and its effects on its interlocutors.

Preamplifier stage: The stage where the signal received from the microphone is amplified.

Predicament: The relevant aspects of a patient's state and situation, including disabilities, participation limitations, environments, demands, resources, attitudes, and behaviors.

Prelingual: Hearing loss incurred before the acquisition of spoken language.

Prenatal: Before birth.

Presbycusis: Age-related hearing loss.

Prescribed gain: Gain and frequency response of a hearing aid that are determined by use of a prescriptive formula.

Prescription procedures: Strategies for fitting hearing aids by using a formula to calculate the desired gain and frequency response.

Prescriptive hearing aid fitting: Strategy for fitting hearing aids by using a formula to calculate the desired gain and frequency response; formula incorporates pure-tone audiometric thresholds and, usually, information about uncomfortable loudness levels.

Prevalence: The percentage of a population that experiences a particular health problem at a point in time.

Probe microphone: Microphone transducer that is inserted into the external ear canal for the purpose of measuring sound near the tympanic membrane.

Processing speed: In cognition, the rate at which information is conducted and manipulated throughout the nervous system.

Processing strategy: Strategy used by cochlear implants to determine how the input signal is processed, including the degree of amplification of different frequency bands and the manner in which the signal is delivered by different electrodes in the electrode array; process used to transform the speech signal into a pattern of electrical stimulation.

Program: The setting of a speech processor or hearing aid according to the user's measured thresholds, comfort levels, and other subjective responses to stimulation.

Programmability: Refers to a feature of some hearing aids, wherein several parameters, such as gain, may be adjusted and controlled by a computer.

Programmable hearing aid: Hearing aid in which several parameters of the instrument, such as gain, are under computer control.

Progressive hearing loss: Advancing; hearing loss that is occurring over time.

Prompting: A procedure, sometimes used during role-playing, that serves to inspire a behavior or an utterance; a technique designed to assist an individual in formulating a remark.

Prosodic cues: Cues provided by intonation, rate, and duration of speech sounds.

Prosody: Suprasegmental aspects of the speech signal, including fluctuations in voice pitch, rhythm, rate, intensity, and stress patterns; intonation.

Psychological factors: Factors that pertain to an individual's attitudes, self-image, motivation, and assertiveness.

Psychosocial support: When provided to persons who have hearing loss (or their family members), a means by which speech and hearing professionals help patients achieve long-term self-sufficiency in managing the psychological and social challenges that result from hearing loss.

Psychotherapy: A treatment for an emotional or behavioral problem in which a mental health expert (e.g., psychiatrist, psychologist, counselor) discusses feelings and problems with a patient, with the goals being the relief of symptoms, changes in behavior leading to improved social, emotional, and vocational functioning, and personality growth.

PTA: Pure-tone average.

Pure-tone average: PTA; average of hearing thresholds at 500 Hz, 1,000 Hz, and 2,000 Hz.

Quest?AR: A structured communication procedure used to assess communication difficulties.

Questionnaires: Instruments designed to obtain subjective information from a patient, such as information about a patient's perceived benefit from hearing aid use; a procedure to assess conversational fluency and participation limitations, in which respondents provide subjective information about their listening and communication difficulties.

Randomized controlled trial: Research participants are randomly assigned into treatment and control groups and then outcomes are compared.

Rational emotive behavior therapy: REBT; a solution-oriented counseling (or therapy) approach that focuses on resolving specific problems using cognitive, behavioral, and affective elements; key to the approach is the idea that emotions result from beliefs rather than events or circumstances.

Reactive procedure: Self-monitoring that influences how a person uses communication behaviors and strategies.

Real-ear gain: Gain of a hearing aid at the tympanic membrane, measured with a probe-microphone; the difference between the SPL in the external ear canal and the SPL at the field reference point for a specified sound field.

Real-ear measures: The use of a probe microphone to measure hearing aid gain and frequency response delivered by a hearing aid at the tympanic membrane.

Real-time captioning: Captioning of a person's speech in real time using computer technology.

Real-world practice: The third stage in a communication strategies training program; practice of a new skill or behavior in an everyday environment.

REBT: Rational emotive behavior therapy.

Receiver: Component that converts electrical energy into acoustic energy, as in a hearing aid; a component of an FM system worn by the listener that receives FM signals from a transmitter; an individual who receives a message from a sender.

Receptive language: The language that we hear or receive via sign.

Receptive repair strategy: Tactic taken by an individual when he or she has not understood a message presented by a communication partner.

Recorded stimuli: Test items presented via a tape recorder or a compact disc player or other playback system such as an iPod.

Referential communication interaction: An interaction in which one communication partner is expected to convey information to another partner by means of an interactive exchange.

Reflection: A counseling technique whereby clinicians paraphrase or summarize what their patient has just said, and thus demonstrate that they are listening carefully and accurately, and also provide their patients with an opportunity to examine their own views or feelings by hearing them expressed by another person.

Rehabilitation: Intervention designed for the reteaching or recovery of particular skills.

Reinforcement: Something desirable, such as a sticker or privilege, provided to a student after he or she performs a training activity or behaves in a desired manner.

Relay system: System used by persons with significant hearing loss to use the telephone; individual contacts a relay operator who serves to transmit messages between caller and person called by means of teletype and/or voice.

Release time: The time it takes for an amplifier to return to its steady state after a loud sound ends.

Reliability: Extent to which a test yields similar results with repeated administration.

Remote control: Hand-held device that permits adjustments in the volume or changes in the program of a programmable hearing aid.

Repair strategies: Tactics implemented by a participant in a conversation to rectify breakdowns in communication.

Residual hearing: The hearing remaining in a person who has hearing loss.

Resource rooms: Classroom wherein children who spend part of their day in regular classrooms receive special or focused instruction.

Retinitis pigmentosa: Any number of inherited, progressive conditions that cause abnormal pigmentation on the retina; often impairs vision, with first a loss of night vision, then a loss of peripheral vision, and then the development of "tunnel vision," and finally causing blindness.

Reverberation: Prolongation of an auditory signal by multiple reflections in a closed environment; amount of echo in an enclosed space.

Role-play: An aural rehabilitation intervention wherein individuals participate in simulated real-world situations and communication interactions.

Round window: Membrane-covered opening between the middle ear space and the scala tympani section of the cochlea in the inner ear.

S/N ratio: Signal-to-noise ratio.

Sales orientation: An orientation to providing rehabilitation services in which emphasis is placed on persuading the patient to pursue and procure services, interventions, and listening devices.

Saturation level: Point at which an amplifier no longer provides an increase in output compared to input.

Saturation sound pressure level: SSPL; the maximum sound pressure level that can be delivered by a hearing aid with its volume at full on.

Screening: The use of tests that are quick and easy to administer to a large group for the purpose of identifying individuals who require further diagnostic testing.

SDT: Speech detection threshold.

Seeing Essential English: SEE1; a manual communication system that incorporates some signs of American Sign Language and some English syntax.

Segmental errors: Errors in articulation pertaining to the sounds of speech.

Self-concept: How persons view themselves.

Self-contained classrooms: Classrooms that contain only children who have disabilities.

Self-efficacy: A patient's estimate or personal judgment of his or her ability to succeed at a particular task or in a particular communication interaction.

Self-image: An individual's awareness of his or her biological or physical self and personality in addition to the individual's sense of identity and self-worth.

Self-stigma: Occurs when a person stigmatizes one's own condition by feelings of shame and embarrassment, and develops a spoiled self-identity by virtue of having a shortcoming or disability.

Self-sufficiency and independence: Whether a person can conduct day-to-day activities without undue reliance on others.

Self-talk: Language stimulation technique in which an adult describes what he or she is doing or thinking for the purpose of promoting language development in a child.

Semantic: Related to meaning, and the relationship between units of language and their referents.

Semantics: The study of the relationships between words, signs, and symbols and what they represent.

Sender: Individual who presents a message, as opposed to a receiver.

Sensation level: SL; the intensity level of a sound in dB expressed in reference to the individual's threshold for the sound.

Sensorineural hearing loss: SNHL; hearing loss with a cochlear or retrocochlear origin.

Service coordinator: A designated person who helps the family during the development, implementation, and the evaluation of the IFSP.

Shaping: A procedure, sometimes used during role-playing, that serves to reinforce those conversational turns that increasingly approximate sought-after behaviors.

Sign language: System of manual communication in which hand configurations, positions, and movements are used to express concepts and linguistic information.

Signal processing: Manipulation of various parameters of the signal.

Signal-processing stage: Stage where the acoustic signal is manipulated to enhance or extract component information.

Signal-to-noise ratio: S/N ratio; the level of a signal relative to a background of noise, usually expressed in dB.

Signed English: Manual communication system that utilizes English word order and syntax.

Signing Exact English: SEE2; a simplified version of Seeing Essential English.

Silica gel: Agent that absorbs moisture, often used in the storage of hearing aids.

Simple amplification systems: Systems that merely amplify the audio signal so that it is more audible to a person with hearing loss.

Simultaneous communication: Educational approach used with individuals with severe and profound hearing loss that integrates spoken language and manual communication; total communication.

SL: Sensational level.

SLP: Speech-language pathologist.

SNHL: Sensorineural hearing loss.

Social factors: The prevailing viewpoints of one's society.

Social stigma: A condition that is devalued because it deviates from a societal norm and results in a negative status being placed on a person or group of persons.

Sociolinguistics: The branch of linguistics that concerns the effects of social and cultural differences within a language community on its use of language and conversational patterns.

Sound awareness: The most basic auditory skill level; awareness of when a sound is present and when it is not.

Sound discrimination: A basic auditory skill level in which the listener is able to tell whether two sounds are different or the same.

Sound field: A free-field environment where sound is propagated.

Sound field FM system: A listening system, similar to an FM trainer, in which sound from a microphone is transmitted to loudspeakers that are positioned throughout the room.

Sound field testing: Determination of hearing sensitivity or speech recognition ability with the stimuli presented through loudspeakers, which is often used in pediatric testing or hearing aid evaluations.

Sound level: The intensity of a sound expressed in decibels.

Sound level meter: An instrument designed to measure the intensity of sound in dB according to an accepted standard.

Sound pressure level: SPL; magnitude of sound energy relative to a reference pressure, 0.0002 dynes/cm^2.

Soundproof: Impenetrable by acoustic energy.

Specific repair strategy: Repair strategy used to rectify a communication breakdown that provides explicit instruction to the communication partner about what to do next.

Speech: Coordination of respiration, phonation, articulation, and resonation for the purpose of producing spoken language.

Speech audiometry: Measurement of speech-listening skills, including speech awareness and speech recognition.

Speech detection threshold: SDT; the level at which speech is just audible.

Speech discrimination score: The percentage of monosyllabic words presented at a comfortable listening level that can be correctly repeated; a term not often used.

Speech features: Categorical properties of phonemes; a phoneme can be described as a bundle of speech features.

Speech-language pathologist: SLP; professional who provides diagnosis and treatment of speech and language disorders.

Speech-language pathology: Professional discipline related to the study, diagnosis, and treatment of speech and language disorders.

Speech processor: The component of a cochlear implant where the input signal is modified for presentation to the electrodes in the electrode array.

Speech reception threshold: SRT; threshold level for speech recognition, which is the lowest presentation level for spondee words at which 50% can be identified correctly.

Speech recognition: The ability to perceive a spoken message and make decisions about its lexical composition using auditory and sometimes visual information.

Speech recognition testing: Testing performed in order to determine how well an individual can recognize speech units.

Speechreading: Speech recognition using auditory and visual cues.

Speechreading enhancement: The difference or ratio between speech recognition performance in a vision-only condition and an audition-plus-vision condition; auditory enhancement.

Spiral ganglion: Comprised of the nuclei of the nerve fibers that connect to the hair cells and meet in the central core (which is called the modiolus) of the cochlea.

SPL: Sound pressure level.

Spondee: Two-syllable word with equal stress on each syllable.

SRT: Speech reception threshold.

SSPL: Saturation sound pressure level.

SSPL-90 curve: Saturation sound pressure level 90; electroacoustic assessment of a hearing aid's maximum level of output signal, expressed as a frequency response curve to a 90-dB signal, with the hearing aid volume control set to full on.

Stage of life: Phases in the life cycle, including childhood, young adulthood, middle age, and old age.

Stetoclip: A nonelectric device that resembles a stethoscope, which enables someone to perform a listening check on a hearing instrument.

Stimulus: Something that can evoke or elicit a response.

Stop consonant: Plosive; speech sound produced by building up air pressure behind a closure in the oral cavity and then releasing it; for example /p, t, k/.

Structured communication interaction: Simulated conversation that reflects some of the communication difficulties a person with hearing loss may experience during everyday conversation; for example, TOPICON.

Sudden hearing loss: Hearing loss that is incurred suddenly; acute and rapid onset.

Suprasegmentals: Prosodic aspects of speech, including variations in pitch, rate, intensity, and duration, that are superimposed on phonemes and words.

Suprasegmental errors: Prosodic errors; for example, inappropriate syllable stress.

Syndrome: Collection of conditions that co-occur as a result from a single cause and constitute a distinct clinical entity.

Syntax: Rules by which words and other elements of sentence structure are combined and manipulated to form grammatical sentences.

Synthesized speech: Speech generated by computer.

Synthetic sentences: Syntactically correct but meaningless sentences, which usually include a noun, verb, and object.

Synthetic training: Speechreading or auditory training that emphasizes the understanding of meaning and not necessarily the identification and comprehension of every word spoken in an utterance.

T-switch: Telecoil switch.

Tactile aid: Vibrotactile aid; aid that transduces sound to vibration and delivers it to the skin for the purpose of sound awareness and gross sound identification.

Target gain: In hearing aid fitting, the prescribed gain for each frequency against which the actual hearing aid output is compared.

Telecoil: T-coil; induction coil often in a hearing aid that receives electromagnetic signals from a telephone or a loop amplification system.

Telecoil switch: T-switch; switch on a hearing aid that activates the telecoil.

Telecommunication device for the deaf: TDD; TT (text telephone); TTY; telephone device for persons wih deafness or significant hearing loss in which messages are typed on a keyboard, transmitted over telephone wires, and displayed on a small monitor screen.

Telegraphic speech: Spoken-language patterns that are characterized by the omission of function words and, sometimes, incorrect word order.

Telephone amplifier: Assistive listening device that increases the intensity of a signal emanating from a telephone receiver.

Television Decoder Circuitry Act: U.S. Public Law 101-336 of 1990; act that requires all televisions with a 13-inch diagonal screen or wider to contain circuitry necessary for closed captioning.

Temperament: Stable personality traits; a person's characteristic manner of thinking, behaving, or reacting.

TEOAE: Transient evoked otoacoustic emission.

Test–retest reliability: Measure of test consistency from one presentation to the next; sometimes called test–retest variability.

Threshold: Level at which sound can be detected only 50% of the time.

Threshold shift: Change in hearing sensitivity expressed in dB.

Time-compressed speech: Speech that has been accelerated by means of removing segments from the waveform and compressing the remaining segments together, without changing its frequency composition.

Time-talk: A language-stimulation technique wherein an adult purposely incorporates time-related language into conversation.

Tinnitus: Sensation of noise in the head without an external cause.

Tinnitus masker: Electronic hearing aid that generates and outputs noise at low levels for the purpose of masking an individual's tinnitus.

T-level: Term used for threshold, especially in reference to cochlear implants.

Tone-decay test: A test of auditory adaptation during which a continuous tone is presented at about threshold and any change in perception is monitored over a set time interval; an abnormal adaptation may indicate a retrocochlear site of lesion.

Tonotopic organization: Structures within the peripheral and central auditory nervous system are arranged topographically according to tonal frequency.

TOPICON: An example of a structured communication interaction activity.

Topic-shading: Occurs when a new topic is derived from a preceding topic in such as way that the flow of conversation is preserved.

Total communication: Simultaneous communication; a communication mode that entails the combined use of sign and speech.

Toxemia: A condition during pregnancy that is characterized by hypertension, or a sharp spike in blood pressure, and edema, or a swelling of the hands and feet as a result of excessive body fluid.

Transient evoked otoacoustic emission: TEOAE; a means to access the integrity and function of the outer hair cells by presenting brief clicks, where the low-level acoustic response emitted by the cochlea is measured.

Translater: A person specially trained to translate written text from one language to another.

Transmitter: A device that emits electromagnetic rays; a component of an FM system that modulates the frequency of a radio signal in an audio frequency signal and transmits the waves through air to an amplifier/receiver.

Troubleshoot: A series of steps to follow when a listening device will not turn on, if the sound is faint or distorted, or feedback occurs, the objective being to locate and correct the source of malfunction.

Tune-up: Mapping; establishing a map for a cochlear implant speech processor.

Tx: Therapy or treatment.

Tympanogram: Graph of middle ear immittance as a function of air pressure in the external auditory canal.

UCL: Uncomfortable loudness level.

UL: Uncomfortable level.

ULL: Uncomfortable loudness level.

Uncomfortable level: UL; level at which sound is judged to be so loud as to be uncomfortable to the listener.

Uncomfortable loudness level: ULL or UCL; intensity level at which a listener judges a sound to be uncomfortably loud; loudness discomfort level (LDL).

Unconditional positive regard: Tenet of person-centered counseling, in which clinicians assume that patients know best and assume that they have the inner resources to overcome their conversational difficulties.

Underserved: A group of patients receiving less than ideal services.

UNHS: Universal newborn hearing screening.

Unilateral: Pertaining to one side.

Unisensory approach: Use of only residual hearing to receive spoken messages.

Universal newborn hearing screening: UNHS; the screening for hearing loss for all newborn infants.

Unserved: Refers to a group of patients in need of but not receiving services.

Use gain: Amount of gain provided by a hearing aid when the volume control is set where it is commonly used.

Validation: To confirm or establish the soundess or correct functioning of a hearing aid or other listening device.

Validity: The extent to which a test measures what it is assumed to measure.

Vent: Bore drilled into an earmold that permits the passage of sound and air; used for aeration of the external auditory canal or for acoustic modification of the amplified sound.

Verification: Determination of whether a hearing aid meets a set of standards, including standards of basic electroacoustics, real-ear electroacoustic performance, and comfortable fit.

Vertigo: Dizziness, including a sensation of spinning or whirling.

Vibrotactile: Pertaining to the detection of vibrations through the sense of touch.

Vibrotactile aid: Tactile aid; an assistive listening device that converts acoustic energy into vibratory patterns that are delivered to the skin.

Vicarious consequences: Students observe the consequences of a model's behaviors.

Videotaped scenarios: Videotaped examples of communication interactions, which may include use of communication strategies and language stimulation techniques.

Viseme: Groups of speech sounds that appear identical on the lips; for example, /p, m, b/.

Vision-only: Presentation of only a visual stimulus in testing or training.

Visual alerting systems: Assistive devices that include alarm clocks, doorbells, and smoke detectors in which the alerting mechanism is a flashing light.

Visual impairment: A vision loss that cannot be compensated through corrective lenses.

Visual lexical neighborhood: A set of words that are visually similar and have approximately the same frequency of occurrence.

Visual reinforcement audiometry: VRA; audiometric technique used with young children in which a correct response to a stimulus presentation is reinforced by a visual reward, such as the activation of a lighted toy.

Voicing: Classification of a speech sound according to whether it is produced with or without voice; for example, /b/ vs. /p/.

Volume control: Manual or automatic control used to adjust the output of a listening device.

Vowel formants: Resonances in the vocal tract that cause some frequencies to have more energy than other frequencies.

VRA: Visual reinforcement audiometry.

WATCH: A brief communication strategies training program.

Well-being: An intangible concept that encompasses both a physical aspect (e.g., health, protection against pain and disease) and a psychological aspect (e.g., stress, worry, pleasure); state or condition of being well.

White noise: Noise having energy at all frequencies audible to the human ear.

Wide-band noise: White noise.

Wireless system: An assistive listening device in which wires are not necessary to connect the sound source to the listener; includes FM and infrared systems.

Word decoding: The ability to apply one's knowledge of letter–sound relationships, including a knowledge of letter patterns, to the task of recognizing and interpreting written words.

Word recognition: Ability to perceive and identify a word.

Word recognition score: Percentage of words correctly identified in a speech recognition test.

Working memory: The ability to store simultaneously and manipulate or transform items in memory.

X-linked: Refers to a trait related to the X chromosome; transmitted by mothers to 50% of their sons who will be affected and to 50% of their daughters who will be carriers and transmitted by fathers to 100% of their daughters.

REFERENCES

A timeline of the hearing industry. (1991). *The Hearing Journal*, 50, 54–72.

Abrahamson, J. A. (1991). Teaching coping strategies: A client education approach to aural rehabilitation. *Journal of the Academy of Rehabilitative Audiology*, 24, 43–54.

Abrahamson, J. A. (2000). Group audiologic rehabilitation. *Seminars in Hearing*, 21, 227–233.

Abrams, H., Chisolm, T. H., Guerreiro, S., & Ritterman, S. (1992). The effects of intervention strategy on self-perception of hearing handicap. *Ear and Hearing*, 13, 371–377.

Abrams, H., Chisolm, T. H., & McArdle, R. (2002). A cost–utility analysis of adult group audiologic rehabilitation: Are the benefits worth the cost? *Journal of Rehabilitation Research and Development*, 39, 549–558.

Adler, J. (2005, November 14). Hitting 60. *Newsweek*, 51–58.

Alcantara, J. I., Cowan, R. S. C., Blamey, P. J., & Clark, G. M. (1990). A comparison of two training strategies for speech recognition with an electrotactile speech processor. *Journal of Speech and Hearing Research*, 33, 195–204.

Alexander Graham Bell Association for the Deaf and Hard of Hearing. (1988). *Speechreading for Better Communication*. Washington, DC: Alexander Graham Bell Association for the Deaf and Hard of Hearing.

Allen, T. E. (1986). Patterns of academic achievement among hearing impaired students: 1974 and 1983. In A. N. Schildroth & M. A. Karchmer (Eds.), *Deaf Children in America* (pp. 161–206). San Diego, CA: College-Hill Press.

Alpiner, J. G., & Garstecki, D. C. (1996). Audiologic rehabilitation for adults: Assessment and management. In R. L. Schow & M. A. Nerbonne (Eds.), *Introduction to Audiologic Rehabilitation* (3rd Ed.) (pp. 361–412). Needham Heights, MA: Allyn & Bacon.

Alzheimer's Association. (2007). *Every 72 Seconds Someone in America Develops Alzheimer's.* Chicago: Alzheimer's Association.

American Academy of Audiology. (2004). Pediatric amplification guidelines. *Audiology Today*, 16, 46–53.

American Academy of Audiology. (2006). Audiologic management of adult hearing impairment: Summary guidelines. *Audiology Today*, 18, 32–36.

American Speech-Language-Hearing Association. (1993). Guidelines for audiology services in the schools. *ASHA*, 35(Suppl. 10), 24–32.

American Speech-Language-Hearing Association. (2002a). Knowledge and skills required for the practice of audiologic/aural rehabilitation: Executive summary. *ASHA Supplement*, 22.

American Speech-Language-Hearing Association. (2002b). Technical Report: Appropriate school facilities for students with speech-language-hearing disorders. *ASHA Supplement*, 23.

American Speech-Language-Hearing Association. (2003). *2003 Omnibus Survey Caseload Report: SLP.* Rockville, MD: American Speech-Language-Hearing Association.

American Speech-Language-Hearing Association (2004a). *Evidence-based practice in communication disorders: An introduction* [Technical report]. Retrieved 07/07/07, from http://www.asha.org/members/deskref-journals/deskref/default.

American Speech-Language-Hearing Association. (2004b). Knowledge and skills needed by speech-language pathologists and audiologists to provide culturally and linguistically appropriate services. *ASHA Supplement*, 24, 152–158.

American Speech-Language-Hearing Association. (2004c). Roles of speech-language pathologists and teachers of children who are deaf and hard of hearing in the development of communicative and linguistic competence. *ASHA Supplement*, 24.

American Speech-Language-Hearing Association. (2005a). *Evidence-based practice in communication disorders: An introduction* [Position paper]. Retrieved 07/07/07 from http://www.asha.org/members/deskref-journals/deskref/default.

American Speech-Language-Hearing Association. (2005b). *(Central) auditory processing disorders.* Retrieved 10/15/07, from http://www.asha.org/members/deskref-journals/deskref/default.

American Speech-Language-Hearing Association. (2005c). *Acoustics in educational settings: Technical report.* Retrieved 09/17/07, from http://www.asha.org/members/deskref-journals/deskref/default.

American Speech-Language-Hearing Association. (2007). *Causes of Hearing Loss in Children.* Retrieved 03/07/07, from http://www.asha.org/public/hearing/disorders/causes.html.

Anderson, I., Baumgartner, W. D., Koheim, K., Nahler, A., Arnolder, C., & D'Haese, P. (2006). Telephone use: What benefit do cochlear implant users receive? *International Journal of Audiology*, 45, 446–453.

Anderson, K. L. (2002). ELF—*Early Listening Function.* Retrieved 04/20/07, from http://www.Phonak.com/

Anderson, K. L. (2004). The problem of classroom acoustics: The typical classroom soundscape is a barrier to learning. *Seminars in Hearing*, 25, 117–129.

Anderson, K. L., & Matkin, N. D. (1991). Relationship of degree of long-term hearing loss to psychosocial impact and educational needs. *Educational Audiology Association Newsletter*, 8, 17–18.

Anderson, K. L., & Smaldino, J. (1998). *Listening Inventory for Education (L.I.F.E.).* Tampa, FL: Educational Audiology Association.

Anderson, K. L., & Smaldino, J. (1999). Listening inventories for education: A classroom measurement tool. *The Hearing Journal*, 52, 74–76.

Anderson, M., Boren, N. J., Kilgore, J., Howard, W., & Krohn, E. (1999). *The Apple Tree Curriculum for Developing Written Language—Second Edition.* Austin, TX: Pro-Ed.

Andersson, G., Melin, L., Lindberg, P., & Scott, B. (1995). Development of a short scale for self-assessment of experiences of hearing loss: The hearing coping assessment. *Scandinavian Audiology*, 24, 147–154.

Andersson, U., & Lidestam, B. (2005). Bottom-up driven speechreading in a speechreading expert: The case of AA. *Ear and Hearing*, 26, 214–224.

Andersson, U., Lyxell, B., Rönnberg, J., & Spens, K. E. (2001). Cognitive correlates of visual speech understanding in hearing-impaired individuals. *Journal of Deaf Studies and Deaf Education*, 6, 103–115.

Antia, S. D. (1982). Social interaction of partially mainstreamed hearing impaired children. *American Annals of the Deaf*, 127, 8–25.

Antia, S. D., & Levine, L. M. (2001). Educating deaf and hearing children together: Confronting the challenges of inclusion. In M. J. Guralnick (Ed.), *Early Childhood Inclusion: Focus on Change.* Baltimore: Paul H. Brooks.

Antia, S. D., Stinson, M. S., & Gaustad, M. G. (2002). Developing membership in the education of deaf and hard-of-hearing students in inclusive settings. *Journal of Deaf Studies and Deaf Education*, 7, 214–229.

Arehart, K. H., Yoshinaga-Itano, C., Thomson, V., Gabbard, S. A., & Brown, A. S. (1998). State of the states: The status of universal newborn hearing screening, assessment, and intervention systems in 16 states. *American Journal of Audiology*, 7, 101–114.

Arlinger, S., Billermark, E., Oberg, M., Lunner, T., & Hellgren, J. (1998). Clinical trial of a digital hearing aid. *Scandinavian Audiology*, 27, 51–61.

Armstrong, T. L. (1991). *The relationship between gender and psychological distress in hard-of-hearing people*. Paper presented to the American Public Health Association, Washington, DC.

Arnold, P., & Hill, F. (2001). Bisensory augmentation: A speechreading advantage when speech is clearly audible and intact. *British Journal of Psychology*, 92, 339–355.

Auer, E. T., & Bernstein, L. E. (1997). Speechreading and the structure of the lexicon: Computationally modeling the effects of reduced phonetic distinctiveness on lexical uniqueness. *Journal of the Acoustical Society of America*, 102, 3704–3710.

Axelsson, A., & Ringdahl, A. (1989). Tinnitus: A study of its prevalence and characteristics. *British Journal of Audiology*, 23, 53–62.

Backenroth, G. A. M., & Ahlner, B. H. (2000). Quality of life of hearing-impaired persons who have participated in audiological rehabilitation counseling. *International Journal for the Advancement of Counseling*, 22, 225–240.

Bader, L. A. (1998). *Bader Reading and Language Inventory* (3rd Ed.). Upper Saddle River, NJ: Prentice-Hall.

Baguley, D. M., Davies, E., & Hazell, J. W. P. (2003). A vision for tinnitus research. *International Journal of Audiology*, 42, 2–3.

Baker, C. (1993). *Foundations of Bilingual Education and Bilingualism*. Clevedon, Avon, ENG: Multicultural Matters.

Bamford, J., & Saunders, E. (1985). *Hearing Impairment, Auditory Perception, and Language Disability*. London, ENG: Edward Arnold.

Bandura, A. (1997). *Self-Efficacy: The Exercise of Control*. New York, NY: Freeman.

Banks, W. A. & Morley, J. E. (2003). Memories are made of this: Recent advances in understanding, cognitive impairment, and dementia. *Journal of Gerontologic Medical Science*, 58A, 314–321.

Barcham, L. J., & Stephens, S. D. (1980). The use of an open-ended problems questionnaire in auditory rehabilitation. *British Journal of Audiology*, 14, 49–54.

Bauman, S. L., & Hambrecht, G. (1995). Analysis of view angle used in speechreading training of sentences. *American Journal of Audiology*, 4, 67–70.

Baylock, R. L., Scudder, R. R., & Wynne, M. K. (1995). Repair behaviors used by children with hearing loss. *Language, Speech, and Hearing Services in Schools*, 26, 278–285.

Bazargan, M., Baker, R. S., & Bazargan, S. H. (2000). Sensory impairments and subjective well-being among aged African American persons. *Journal of Gerontology: Psychological Sciences*, 56B, 268–278.

Beck, A. T., & Emery, G. (1985). *Anxiety Disorders and Phobias*. New York, NY: Basic Books.

Beck, P. H. (2006). Cued speech across cultures. *Volta Voices*, September/October, 26–28.

Bellis, T. J. (1996). *Assessment and Management of Central Auditory Processing Disorders in the Educational Setting: From Science to Practice*. Clifton Park, NY: Delmar Learning.

Bench, J., & Bamford, J. (1979). *Speech-Hearing Tests and the Spoken Language of Hearing-Impaired Children*. London, ENG: Academic Press.

Bench, J., Daly, N., Doyle, J., & Lind, C. (1995). Choosing talkers for the BKB/A speechreading test: A procedure with observations on talker age and gender. *British Journal of Audiology*, 29, 172–187.

Benitez, L., & Speaks, C. (1968). A test of speech intelligibility in the Spanish language. *International Audiology*, 7, 16–22.

Benson, V., & Marano, M. A. (1998). Current estimates from the National Health Interview Survey, 1995, National Center for Health Statistics. Vital Health Statistics, 10 [1991].

Bentler, R. A. (2005). Effectiveness of directional microphones and noise reduction schemes in hearing aids: A systematic review of the evidence. *Journal of the American Academy of Audiology*, 16, 473–484.

Bentler, R. A., & Kramer, S. E. (2000). Guidelines for choosing a self-report outcome measure. *Ear and Hearing*, 21, 37S–49S.

Bentler, R. A., Palmer, C., & Mueller, H. G. (2006). Evaluation of a second-order directional microphone hearing aid: I. speech perception outcomes. *Journal of the American Academy of Audiology*, 27, 179–189.

Benyon, G., Thornton, F., & Pool, C. (1997). A randomized, controlled trial of the efficacy of a communication course for first time hearing aid users. *British Journal of Audiology*, 31, 345–351.

Berger, K. W. (1972). *Speechreading: Principles and Methods*. Baltimore: National Education Press.

Bergman, B., & Rosenhall, U. (2001). Vision and hearing in old age. *Scandinavian Audiology*, 30, 255–263.

Berko, J. (1984). The child's learning of English morphology. *Word*, 14, 150–177.

Bernstein, L. E., Auer, E. T., & Moore, J. K. (2004). Audiovisual speech binding: Convergence or association? In G. A. Calvert, C. Spence, & Stein, B. E. (Eds.), *The Handbook of Multisensory Processes* (pp. 203–223). Boston, MA: MIT Press.

Bernstein, L. E., Auer, E. T., & Tucker, P. E. (2001). Enhanced speechreading in deaf adults: Can short-term training/practice close the gap for hearing adults? *Journal of Speech, Language, and Hearing Research*, 44, 5–18.

Bernstein, L. E., Demorest, M. E., Coulter, D. C., & O'Connell, M. P. (1991). Lipreading sentences with vibrotactile vocoders: Performance of normal-hearing and hearing-impaired subjects. *Journal of the Acoustical Society of America*, 90, 2971–2984.

Bernstein, L. E., Demorest, M. E., & Tucker, P. E. (2000). Speech perception without hearing. *Perception and Psychophysics*, 62, 233–252.

Berry, J. A., Gold, S. L., Frederick, E. A., Gray, W. C., & Staecker, H. (2002). Patient-based outcomes in patients with primary tinnitus undergoing tinnitus retraining therapy. *Archives of Otolaryngology—Head and Neck Surgery*, 128, 1153–1157.

Berry, S. (1981). *Written Language Syntax Test*. Washington, DC: Gallaudet College Press.

Bess, F. H. (2000). The role of generic health-related quality of life measures in establishing audiological rehabilitation. *Ear and Hearing*, 21, 74S–79S.

Beyer, C. M., & Northern, J. L. (2000). Audiologic rehabilitation support programs: A network model. *Seminars in Hearing*, 21, 257–265.

Bilger, R. C., Nuetzel, J. M., Rabinowitz, W. M., & Rzeczkowski, C. (1984). Standardization of a test of speech perception in noise. *Journal of Speech and Hearing Research*, 27, 32–48.

Binnie, C. A. (1977). Attitude changes following speechreading training. *Scandinavian Audiology*, 6, 13–19.

Blackwood, M. J. (2006). Rediscover sounds of life. *Ladue News*, 5, 25.

Blamey, P. J., & Alcantara, J. I. (1994). Research in auditory training. *Journal of the Academy of Rehabilitative Audiology*, 27(Suppl.), 161–192.

Blamey, P. J., Barry, J. G., & Jacq, P. (2001). Phonetic inventory development in young cochlear implant users 6 years post-operation. *Journal of Speech, Language, and Hearing Research*, 44, 73–79.

Blamey, P. J., Cowan, R. S. C., Alcantara, J. I., Whitford, L. A., & Clark, G. M. (1989). Speech perception using combinations of auditory, visual, and tactile information. *Journal of Rehabilitation Research and Development*, 26, 15–24.

Blamey, P. J., Fiket, H. J., & Steele, B. R. (2006). Improving speech intelligibility in background noise with an adaptive directional microphone. *Journal of the American Academy of Audiology*, 17, 519–530.

Blanchfield, B. B., Feldman, J. J., Dunbar, J. L., & Gardner, E. N. (2001). The severely to profoundly hearing-impaired population in the United States: Prevalence estimates and demographics. *Journal of the American Academy of Audiology*, 12, 183–189.

Blood, G. W., Blood, I. M., & Danhauer, J. L. (1978). Listeners' impression of normal-hearing and hearing-impaired children. *Journal of Communication Disorders*, 11, 513–518.

Bloom, S. (1999). Marketing to baby boomers: Challenges and opportunities are greater than ever. *The Hearing Journal*, 52, 23–30.

Blumsack, J. T. (2003). Audiological assessment, rehabilitation, and spatial hearing considerations associated with visual impairment in adults: An overview. *American Journal of Audiology*, 12, 76–83.

Bode, D., & Oyer, H. (1970). Auditory training and speech discrimination. *Journal of Speech and Hearing Research*, 13, 839–855.

Bodrova, E., Leong, D. J., Paynter, D. E., & Semenov, D. (2000). *A Framework for Early Literacy Instruction: Aligning Standards to Developmental Accomplishments and Student Behaviors*. Aurora, CO: Mid-continent Research for Education and Learning.

Boettcher, F. A. (2002). Presbycusis and the auditory brainstem response. *Journal of Speech, Language, and Hearing Research*, 45, 1249–1262.

Boothroyd, A. (1984). Auditory perception of speech contrasts by subjects with sensorineural hearing loss. *Journal of Speech and Hearing Research*, 27, 134–144.

Boothroyd, A., Hanin, L., & Hnath-Chisholm, T. (1985). *The CUNY Sentence Test*. New York, NY: City University of New York.

Boothroyd, A., Hnath-Chisholm, T., Hanin, L., & Kishon-Rabin, L. (1988). Voice fundamental frequency as an auditory supplement to the speechreading of sentences. *Ear and Hearing*, 9, 306–312.

Borg, E., Danermark, B., & Borg, B. (2002). Behavioral awareness, interaction and counseling education in audiological rehabilitation: Development of methods and application in a pilot study. *International Journal of Audiology*, 41, 308–322.

Borrel-Carrio, F., Suchman, A. L., & Epstein, R. M. (2004). The biopsychosocial model 25 years later: Principles, practice, and scientific inquiry. *Annals of Family Medicine*, 2, 576–582.

Boswell, S. (2007). Jane K. Fernandes. *ASHA Leader*, 12, 14–15.

Braida, L. (1991). Crossmodal integration in the identification of consonant segments. *Psychological Quarterly Journal of Experimental Psychology*, 43, 647–677.

Brainerd, S. H., & Frankel, B. G. (1985). The relationship between audiometric and self-report measures of hearing handicap. *Ear and Hearing*, 6, 89–92.

Brennan, M. (2002). When vision and hearing fail: Dual sensory impairment among older adults. *Lighthouse International Aging and Vision Newsletter, Fall,* 2-3.

Brewer, D. (2001). Considerations in measuring effectiveness of group audiologic rehabilitation classes. *Journal of the Academy of Rehabilitative Audiology*, 34, 53–60.

Brigance, A. H. (1999). *Brigance Comprehensive Inventory of Basic Skills-Revised (CIBS–R)*. North Billerica, MA: Curriculum Associates.

Bromwich, R. (1981). *Working with Parents and Infants: An Interactional Approach*. Baltimore, MD: University Park Press.

Brooks, D. N. (1979). Counseling and its effect on hearing aid use. *Scandinavian Audiology*, 8, 101–107.

Brooks, D. N. (1990). Measures for the assessment of hearing aid provision and rehabilitation. *British Journal of Audiology*, 24, 229–233.

Brooks, D. N., & Hallam, R. S. (1998). Attitudes to hearing difficulty and hearing aids and the outcome of audiological rehabilitation. *British Journal of Audiology*, 24, 229–233.

Brown, G. R. (2004). Tinnitus: The ever-present tormentor. *The Hearing Journal*, 57, 52–54.

Bruce, R. V. (1973). *Bell: Alexander Graham Bell and the Conquest of Solitude*. Ithaca, NY: Cornell University Press.

Bryant, B., & Wiederhold, J. L. (1991). *Gray Oral Reading Test-Diagnostic (GORT-D)*. Austin, TX: Pro-Ed.

Budd, R. J., & Pugh, R. (1995). The relationship between locus of control, tinnitus severity, and emotional distress in a group of tinnitus sufferers. *Journal of Psychosomatic Research*, 39, 1015–1018.

Burk, M. H., & Humes, L. E. (2007). Effects of training on speech recognition performance in noise using lexically hard words. *Journal of Speech, Language, and Hearing Research,* 50, 25–40.

Burk, M. H., Humes, L. E., Amos, N., & Strauser, L. (2006). Effect of training on word-recognition performance in noise for young normal-hearing and older hearing-impaired listeners. *Ear and Hearing*, 27, 263–278.

Burns, E. (2004). *The Special Education Consultant Teacher: Enabling Children with Disabilities to be Educated with Nondisabled Children to the Maximum Extent Appropriate.* Springfield, IL: Thomas.

Busa, J. (2005). A mother's unexpected role. *Volta Voices,* November/December, 9.

Caissie, R. (2001). Conversational topic shifting and its effect on communication breakdowns. *Volta Review*, 102, 45–56.

Caissie, R., Campbell, M. M., Grenette, W., Scott, L., Howell, I., & Roy, A. (2005). Clear speech for adults with a hearing loss: Does intervention with communication partners make a difference? *Journal of the American Academy of Audiology*, 16, 157–171.

Caissie, R., & Gibson, C. L. (1997). The effectiveness of repair strategies used by people with hearing losses and their conversational partners. *Volta Review,* 99, 203–218.

Caissie, R., & Rockwell, E. (1994). Communication difficulties experienced by nursing home residents with a hearing loss during conversation with staff members. *Journal of Speech-Language Pathology and Audiology*, 18, 127–134.

Campbell, R. (1998). How brains see speech: The cortical localization of speechreading in hearing people. In R. Campbell, B. Dodd, & D. Burnham (Eds.), *Hearing by Eye II* (pp. 177–194). East Sussex, ENG: Psychology Press.

Canadian Cochrane Network/Centre Affiliate Representatives. (2003). *A Primer on Evidence-Based Clinical Practice.* Retrieved 05/09/07, from http://cochrane.mcmaster.ca/pdf/presentations/EBCPPrimer.

Carrow-Woolfolk, E. (1996). *Oral and Written Language Scales (OWLS).* Circle Pines, MN: American Guidance Services.

Carrow-Woolfolk, E. (1999). *Test for Auditory Comprehension of Language-III.* Austin, TX: Pro-Ed.

Carter, C. J. (2008, March 8). Sounds of war can leave soldiers in silence. *The St. Louis Post Dispatch*, p. A18.

Cassell, J. (2001). Nudge nudge wink wink: Elements of face-to-face conversation for embodied conversational agents. In J. Cassell (Ed.), *Embodied Conversational Agents* (pp. 1–27), Cambridge, MA: MIT Press.

Castle, D. (1988). The oral interpreter. *Volta Review*, 90, 307–313.

Ceasar, L. G., & Williams, D. R. (2002). Socioculture and the delivery of health care: Who gets what and why. *ASHA Leader*, 7, 6–8.

Centers for Disease Control and Prevention. (2001). Trends in vision and hearing among older Americans. *Aging Trends*, 2, 1–8.

Centers for Disease Control and Prevention. (2007). *Early hearing detection and intervention program*. Retrieved 01/03/07, from http://www.cdc.gov/ncbddd/ehdi/ehdi.htm.

Cheesman, M. G. (1997). Speech perception by elderly listeners: Basic knowledge and implications for audiology. *Journal of Speech Language Patholody and Audiology*, 21, 104–110.

Cherry, R., & Rubinstein, A. (1988). Speechreading instruction for adults: Issues and practices. *Volta Review*, 90, 289–306.

Chin, S. B. (2003). Children's consonant inventories after extended cochlear implant use. *Journal of Speech, Language, and Hearing Research*, 46, 849–862.

Ching, T. Y., Incerti, P., & Hill, M. (2004). Binaural benefits for adults who use hearing aids and cochlear implants in opposite ears. *Ear and Hearing*, 25, 9–21.

Chisolm, T. H., Abrams, H., & McArdle, R. (2004). Short and long-term outcomes of adult audiologic rehabilitation. *Ear and Hearing*, 25, 464–477.

Chisolm, T. H., Johnson, C. E., Danhauer, J., Portz, L., Abrams, H., Lesner, S., et al. (2007). A systematic review of health-related quality of life and hearing aids: Final report of the American Academy of Audiology task force on the health-related quality of life benefits of amplification in adults. *Journal of the American Academy of Audiology*, 18, 151–183.

Chisolm, T. H., Willott, J. F., & Lister, J. J. (2003). The aging auditory system: Anatomic and physiologic changes and implications for rehabilitation. *International Journal of Audiology*, 42, 2S3–2S10.

Christopherson, L. A., & Humes, L. E. (1992). Some psychometric properties of the Test of Basic Auditory Capabilities (TBAC). *Journal of Speech and Hearing Research*, 35, 929–935.

Cienkowski, K. M., & Carney, A. E. (2002). Auditory-visual speech perception and aging. *Ear and Hearing*, 23, 439–449.

Ciocci, S., & Baran, J. (1998). The use of conversational repair strategies by children who are deaf. *American Annals of the Deaf*, 143, 235–245.

Clark, H. H., & Brennan, S. E. (1991). Grounding in communication. In L. B. Resnick, J. Levine, & S. D. Teasley (Eds.), *Perspectives on Socially Shared Cognition* (pp. 127–149), Washington, DC: APA.

Clark, J. G. (1994). *Effective Counseling in Audiology: Perspectives and Practice*. Englewood Cliffs, NJ: Prentice-Hall.

Clark, J. G., & English, K. M. (2004). *Counseling in Audiologic Practice: Helping Patients and Families Adjust to Hearing Loss*. Boston, MA: Pearson.

Clark, T. (1994). SKI*HI: Applications for home-based intervention. In J. Rousch & N. Matkin (Eds.), *Infants and toddlers with hearing loss: Family-centered assessment and intervention* (pp. 237–251). Baltimore, MD: York Press.

Code of Ethics. (1984). In W. H. Northcott (Ed.), *Oral Interpreting: Principles and Practices* (pp. 266–269). Baltimore, MD: University Park Press.

Cole, E. B. (1993). *Listening and Talking: A Guide to Promoting Spoken Language in Young Hearing-Impaired Children*. Washington, DC: Alexander Graham Bell Association for the Deaf.

Connor, C. M., Craig, H. K., Raudenbush, S. W., Heavner, K., & Zwolan, T. A. (2006). The age at which young deaf children receive cochlear implants and their vocabulary and speech-production growth: Is there an added value for early implantation? *Ear and Hearing*, 27, 628–644.

Connor, C. M., Hieber, S., Arts, H. A., & Zwolan, T. A. (2000). Speech, vocabulary and the education of children using cochlear implants: Oral or total communication? *Journal of Speech, Language, and Hearing Research*, 43, 185–204.

Connor, C. M., & Zwolan, T. A. (2004). Examining multiple sources of influence on the reading comprehension skills of children who use cochlear implants. *Journal of Speech, Language, and Hearing Research*, 47, 509–526.

Cornett, R. O. (1967). Cued speech. *American Annals of the Deaf*, 112, 313.

Cowie, R., & Douglas-Cowie, E. (1992). *Postlingually Acquired Deafness: Speech Deterioration and the Wider Consequences*. New York, NY: Mouton de Gruyter.

Cox, R. M. (2003). Assessment of subjective outcome of hearing aid fitting: Getting the client's point of view. *International Journal of Audiology*, 42, S90–S96.

Cox, R. M. (2005). Evidence-based practice in provision of amplification. *Journal of the American Academy of Audiology*, 16, 419–438.

Cox, R. M., & Alexander, G. C. (1991). Hearing aid benefit in everyday environments. *Ear and Hearing*, 12, 127–139.

Cox, R. M., & Alexander, G. C. (1995). The abbreviated profile of hearing aid benefit. *Ear and Hearing*, 16, 176–183.

Cox, R. M., & Alexander, G. C. (1999). Measuring satisfaction with amplification in daily life: The S\ADL scale. *Ear and Hearing*, 20, 306–320.

Cox, R. M., Alexander, G. C., & Gilmore, C. (1987). Development of the connected speech test (CST). *Ear and Hearing*, 9, 198–207.

Cox, R. M., & Gilmore, C. (1990). Development of the profile of hearing aid performance (PHAP). *Journal of Speech and Hearing Research*, 33, 343–357.

Cox, R. M., Gilmore, C. G., & Alexander, G. C. (1991). Comparison of two questionnaires for patient-assessed hearing aid benefit. *Journal of the American Academy of Audiology*, 2, 134–145.

Cox, R. M., Hyde, M., Gatehouse, S., Noble, W., Dillon, H., Bentler, R., et al. (2000). Optimal outcome measures, research priorities, and international cooperation. *Ear and Hearing*, 21, 106S–115S.

Cox, R. M., & Rivera, I. M. (1992). Predictability and reliability of hearing aid benefit measured using the PHAP. *Journal of the American Academy of Audiology*, 3, 242–254.

Craig, W. N. (1964). Effects of preschool training on the development of reading and lip-reading skills of deaf children. *American Annals of the Deaf*, 109, 280–296.

Crandell, C. C. (1992). Classroom acoustics for hearing-impaired children. *Journal of the Acoustical Society of America*, 92, 2470.

Crandell, C. C. (1993). Noise effects on the speech recognition of children with minimal hearing loss. *Ear and Hearing*, 14, 210–216.

Crandell, C. C., & Bess, F. (1986). Speech recognition of children in "typical" classroom settings. *ASHA*, October, 82.

Crandell, C. C., & Smaldino, J. J. (1995). An update of classroom acoustics for children with hearing impairment. *Volta Review*, 97, 4–12.

Crandell, C. C., & Smaldino, J. J. (2000). Classroom acoustics for children with normal hearing and with hearing impairment. *Language, Speech, and Hearing Services in Schools*, 31, 362–370.

Cray, J. W., Allen, R. L., Stuart, A., Hudson, S., Layman, E., & Givens, G. D. (2004). An investigation of telephone use among cochlear implant recipients. *American Journal of Audiology*, 13, 200–212.

Cruickshanks, K. J., Tweed, T. S., Wiley, T. L., Klein, B. E., Klein, R., Chappell, R., et al. (2003). The 5-year incidence and progression of hearing loss: The epidemiology of hearing loss study. *Archives of Otolaryngology—Head and Neck Surgery*, 129, 1041–1046.

Cruickshanks, K. J., Wiley, T. L., Tweed, T. S., Klein, B. E., Klein, R., Mares-Perlman, J. A., et al. (1998). Prevalence of hearing loss in older adults in Beaver Dam, Wisconsin. *American Journal of Epidemiology*, 148, 879–886.

Dagenais, P., & Critz-Crosby, P. (1992). Comparing tongue positioning by normal hearing and hearing-impaired children during vowel production. *Journal of Speech and Hearing Research*, 35, 5–44.

Dalton, D., Cruickshanks, K., Klein, B., Klein, R., Wiley, T., & Nondahl, D. (2003). The impact of hearing loss on quality of life in older adults. *Gerontologist*, 43, 661–668.

Daly, N., Bench, J., & Chappell, H. (1996). Gender differences in speechreadability. *Journal of the Academy of Rehabilitative Audiology*, 29, 27–40.

Dancer, J. (2001). Arkansas tinnitus survey reflects national picture. *Advance for Speech-Language Pathologists and Audiologists*, September, 10–11.

Dancer, J. (2006). Celebrate Diversity. *Advance for Audiologists*, July/August, 24–26.

Dancer, J., & Gener, J. (1999). Survey on the use of adult hearing assessment scales. *Hearing Review*, 6, 26–35.

Dancer, J., Krain, M., Thompson, C., Davis, P., & Glenn, J. (1994). A cross-sectional investigation of speechreading in adults: Effects of gender, practice, and education. *Volta Review*, 96, 31–40.

Danermark, B., & Gellerstedt, L. C. (2004). Psychosocial work environment, hearing impairment and health. *International Journal of Audiology*, 43, 383–389.

Danhauer, J. L., Johnson, C. E., Kasten, R. N., & Brimacombe, J. A. (1985). The hearing aid effect: Summary, conclusions and recommendations. *The Hearing Journal*, March 12–14.

Danz, A. D., & Binnie, C. A. (1983). Quantification of the effects of training the auditory-visual reception of connected speech. *Ear and Hearing*, 4, 146–151.

Data snapshot and quick facts. (2002). *ASHA Leader, 7,* 10, 32.

Davis, A. (1989). The prevalence of hearing impairment and reported hearing disability among adults in Great Britain. *International Journal of Epidemiology*, 18, 911–917.

Davis, A. (1994). *Hearing in Adults.* London, ENG: Whurr.

Davis, A., & Refaie, A. E. (2000). Epidemiology of tinnitus. In R. Tyler (Ed.), *Tinnitus Handbook* (pp. 1–23). Clifton Park, NY: Delmar Learning.

Davis, H., & Silverman, R. (1978). *Hearing and Deafness* (4th Ed.). New York, NY: Holt Rinehart & Winston.

Davis, J. M., Elfenbein, J., Schum, R., & Bentler, R. (1986). Effects of mild and moderate hearing impairments on language, educational, and psychosocial behavior of children. *Journal of Speech and Hearing Disorders*, 51, 53–62.

De Fillipo, C. L., & Scott, B. L. (1978). A method for hearing and evaluating the reception of ongoing speech. *Journal of the Acoustical Society of America*, 63, 1186–1192.

De Fillipo, C. L., Sims, D. G., & Gottermeier, L. (1995). Linking visual and kinesthetic imagery in lipreading instruction. *Journal of Speech and Hearing Research*, 38, 244–256.

Demorest, M. E., & Erdman, S. A. (1987). Development of the communication profile for the hearing impaired. *Journal of Speech and Hearing Disorders*, 52, 129–143.

Demorest, M. E., & Walden, B. E. (1984). Psychometric principles in the selection, interpretation, and evaluation of communication self-assessment inventories. *Journal of Speech and Hearing Disorders*, 54, 180–188.

Desai, M., Pratt, L., Lentzner, H., & Robinson, K. (2001). Trends in vision and hearing among older Americans. *Aging Trends*, 2, 1–8.

Di Francesca, S. (1972). *Academic Achievement Test Results of a National Testing Program for Hearing-Impaired Students—United States, Spring 1971* (Series D, No. 9). Washington, DC: Gallaudet University, Office of Demographic Studies.

Dillon, H. (2001). *Hearing Aids.* Sydney, AUS: Boomerang Press Thieme.

Dillon, H., Birtles, G., & Lovegrove, R. (1999). Measuring the outcomes of a national rehabilitation program: Normative data for the client oriented scale of improvement (COSI) and the hearing aid user's questionnaire (HAUQ). *Journal of the American Academy of Audiology*, 10, 67–79.

Dillon, H., James, A., & Ginis, J. (1997). Client oriented scale of improvement (COSI) and its relationship to several other measurements of benefit and satisfaction provided by hearing aids. *Journal of the American Academy of Audiology*, 8, 27–43.

Directors of Health Promotion and Education. (2007). Cytomegalovirus. Retrieved 07/10/07, from http://dhpe.org/infect/cytomegalo.html.

Dodd, B., Plant, G., & Gregory, M. (1989). Teaching lip-reading: The efficacy of lessons on video. *British Journal of Audiology*, 23, 229–238.

Doman, D., Hickson, L., Murdoch, B., & Houston, T. (2008). Outcomes of an auditory-verbal program for children with hearing loss: A comparative study with a matched group of children with normal hearing. *Volta Review, 107,* 37–54.

Donaldson, N., Worrall, L., & Hickson, L. (2004). Older people with hearing impairment: A literature review of the spouse's perspective. *The Australian and New Zealand Journal of Audiology*, 26, 30–39.

Dowell, R. (2005). Evaluating cochlear implant candidacy: Recent developments. *The Hearing Journal*, 9–23.

Downs, M. (1974). Deafness management quotient (DMQ). *Hearing and Speech News*, 42, 26–28.

Dubno, J. R., Lee, F. S., Matthews, L. J., & Mills, J. H. (1997). Age-related and gender-related changes in monaural speech recognition. *Journal of Speech, Language, and Hearing Research*, 40, 444–452.

Dunn, L., & Dunn, L. (1981). *Peabody Picture Vocabulary Test-Revised*. Circle Pines, MN: American Guidance Service.

Dunst, C. (1985). Rethinking early intervention. *Analysis and Intervention in Developmental Disabilities*, 5, 165–201.

Durrell, D., & Catterson, J. (1980). *Durrell Analysis of Reading Difficulty* (3rd Ed.). San Antonio, TX: Harcourt Brace Educational Measurement.

Dworkin, M. (2004). Soaring high in the mainstream. *Volta Voices*, November/December, 12.

Dye, C., & Peak, M. (1983). Influence of amplification on the psychological functioning of older adults with neurosensory hearing loss. *Journal of the Academy of Rehabilitative Audiology*, 16, 210–220.

Dykman, J. (2006, October 30). America by the numbers: How we spend time. *Time*, 52–53.

Edgerton, B. J., & Danhauer, J. L. (1979). *Clinical Implications of Speech Discrimination Testing Using Nonsense Stimuli*. Baltimore, MD: University Park Press.

Edwards, C. (2003). Reflections on counseling: Families and hearing loss. *Loud & Clear*, 2, 1–8.

Eggermont, J. J. (2005). Tinnitus: Neurobiological substrates. *Drug Discovery Today*, 10, 1283–1290.

El Nasser, H., & Overberg, P. (2007, May 17). Nation's minority numbers top 100 M. *USA Today*, 1–2.

Elfenbein, J. (1992). Coping with communication breakdown: A program of strategy development for children who have hearing losses. *American Journal of Audiology*, 1, 25–29.

Elfenbein, J. (1994). Communication breakdowns in conversations: Child-initiated repair strategies. In N. Tye-Murray (Ed.), *Let's Converse: A How-to Guide to Develop and Expand the Conversational Skills of Children and Teenagers Who Are Hearing Impaired* (pp. 123–146). Washington, DC: Alexander Graham Bell Association for the Deaf.

Elfenbein, J., Hardin-Jones, M. A., & Davis, J. M. (1994). Oral communication skills of children who are hard of hearing. *Journal of Speech and Hearing Research*, 37, 216–226.

Elkayam, J., & English, K. (2003). Counseling adolescents with hearing loss with the use of self-assessment/significant other questionnaires. *Journal of the American Academy of Audiology*, 14, 485–499.

Elliott, L., & Katz, D. (1980). *Development of a New Children's Test of Speech Recognition.* St. Louis, MO: Audiotec.

Ellis, A. (2001). *Overcoming Destructive Beliefs, Feelings, and Behaviors.* Amhurst, NY: Prometheus Books.

Ellis, A., & Grieger, R. (1977). *Handbook of Rational-Emotive Therapy.* New York, NY: Springer.

Ellis, A., & MacLaren, C. (1998). *Rational Emotive Behavior Therapy: A Therapist's Guide.* Atascadero, CA: Impact.

Elman, R. J. (2006). Evidence-based practice: What evidence is missing? *Aphasiology,* 20, 103–109.

Engel, C. (2007). Baby boomers: The next generation. *Advance for Audiologists,* January/February, 40–44.

Engen, E., & Engen, T. (1983). *Rhode Island Test of Language Structure Manual.* Baltimore, MD: University Park Press.

English, K. (2004). Informing parents of their child's hearing loss: Breaking bad news guidelines for audiologists. *Audiology Today,* March/April, 10–12.

English, K., Mendel, L. L., Rojeski, T., & Hornak, J. (1999). Counseling in audiology, or learning to listen: Pre- and post-measures from an audiology counseling course. *American Journal of Audiology,* 8, 34–39.

Erber, N. P. (1971). Effects of distance on the visual reception of speech. *Journal of Speech and Hearing Research,* 17, 99–112.

Erber, N. P. (1974). Visual perception of speech by deaf children: Recent developments and continuing needs. *Journal of Speech and Hearing Disorders,* 39, 178–185.

Erber, N. P. (1982). *Auditory Training.* Washington, DC: Alexander Graham Bell Association for the Deaf.

Erber, N. P. (1985). *Telephone Communication and Hearing Impairment.* San Diego, CA: College-Hill Press.

Erber, N. P. (1988). *Communication Therapy for Hearing Impaired Adults.* Abbotsford, Victoria, AUS: Clavis.

Erber, N. P. (1996). *Communication Therapy for Adults with Sensory Loss* (2nd Ed.). Melbourne, AUS: Clavis.

Erber, N. P. (1998). Dyalog: A computer-based measure of conversational performance. *Journal of the Academy of Rehabilitative Audiology*, 31, 69–76.

Erber, N. P., & Lind, C. (1994). Communication therapy: Theory and practice. *Journal of the Academy of Rehabilitative Audiology*, 27 (Suppl.), 267–287.

Erber, N. P., & Yelland, J. (1998). CONAN: A system for analysis of temporal factors in conversation. *Journal of Academy of Rehabilitative Audiology*, 31, 77–86.

Erdman, S. A. (1994). Self-assessment: From research focus to research tool. *Journal of the Academy of Rehabilitative Audiology*, 27 (Suppl.), 67–92.

Erdman, S. A. (2000). Counseling hearing impaired adults. In J. Alpiner & P. McCarthy (Eds.), *Rehabilitative Audiology: Children and Adults* (3rd Ed.) (pp. 435–470). Baltimore: Williams & Wilkins.

Eriks-Brophy, A., Durieux-Smith, A., Olds, J., Fitzpatrick, E., Duquette, C., & Whittingham, J. (2006). Facilitators and barriers to the inclusion of orally educated children and youth with hearing loss in schools: Promoting partnerships to support inclusion. *Volta Review*, 106, 53–88.

Eriks-Brophy, A., Durieux-Smith, A., Olds, J., Fitzpatrick, E., Duquette, C., & Whittingham, J. (2007). Facilitators and barriers to the integration of orally educated children and youth with hearing loss into their families and communities. *Volta Review*, 107, 5–36.

Erlandsson, S. I., Hallberg, L., & Axelsson, A. (1992). Psychological and audiological correlates of perceived tinnitus severity. *Audiology*, 31, 168–179.

Erler, S. F., & Garstecki, D. C. (2002). Hearing loss-and hearing-related stigma: Perceptions of women with age-normal hearing. *American Journal of Audiology*, 11, 83–91.

Ertmer, D. J., Leonard, J. S., & Pachuilo, M. L. (2002). Communication intervention for children with cochlear implants: Two case studies. *Language, Speech, and Hearing Services in Schools*, 33, 205–217.

Espmark, A. K., & Scherman, M. H. (2003). Hearing confirms existence and identity—experiences from persons with presbycusis. *International Journal of Audiology*, 42, 106–115.

Etymotic Research (2001). *Quick Speech in Noise Test (QuickSIN)*. Elk Grove Village, IL: Etymotic Research.

Farrimond, T. (1959). Age differences in the ability to use visual codes in auditory communication. *Language and Speech*, 2, 179.

Ferguson, N. M., & Nerbonne, M. A. (2003). Status of hearing aids in nursing homes and retirement centers in 2002. *Journal of the Academy of Rehabilitative Audiology*, 36, 37–44.

Fey, M. E., Warr-Leeper, G., Webber, S. A., & Disher, L. M. (1988). Repairing children's repairs: Evaluation and facilitation of children's clarification requests and responses. *Topics in Language Disorders*, 8, 63–84.

Fitch, J. L., & Holbrook, A. (1970). Modal vocal frequency of young adults. *Archives of Otolaryngology*, 92, 379–382.

Fitzgibbons, P. J., & Gordon-Salant, S. (1996). Auditory temporal processing in elderly listeners. *Journal of the American Academy of Audiology*, 7, 183–189.

Flanders, J. (2006). Advocating for classroom acoustics: Connecticut's story. *Volta Voices*, May/June, 12–14.

Flexer, C. (1997). Sound-field FM systems: Questions most often asked about classroom amplification. *Hearsay*, 11, 514.

Flexer, C. (1999). *Facilitating Hearing and Listening in Young Children* (2nd Ed). Clifton Park, NY: Delmar Learning.

Focus on multiculturalism: Data snapshots. (2002). *ASHA Leader,* 7, 32.

Folstein, M. F., Folstein, S. E., & McHugh, P. R. (1975). Mini-mental state: A practical method for grading the cognitive state of patients for the clinician. *Journal of Psychiatric Research*, 12, 189–198.

Fountain, H. (2007, May 29). For babies and language, seeing is believing, even without hearing. *The New York Times*, C-1.

Forner, L., & Hixon, T. (1977). Respiratory kinematics in profoundly hearing-impaired speakers. *Journal of Speech and Hearing Research*, 66, 373–408.

Fryauf-Bertschy, H., Tyler, R. S., Kelsay, D., Gantz, B., & Woodworth, G. (1997). Cochlear implant use by prelingually deafened children: The influences of age at implant and length of device use. *Journal of Speech, Hearing, and Language Research*, 40, 183–199.

Fu, Q. J., & Galvin, J. J. (2007). Computer-assisted speech training for cochlear implant patients: Feasibility, outcomes, and future directions. *Seminars in Hearing,* 28, 142–150.

Gabrel, C. (2000). Characteristics of elderly nursing home current residents and discharges: Data from the 1997 National Nursing Home Survey, National Center for Health Statistics. *Advance Data from Vital and Health Statistics*, 312.

Gagné, J. P. (2000). What is treatment evaluation research? What is its relationship to the goals of audiological rehabilitation? Who are the stakeholders of this type of research? *Ear and Hearing*, 21, S60–S73.

Gagné, J. P. (2003). Treatment effectiveness research in audiological rehabilitation: Fundamental issues related to dependent variables. *International Journal of Audiology*, 42, S104–S111.

Gagné, J. P., & Boutin, L. (1997). The effects of speaking rate on visual speech intelligibility. In C. Benoit & R. Campbell (Eds.), *Proceedings of the Workshop on Audio-visual Speech Processing* (pp. 29–32).

Gagné, J. P., Charest, M., Monday, K. L., & Desbiens, C. (2006). Evaluation of an audiovisual-FM system: Speechreading performance as a function of distance. *International Journal of Audiology*, 45, 295–300.

Gagné, J. P., Dinon, D., & Parsons, J. (1991). An evaluation of CAST: A computer-aided speechreading training program. *Journal of Speech and Hearing Research*, 34, 213–221.

Gagné, J. P., & Jennings, M. B. (2000). Audiological rehabilitation intervention services for adults with acquired hearing impairment. In M. Valente, H. Hosford-Dunn, & R. J. Roeser (Eds.), *Audiology Treatment* (pp. 547–579), New York, NY: Thieme.

Gagné, J. P., Laplante-Levesque, A., & Labelle, M. (2006). Evaluation of an audiovisual-FM system: Investigating the interaction between illumination level and a talker's skin color on speech-reading performance. *Journal of Speech, Language, and Hearing Research*, 49, 628–635.

Gagné, J. P., McDuff, S., & Getty, L. (1999). Some limitations of evaluative investigations based solely on normed outcome measures. *Journal of the American Academy of Audiology*, 10, 46–62.

Gagné, J. P., Stelmacovich, P., & Yovetich, W. (1991). Reactions to requests for clarification used by hearing-impaired individuals. *Volta Review*, 93, 129–143.

Gagné, J. P., Tugby, K. G., & Michoud, J. (1991). Development of a speechreading test on the utilization of contextual cues (STUCC): Preliminary findings with normal-hearing subjects. *Journal of the Academy of Rehabilitative Audiology*, 24, 157–170.

Gagné, J. P., & Wyllie, K. M. (1989). Relative effectiveness of three repair strategies on the visual-identification of misperceived words. *Ear and Hearing*, 10, 368–374.

Gallaudet Research Institute. (2003). *Regional and National Summary Report of Data from the 2001–2002 Annual Survey of Deaf and Hard of Hearing Children and Youth*. Washington, DC: Gallaudet University Press.

Garahan, M. B., Waller, J. A., Houghton, M., Tisdale, W. A., & Runge, C. F. (1992). Hearing loss prevalence and management in nursing home residents. *Journal of the American Geriatric Society*, 40, 130–134.

Gardner, E., Rudman, H., Karlsen, B., & Merwin, J. (1982). *Stanford Achievement Test*. San Antonio, TX: The Psychological Corp.

Garstecki, D. C., & Erler, S. F. (1998). Hearing loss, control, and demographic factors influencing hearing aid use among older adults. *Journal of Speech, Language, and Hearing Research*, 41, 527–537.

Garstecki, D. C., & Erler, S. F. (1999). Older adult performance on the communication profile for the hearing impaired: Gender difference. *Journal of Speech, Language, and Hearing Research,* 42, 785–796.

Garstecki, D. C., & O'Neill, J. J. (1980). Situational cue strategy influence on speechreading. *Scandinavian Audiology*, 9, 147–151.

Gatehouse, S. (1999). Glasgow hearing aid benefit profile: Derivation and validation of a client-centered outcome measure for hearing aid services. *Journal of American Academy of Audiology*, 10, 80–103.

Gatehouse, S. (2003). Rehabilitation: Identification of needs, priorities and expectations, and the evaluation of benefit. *International Journal of Audiology*, 42, 2S77–2S83.

Gatehouse, S. (2005). There's more than you thought to hearing and hearing aid effects. *The Hearing Journal*, August, 10–15.

Gatehouse, S., & Noble, W. (2004). The speech, spatial and qualities of hearing scale. *International Journal of Audiology*, 43, 85–99.

Geers, A. E. (2003). Predictors of reading skill development in children with early cochlear implantation. *Ear and Hearing*, 24, 59S–68S.

Geers, A. E., & Moog, J. S. (1992). Speech perception and production skills of students with impaired hearing from oral and total communication education settings. *Journal of Speech and Hearing Research*, 35, 1384–1393.

Geers, A. E., Nicholas, J., & Sedey, A. L. (2003). Language skills of children with early cochlear implantation. *Ear and Hearing*, 24, 46S–58S.

Gesi, A. T., Massaro, D., & Cohen, M. M. (1992). Discovery and expository methods in teaching visual consonant and word identification. *Journal of Speech and Hearing Research*, 35, 1180–1188.

Getty, L., & Hétu, R. (1991). Development of a rehabilitation program for people affected with occupational hearing loss. *Audiology,* 30, 317–329.

Gfeller, K., Christ, A., Knutson, J. F., Witt, S., & Mehr, M. (2003). The effects of familiarity and complexity on appraisal of complex songs by cochlear implant recipients and normal hearing adults. *Journal of Music Therapy*, 40, 78–112.

Gfeller, K., Mehr, M. A., & Witt, S. (2001). Aural rehabilitation of music perception and enjoyment of adult cochlear implant users. *Journal of the Academy of Aural Rehabilitation,* 34, 17–27.

Gfeller, K., Olszewski, C., Rychener, M., Sena, K., Knutson, J. F., Witt, S., et al. (2005). Recognition of "real world" musical excerpts by cochlear implant recipients and normal-hearing adults. *Ear and Hearing*, 26, 237–250.

Gfeller, K., & Schum, R. (1994). Requisites for conversation: Engendering world knowledge. In N. Tye-Murray (Ed.), *Let's Converse: A How-to Guide to Develop and Expand Conversational Skills of Children and Teenagers Who are Hearing Impaired* (pp. 177–212). Washington, DC: Alexander Graham Bell Association for the Deaf.

Giolas, T. G., Owens, E., Lamb, S. H., & Schubert, E. D. (1979). Hearing performance inventory. *Journal of Speech and Hearing Disorders*, 44, 169–195.

Gitles, T. (1999). Re-inventing the profession: The relationship model of hearing care. *The Hearing Journal*, 52, 53–56.

Givens, G. D., & Greenfeld, D. (1982). Revision behaviors of normal and hearing-impaired children. *Ear and Hearing*, 3, 274–279.

Glennon, S. L. (1990). Homework activities for social skills training. In P. J. Schloss & M. A. Smith (Eds.), *Teaching Social Skills to Hearing-Impaired Students* (pp. 85–90). Washington, DC: Alexander Graham Bell Association for the Deaf.

Golding-Meadow, S., & Mayberry, R. I. (2001). How do profoundly deaf children learn to read? *Learning Disabilities Research and Practice*, 16, 222–229.

Goldman, R., & Fristoe, M. (1969). *Test of Articulation*. Circle Pines, MN: American Guidance Service.

Golz, A., Netzer, A., & Westerman, S. T. (2005). Reading performance in children with otitis media. *Otolaryngology Head & Neck Surgery*, 132, 495–499.

Goodale, C. (2003). Redefining the baby boomer image. *Advance for Audiologists,* 5, 51–52.

Gordon-Salant, S,. & Fitzgibbons, P. J. (1999). Profile of auditory processing in older listeners. *Journal of Speech, Language, and Hearing Research,* 42, 300–310.

Grant, K. W., & Seitz, P. F. (2000). The recognition of isolated words and words in sentences: Individual variability in the use of sentence context. *Journal of the Acoustical Society of America*, 107, 1000–1011.

Grant, K. W., Walden, B. E., & Seitz, P. F. (1998). Auditory-visual speech recognition by hearing-impaired subjects: Consonant recognition, sentence recognition, and auditory-visual integration. *Journal of the Acoustical Society of America*, 103, 2677–2690.

Green, W., & Shephard, D. (1975). The semantic structure in deaf children. *Journal of Communication Disorders*, 8, 357–365.

Greenberg, S. (1999). Speaking in shorthand: A syllable-centric perspective for understanding pronunciation variability. *Speech Communication*, 29, 159–176.

Greenburg, J. H., & Jenkins, J. J. (1964). Studies in the psychological correlates of the sound system of American English. *Word*, 20, 157–177.

Grice, H. P. (1975). Logic and conversation. In P. Cole & J. Morgan (Eds.), *Syntax and Semantics 3: Speech Acts* (pp. 41–58). New York, NY: Academic Press.

Griswold, E., & Cummings, J. (1974). The expressive vocabulary of preschool deaf children. *American Annals of the Deaf*, 119, 16–28.

Groher, M. E. (1989). Modifications in assessment and treatment for the communicatively impaired elderly. In R. Hull & K. Griffin (Eds.), *Communication Disorders in Aging* (pp. 50–72). Newbury Park, CA: Sage.

Hager, R. M. (2007). Obtaining hearing aids for children. *Volta Voices*, July/August, 20–24.

Hale, S., & Myerson, J. (1996). Experimental evidence for differential slowing in the lexical and nonlexical domains. *Aging, Neuropsychology, and Cognition*, 3, 154–165.

Halford, J., & Aderson, S. (1991). Tinnitus severity measured by a subjective scale, audiometry and clinical judgment. *Journal of Laryngology and Otology*, 105, 89–93.

Hall, J. W., Smith, S. D., & Popelka, G. R. (2004). Newborn hearing screening with combined otoacoustic emissions and auditory brainstem responses. *Journal of the American Academy of Audiology*, 15, 414–425.

Hallam, R. S., & Brooks, D. N. (1996). Development of the hearing attitudes in rehabilitation questionnaire (HARQ). *British Journal of Audiology*, 30, 199–213.

Hallam, R. S., Jakes, S. C., & Hinchcliffe, R. (1988). Cognitive variables in tinnitus annoyance. *British Journal of Clinical Psychology*, 27, 213–222.

Hallberg, L. R.-M. (1996). Occupational hearing loss: Coping and family life. *Scandinavian Audiology*, 25, 25–33.

Hallberg, L. R.-M. (1998). Evaluation of a Swedish version of the hearing disabilities and handicaps scale, based on a clinical sample of 101 men with noise-induced hearing loss. *Scandinavian Audiology*, 27, 21–29.

Hallberg, L. R.-M. (1999). Hearing impairment, coping, and consequences on family life. *Journal of the Academy of Rehabilitative Audiology*, 32, 45–59.

Hallberg, L. R.-M., & Barrenäs, M.-L. (1995). Coping with noise-induced hearing loss: Experiences form the perspective of middle-aged male victims. *British Journal of Audiology*, 29, 219–230.

Hallberg, L. R.-M., & Jansson, G. (1996). Women with noise-induced hearing loss: An invisible group? *British Journal of Audiology*, 30, 340–345.

Hallman, R. S., McKenna, L., & Shurlock, L. (2004). Tinnitus impairs cognitive efficiency. *International Journal of Audiology*, 43, 218–226.

Hampton, D. (2005). Desertion or retention? *Advance for Audiologists*, September/October, 59–79.

Hanin, L. (1988). *The effects of experience and linguistic context on speechreading*. Unpublished doctoral dissertation, City University Graduate School, New York, NY.

Hanratty, V., & Lawlor, D. A. (2000). Effective management of the elderly hearing impaired: A review. *Journal of Public Health Medicine*, 22, 512–517.

Hansen, D., & Howard, S. R. (1992). *Facilitating Early Language*. Vero Beach, FL: The Speech Bin.

Harker, L. A., Vanderheiden, S., Veazey, D., Gentile, N., & McCleary, E. (1999). Multichannel cochlear implantation in children with large vestibular aqueduct syndrome. *Annals of Otology, Rhinology, and Laryngology*, 108, 39–43.

Harless, E., & McConnell, F. (1982). Effects of hearing aid use on self concept in older persons. *Journal of Speech and Hearing Disorders*, 47, 305–309.

Harvey, M. A. (2003). *Psychotherapy with Deaf and Hard-of-Hearing Persons: A Systematic Model* (2nd Ed.). Mahwah, NJ: Erlbaum.

Hasenstab, M. S., & Tobey, E. A. (1991). Language development in children receiving Nucleus multichannel cochlear implants. *Ear and Hearing*, 12, 55S–65S.

Haskins, H. (1949). *A phonetically balanced test of speech discrimination for children*. Unpublished master's thesis, Northwestern University, Evanston, IL.

Hawkins, D. B. (2005). Effectiveness of a counseling-based adult group aural rehabilitation programs: A systematic review of the evidence. *Journal of the American Academy of Audiology*, 16, 485–493.

Haycock, G. S. (1933). *The Teaching of Speech*. Washington, DC: Alexander Graham Bell Association for the Deaf.

Hayes, D. (2003). Screening methods: Current status. *Mental Retardation and Developmental Disabilities Research Reviews*, 9, 65–72.

Haynes, W., Moran, M., & Pindzola, R. (2006). *Communication Disorders in the Classroom* (4th Ed.). Sudbury, ENG: Jones & Bartlett.

Hayward, M. D., Crimmins, E. M., Miles, T. P., & Yang, Y. (2000). The significance of socioeconomic status in explaining the racial gap in chronic health conditions. *American Sociological Review*, 65, 910–930.

Hazard, W. R., Andrews, R., Bierman, E. L., & Blass, J. P. (1990). *Principles of Geriatric Medicine and Gerontology* (2nd Ed.). New York, NY: McGraw-Hill.

He, W., Sengupta, M., Velkoff, V. A., & DeBarros, K. A. (2005). *65+ in the United States: 2005*. Issued December 2005. Washington, DC: U.S. Department of Health and Human Services.

Hear-It Organization. (2003). *Costly for the individual—expensive for society*. Retrieved 01-20-07, from http://www.press.hear-it.org.

Heide, V. H. (2005). Can your patients pass the road test? *Advance for Audiologists*, March/April, 63–65.

Helfer, K. S. (1997). Auditory and auditory-visual perception of clear and conversational speech. *Journal of Speech Language Hearing Research*, 40, 432–443.

Helfer, K. S. (2001). Gender issues in audiologic rehabilitation. *Journal of the Academy of Rehabilitative Audiology*, 34, 41–52.

Heller, P. J. (1990). Psycho-educational assessment. In M. Ross (Ed.), *Hearing-Impaired Children in the Mainstream* (pp. 45–60). Baltimore, MD: York Press.

Henry, J. A., Dennis, K. C., & Schechter, M. A. (2005). General review of tinnitus: Prevalence, mechanisms, effects, and management. *Journal of Speech, Language, and Hearing Research*, 48, 1204–1235.

Henry, J. A., Zaug, T. L., & Schechter, M. A. (2005). Clinical guide for audiologic tinnitus management I: Assessment. *American Journal of Audiology*, 14, 21–48.

Herbert, S., & Carrier, J. (2007). Sleep complaints in elderly tinnitus patients: A controlled study. *Ear & Hearing*, 28, 649–655.

Hergils, L., & Hergils, A. (2000). Universal neonatal hearing screening—parental attitudes and concern. *British Journal of Audiology*, 34, 321–327.

Hermann, B. S., Thornton, A. R., & Joseph, J. M. (1995). Automated infant hearing screening using the ABR: Development and validation. *American Journal of Audiology*, 4, 6–14.

Hernandez, D., & Amlani, A. M. (2004). Patient, client or consumer? *Audiology Today*, September/October, 32–35.

Hétu, R. (1996). The stigma attached to hearing impairment. *Scandinavian Audiology*, 43, 12–24.

Hétu, R., Getty, L., Philibert, L., Desilets, F., Noble, W., & Stephens, D. (1994). Development of a clinical tool for the measurement of the severity of hearing disabilities and handicaps. *Journal of Speech-Language Pathology and Audiology* [French], 18, 82–95.

Hétu, R., Jones, L., & Getty, L. (1993). The impact of acquired hearing impairment on intimate relationships: Implications for rehabilitation. *Audiology*, 32, 363–381.

Hétu, R., Lalande, M., & Getty, L (1987). Psychological disadvantages associated with occupational hearing loss as experienced in the family. *Audiology*, 26, 141–152.

Hétu, R., Reverin, L., Lalande, N., Getty, L. & St-Cyr, C. (1988). Qualitative analysis of the handicap associated with occupational hearing loss. *British Journal of Audiology*, 22, 251–264.

Hétu, R., Reverin, L., Getty, L., Lalande, N. M., & St-Cyr, C. (1990). The reluctance to acknowledge hearing difficulties among hearing-impaired workers. *British Journal of AudiAudiology*, 24, 265–276.

Heydebrand, G., Mauzé, E., Tye-Murray, N., Binzer, S. & Skinner, M. (2005). The efficacy of a structured group therapy intervention for adult cochlear implant recipients. *International Journal of Audiology*, 44, 272–280.

Hickson, L. & Worrall, L. (2003). Beyond hearing aid fitting: Improving communication for older adults. *International Journal of Audiology*, 42 (Suppl. 2), 2S84–91.

Hickson, L., Worrall, L., & Scarinci, N. (2006a). *Active Communication Education (ACE): A Program for Older Persons with Hearing Impairment.* Brackley, ENG: Speechmark.

Hickson, L., Worrall, L., & Scarinci, N. (2006b). Measuring outcomes of a communication program for older people with hearing impairment using the International Outcome Inventory. *International Journal of Audiology*, 45, 238–246.

Higgins, M. B., McCleary, E. A., Carney, A. E., & Schulte, L. (2003). Longitudinal changes in children's speech and voice physiology after cochlear implantation. *Ear and Hearing*, 24, 48–70.

High, W. S., Fairbanks, G., & Glorig, A. (1964). Scale for self-assessment of hearing handicap. *Journal of Speech and Hearing Disorders,* 29, 215–230.

Hirsh, I. J., Davis, H., Silverman, S. R., Reynolds, E. G., Eldert, E., & Benson, R. W. (1952). Development of materials for speech audiometry. *Journal of Speech and Hearing Disorders,* 17, 321–337.

Hnath-Chisolm, T. E. (1997). Context effects in auditory training with children. *Scandinavian Audiology*, 26, 64–69.

Hnath-Chisolm, T. E., Laipply, E., & Boothroyd, A. (1998). Age-related changes on a children's test of sensory-level speech perception capacity. *Journal of Speech, Language, and Hearing Research*, 41, 94–106.

Hogan, A. (2001). *Hearing Rehabilitation for Deafened Adults: A Psychosocial Approach.* Philadelphia, PA: Whurr.

Holgers, K.-M., & Juul, J. (2006). The suffering of tinnitus in childhood and adolescence. *International Journal of Audiology*, 45, 267–272.

Holgers, K.-M., Zöger, S., & Svedlund, K. (2005). Predictive factors for development of severe tinnitus suffering: Further characterization. *International Journal of Audiology*, 44, 584–592.

Honnell, S., Dancer, J., & Gentry, B. (1991). Age and speechreading performance in relation to percent correct, eye blinks, and written responses. *Volta Review*, 93, 207–231.

Hoover, B. M. (2001). Hearing aid fitting in infants. *Volta Review*, 102, 57–73.

Horii, Y. (1982). Some voice fundamental frequency characteristics of oral reading and spontaneous speech by hard-of-hearing young women. *Journal of Speech and Hearing Research,* 25, 608–610.

Horowitz, A., Teresi, J. A., & Cassels, L. A. (1991). Development of a vision screening questionnaire for older people. *Journal of Gerontological Social Work*, 17, 37–56.

Houle, C. O. (1997). *Governing Boards.* San Francisco, CA: Jossey-Bass.

House, J., Lanids, K., & Umberson, D. (1988). Social relationships and health. *Science*, 241, 540–545.

Hull, R. H. (1995). *Hearing in Aging.* Clifton Park, NY: Delmar Learning.

Hull, R. H. (1997). Hearing loss in older adulthood. In R. H. Hull (Ed.), *Aural Rehabilitation: Serving Children and Adults* (3rd Ed.) (pp. 373–392). Clifton Park, NY: Delmar Learning.

Hull, R. H., & Griffin, K. (1992). *Communication Disorders in Aging.* Beverly Hills, CA: Sage.

Humes, L. E. (1996). Speech understanding in the elderly. *Journal of the American Academy of Audiology*, 7, 161–167.

Humes, L. E. (1999). Dimensions of hearing aid outcome. *Journal of the American Academy of Audiology*, 10, 26–39.

Humes, L. E. (2004). As outcome measures proliferate, how do you choose which ones to use? *The Hearing Journal*, 57, 10–17.

Humes, L. E. (2005). Do "auditory processing" tests measure auditory processing in the elderly? *Ear and Hearing*, 26, 109–119.

Humes, L. E., Coughlin, M., & Talley, L. (1996). Evaluation of the use of a new compact disc for auditory perceptual assessment in the elderly. *Journal of the American Academy of Audiology*, 7, 419–427.

Hutton, C. L. (1980). Responses to a hearing problem inventory. *Journal of the Academy of Rehabilitative Audiology*, 13, 133–154.

Huttunen, K. H. (2001). Educational needs of speech and language therapists in the field of audiology. *Scandinavian Audiology*, 30, 88–89.

Hyde, M. L., & Riko, K. (1994). A decision-analytic approach to audiological rehabilitation. *Journal of the Academy of Rehabilitative Audiology*, 27, 337–374.

Hygge, S., Rönnberg, J., Larsby, B., & Arlinger, S. (1992). Normal and hearing-impaired subjects' ability to just follow conversation in competing speech, reversed speech, and noise backgrounds. *Journal of Speech and Hearing Research*, 35, 208–215.

Ijsseldijk, F. J. (1992). Speechreading performance under different conditions of video image, repetition, and speech rate. *Journal of Speech and Hearing Research*, 35, 466–471.

Israelite, N., Ower, J., & Goldstein, G. (2002). Hard-of-hearing adolescents and identity construction: Influences of school experiences, peers, and teachers. *Journal of Deaf Studies and Deaf Education*, 7, 134–148.

Itoh, M., Horii, Y., Daniloff, R., & Binnie, C. (1982). Selected aerodynamic characteristics of deaf individuals' various speech and nonspeech tasks. *Folia Phoniatrica*, 34, 191–209.

Janota, J. (1999). Otitis media. ASHA, May/June, 48.

Jastreboff, M. M., & Jastreboff J. (1999). *Questionnaires for the assessment of patients and treatment outcome.* Paper presented at the Sixth International Tinnitus Seminar, Cambridge, England.

Jastreboff, P. J. (1990). Phantom auditory perception (tinnitus): Mechanisms of generation and perception. *Neuroscience Research*, 8, 221–254.

Jastreboff, P. J. (2000). Tinnitus habituation therapy (THT) and tinnitus retraining therapy (TRT). In R. Tyler (Ed.), *Tinnitus Handbook* (pp. 357–376). Clifton Park, NY: Delmar Learning.

Jastreboff, P. J., Gray, W. C., & Gold, S. L. (1996). Neurophysiological approach to tinnitus patients. *American Journal of Otology*, 17, 236–240.

Jeffers, J., & Barley, M. (1971). *Speechreading (Lipreading)*. Springfield, IL: Thomas.

Jenkins, L., Myerson, J., Joerding, J. A., & Hale, S. (2000). Converging evidence that visuospatial cognition is more age-sensitive than verbal cognition. *Psychology and Aging*, 15, 157–175.

Jennings, M. B. (1993). *Aural Rehabilitation Curriculum Series: Hearing Help Class II: Coping with Hearing Loss*. Toronto, Ontario, CAN: Canadian Hearing Society.

Jensema, C., & Trybus, R. (1978). *Communication patterns and educational achievement of hearing impaired students* (Series T, No. 2). Washington, DC: Gallaudet College, Office of Demographic Studies.

Jerger, J., Speaks, C., & Trammell, J. L. (1968). A new approach to speech audiometry. *Journal of Speech and Hearing Disorders*, 33, 318–329.

Jerram, J. C., & Purdy, S. C. (2001). Technology, expectations, and adjustment to hearing loss: Predictions of hearing-aid outcome. *Journal of the American Academy of Audiology*, 12, 64–75.

Jiménez-Sánchez, C., & Antia, S. (1999). Team-teaching in an integrated classroom: Perceptions of deaf and hearing teachers. *Journal of Deaf Studies and Deaf Education*, 4, 215–224.

John, J., & Howarth, J. (1976). The effect of time distortions on the intelligibility of deaf children's speech. *Language and Speech*, 8, 127–134.

Johnson, C. D. (2006). *How the Individuals with Disabilities Education Act (IDEA) Applies to Deaf and Hard of Hearing Students*. Washington, DC: Laruent Clerc National Deaf Education Center.

Johnson, D. D. (1975). Communication characteristics of NTID students. *Journal of the Academy of Rehabilitative Audiology*, 8, 17–32.

Johnson, S. M., & Wilhite, G. (1971). Self-observation as an agent of behavioral change. *Behavior Therapy*, 2, 488–497.

Joint Committee on Infant Hearing (1994). 1994 Position statement. *International Journal of Pediatric Otorhinolaryngology*, 32, 265–274.

Joint Committee on Infant Hearing (2000). 2000 Position statement, principles, and guidelines for early hearing detection and intervention programs. *Pediatrics*, 106, 798–817.

Jones, D. L., Gao, S., & Svirsky, M. A. (2003). The effect of short-term auditory deprivation on the control of intraoral pressure in pediatric cochlear implant users. *Journal of Speech, Language, and Hearing Research*, 46, 658–669.

Jones, L., Kyle, J., & Wood, P. (1987). *Words Apart: Losing Your Hearing as an Adult*. New York, NY: Tavistock.

Jordan, T. R., & Bevan, K. (1997). Seeing and hearing rotated faces: Influences of facial orientation on visual and audiovisual speech recognition. *Journal of Experimental Psychology: Human Perception and Performance*, 23, 288–403.

Jordan, T. R., & Sergeant, P. (2000). Effects of distance on visual and audiovisual speech recognition. *Language and Speech*, 43, 107–124.

Jorgensen, B. (2005). Sound effects. *Advance for Audiologists*, March/April, 25–29.

Kaiser, A., Hancock, T., & Nietfeld, J. (2000). The effects of parent implemented enhanced milieu teaching on the social communication of children who have autism. *Early Education and Developmental Disorders*, 11, 423–446.

Kaiser, A. R., Kirk, K. I., Lachs, L., & Pisoni, D. B. (2003). Talker and lexical effects on audiovisual word recognition by adults with cochlear implants. *Journal of Speech, Language, and Hearing Research*, 46, 390–404.

Kantrowitz, B., & Springen, K. (2007, June 18). Confronting Alzheimer's. *Newsweek*, 55–64.

Kaplan, H. (1996). Assistive devices for the elderly. *Journal of the American Academy of Audiology*, 7, 203–211.

Kaplan, H., Bally, S. J., & Brandt, F. (1995). Revised communication self-assessment scale inventory for deaf adults (CSDA). *Journal of the American Academy of Audiology*, 6, 311–329.

Kaplan, H., Bally, S. J., Brandt, F., Busacco, D., & Pray, J. (1997). Communications scale for older adults (CSOA). *Journal of the American Academy of Audiology*, 8, 203–217.

Kaplan, H., Bally, S. J., & Garretson, C. (1985). *Speechreading: A Way to Improve Understanding*. Washington, DC: Gallaudet University Press.

Kaplan, H., Feeley, J., & Brown, J. (1978). A modified Denver scale: Test–retest reliability. *Journal of the Academy of Rehabilitation Audiology*, 11, 15–32.

Kashinath, S., Woods, J., & Goldstein, H. (2006). Enhancing generalized teaching strategy use in daily routines by parents of children with autism. *Journal of Speech, Language, and Hearing Research*, 49, 466–485.

Katz, S. (1983). Assessing self-maintenance: Activities of daily living, mobility, and instrumental activities of daily living. *Journal of the American Geriatric Society*, 31, 721–727.

Kaufman, A., & Kaufman, N. (1983). *Kaufman Assessment Battery for Children (K-ABC)*. Circle Pines, MN: American Guidance Service.

Keate, B. (2006). Diet and tinnitus. *Advance for Audiologists*, September/October, 55–58.

Kempter, S. (1986). Imitation of complex syntactic constructions by elderly adults. *Applied Psycholinguistics*, 7, 277–288.

Kentish, R. C., Crocker, S. R., & McKenna, L. (2000). Children's experience of tinnitus: A preliminary survey of children presenting to a psychology department. *British Journal of Audiology*, 34, 335–340.

Keogh, T., Kei, J., Driscoll, C., Cahill, L., Hoffmann, A., Wilce, E., et al. (2005). Measuring the ability of school children with a history of otitis media to understand everyday speech. *Journal of the American Academy of Audiology*, 16, 301–311.

Kerr, P. C., & Cowie, R. I. D. (1997). Acquired deafness: A multi-dimensional experience. *British Journal of Audiology*, 31, 177–188.

Kessels, R. P. C. (2003). Patients' memory for medical information. *Journal of the Royal Society of Medicine*, 96, 219–222.

Kiese-Himmel, C., & Reeh, M. (2006). Assessment of expressive vocabulary outcomes in hearing-impaired children with hearing aids: Do bilaterally hearing-impaired children catch up? *The Journal of Laryngology & Otology*, 120, 619–626.

Kileny, P. R., Zwolan, T. A., & Ashbaugh, C. (2001). The influence of age at implantation on performance with a cochlear implant in children. *Otology and Neurotology*, 22, 42–46.

Killion, M. C., & Villchur, E. (1993). Kessler was right—partly: But SIN test shows some aids improve hearing in noise. *Hearing Journal*, 46, 31–35.

Kirchner, R., & Peterson, R. (1980). Multiple impairments among noninstitutionalized blind and visually impaired persons. *Journal of Visual Impairment and Blindness*, 74, 42–44.

Kirk, K. I. (1998). Assessing speech perception in listeners with cochlear implants: The development of the lexical neighborhood tests. *Volta Review*, 100, 63–86.

Kirk, K. I., Firszt, J. B., Hood, L. J., & Holt, R. F. (2006). New directions in pediatric cochlear implantation: Effects on candidacy. *ASHA Leader*, 11, 6–7,14–15.

Kirk, K. I., Miyamoto, R. T., Ying, E. A., Perdew, A. E., & Zuganelis, H. (2002). Cochlear implantation in young children: Effects of age at implantation and communication mode. *Volta Review*, 102, 123–126.

Kirk, K. I., Pisoni, D. B., & Osberger, M. J. (1995). Lexical effects on spoken word recognition by pediatric cochlear implant users. *Ear and Hearing*, 16, 470–481.

Kirkwood, D. H. (1999). Dispensers in survey take satisfaction in their work, but many feel unappreciated. *The Hearing Journal*, 52, 19–32.

Kishon-Rabin, L., Haras, N., & Bergman, M. (1997). Multisensory speech perception of young children with profound hearing loss. *Journal of Speech, Language, and Hearing Research*, 40, 1135–1150.

Kishon-Rabin, L., & Henkin, Y. (2000). Age-related changes in the visual perception of phonologically significant contrasts. *British Journal of Audiology*, 34, 363–374.

Kishon-Rabin, L., Taitelbaum, R., Tobin, Y., & Hildesheimer, M. (1999). The effect of partially restored hearing on speech production of postlingually deafened adults with multi-channel cochlear implants. *Journal of the Acoustical Society of America*, 106, 2843–2857.

Kitano, Y., Siegenthaler, B. M., & Stoker, R. G. (1985). Facial hair as a factor in speechreading performance. *Journal of Communication Disorders*, 18, 373–381.

Kluwin, T. N. (1999). Co-teaching deaf and hearing students: Research on social integration. *American Annals of the Deaf*, 144, 339–344.

Knutson, J. F., & Lansing, C. R. (1990). The relationship between communication problems and psychological difficulties in persons with profound acquired hearing loss. *Journal of Speech and Hearing Disorders*, 55, 656–664.

Kochkin, S. (1999). Baby boomers spur growth in potential market, but penetration rate declines. *The Hearing Journal*, 52, 33–48.

Kochkin, S. (2000). MarkeTrakV: Why my hearing aids are in the drawer: The consumer perspective. *The Hearing Journal*, 53, 34–42.

Kochkin, S. (2002). Factors impacting consumer choice of dispenser and hearing aid brand. *The Hearing Review*, 9, 14–23.

Kochkin, S. (2005a). Customer satisfaction with hearing instruments in digital age. *The Hearing Journal*, 58, 30–43.

Kochkin, S. (2005b). MarkeTrak VII: Hearing loss population tops 31 million people. *The Hearing Review*, July, 16–29.

Kochkin, S. (2007). MarkeTrak VII: Obstacles to adult non-user adoption of hearing aids. *The Hearing Journal*, 60, 24–51.

Kopun, J. G., & Stelmachowicz, P. G. (1998). Perceived communication difficulties of children with hearing loss. *American Journal of Audiology*, 7, 30–38.

Kosky, C., & Boothroyd, A. (2001). Perception and production of sibilants by children with hearing loss: A training study. *Volta Review*, 103, 71–98.

Kozak, V. J., & Brooks, B. M. (2001). *Baby Talk: Helping Your Hearing-Impaired Baby Listen and Talk*. St. Louis, MO: Central Institute for the Deaf.

Kraaij, V., Arensman, E., & Spinhoven, P. (2002). Negative life events and depression in elderly persons. *Journal of Gerontology Series B: Psychological Sciences and Social Sciences*, 57, 87–94.

Kramer, S. E., Allessie, H. M., Dondorp, A. W., Zekveld, A. A., & Kapteyn, T. S. (2005). A home education program for older adults with hearing impairment and their significant others: A randomized clinical trial evaluating short- and long-term effects. *International Journal of Audiology*, 44, 255–264.

Kramer, S. E., Kapteyn, T. S., & Festen, J. M. (1998). The self-reporting handicapping effect of hearing disabilities. *Audiology*, 37, 302–310.

Kramer, S. E., Kapteyn, T. S., Festen, J. M., & Tobi, H. (1995). Factors in subjective hearing disability. *Audiology*, 34, 167–199.

Kramer, S. E., Kapteyn, T. S., Festen, J. M., & Tobi, H. (1996). The relationships between self-reported hearing disability and measurements of auditory disability. *Audiology*, 35, 277–287.

Krantz, P., MacDuff, M., & McClannahan, L. (1993). Programming participation in family activities for children with autism: Parents' use of photographic activity schedules. *Journal of Applied Behavior Analysis*, 26, 137–138.

Kraus, N., McGee, T., Carrell, T., King, C., Tremblay, K., & Nicol, T. (1995). Central auditory system plasticity associated with speech discrimination training. *Journal of Cognitive Neuroscience*, 7, 25–32.

Kravitz, L., & Selekman, J. (1992). Understanding hearing loss in children. *Pediatric Nursing*, 18, 591–594.

Kretschmer, R., & Kretschmer, L. (1978). *Language Development and Intervention with the Hearing Impaired*. Baltimore, MD: University Park Press.

Kretschmer, R., & Kretschmer, L. (1994). Discourse and hearing impairment. In D. Ripich & N. Creaghead (Eds.), *School Discourse Problems* (p. 263–296). San Diego, CA: Singular.

Kricos, P. B. (2006). Audiologic management of older adults with hearing loss and compromised cognitive/psychoacoustic auditory processing capabilities. *Trends in Amplification*, 10, 1–28.

Kricos, P. B., Erdman, S., Bratt, G. W., & Williams, D. W. (2007). Psychosocial correlates of hearing aid adjustment. *Journal of the American Academy of Audiology*, 18, 304–322.

Kricos, P. B., & Holmes, A. E. (1996). Efficacy of audiologic rehabilitation for older adults. *Journal of the American Academy of Audiology*, 7, 219–229.

Kricos, P. B., Holmes, A. E., & Doyle, D. (1992). Efficacy of a communication training program for hearing-impaired elderly adults. *Journal of the Academy of Rehabilitative Audiology*, 25, 69–80.

Kricos, P. B., & Lesner, S. A. (1995). *Hearing Care for the Older Adult: Audiologic Rehabilitation*. Boston, MA: Butterworth-Heinemann.

Kricos, P. B., Lesner, S. A., Sandridge, S. A., & Yanke, R. B. (1987). Perceived benefits of amplification as a function of central auditory status in the elderly. *Ear and Hearing*, 8, 337–342.

Kricos, P. B., & McCarthy, P. (2007). From ear to there: A historical perspective on auditory training. *Seminars in Hearing*, 28, 89–98.

Kuhl, P. K., & Meltzoff, A. N. (1982). The bimodal perception of speech in infancy. *Science*, 218, 1138–1141.

Kuk, F. K., Tyler, R. S., Russell, D., & Jordan, H. (1990). The psychometric properties of a tinnitus handicap questionnaire. *Ear and Hearing*, 11, 434–445.

Kynette, D., & Kemper, S. (1986). Aging and loss of grammatical forms: A cross-sectional study of language performance. *Language and Communication*, 6, 65–72.

Lach, R., Ling, D., Ling, L., & Ship, N. (1970). Early speech development in deaf infants. *American Annals of the Deaf*, 115, 522–526.

Lachs, L., Pisoni, D. B., & Kirk, K. I. (2001). Use of audiovisual information in speech perception by prelingually deaf children with cochlear implants: A first report. *Ear and Hearing*, 22, 236–251.

Lansing, C. R., & Davis, J. M. (1988). Early versus delayed speech perception training for adult cochlear implant users: Initial results. *Journal of the Academy of Rehabilitative Audiology*, 21, 29–41.

Lansing, C. R., & Helgeson, C. L. (1995). Priming the visual recognition of spoken words. *Journal of Speech and Hearing Research*, 38, 1377–1386.

Lansing, C. R., & McConkie, G. W. (1999). Attention to facial regions in segmental and prosodic visual speech perception tasks. *Journal of Speech, Language, and Hearing* Research, 42, 526–539.

Laski, K., Charlop, M., & Schreibman, L. (1988). Training parents to use the natural language paradigm to increase their autistic children's speech. *Journal of Applied Behavior Analysis*, 21, 391–400.

Lawton, M. P. & Brody, E. M. (1969). Assessment of older people: Self-maintaining and instrumental activities of daily living. *Gerontology*, 19, 179–185.

Lee, D. J., Gómez-Marín, O. & Lee, H. M. (1996). Sociodemographic correlates of hearing loss and hearing aid use in Hispanic adults. *Epidemiology*, 7, 443–446.

Lee, L. (1974). *Developmental Sentence Analysis*. Evanston, IL: Northwestern University Press.

Leigh, I. W. (1999). Inclusive education and personal development. *Journal of Deaf Studies and Deaf Education*, 4, 236–245.

Lesinski-Schiedat, A., Illg, A., Heermann, R., Bertram B., & Lenarz, T. (2004). Paediatric cochlear implantation in the first and in the second year of life: A comparative study. *Cochlear Implants International*, 5, 146–159.

Lesner, S. (1996). Group hearing care for older adults. In P. Kricos & S. Lesner (Eds.), *Hearing Care for the Older Adult: Audiologic Rehabilitation* (pp. 203–277). Newton, MA: Butterworth-Heinemann.

Lesner, S. (2003). Candidacy and management of assistive listening devices: Special needs of the elderly. *International Journal of Audiology*, 42, S68–S76.

Lesner, S., & Kricos, P. (1981). Visual vowel and diphthong perception across speakers. *Journal of the Academy of Rehabilitative Audiology*, 14, 252–258.

Lesner, S., Sandridge, S., & Kricos, P. (1987). Training influences on visual consonant and sentence recognition. *Ear and Hearing*, 8, 283–287.

Leung, J., Wang, N., Yeagle, J., Chinnici, J., Bowditch, S., Francis, H., et al. (2005). Predictive models for cochlear implantation in elderly candidates. *Archives of Otolaryngology—Head & Neck Surgery*, 131, 1049–1054.

Levitt, H. (1987). *Fundamental Speech Skills Test*. New York, NY: City University of New York.

Levitt, H., McGarr, N. S., & Geffner, D. (Eds.). (1987). *Development of Language and Communication Skills in Hearing-Impaired Children*. Washington, DC: American Speech-Language-Hearing Association.

Lictman, W. (2005, May). Seeing kids clearly. *Good Housekeeping*, 120.

Light, L., & Capps, J. (1986). Comprehension of pronouns in young and older adults. *Developmental Psychology*, 22, 580–585.

Lind, C., Hickson, L., & Erber, N. P. (2006). Conversation repair and adult cochlear implantation: A qualitative case study. *Cochlear Implants International*, 7, 33–48.

Ling, D. (1976). *Speech and the Hearing-Impaired Child: Theory and Practice*. Washington, DC: Alexander Graham Bell Association for the Deaf.

LitConn, Inc. (2000). *Reading and Oral Language Assessment (ROLA)*. Fresno, CA: LitConn, Inc.

Litovsky, R., Parkinson, A., Arcaroli, J., & Sammeth, C. (2006). Simultaneous bilateral cochlear implantation in adults: A multicenter clinical study. *Ear and Hearing, 27,* 714–731.

Lloyd, J. (1999). Hearing-impaired children's strategies for managing communication breakdowns. *Deafness and Education International, 1,* 188–199.

Lloyd, P., Boada, H., & Forns, M. (1992). New directions in referential communication research. *British Journal of Developmental Psychology, 10,* 385–403.

Lonka, E. (1995). Speechreading instruction for hard-of-hearing adults: Effects of training face-to-face and with a video programmer. *Scandinavian Audiology, 24,* 193–198.

Luce, P. A. (1986). A computational analysis of uniqueness points in auditory word recognition. *Perception and Psychophysics, 39,* 155–159.

Luce, P. A., & Pisoni, D. B. (1998). Recognizing spoken words: The neighborhood activation model. *Ear and Hearing, 19,* 1–36.

Luterman, D. (1987). *Deafness in the Family.* Washington, DC: Alexander Graham Bell Association for the Deaf.

Luterman, D. (2001). *Counseling Parents of Hearing-Impaired Children* (4th Ed.). Boston, MA: Little, Brown.

Luterman, D. (2004). Counseling families of children with hearing loss and special needs. *Volta Review, 104,* 215–220.

Luterman, D., & Kurtzer-White, E. (1999). Identifying hearing loss: Parents' needs. *American Journal of Audiology, 8,* 13–18.

Luterman, D., & Ross, M. (1991). *When Your Child Is Deaf.* Parkton, MD: York Press.

Luxford, W. M., & Brackmann, D. E. (1985). The history of cochlear implants. In R. F. Gray (Ed.), *Cochlear Implants* (pp. 1–26). San Diego, CA: College-Hill Press.

Lyman, R. (2006, March 10). Census report foresees no crisis over aging generation's health. *The New York Times,* 1, 17.

Lyxell, B. (1994). Skilled speechreading: A single-case study. *Scandinavian Journal of Audiology, 35,* 212–219.

Lyxell, B., & Rönnberg, J. (1987). Guessing and speechreading. *British Journal of Audiology, 21,* 13–20.

Lyxell, B., & Rönnberg, J. (1989). Information-processing skills and speechreading. *British Journal of Audiology, 23,* 339–347.

MacLeod, A., & Summerfield, Q. (1987). Quantifying the contribution of vision to speech perception in noise. *British Journal of Audiology*, 21, 131–141.

Madell, J. R. (2000). Counseling for diagnosis and management of auditory disorders in infants, children, and adults. In M. Valente, H. Hosford-Dunn, & R. J. Roeser (Eds.), *Audiology Treatment* (pp. 291–305). New York, NY: Thieme.

Mak, M., Grayden, D., Dowell, R. C., & Lawrence, D. (2006). Speech perception for adults who use hearing aids in conjunction with cochlear implants in opposite ears. *Journal of Speech, Language, and Hearing Research*, 49, 338–351.

Maki-Torkko, E., Brorsson, B., Davis, A., Mair, W., Myhre, K., Parving, A., et al. (2001). Hearing impairment among adults—Extent of the problem and scientific evidence on the outcome of hearing aid rehabilitation. *Scandinavian Audiology*, 30, 8–15.

Marcian, E., Carrabba, L., Giannini, P., Sementina, C., Verde, P., Bruno, C., et al. (2003). Psychiatric comorbidity in a population of outpatients affected by tinnitus. *International Journal of Audiology*, 42, 4–9.

Margolis, R. H. (2004). Audiology information counseling: What do patients remember? *Audiology Today*, March/April, 14–15.

Markides, A. (1970). The speech of deaf and partially hearing children with special reference to factors affecting intelligibility. *British Journal of Disordered Communication*, 5, 126–140.

Marmor, G., & Petitito, L. (1979). Simultaneous communication in the classroom: How well is English grammar represented? *Sign Language Studies*, 23, 99–136.

Marmor, M. F. (1998). Normal age-related vision changes and their effects on vision. *Aging & Vision Newsletter*, Spring, 1–7.

Marschark, M. (2003). Interactions of language and cognition in deaf learners: From research to practice. *International Journal of Audiology*, 42, S41–S48.

Marschark, M., Young, A., & Lukomski, J. (2002). Perspectives in inclusion. *Journal of Deaf Studies and Deaf Education*, 7, 187–188.

Marslen-Wilson, W. D., Moss, H. E., & van Halen, S. (1996). Perceptual distance and completion in lexical access. *Journal of Experimental Psychology: Human Perception and Performance*, 22, 1376–1392.

Martin, F. N., & Clark, J. G. (2006). *Introduction to Audiology* (9th Ed.). Boston, MA: Allyn & Bacon.

Martin, R. (2004). Wear your hearing aids or your brain will rust. *The Hearing Journal*, 57, 46.

Massaro, D. (1998). *Perceiving Talking Faces: From Speech Perception to a Behavioral Principle*. Cambridge, MA: MIT Press.

Massaro, D., & Cohen, M. M. (2000). Tests of auditory-visual integration efficiency within the framework of the fuzzy logical model of perception. *Journal of the Acoustical Society of America*, 108, 784–789.

Massaro, D., & Light, J. (2004). Using visible speech to train perception and production of speech for individuals with hearing loss. *Journal of Speech, Language, and Hearing Research*, 47, 304–320.

Mattys, S. L., Bernstein, L. E., & Auer, E. T. (2002). Stimulus-based lexical distinctiveness as a general word-recognition mechanism. *Perception and Psychophysics*, 64, 667–679.

Mauzé, E. Tye-Murray, N., & Jerger, S. (2007, October 21). *Effects of hearing loss and maturation on children's speechreading performance.* Paper presented at the Academy of Rehabilitative Audiology, St. Louis, MO.

McCullough, J. A., & Wilson, R. H. (2001). Performance on a Spanish picture-identification task using a multimedia format. *Journal of the American Academy of Audiology*, 12, 254–260, October 19–20.

McCracken, W., Young, A., & Tattersall, H. (2008). Universal newborn hearing screening: Parental reflections on very early audiological management. *Ear and Hearing*, 29, 54–64.

McCullough, J. A., Wilson, R. H., Birck, J. D., & Anderson, L. G. (1995). A multimedia approach for estimating speech recognition of multilingual clients. *American Journal of Audiology*, 3, 19–22.

McDowd, J. M., & Shaw, R. J. (2000). Attention and aging: A functional perspective. In F. Craik & T. Salthouse (Eds.), *The Handbook of Aging and Cognition* (2nd Ed.) (pp. 221–292). Mahwah, NJ: Erlbaum.

McFall, R. M. (1970). Effects of self-monitoring on normal smoking behavior. *Journal of Consulting and Clinical Psychology*, 35, 135–142.

McGarr, N. (1987). Communication skills of hearing-impaired children in schools for the deaf. In H. Levitt, N. McGarr, & D. Geffner (Eds.), Development of language and communication in hearing-impaired children. *ASHA Monographs*, 26, 91–107.

McGuire, R. (2002). Marketing to the baby boomer. *The Hearing Review*, September, 44–46.

McGukian, M., & Henry A. (2007). The grammatical morpheme deficit in moderate hearing impairment. *International Journal of Language and Communication Disorders*, 42 (Suppl. 1), 17–36.

McGurk, H., & MacDonald, J. (1976). Hearing lips and seeing voices. *Nature*, 264, 746–748.

Meister, H., Lausberg, I., Kiessling, J., von Wedel, H., & Walger, M. (2003). Modeling relationships between various domains of hearing aid provision. *Audiology & Neuro*-Otology, 8, 153–165.

McKenna, L. (1987). Goal planning in audiological rehabilitation. *British Journal of Audiology*, 21, 5–11.

Mellon, N. (2005). The River School: Educating children with hearing loss in an inclusion model. *ASHA Leader*, 3, 6–24.

Mendel, L., & Danhauer, J. (1997). *Audiologic Evaluation and Management and Speech Perception Assessment*. San Diego, CA: Singular.

Messina, J. J., & Messina, C. M. (2004). The Federal Laws Governing Education for Exceptional Students. Retrieved 02/11/04, from http://www.copying.org/involvepar/laws.htm.

Metz, D., Whitehead, R., & Whitehead, B. (1984). Mechanics of vocal fold vibration and laryngeal articulatory gestures produced by hearing-impaired speakers. *Journal of Speech and Hearing Research*, 27, 62–69.

Miller, D. A., & Fredrickson, J. M. (2000). Implantable hearing aids. In M. Valente, H. Hosford-Dunn, & R. J. Roeser (Eds.), *Audiology Treatment* (pp. 489–510). New York, NY: Thieme.

Miller, G. A., & Nicely, P. E. (1955). An analysis of perceptual confusions among some English consonants. *Journal of the Acoustical Society of America*, 27, 338–352.

Mills, J. H., Schmiedt, R. A., & Dubno, J. R. (2006). Older and wiser, but losing hearing nonetheless. *Hearing Health*, Summer, 12–19.

Miyamoto, R., Kirk, K. I., Svirsky, M. A., & Sehgal, S. T. (1999). Communication skills of pediatric cochlear implant recipients. *Acta Otolaryngologica*, 119, 219–224.

Mize, J., & Wigley, H. (2002, November). *Hearing the truth about pediatric audiology.* Paper presented at the American Speech-Language-Hearing Association Convention, Atlanta, GA.

Mohammed, T., Campbell, R., MacSweeney, M., Mine, E., Hansen, P., & Coleman, M. (2005). Speechreading skill and visual movement sensitivity are related in deaf speechreaders. *Perception*, 34, 205–216.

Monsen, R. (1976). The production of English stop consonants in the speech of deaf children. *Journal of Phonetics*, 4, 29–42.

Monsen, R. (1978). Toward measuring how well hearing-impaired children speak. *Journal of Speech and Hearing Research*, 21, 197–219.

Monsen, R. (1981). A usable test for the speech intelligibility of deaf talkers. *American Annals of the Deaf*, 126, 845–852.

Montgomery, A. A. (1994). WATCH: A practical approach to brief auditory rehabilitation. *The Hearing Journal*, 10, 10–55.

Montgomery, A.A., Walden, B. E., & Prosek, R. A. (1987). Effects of consonantal context on vowel lipreading. *Journal of Speech and Hearing Research*, 30, 50–59.

Montgomery, A., Walden, B., Schwartz, D., & Prosek, R. (1984). Training auditory-visual speech recognition in adults with moderate sensorineural hearing loss. *Ear and Hearing*, 5, 30–36.

Montoya, L. A. (2007, April). *The elephant in the room: Parental grief.* Paper presented at the American Academy of Audiology Convention, Denver, CO.

Moog, J. (1988). *The CID Phonetic Inventory.* St. Louis, MO: Central Institute for the Deaf.

Moog, J., Biedenstein, J., & Davidson, L. (1995). *SPICE: The Speech Perception Instructional Curriculum and Evaluation.* St. Louis, MO: Central Institute for the Deaf.

Moog, J., & Geers, A. E. (1979). *Grammatical Analysis of Elicited Language: Simple Sentence Level.* St. Louis, MO: Central Institute for the Deaf.

Moog, J., & Geers, A. E. (1990). *Early Speech Perception Test.* St. Louis, MO: Central Institute for the Deaf.

Moog, J. S., Kozak, V. J., & Geers, A. E. (1983). *Grammatical Analysis of Elicited Language (GAEL-p).* St. Louis, MO: Central Institute for the Deaf.

Moran, D., & Whitman, T. (1991). Developing generalized teaching skills in mothers of autistic children. *Child and Family Behavior Therapy*, 13, 13–37.

More, L. A. (2006). Empathy: A clinician's perspective. *ASHA Leader*, 7, 16–17, 35.

Most, T. (2002). The use of repair strategies by children with and without hearing impairment. *Language, Speech, and Hearing in Schools*, 33, 112–123.

Most, T. (2003). The use of repair strategies: Bilingual deaf children using sign language and spoken language. *American Annals of the Deaf*, 148, 308–314.

Moxley, A., Mahendra, N., & Vega-Barachowitz, C. (2004). Cultural competence in health care. *ASHA Leader*, 4, pp. 6–22.

Mueller, H. G. (1994). CIC hearing aids: What is their impact on the occlusion effect? *The Hearing Journal*, 47, 29–30, 32–35.

Mueller, H. G. (2001). Speech audiometry and hearing aid fittings: Going steady or casual acquaintances? *The Hearing Journal*, 54, 19–29.

Mueller, H. G., (2005). Fitting hearing aids to adults using prescriptive methods: An evidence-based review of effectiveness. *Journal of the American Academy of Audiology*, 16, 448–460.

Mueller, H. G., & Bentler, R. A. (2005). Fitting hearing aids using clinical measures of loudness discomfort levels: An evidence-based review of effectiveness. *Journal of the American Academy of Audiology*, 461–472.

Mueller, H. G., Bryant, M., Brown, W., & Budinger, A. (1991). Hearing aid selection for high-frequency hearing loss. In G. Studebaker, F. Bess, & L. Beck (Eds.), *The Vanderbilt Hearing-Aid Report II* (pp. 35–51). Parkton, MD: York Press.

Mueller, H. G., & Grimes, A. (1987). Amplification systems for the hearing impaired. In J. G. Alpiner & P. A. McCarthy (Eds.), *Rehabilitative Audiology: Children and Adults* (pp. 116–162). Baltimore, MD: Williams & Wilkins.

Mueller, H. G., & Palmer, C. V. (1998). The profile of aided loudness: A new "PAL" for 98. *The Hearing Journal*, 51, 10–19.

Mulrow, C., Aguilar, C., & Endicott, J. (1990). Association between hearing impairment and the quality of life of elderly individuals. *Journal of the American Geriatric Society*, 38, 45–50.

National Association of the Deaf. (1991). *Cochlear implants in children: A position paper of the National Association of the Deaf.* Silver Springs, MD: National Association of the Deaf.

National Center for Health Statistics. (1987). *Current Estimates From the National Health Interview Survey: United States, 1987* (Vital and Health Statistics, Series 10). Washington, DC: U.S. Government Printing Office.

National Center for Health Statistics (2002). *Chartbook on Trends in the Health of Americans, Excepted from Health United States, 2002* (Centers for Disease Control and Prevention/National Center for Health Statistics, Vital Health Statistics, Series 10, No. 209). Washington, DC: U.S. Government Printing Office.

National Council on Aging. (1999). *The Consequences of Untreated Hearing Loss in Older Persons.* Washington, DC: National Council on Aging.

National Dissemination Center for Children with Disabilities. (2003, October). *Deafness and Hearing Loss* (Disability Fact Sheet, No. 3). Washington, DC: National Dissemination Center for Children with Disabilities.

National Eye Institute Visual Functioning Questionnaire-25 (VFQ-25) (2000). Retrieved 07/06/07, from http://www.nei.nih.gov/resources/visionfunction/vfq_ia.pdf.

National Institute on Aging. (2002). *Alzheimer's Disease: Unraveling the Mystery* (National Institutes of Health Publication No. 02-3782, Department of Health and Human Services). Washington, DC: U.S. Government Printing Office.

National Institute of Deafness and Communication Disorders. (2002). *Report of the Ad Hoc Committee on Epidemiology and Statistics in Communication.* Washington, DC: NIDCD.

National Institutes of Health. (2006). *Fact Sheet: Newborn Hearing Screening.* Washington, DC: U.S. Department of Health and Human Services.

National Mental Health Association. (2003). *Depression and Older Americans.* Retrieved 03/07/07, from http://secured.nmha.org/ccd/support/factsheet.older.cfm/.

Neely, K. K. (1956). Effects of visual factors on the intelligibility of speech. *Journal of the Acoustical Society of America*, 28, 1275–1277.

Newby, H. A., & Popelka, G. R. (1992). *Audiology* (6th Ed.). Englewood Cliffs, NJ: Prentice-Hall.

Newman, C. W., Jacobson, G. P., & Spitzer, J. B. (1996). Development of the tinnitus handicap inventory. *Archives of Otolaryngology—Head & Neck Surgery*, 122, 143–148.

Newman, C. W., Weinstein, B. E., Jacobson, G. P., & Hug, G. A. (1990). The hearing handicap inventory for adults: Psychometric adequacy and audiometric correlates. *Ear and Hearing*, 11, 430–433.

Nicholas, M., Barth, C., Obler, L. K., Au, R., & Albert, M. L. (1997). Naming in normal aging and dementia of the Alzheimer's type. In H. Goodlass & A. Wingfield (Eds.), *Neuroanatomical and Cognitive Correlates* (pp. 166–188). San Diego, CA: Academic Press.

Nidday, K. J., & Elfenbein, J. L. (1991). The effects of visual barriers used during auditory training on sound transmission. *Journal of Speech and Hearing Research*, 34, 694–696.

Nilsson, M., Soli, S. D., & Sullivan, J. A. (1994). Development of the hearing in noise test for the measurement of speech reception thresholds in quiet and in noise. *Journal of the Acoustical Society of America*, 95, 1085–1099.

Niskar, A. S., Kieszak, S. M., Holmes, A., Esteban, E., Rubin, C., & Brody, D. J. (1998). Prevalence of hearing loss among children 6 to 19 years of age. *Journal of the American Medical Association*, 279, 1071–1075.

Nix, G. W. (1983). How total is total communication? *Journal of British Association for Teachers of the Deaf*, 7, 177–181.

Noble, W. (1996). What is a psychosocial approach to hearing loss? *Scandinavian Audiology*, 25, 6–11.

Noffsinger, D., Wilson, R. H., & Musiek, F. E. (1994). Department of Veterans Affairs Compact Disc (VA-CD) recording for auditory perceptual assessment: Background and introduction. *Journal of the American Academy of Audiology*, 5, 231–235.

Nondahl, D. M., Cruickshanks, K. J., Dalton, D. S., Klein, B., Klein, R., Schubert, C. R., et al. (2007). The impact of tinnitus on quality of life in older adults. *Journal of the American Academy of Audiology*, 18, 257–266.

Northern, J., & Beyer, C. M. (1999). Reducing hearing aid returns through patient education. *Audiology Today*, 11, 10–11.

Northern, J., & Downs, M. P. (1991). *Hearing in Children* (4th Ed.). Baltimore, MD: Williams and Wilkins.

Nusbaum, N. J. (1999). Aging and sensory senescence. *Southern Medical Journal*, 92, 267–275.

Nussbaum, J. F., Thompson, T., & Robinson, J. D. (1989). *Communication and Aging*. New York, NY: Harper & Row.

Odom, S. L., Blanton, R. L., & Laukhuf, C. (1973). Facial expression and interpretation of emotion-arousing situations in deaf and hearing children. *Journal of Abnormal Psychology*, 1, 139–151.

O'Donoghue, G. M., Nikolopoulos, T. P., & Archbold, S. M. (2000). Determinants of speech perception in children after cochlear implantation. *The Lancet*, 9228, 466–468.

Ohna, S. E. (2003). Education of deaf children and the politics of recognition. *Journal of Deaf Studies and Deaf Education*, 8, 5–10.

Osberger, M. J., & Fischer, L. M. (2000). Preoperative predictors of postoperative implant performance in children. *Annals of Otology, Rhinology, and Laryngology*, 109, 44–46.

Oticon (2006). *Teacher's Guide*. Denmark: Oticon.

Ouni, S., Cohen, M. Ishak, H., & Massaro, D. (2007). Visual contribution to speech perception: Measuring the intelligibility of animated talking heads. *Eurasip Journal of Audio Speech Music Process*, Article ID 47891.

Paatsch, L. E., Blamey, P. J., & Sarant, J. Z. (2001). Effects of articulation training on the production of trained and untrained phonemes in conversations and formal tests. *Journal of Deaf Studies and Deaf Education*, 6, 32–42.

Pakulski, L. A. & Kaderavek, J. N. (2001). Narrative production by children who are deaf or hard of hearing: The effect of role-play. *Volta Review*, 103, 127–139.

Pallarito, K. (2006). Overburdened and under-appreciated, school audiologists forge ahead. *The Hearing Journal*, 59, 19–24.

Palmer, C., Bentler, R., & Mueller, H. G. (2006). Evaluation of a second-order directional microphone hearing aid: II. Self-report outcomes. *Journal of the American Academy of Audiology*, 27, 190–201.

Palmer, C. V., Mueller, H. G., & Moriarty, M. (1999). Profile of aided loudness: A validation procedure. *The Hearing Journal*, 52, 34–42.

Palmer, C., Nelson, C., & Lindley, G. (1998). The functionally and physiologically plastic adult auditory system. *Journal of the Acoustical Society of America*, 103, 1705–1721.

Pascoe, D. P. (1995). Post-fitting and rehabilitative management of the adult hearing-aid user. In R. E. Sandlin (Ed.), *Handbook of Hearing Aid Amplification (Vol. 2,)* (pp. 61–86). Clifton Park, NY: Delmar Learning.

Paul, P. V., & Jackson, D. W. (1993). *Toward a Psychology of Deafness*. Boston, MA: Allyn & Bacon.

Paul, R. G., & Cox, R. M. (1995). Measuring hearing aid benefit with the APHAB: Is this as good as it gets? *American Journal of Audiology*, 4, 10–13.

Pederson, K. E., Rosenthal, U., & Moller, M. B. (1991). Longitudinal study of changes in speech perception between 70 and 81 years of age. *Audiology*, 30, 201–211.

Pedley, K., Giles, E., & Hogan, A. (2005). *Adult Cochlear Implant Rehabilitation*. London, ENG: Whurr.

Pedley, K., Tari, S., & Drinkwater, T. (2003). Cochlear implantation in older adults. *Hear Now*, August, 1–6.

Pelli, D., Robson, J., & Wilkins, A. (1998). The design of a new letter chart for measuring contrast sensitivity. *Clinical Vision Science, 2,* 187–199.

Peng, S., Spencer, L. J., & Tomblin, J. B. (2004). Speech intelligibility of pediatric cochlear implant recipients with 7 years of device experience. *Journal of Speech, Language, and Hearing Research*, 47, 1227–1236.

Picheny, M. A., Durlach, N., & Braida, L. D. (1985). Speaking clearly for the hard of hearing I: Intelligibility differences between clear and conversational speech. *Journal of Speech and Hearing Research*, 28, 96–103.

Picheny, M. A., Durlach, N., & Braida, L. D. (1986). Speaking clearly for the hard of hearing II: Acoustic characteristics of clear and conversational speech. *Journal of Speech and Hearing Research*, 29, 434–446.

Pichora-Fuller, M. K. (1997). Language comprehension in older listeners. *Journal of Speech-Language Pathology and Audiology,* 21, 125–142.

Pichora-Fuller, M. K., & Benguerel, A.-P. (1990). Development of CAST: A computer-aided speechreading training program. *Journal of Speech and Hearing Research*, 34, 202–212.

Pichora-Fuller, M. K., & Carson, A. J. (2001). Hearing health and the listening experiences of older communicators. In M. L. Hummert & J. F. Nussbaum (Eds.), *Aging, Communication, and Health: Linking Research and Practice for Successful Aging* (pp. 44–74). Mahwah, NJ: Erlbaum.

Pichora-Fuller, M. K., & Cicchelli, M. (1986). *Computer Aided Speechreading Training (CAST) owner's manual.* Mississauga, Ontario, CAN: Department of Psychology, University of Toronto.

Pichora-Fuller, M. K., Schnieder, B., & Daneman, M. (1995). How young and old adults listen to and remember speech in noise. *Journal of the Acoustical Society of America*, 97, 593–607.

Pichora-Fuller, M. K., & Singh, G. (2006). Effects of age on auditory and cognitive processing: Implications for hearing aid fitting and audiologic rehabilitation. *Trends in Amplification*, 10, 29–59.

Pichora-Fuller, M. K., & Souza, P. E. (2003). Effects of aging in auditory processing of speech. *International Journal of Audiology*, 42, 2S11–2S16.

Pipp-Siegel, S., & Biringen, Z. (2000). Assessing the quality of relationships between parents and children: The emotional availability scales. *Volta Review*, 100, 237–249.

Pittman, A. L., Lewis, D. E., Hoover, B. M., & Stelmachowicz, P. G. (2005). Rapid word-learning in normal-hearing and hearing-impaired children: Effects of age, receptive vocabulary, and high-frequency amplification. *Ear and Hearing*, 26, 619–629.

Plant, G. (1998). Training in the use of a tactile supplement to lipreading: A long-term case study. *Ear and Hearing*, 19, 394–406.

Plath, P. (1991). Speech recognition in the elderly. *Acta Otolaryngology*, 476 (Suppl.), 127–130.

Pollack, D. (1970). *Educational Audiology For the Limited Hearing Infant.* Springfield, IL: Thomas.

Pratt, S. (2003). Reducing consonant voicing inconsistency in a child with a severe-to-profound hearing loss with computer-based visual feedback. *Journal of the Academy of Rehabilitative Audiology*, 36, 45–65.

Preminger, J. (2003). Should significant others be encouraged to join adult group audiologic rehabilitation classes? *Journal of the American Academy of Audiology*, 14, 545–555.

Prendergast, S. G., & Kelley, L. A. (2002). Aural rehab services: Survey reports who offers which ones and how often. *The Hearing Journal*, 55, 30–35.

Primeau, R. L. (1997). Hearing aid benefit in adults and older adults. *Seminars in Hearing*, 18, 29–36.

Prince Market Research. (2006). *Clarity Final Report: Baby Boomer Hearing Loss Study*. Nashville, TN: Prince Market Research.

Psychological Corporation (1994). *GOALS: A Performance Based Measure of Achievement*. San Antonio, TX: Psychological Corporation.

Psychological Corporation. (1997). *The Wechsler Adult Intelligence Scale*. San Antonio, TX: Psychological Corporation.

Quigley, S. P., & Kretschmer, R. E. (1982). *The Education of Deaf Children*. Austin, TX: Pro-Ed.

Quigley, S. P., Monranelli, D. S., & Wilbur, R. B. (1976). Some aspects of the verb system in the language of deaf students. *Journal of Speech and Hearing Research*, 19, 536–550.

Quigley, S. P., & Paul, P. V. (1984). *Language and Deafness*. London, ENG: Croom Helm.

Rabinowitz, P. M., Slade, M. D., Galusha, D., Dixon-Ernst, C., & Cullen, M. R. (2006). Trends in the prevalence of hearing loss among young adults entering an industrial workforce 1985–2004. *Ear and Hearing*, 27, 369–375.

Rall, E., & Montoya, L.A. (2005). *Pediatric Audiology Counseling Guidelines: Birth-Adolescence*. [Handout]. Philadelphia, PA: Children's Hospital of Philadelphia.

Rance, G., McKay, C., & Grayden, D. (2004). Perceptual characterization of children with auditory neuropathy. *Ear and Hearing*, 25, 34–46.

Reese, J. L., & Hnath-Chisolm, T. (2005). Recognition of hearing aid orientation content by first-time users. *American Journal of Audiology*, 14, 94–104.

Reich, G. E. (2000). American Tinnitus Association and self-help groups. In R. S. Tyler (Ed.), *Tinnitus Handbook* (pp. 419–436). Clifton Park, NY: Delmar Learning.

Reid, K., Hresko, W., Hammill, D., & Wiltshire, S. (1991). *Test of Early Reading Ability—Deaf and Hard of Hearing (TERA-D/HH)*. Austin, TX: Pro-Ed.

Reisberg, D., McLean, J., & Goldfield, A. (1987). Easy to hear but hard to understand: A speechreading advantage with intact stimuli. In R. Campbell & B. Dodd (Eds.), *Hearing by Eye: The Psychology of Lip-reading* (pp. 97–113). London, ENG: Erlbaum.

Reynell, J. K. (1977). *Reynell Development Language Scale*. Windsor, Ontario, CAN: NFER Nelson.

Ries, P. W. (1991). The demography of hearing loss. In H. Orlans (Ed.), *Adjustment to Adult Hearing Loss* (2nd Ed.) (pp. 3–22.), Clifton Park, NY: Delmar Learning.

Ringdahl, A., Eriksson-Mangold, M., & Andersson, G. (1998). Psychometric evaluation of the Gothenburg profile for measurement of experienced hearing disability and handicap: Applications with new hearing aid candidates and experienced hearing aid users. *British Journal of Audiology*, 32, 375–385.

Rivera, L., Boppana, S., Fowler, K., Britt, W., Stagno, S., & Pass, R. (2002). Predictors of hearing loss in children with symptomatic congenital cytomegalovirus infection. *Pediatrics*, 110, 762–767.

Robb, M., & Pang-Ching, G. (1992). Relative timing characteristics of hearing-impaired speakers. *Journal of the Acoustical Society of America*, 91, 2954–2960.

Robbins, A. M., Koch, D., Osberger, M. J., Zimmerman-Phillips, S., & Kishon-Rabin, L. (2004). Effect of age at cochlear implantation on auditory skill development in infants and toddlers. *Archives of Otolaryngology-Head & Neck Surgery*, 130, 570–574.

Robbins, A. M., Renshaw, J. J., Miyamoto, R. T., Osberger, M. J., & Pope, M. L. (1988). *Minimal Pairs Test*. Indianapolis, IN: Indiana University School of Medicine.

Roberts, S. (2007, June 12). Suburbs are graying faster than big cities. *The New York Times*, A12.

Rogers, C. R. (1980). *A Way of Being*. Boston, MA: Houghton Mifflin.

Rönnberg, J. (1995). What makes a skilled speechreader? In G. Plant & K. Spens (Eds.), *Profound Deafness and Speech Communication* (pp. 393–416). London, ENG: Whurr.

Rönnberg, J. (1996). Speech gestures and facial expression in speechreading. *Scandinavian Journal of Psychology*, 37, 132–139.

Rönnberg, J., Andersson, J., Samuelsson, S. Södderfeldt, B., Lyxell, B., & Risberg, J. (1999). A speechreading expert: The case of MM. *Journal of Speech, Language, and Hearing Research*, 42, 5–20.

Rönnberg, J., Arlinger, S., Lyxell, B., & Kinnefors, C. (1989). Visual evoked potentials: Relation to adult speechreading and cognitive function. *Journal of Speech and Hearing Research*, 32, 725–735.

Rönnberg, J., Öhngren, G., & Nilsson, L. G. (1982). Hearing deficiency, speechreading and memory functions. *Scandinavian Audiology*, 11, 261–268.

Rönnberg, J., Öhngren, G., & Nilsson, L. G. (1983). Speechreading performance evaluated by means of TV and real-life presentation: A comparison between a normally hearing, moderately impaired and profoundly hearing-impaired group. *Scandinavian Audiology*, 12, 71–77.

Rose, S., McAnally, P. L., & Quigley, S. P. (2004). *Language Learning Practices with Deaf Children*. Austin, TX: Pro-Ed.

Rosen, S. M., Fourcin, A. J., & Moore, B. C. J. (1981). Voice pitch as an aid to lipreading. *Nature*, 291, 150–152.

Rosenbloom, S. (2007, July 12). The day the music died. *The New York Times*, E1–E6.

Ross, M. (1990). Definitions and descriptions. In J. Davis (Ed.), *Our Forgotten Children: Hard of Hearing Pupils in the Schools*. Washington, DC: Self Help for Hard of Hearing People.

Ross, M., & Lerman, J. (1971). *Word Intelligibility by Picture Identification*. Pittsburgh, PA: Stanwix House.

Rossiter, S., Stevens, C., & Walker, G. (2006). Tinnitus and its effect on working memory and attention. *Journal of Speech, Language, and Hearing Research*, 49, 150–160.

Rothman, H. (1976). A spectrographic investigation of consonant-vowel transitions in the speech of deaf adults. *Phonetica*, 4, 129–136.

Roup, C. M., Wiley, T. L., & Wilson, R. H. (2006). Dichotic word recognition in young and older adults. *Journal of the American Academy of Audiology*, 17, 230–240.

Rousey, C. (1976). Psychological reactions to hearing loss. *Journal of Speech and Hearing Disorders*, 36, 382–389.

Roush, J. (1994). Strengthening family–professional relations: Advice from parents. In J. Rousch & N. D. Matkin (Eds.), *Infants and Toddlers with Hearing Loss* (pp. 337–350). Baltimore, MD: York Press.

Roush, J., & McWilliam, R. (1990). A new challenge for pediatric audiology: Public Law 99–457. *Journal of the American Academy of Audiology*, 1, 196–208.

Rubinstein, A., & Boothroyd, A. (1987). Effects of two approaches to auditory training on speech recognition by hearing-impaired adults. *Journal of Speech and Hearing Research*, 30, 153–160.

Rubinstein, A., Cherry, R., Hecht, P., & Idler, C. (2000). Anticipatory strategy training: Implications for the postlingually hearing-impaired adult. *Journal of the American Academy of Audiology*, 11, 52–55.

Russell, K., Quigley, S., & Power, D. (1976). *Linguistics and Deaf Children: Transformational Syntax and Its Applications.* Washington, DC: Alexander Graham Bell Association for the Deaf.

Russo, N. M., Nicol, T. G., Zecker, S. G., Hayes, E. A., & Kraus, N. (2005). Auditory training improves neural responses in the human brainstem. *Behavioral Brain Research,* 156, 95–103.

Sackett, D. L., Roenberg, W. M., Gray, J. A., Haynes, R. B., & Richardson, W. S. (1996). Evidence-based medicine: What it is and what it isn't. *British Medical Journal,* 312, 71–72.

Salthouse, T. A. (1994). The aging of working memory. *Neuropsychology,* 8, 535–543.

Samar, V. J., & Metz, D. (1988). Criterion validity of speech intelligibility rating-scale procedures for the hearing-impaired population. *Journal of Speech and Hearing Research,* 31, 307–316.

Samar, V. J., & Sims, D. G. (1983). Visual evoked response correlates of speechreading performance in normal-hearing adults: A replication and factor analytic extension. *Journal of Speech and Hearing Research,* 26, 2–9.

Sass-Lehrer, M. (2004). Early detection of hearing loss: Maintaining a family-centered perspective. *Seminars in Hearing,* 24, 295–307.

Scarborough, H. (1990). Index of productive syntax. *Applied Psycholinguistics,* 11, 122.

Scarola, D. (2005). Learning to listen: An interview with Warren Estabrooks. *Volta Voices,* November/December, 38–40.

Schafer, D., & Lynch, J. (1980). Emergent language of six prelingually deaf children. *Teachers of the Deaf,* 5, 94–111.

Schafer, E. C., & Thibodeau, L. M. (2004). Speech recognition abilities of adults using cochlear implants with FM systems. *Journal of the American Academy of Audiology,* 15, 678–691.

Scheetz, N. (1993). *Orientation to Deafness.* Needham Heights, MA: Allyn & Bacon.

Scheikh, J. I., & Yesavage, J. A. (1986). Geriatric depression scale (GDS): Recent evidence and development of a shorter version. *Clinical Gerontology,* 5, 165–172.

Schloss, P. J., & Smith, M. A. (1990). *Teaching Social Skills to Hearing-Impaired Students.* Washington, DC: Alexander Graham Bell Association for the Deaf.

Schmida, M. J., Peterson, H. J., & Tharpe, A. M. (2003). Visual reinforcement audiometry using digital video disc and conventional reinforcers. *American Journal of Audiology,* 12, 35–40.

Schneider, B. (1997). Psychoacoustics and aging: Implications for everyday listening. *Journal of Speech-Language Pathology and Audiology*, 21, 111–124.

Schow, R. L. (2001). A standardized AR battery for dispensers is proposed. *The Hearing Journal*, 54, 10–20.

Schow, R. L., & Nerbonne, M. (1980). Hearing levels among elderly nursing home residents. *Journal of Speech and Hearing Disorders*, 45, 124–132.

Schow, R. L., & Nerbonne, M. A. (1982). Communication screening profile: Use with elderly adults. *Ear and Hearing*, 3, 135–147.

Schum, D. J. (1989, November). *Clear and conversational speech by untrained talkers: Intelligibility*. Paper presented at the American Speech-Language-Hearing Association convention, Seattle, WA.

Schum, D. J. (1997). Beyond hearing aids: Clear speech training as an intervention strategy. *The Hearing Journal*, 50, 36–38.

Schum, D. J. (1999). Perceived hearing aid benefit in relation to perceived needs. *Journal of the American Academy of Audiology*, 10, 40–45.

Schum, L. K., & Tye-Murray, N. (1995). Alerting and assistive systems: Counseling implications for cochlear implant users. In R. S. Tyler & D. J. Schum (Eds.), *Assistive Devices for Persons With Hearing Impairment* (pp. 86–122). Needham Heights, MA: Allyn & Bacon.

Schum, R. L. (1991). Communication and social growth: A developmental model of social behavior in deaf children. *Ear and Hearing*, 12, 320–327.

Schum, R. L., & Gfeller, K. (1994). Requisites for conversation: Engendering social skills. In N. Tye-Murray (Ed.), *Let's Converse: A How-to Guide to Develop and Expand Conversational Skills of Children and Teenagers Who Are Hearing Impaired* (pp. 147–176). Washington, DC: Alexander Graham Bell Association for the Deaf.

Scott, A. O. (2007). Kiss, kiss, talk, talk. *NY Times Book Review*, March 4, 11.

Seaver, L. & DesGeorges, J. (2004). Special education law: A new IDEA for students who are deaf and hard of hearing. In R. J. Roeser & M. P. Downs (Eds.), *Auditory Disorders in School Children* (4th Ed.) (pp. 2–24). New York, NY: Thieme.

Secord, W. (1981). *T-MAC: Test of Minimal Articulation Competence*. Columbus, OH: Merrill.

Sensimetrics. (2006). *Seeing and Hearing Speech*. Retrieved 04/24/07, from http://www.seeingspeech.com.

Serry, T. A., & Blamey, P. J. (1999). A 4-year investigation into phonetic inventory development in young cochlear implant users. *Journal of Speech, Language, and Hearing Research*, 42, 141–154.

Setiz, P. R. (2002). French origins of the cochlear implant. *Cochlear Implants International*, 3, 77–86.

Seyfried, D. N., & Kricos, P. B. (1996). Language and speech of the deaf and hard of hearing. In R. L. Schow & M. A. Nerbonne (Eds.), *Introduction to Audiologic Rehabilitation* (3rd Ed.) (pp. 168–228). Boston, MA: Allyn & Bacon.

Shatner, W. (1997). Sound of silence. *People*, 47, 153–155.

Shepherd, D. (1982). Visual-neural correlates of speech-reading ability in normal-hearing adults: Reliability. *Journal of Speech and Hearing Research*, 25, 521–527.

Shepherd, D., DeLavergne, R. W., Frueh, F. X., & Colbridge, C. (1977). Visual-neural correlate of speech-reading abilities in normal-hearing adults. *Journal of Speech and Hearing Research*, 20, 752–765.

Shestok, J. (2006). Amplification's makeover. *Advance for Audiologists*, January/February, 31–34.

Shibuya, L. (2006). One family's journey into the hearing world. *Volta Voices*, January/February, 20–21.

Shimon, D. A. (1992). *Coping with Hearing Loss and Hearing Aids*. Clifton Park, NY: Delmar Learning.

Shriberg, L., Flipsen, P., Thielke, H., Kwiatkowski, J., Kertoy, M., Katcher, M., et al. (2000). Risk for speech disorder associated with early recurrent otitis media with effusion: Two retrospective studies. *Journal of Speech, Language, and Hearing Research*, 43, 79–99.

Shultz, D., & Mowry, R. B. (1995). Older adults in long-term care facilities. In P. B. Kricos & S. A. Lesner (Eds.), *Hearing Care For the Older Adults: Audiologic Rehabilitation* (pp. 167–179). Newton, MA: Butterworth-Heinemann.

Siebein, G. W., Gold, M. A., Siebein, G. W., & Ermann, M. G. (2000). Ten ways to provide a high-quality acoustical environment in schools. *Language, Speech, and Hearing Services in Schools*, 31, 376–384.

Siemens Audiology Group. (2000, March). *Hearing training against hearing frustration: When high-tech alone is not enough*. Proceedings of the Beethoven Discussions 2000, Bonn, Germany.

Silverman, R. S., & Hirsh, I. (1955). Problems related to the use of speech in clinical audiometry. *Annals of Otology, Rhinology, and Laryngology*, 64, 1234–1244.

Silwa, L., Kochanek, K., Durrant, J., & Smurzynski, J. (2008). Audiology makes rapid advances in Poland. *The Asha Leader*, February 12, 28–30.

Sims, D., Dorn, C., Clark, C., Bryant, L., & Mumford, B. (2002, November). *New developments in computer assisted speechreading and auditory training.* Paper presented at the American Speech-Language-Hearing Association convention, Atlanta, GA.

Sims, D., & Gottermeier, L. (2000). Computer applications in audiologic rehabilitation. In J. G. Alpiner & P. A. McCarthy (Eds.), *Rehabilitative Audiology: Children and Adults* (3rd Ed.) (pp. 556–571). Baltimore, MD: Lippincott, Williams & Wilkins.

Sindhusake, D., Mitchell, P., Golding, M., Rochtchina, E., & Rubin, G. (2003). Prevalence and characteristics of tinnitus in older adults: The Blue Mountains hearing study. *International Journal of Audiology*, 42, 289–294.

Sininger, Y. S. (2002). Otoacoustic emissions in the diagnosis of hearing disorder in infants. *The Hearing Journal*, 55, 22–26.

Skinner, B. F. (1953). *Science and Human Behavior.* New York, NY: Macmillan.

Skinner, B. F. (1971). *Beyond Freedom and Dignity.* New York, NY: Knopf.

Small, L. H., & Infante, A. A. (1988). Effects of training and visual distance on speechreading. *Perception and Motor Skills*, 66, 415–418.

Smith, C. (1975). Residual hearing and speech production in the deaf. *Journal of Speech and Hearing Research*, 19, 795–811.

Smith, R. J. H,. & Van Camp, G. (2007). Deafness and hereditary hearing loss overview. *Gene Reviews.* Retrieved 07/10/07 from http://www.genetests.org.

Smith, S. L., & West, R. L. (2006). The application of self-efficacy principles to audiologic rehabilitation: A tutorial. *American Journal of Audiology*, 15, 46–56.

Smith, S. M., & Ample, C. M. (1997). Interpersonal relationship implications of hearing loss in persons who are older. *The Journal of Rehabilitation*, 63, 15–21.

Sommers, M., Tye-Murray, N., & Spehar, B. (2005a). Audiovisual integration and aging. *Ear and Hearing*, 26, 263–275.

Sommers, M., Tye-Murray, N., & Spehar, B. (2005b). The effects of signal-to-noise ratio on auditory-visual integration: Integration and encoding are not independent. *Journal of the Acoustical Society of America*, 117, 2574.

Sonnenschein, E., & Cascella, P. W. (2004). Pediatricians' opinions about otitis media and speech-language-hearing development. *Journal of Communication Disorders*, 37, 313–323.

Sorkin, D. (2002). Cochlear implant candidacy and outcomes: 2002 update. *Hearing Loss*, July/August, 12–17.

Sorkin, D. (2004). Disability law and people with hearing loss: We've come a long way (but we're not there yet). *Hearing Loss*, May/June, 13–17.

Southall, K., Gagné, J. P., & Leroux, T. (2006). Factors that influence the use of assistance technologies by older adults who have a hearing loss. *International Journal of Audiology*, 45, 252–259.

Souza, P. (2004). New hearing aids for older listeners. *The Hearing Journal*, 57, 10–17.

Speaks, C., & Jerger, J. (1965). Performance-intensity characteristics of synthetic sentences. *Journal of Speech and Hearing Research*, 9, 305–312.

Speaks, C. S., Jerger, J., & Trammell, J. (1970). Measurement of hearing handicap. *Journal of Speech and Hearing Research*, 13, 768–776.

Spencer, L. (1994). Some ways to nurture children's conversational and language skills. In N. Tye-Murray (Ed.), *Let's Converse: A How-to Guide to Develop and Expand the Conversational Skills of Children and Teenagers Who Are Hearing Impaired* (pp. 51–84). Washington, DC: Alexander Graham Bell Association for the Deaf.

Spencer, L., Barker, B., & Tomblin, J. B. (2003). Exploring the language and literacy outcomes of pediatric cochlear implant users. *Ear and Hearing*, 24, 236–247.

Spencer, L., Tomblin, J. B., & Gantz, B. J. (1997). Reading skills in children with multi-channel cochlear implant experience. *Volta Review*, 99, 193–202.

Spencer, P., & Lederberg, A. (1997). Different modes, different models: Communication and language of young deaf children and their mothers. In L. Adamson & M. Romski (Eds.), *Communication and Language: Discoveries from Atypical Development* (pp. 203–230). Baltimore, MD: Brookes.

Stach, B. A. (2000). *Comprehensive Dictionary of Audiology* (2nd Ed.). Clifton Park, NY: Delmar Learning.

Stanton, J. F. (2005). Captioning in theaters: What will it take? *Volta Voices*, May/June, 28–30.

Stapells, D. R. (2002). The tone-evoked ABR: Why it's the measure of choice for young infants. *The Hearing Journal*, 55, 14–18.

Stark, P., & Hickson, L. (2004). Outcomes of hearing aid fitting for older people with hearing impairment and their significant others. *International Journal of Audiology*, 43, 390–398.

Stelmachowicz, P. G., Pittman, A. L., Hoover, B. M., & Lewis, D. E. (2004). Novel-word learning in children with normal hearing and hearing loss. *Ear and Hearing*, 25, 47–56.

Stephens, S. D., Jaworski, A., Kerr, P., & Zhao, F. (1998). Use of patient-specific estimates in patient evaluation and rehabilitation. *Scandinavian Audiology (Suppl.)*, 49, 61–68.

Stephens, S. D., Jaworski, A., Lewis, P., & Aslan, S. (1999). An analysis of the communication tactics used by hearing-impaired adults. *British Journal of Audiology*, 33, 17–27.

Stika, C.J., Ross, M., & Cuevas, C. (2002). Hearing aid services and satisfaction: The consumer viewpoint. *Hearing Loss*, May/June, 25–31.

Stine, E. A., Wingfield, A., & Poon, L. W. (1986). How much and how fast: Rapid processing of spoken language in later adulthood. *Psychology & Aging*, 1, 303–311.

Stinson, M. S., & Antia, S. D. (1999). Considerations in educating deaf and hard-of-hearing students in inclusive settings. *Journal of Deaf Studies and Deaf Education*, 4, 163–175.

Stoel-Gammon, C. (1988). Prelinguistic vocalizations of hearing-impaired and normally hearing subjects: A comparison of consonantal inventories. *Journal of Speech and Hearing Disorders*, 53, 302–315.

Stout, G., & Windel, J. (1992). *Developmental Approach to Successful Listening II*. Englewood, CO: Resource Point.

Strawbridge, W. J., Cohen, R. D., Shema, S. J., & Kaplan, G. A. (1996). Successful aging: Predictors and associated activities. *American Journal of Epidemiology*, 144, 135–141.

Strinivasan, R. J., & Massaro, D. W. (2003). Perceiving prosody from the face and voice: Distinguishing statements from echoic questions in English. *Language and Speech*, 46, 1–22.

Suárez, M. (2000). Promoting social competence in deaf students: The effect of an intervention program. *Journal of Deaf Studies and Deaf Education*, 5, 323–336.

Suárez, M., & Torres, E. (1996). Dyadic interactions between deaf children and their communication partners. *American Annals of the Deaf*, 141, 245–251.

Subtelny, J. D., Orlando, N. A., & Whitehead, R. L. (1981). *Speech and Voice Characteristics of the Deaf*. Washington, DC: Alexander Graham Bell Association for the Deaf.

Sumby, W. H., & Pollack, I. (1954). Visual contribution to speech intelligibility in noise. *Journal of the Acoustical Society of America*, 26, 212–215.

Summerfield, Q. (1989). Visual perception of phonetic gestures. In I. G. Mattingly (Ed.), *Modularity and the Motor Theory of Speech Perception* (pp. 117–137). Hillsdale, NJ: Erbaum.

Summerfield, Q. (1992). Lipreading and audiovisual speech perception. *Philosophical Transactions of the Royal Society of London*, 5, 71–78.

Summerfield, Q., Barton, G. R., Toner, J., McAnallen, C., Proops, D., Harries, C., et al. (2006). Self-reported benefits from successive bilateral cochlear implantation in post-lingually deafened adults: Randomized controlled trial. *International Journal of Audiology*, 45(Suppl. 1), S99–S107.

Sutherland, G. (1995). Increasing consumer acceptance of assistive devices. In R. S. Tyler & D. J. Schum (Eds.), *Assistive Devices for Persons with Hearing Impairment* (pp. 251–266). Needham Heights, MA: Allyn & Bacon.

Svirsky, M. A., Chute, P. M., Green, J., Bollard, P., & Miyamoto, R. T. (2002). Language development in children who are prelingually deaf who have used the SPEAK or CIS stimulation strategies. *Volta Review*, 102, 199–214.

Svirsky, M. A., Jones, D., Osberger, M. J., & Miyamoto, R. T. (1998). The effect of auditory feedback on the control of oral-nasal resonance by pediatric cochlear implant users. *Ear and Hearing*, 19, 385–393.

Svirsky, M., Robbins, A. M., Kirk, K. I., Pisoni, D. B., & Miyamoto, R. T. (2000). Language development in profoundly deaf children with cochlear implants. *Psychological Science*, 11, 153–158.

Sweetow, R. (2006a). *Listening Aid Communication Enhancement (LACE)*. Redwood, CA: Neurotone.

Sweetow, R. (2006b, April). *Tinnitus patient management*. Paper presented at the meeting of the American Academy of Audiology, Denver, CO.

Sweetow, R., & Barrager, D. (1980). Quality of comprehensive audiological care: A survey of parents of hearing-impaired children. *ASHA*, 22, 841–847.

Sweetow, R., & Levy, M. C. (1990). Tinnitus severity scaling for diagnostic/therapeutic usage. *Hearing Instruments*, 41, 20–21, 46.

Sweetow, R., & Palmer, C. (2005). Efficacy of individual auditory training in adults: A systematic review of the evidence. *Journal of the American Academy of Audiology*, 16, 494–504.

Sweetow, R., & Sabes, J. (2006). The need for and development of an adaptive listening and communication enhancement (LACE) Program. *Journal of the American Academy of Audiology*, 17, 538–558.

Sweetow, R., & Sabes, J. H. (2007). Listening and communication enhancement (LACE). *Seminars in Hearing*, 28, 133–141.

Takahashi, G., Martinez, C., Beamer, S., Bridges, J., Noffsinger, D., Sugiura, K., et al. (2007). Subjective measures of hearing aid benefit and satisfaction in the NIDCD/VA follow-up study. *Journal of the American Academy of Audiology*, 18, 323–349.

Takeoka, A., & Shimojima, A. (2002). Grounding styles of aged dyads: An exploratory study. In Proceedings of the Third SIGdial Workshop on Discourse and Dialogue (pp. 188–195).

Tambs, K. (2004). Moderate effects of hearing loss on mental health and subjective well-being: Results from the Nord–Trondelag hearing loss study. *Psychosomatic Medicine*, 66, 776–782.

Tannahill, J. C. (1979). The hearing handicap scale as a measure of hearing aid benefit. *Journal of Speech and Hearing Disorders*, 44, 91–99.

Tannen, D. (2000). "Don't just sit there—interrupt!": Pacing and pausing in conversational style. *American Speech*, 75, 393–395.

Task Force on Newborn and Infant Hearing. (1999). Newborn and infant hearing loss: Detection and intervention. *Pediatrics*, 103, 527–530.

Taylor, B. (2004). Recharging your test battery to keep up with the times. *The Hearing Journal*, 57, 20–24.

Taylor, B., & Hansen, V. (2002). To change the industry, we must change, Part 1. *The Hearing Review*, 9, 28–56.

Taylor, K. S., & Jurma, W. E. (1999). Study suggests that group rehabilitation increases benefit of hearing aid fittings. *The Hearing Journal*, 52, 48–54.

Thorn, F., & Thorn, S. (1989). Speechreading with reduced vision: A problem of aging. *Journal of Optometry Society of America*, 6, 491–499.

Tillman, T. W., & Carhart, R. (1966). *An Expanded Test for Speech Discrimination utilizing CNC monosyllabic Words: Northwestern University Auditory Test No. 6* [Tech. Rep. No. SAM-TR-6655. USAF School of Aerospace Medicine]. San Antonio, TX: Brooks Air Force Base.

Tobey, E., Devous, M., Buckley, K., Overson, G., Harris, T., Ringe, W., et al. (2005). Pharmacological enhancement of aural habilitation in adult cochlear implant users. *Ear and Hearing*, 26, 45S–56S.

Tobey, E., Geers, A. E., & Brenner, C. (1994). Speech production results: Speech feature acquisition. *Volta Review*, 96, 109–130.

Tobey, E., Geers, A. E., Brenner, C., Altuna, D., & Gabbert, G. (2003). Factors associated with speech production skills in children implanted by age five. *Ear and Hearing*, 24, 36S–45S.

Tomblin, J. B., Spencer, L., Flock, S., Tyler, R., & Gantz, B. (1999). A comparison of language achievement in children with cochlear implants and children using hearing aids. *Journal of Speech, Language, and Hearing* Research, 42, 497–509.

Tomoeda, C. K., & Bayles, K. A. (2002). Cultivating cultural competence in the workplace, classroom, and clinic. *ASHA Leader*, 7, 4–17.

Touchstone Applied Science Associates (2001). *Signposts Early Literacy Battery and Pre-DRP Test*. Brewster, NY: Touchstone Applied Science Associates.

Tremblay, K. L. (2006). Hearing aids and the brain: What's the connection? *The Hearing Journal*, 59, 10–17.

Tremblay, K. L., & Kraus, N. (2002). Auditory training induces asymmetrical changes in cortical neural activity. *Journal of Speech, Language, and Hearing Research*, 45, 564–572.

Tremblay, K. L., Kraus, N., Carell, T., & McGee, T. (1997). Central auditory system plasticity: Generalization to novel stimuli following listening training. *Journal of the Acoustical Society of America*, 102, 3762–3773.

Tremblay, K. L., Piskosz, M., & Souza, P. (2003). Auditory training induces asymmetrical changes in cortical neural activity. *Journal of Speech, Language, and Hearing Research*, 45, 564–572.

Trybus, R. J., & Krachmer, M. A. (1977). School achievement scores of hearing-impaired children: National data on achievement status and growth patterns. *American Annals of the Deaf*, 122, 62–69.

Trychin, S. (1987). *Did I Do That?* Washington, DC: Gallaudet University Press.

Trychin, S. (1988). *So That's the Problem!* Washington, DC: Gallaudet University Press.

Trychin, S. (1994). Helping people cope with hearing loss. In J. G. Clark & F. N. Martin (Eds.), *Effective Counseling in Audiology: Perspectives and Practice* (pp. 247–277). Englewood Cliffs, NJ: Simon & Schuster.

Trychin, S., & Wright, F. (1989). *Is That What You Think?* Washington, DC: Gallaudet University Press.

Turner, C., Gantz, B.J., Lowder, M., & Gfeller, K. (2003). Benefits seen in acoustic hearing + electric stimulation in same ear. *The Hearing Journal*, 58, 53–55.

Tye-Murray, N. (1987). Effects of vowel context on the articulatory closure postures of deaf speakers. *Journal of Speech and Hearing Research*, 30, 90–104.

Tye-Murray, N. (1991a). The establishment of open articulatory postures by deaf and hearing talkers. *Journal of Speech and Hearing Research*, 34, 453–459.

Tye-Murray, N. (1991b). Repair strategy usage by hearing-impaired adults and changes following communication therapy. *Journal of Speech and Hearing Research*, 34, 921–928.

Tye-Murray, N. (1992a). Auditory training. In N. Tye-Murray (Ed.), *Children with Cochlear Cochlear Implants: A Handbook for Parents, Teachers and Speech and Hearing Professionals* (pp. 91–114). Washington, DC: Alexander Graham Bell Association for the Deaf.

Tye-Murray, N. (1992b). Communication therapy. In N. Tye-Murray (Ed.), *Children with Cochlear Implants: A Handbook for Parents, Teachers and Speech and Hearing Professionals* (pp. 137–168). Washington, DC: Alexander Graham Bell Association for the Deaf.

Tye-Murray, N. (1992c). Preparing for communication interactions: The value of anticipatory strategies for adults with hearing impairment. *Journal of Speech and Hearing Research, 35,* 430–435.

Tye-Murray, N. (1992d). Speechreading training. In N. Tye-Murray (Ed.), *Children with Cochlear Implants: A Handbook for Parents, Teachers and Speech and Hearing Professionals* (pp. 115–136). Washington, DC: Alexander Graham Bell Association for the Deaf.

Tye-Murray, N. (1992e). Teaching speech perception skills: General guidelines. In N. Tye-Murray (Ed.), *Children with Cochlear Implants: A Handbook for Parents, Teachers and Speech and Hearing Professionals* (pp. 79–90). Washington, DC: Alexander Graham Bell Association for the Deaf.

Tye-Murray, N. (1993). *Communication Training for Hearing-Impaired Children and Teenagers: Speechreading, Listening, and Using Repair Strategies.* Austin, TX: Pro-Ed.

Tye-Murray, N. (1994a). Some conversation strategies for adults who interact with hard-of-hearing children. In N. Tye-Murray (Ed.), *Let's Converse! A How-to Guide to Develop and Expand the Conversational Skills of Children and Teenagers Who Are Hearing Impaired* (pp. 11–50). Washington, DC: Alexander Graham Bell Association for the Deaf.

Tye-Murray, N. (1994b). Communication breakdowns in conversations: Adult-initiated repair strategies. In N. Tye-Murray (Ed.), *Let's Converse! A How-to Guide to Develop and Expand the Conversational Skills of Children and Teenagers Who Are Hearing Impaired* (pp. 85–121). Washington, DC: Alexander Graham Bell Association for the Deaf.

Tye-Murray, N. (1994d). Some conversation strategies for adults who interact with hard-of-hearing children. In N. Tye-Murray (Ed.), *Let's converse! A How-to Guide to Develop and Expand the Conversational Skills of Children and Teenagers Who Are Hearing Impaired* (pp. 11–50). Washington, DC: Alexander Graham Bell Association for the Deaf.

Tye-Murray, N. (1997). *Communication Strategies Training for Older Teenagers and Adults.* Austin, TX: Pro-Ed.

Tye-Murray, N. (2002a). *Conversation Made Easy: Speechreading and Conversation Training for Individuals Who Have Hearing Loss (Adults and Teenagers).* St. Louis, MO: Central Institute for the Deaf.

Tye-Murray, N. (2002b). *Conversation Made Easy: Speechreading and Conversation Training for Individuals Who Have Hearing Loss (Children)*. St. Louis, MO: Central Institute for the Deaf.

Tye-Murray, N. (2003). Conversational fluency in children who use cochlear implants. *Ear and Hearing*, 24, 82S–90S.

Tye-Murray, N., & Folkins, J. (1990). Jaw and lip movements of deaf talkers producing utterances with known stress patterns. *Journal of the Acoustical Society of America*, 87, 2675–2683.

Tye-Murray, N., & Fryauf-Bertschy, H. (1992). Auditory training. In N. Tye-Murray (Ed.), *Children with Cochlear implants: A Handbook for Parents, Teachers and Speech and Hearing Professionals* (pp. 91–114). Washington, DC: Alexander Graham Bell Association for the Deaf.

Tye-Murray, N., & Geers, A. E. (2002). *The Children's Audiovisual Enhancement Speech Test (CHIVE)*. St. Louis, MO: Central Institute for the Deaf.

Tye-Murray, N., & Kelsey, D. R. (1993). Communication therapy for parents of cochlear implant users. *Volta Review*, 95, 21–32.

Tye-Murray, N., & Kirk, K. I. (1993). Vowel and diphthong production by young users of cochlear implants and the relationship between the phonetic level evaluation and spontaneous speech. *Journal of Speech and Hearing Research*, 36, 488–502.

Tye-Murray, N., Knutson, J. F., & Lemke, J. (1993). Assessment of communication strategies use: Questionnaires and daily diaries. *Seminars in Hearing*, 14, 338–353.

Tye-Murray, N., Purdy, S. C., & Woodworth, G. (1992). The reported use of communication strategies by members of SHHH and its relationship to client, talker, and situational variables. *Journal of Speech and Hearing Research*, 35, 708–717.

Tye-Murray, N., Purdy, S. C., Woodworth, G., & Tyler, R. S. (1990). Effects of repair strategies on visual identification of sentences. *Journal of Speech and Hearing Disorders*, 55, 621–627.

Tye-Murray, N., & Schum, L. A. (1994). Conversation training for frequent communication partners. *Journal of the Academy Rehabilitative Audiology*, 27, 209–222.

Tye-Murray, N., Sommers, M., & Spehar, B. (2006). *The Build-A-Sentence Test*. St. Louis, MO: Washington University School of Medicine.

Tye-Murray, N., Sommers, M., & Spehar, B. (2007a). Audiovisual integration and lipreading abilities of older adults with normal and impaired hearing. *Ear and Hearing*, 28, 656–668.

Tye-Murray, N., Sommers, M., & Spehar, B. (2007b). Lipreading and aging: Does gender make a difference? *Journal of the American Academy of Audiology*, 18, 883–892.

Tye-Murray, N., Sommers, M., & Spehar, B. (2008). Auditory and visual lexical neighborhoods in audiovisual speech perception. *Trends in Amplification*, 11, 233–241.

Tye-Murray, N., Spencer, L., Bedia, E. G., & Woodworth, G. (1996). Differences in children's sound production when speaking with a cochlear implant turned on and turned off. *Journal of Speech and Hearing Research*, 39, 604–610.

Tye-Murray, N., Spencer, L., & Gilbert-Bedia, E. (1995). Relationships between speech production and speech perception skills in young cochlear-implant users. *Journal of the Acoustical Society of America*, 98, 2454–2460.

Tye-Murray, N., Spencer, L., & Woodworth, G. (1995). Acquisition of speech by children who have prolonged cochlear implant experience. *Journal of Speech and Hearing Research*, 38, 327–337.

Tye-Murray, N., Tomblin, B., & Spencer, L. (1997, November). *Speech and language acquisition over time in children with cochlear implants.* Paper presented at the American Speech-Language Hearing Convention, Boston, MA.

Tye-Murray, N., & Tyler, R. S. (1988). A critique of continuous discourse tracking as a test procedure. *Journal of Speech and Hearing Disorders*, 53, 226–231.

Tye-Murray, N., Tyler, R. S., Woodworth, G., & Gantz, B. (1992). Performance over time with a Nucleus or Ineraid cochlear implant. *Ear and Hearing*, 13, 200–209.

Tye-Murray, N., & Witt, S. (1996). Conversational moves and conversational styles of adult cochlear-implant users. *Journal of the Academy of Rehabilitative Audiology*, 29, 11–25.

Tye-Murray, N., Witt, S., & Schum, L. (1995). Effects of talker familiarity on communication breakdown in conversation with adult cochlear-implant users. *Ear and Hearing*, 16, 459–469.

Tye-Murray, N., Witt, S., Schum, L., & Sobaski, C. (1995). Communication breakdowns: Partner contingencies and partner reactions. *Journal of the Academy of Rehabilitative Audiology*, 25, 1–27.

Tye-Murray, N., Zimmermann, G., & Folkins, J. (1987). Movement timing in deaf and hearing speakers: Comparison of phonetically heterogeneous syllable strings. *Journal of Speech and Hearing Research*, 30, 411–417.

Tyler, R. S., & Baker, L. J. (1983). Difficulties experienced by tinnitus sufferers. *Journal of Speech and Hearing Disorders*, 48, 150–154.

Tyler, R. S., Fryauf-Bertschy, H., & Kelsay, D. (1991). *Audiovisual Feature Test for Young Children.* Iowa City, IA: University of Iowa Hospitals and Clinics.

Tyler, R. S., Preece, J., & Tye-Murray, N. (1986). *The Iowa Phoneme and Sentence Tests.* Iowa City, IA: University of Iowa Hospitals and Clinics.

Uchanski, R., Choi, S. S., Sunkyung, S., Braida, L. D., Reed, C. M., & Durlach, N. I. (1996). Speaking clearly for the hard of hearing IV: Further studies of the role of speaking rate. *Journal of Speech and Hearing Research*, 39, 494–509.

Uhlmann, R., Larson, E., Rees, T., Koepsell, T., & Duckert, L. (1989). Cognitive functioning and health as determinants of mortality in an older population. *American Journal of Epidemiology*, 150, 978–986.

Underwood, A., & Adler, J. (2005, April 25). When cultures clash. *Newsweek*, 68–72.

Underwood, N. (2006). A family's journey through due process. *Volta Voices*, May/June, 40–44.

UK Cochlear Implant Study Group. (2004). Criteria of candidacy for unilateral cochlear implantation in postlingually deafened adults I: Theory and measures of effectiveness. *Ear and Hearing*, 25, 310–335.

U.S. Bureau of the Census (2003). *Current Population Survey, Annual Social and Economic Supplement*, detailed tables. Washington, DC: U.S. Government Printing Office.

U.S. Bureau of the Census. (2004). International Programs Center, International Data Base. Retrieved 05/23/07, from http://www.census.gov/ipc/www/idbnew.html.

U.S. Bureau of the Census. (2007). *Annual Estimates of the Population by Sex, Race, and Hispanic or Latino Origin for the U.S.: April, 2000 to 2006 (NC-EST 2006-03)*. Washington, DC: U.S. Government Printing Office.

U.S. Department of Health and Human Services. (2001). *National standards for Biculturally and Linguistically Appropriate Services in Health Care*. Commerce Bureau of the Census. (1986). Statistical abstract of the U.S. (106th ed.). Washington, DC: U.S. Department of Health and Human Services.

U.S. Department of Education (1998). *19th Annual Report to Congress on the Implementation of the IDEA, Appendix A*. Washington, DC: Government Printing Office.

U.S. Government Printing Office (1942). *Rehabilitation of the Deaf and the Hard of Hearing: A Manual for Rehabilitation Case Workers.* (Vocational Rehabilitation Series, Bulletin No. 26) Washington, DC: U.S. Government Printing Office.

Urbantschitsch, V. (1982). *Auditory Training for Deaf Mutism and Acquired Deafness.* (S. Richard Silverman, Trans.). Washington, DC: Alexander Graham Bell Association for the Deaf. (Original work published 1895)

VandenBrink, R. H. S. (1995). *Attitude and illness behavior in hearing impaired elderly.* Unpublished doctoral thesis, University of Groningen, Netherlands.

Van Hecke, M. (1994). Emotional responses to hearing loss. In J. G. Clark & F. N. Martin (Eds.), *Effective Counseling in Audiology: Perspectives and Practice* (pp. 92–115). Englewood Cliffs, NJ: Prentice-Hall.

Van Uden, A. (1988). Interrelating reception and expression in speechreading training. *Volta Review*, 90, 261–272.

Ventry, I., & Weinstein, B. (1982). The hearing inventory for the elderly: A new tool. *Ear and Hearing*, 3, 128.

Ventry, I., & Weinstein, B. (1983). Identification of elderly people with hearing problems. *ASHA*, 25, 37–47.

Vergara, K. C., & Miskiel, L. W. (1994). *CHATS: The Miami Cochlear Implant, Auditory and Tactile Skills Curriculum*. Miami, FL: Intelligent Hearing Systems.

Vermeulen, A. M., van Bon, W., Schreuder, R., Knoors, H., & Snik, A. (2007). Reading comprehension of deaf children with cochlear implants. *Journal of Deaf Studies and Deaf Education*, 12, 283–302.

Vernon, J. A., & Meikle, M. B. (2000). Tinnitus masking. In R. Tyler (Ed.), *Tinnitus Handbook* (pp. 313–356). Clifton Park, NY: Delmar Learning.

Vinding, T. (1989). Age-related macular degeneration: Macular changes, prevalence, and sex ratio. *Acta Ophthalmology*, 67, 609–616.

Voeks, S., Gallagher, C., Langer, E., & Drinka, P. (1990). Hearing loss in the nursing home: An institutional issue. *Journal of the American Geriatrics Society*, 38, 141–145.

Voelker, C. (1938). An experimental study of the comparative rate of utterances of deaf and normal-hearing speakers. *American Annals of the Deaf*, 83, 274–284.

von Hapsburg, D., & Davis, B. L. (2006). Auditory sensitivity and the prelinguistic vocalizations of early-amplified infants. *Journal of Speech, Language, and Hearing Research*, 49, 809–822.

von Hapsburg, D., & Peña, E. D. (2002). Understanding bilingualism and its impact on speech audiometry. *Journal of Speech, Language, and Hearing Research*, 45, 202–213.

von Hapsburg, D., Champlin, C. A., & Shetty, S. R. (2004). Reception thresholds for sentences in bilingual (Spanish/English) and monolingual (English) listeners. *Journal of the American Academy of Audiology*, 16, 88–98.

Vonlanthen, A. (2000). *Hearing Instrument Technology for the Hearing Healthcare Professional* (2nd Ed.). Clifton Park, NY: Delmar Learning.

Vorce, E. (1971). Speech curriculum. In L. E. Connor (Ed.), *Speech for the Deaf Child* (pp. 221–224). Washington, DC: Alexander Graham Bell Association for the Deaf.

Vorce, E. (1974). *Teaching Speech to Deaf Children.* Washington, DC: Alexander Graham Bell Association for the Deaf.

Vuorialho, A., Karinen, P., & Sorri, M. (2006). Effect of hearing aids on hearing disability and quality of life in the elderly. *International Journal of Audiology*, 45, 400–405.

Wackym, P. A., Runge-Samuelson, C. L., Firszt, J. B., Alkaf, F. M., & Burg, L.S. (2007). More challenging speech-perception tasks demonstrate binaural benefit in bilateral cochlear implant users. *Ear and Hearing*, 28, 80S–85S.

Wake, M., Hughes, E. K., Poulakis, Z., Collins, C., & Rickhards, F. W. (2004). Outcomes of children with mild-profound congenital hearing loss at 7 to 8 years: A population study. *Ear and Hearing*, 25, 1–8.

Walden, B. E., Demorest, M. E., & Helper, E. L. (1984). Test–retest reliability of the hearing handicap inventory for the elderly. *Ear and Hearing*, 7, 295–299.

Walden, B. E., Erdman, S. A., Montgomery, A. A., Schwartz, D. M., & Prosek, R. A. (1981). Effects of training on the visual recognition of consonants. *Journal of Speech and Hearing Research*, 20, 130–145.

Walden, B. E., Prosek, R. A., Montgomery, A. A., Scherr, C. K., & Jones, C. J. (1977). Effects of training on the visual recognition of consonants. *Journal of Speech and Hearing Research*, 20, 130–145.

Wallace, V., Menn, L., & Yoshinaga-Itano, C. (1998). Is babble the gateway to speech for all children? A longitudinal study of children who are deaf or hard of hearing. *Volta Review*, 100, 121–148.

Wallis, D., Musselman, C., & MacKay, S. (2004). Hearing mothers and their deaf children: The relationship between early, ongoing mode match and subsequent mental health functioning in adolescence. *Journal of Deaf Studies and Deaf Education*, 9, 2–14.

Waltzman, S. (2005). Expanding patient criteria for cochlear implantation. *Audiology Today*, September/October, 20–21.

Waltzman, S., Cohen, N., Gomolin, R., Green, J., Shapiro, W., Brackett, D., et al. (1997). Perception and production results in children implanted between 2 and 5 years of age. *Advances in OtoRhino-Laryngology*, 52, 177–180.

Warner-Czyz, A. D., Davis, B. L., & Morrison, H. M. (2005). Production accuracy in a young cochlear implant recipient. *Volta Review*, 105, 151–173.

Warren, S. F., & Yoder, P. J. (1996). Enhancing communication and language development in young children with developmental delays and disorders. *Peabody Journal of Education*, 71, 118–132.

Warren, Y., Dancer, J., Monfils, B., & Pittenger, J. (1989). The practice effect in speechreading distributed over five days: Same versus different CID sentence lists. *Volta Review*, 91, 321–325.

Watson, L. M., Archbold, S. M., & Niolopoulos, T. P. (2006). Children's communication mode five years after cochlear implantation: Changes over time according to age at implant. *Cochlear Implants International*, 7, 77–91.

Wayner, D. S. (2005). Aural rehabilitation adds value, lifts satisfaction, cuts returns. *The Hearing Journal*, 58, 30–38.

Wayner, D. S., & Abrahamson, J. A. (1996). *Learning to Hear Again: An Audiologic Rehabilitation Curriculum Guide*. Austin, TX: Hear Again.

Wayner, D. S., & Abrahamson, J. A. (1998). *Learning to Hear Again With a Cochlear Implant: An Audiologic Rehabilitation Curriculum Guide*. Austin, TX: Hear Again.

Weichbold, V., Nekahm-Heis, D., & Wilzl-Mueller, K. (2007). Universal newborn hearing screening and postnatal hearing loss. *Pediatrics*, 117, e631–e636.

Weikum, W. M., Vouloumanos, A., Navarra, J., Soto-Faraco, S., Sebastian-Galles, N., & Werker, J. (2007). Visual language discrimination in infancy. *Science*, 316, 1159.

Weinstein, B. E., Spitzer, J. B., & Ventry, I. M. (1986). Test–retest reliability of the hearing handicap inventory for the elderly. *Ear and Hearing*, 7, 295–299.

Weinstein, B. E., & Ventry, I. M. (1982). Hearing impairment and social isolation in the elderly. *Journal of Speech and Hearing Disorders*, 25, 593–599.

Weinstein, B. E., & Ventry, I. M. (1983). Audiometric correlates of the hearing handicap inventory for the elderly. *Journal of Speech and Hearing Disorders*, 48, 379–384.

Weisleder, P., & Hodgson, W. R. (1980). Evaluation of four Spanish word-recognition-ability lists. *Ear and Hearing*, 1, 387–393.

White, K.R. (1996). Universal newborn hearing screening using transient-evoked otoacoustic emissions: Past, present, and future. *Seminars in Hearing*, 17, 171–173.

White, K. R. (2004). Newborn hearing screening: Nation's progress plateaus short of goal. *Hearing Health*, Summer, 19–21.

Whitehead, R. L. (1982). Some respiratory and aerodynamic patterns in the speech of the hearing impaired. In I. Hochberg, & M. J. Osberger, (Eds.), *Speech of the Hearing Impaired: Research, Training, and Personnel Preparation*. Baltimore, MD: University Park Press.

Widen, J. E., & O'Grady, G. M. (2002). Using visual reinforcement audiometry in the assessment of hearing in infants. *The Hearing Journal*, 55, 28–36.

Wiley, T. L., Cruickshanks, K. J., Nondahl, D. M., Tweed, T. S., Klein, R., & Klein, B. (1998). Aging and word recognition in competing message. *Journal of the American Academy of Audiology*, 9, 191–198.

Wilkinson, A. S., & Brinton, J. C. (2003). Speech intelligibility rating of cochlear implanted children: Inter-rater reliability. *Cochlear Implants International*, 4, 22–30.

Williams, D. R. (1990). Socioeconomic differentials in health. *Social Psychology Quarterly*, 53, 81–99.

Williams-Scott, B., & Kipila, E. (1987). Cued speech: A professional point of view. In S. Schwartz (Ed.), *Choices in Deafness: A Parent's Guide*. Washington, DC: Woodbine House.

Willott, J. F. (1996). Anatomic and physiologic aging: A behavioral neuroscience perspective. *Journal of the American Academy of Audiology*, 7, 141–151.

Wilson, D. H., Walsh, P. G., Sanchez, L., Davis, A. C., Taylor, A. W., Tucker, G., et al. (1999). The epidemiology of hearing impairment in an Australian adult population. *International Journal of Epidemiology*, 28, 247–252.

Wilson, P. H., & Henry, J. L. (1998). Tinnitus cognitions questionnaire: Development and psychometric properties of a measure of dysfunctional cognitions associated with tinnitus. *International Tinnitus Journal*, 4, 1–7.

Wilson, P. H., & Henry, J. L. (2000). Psychological management of tinnitus. In R. S. Tyler (Ed.), *Tinnitus Handbook* (pp. 263–280). Clifton Park, NY: Delmar Learning.

Wilson, P. H., Henry, J. L., Bowen, M., & Haralambous, G. (1991). Tinnitus reaction questionnaire: Psychometric properties of a measure of distress associated with tinnitus. *Journal of Speech and Hearing Research*, 34, 197–201.

Wingfield, A., Aberdeen, J. S., & Stine, E. A. L. (1991). Word onset gating and linguistic context in spoken word recognition by young and elderly adults. *Journal of Gerontological Psychological Sciences*, 46, 127–129.

Wingfield, A., Poon, L. W., Lombardi, L., & Lowe, D. (1985). Speed of processing in normal aging: Effects of speech rate, linguistic structure, and processing time. *Journal of Gerontology*, 40, 579–585.

Wingfield, A., Stine, E. A., Lahar, C. J., & Aberdden, J. S. (1988). Does the capacity of working memory change with age? *Experimental Aging Research*, 14, 103–107.

Wingfield, A., & Tun, P. A. (2001). Spoken language comprehension in older adults: Interactions between sensory and cognitive change in normal aging. *Seminars in Hearing*, 22, 287–301.

Witt, S. (1997). *Effectiveness of an intensive aural rehabilitation program for adult cochlear implant users; A demonstration project*, unpublished master's thesis, University of Iowa, Iowa City, IA.

Woodcock, R. (1997). *Woodcock Diagnostic Reading Battery (WDRB)*. Itasca, IL: Riverside.

Woodcock, R., & Johnson, M. B. (1989). *Woodcock–Johnson Psycho-Educational Battery (WJ–R)*. Itasca, IL: Riverside.

Woods, D. L., & Yund, E.W. (2007). Perceptual training of phoneme identification for hearing loss. *Seminars in Hearing*, 28, 110–119.

Woods, M. L., & Moe, A. (1999). *Analytical Reading Inventory* (6th Ed.). Columbus, OH: Merrill Education (Prentice Hall).

Woodward, M. F., & Barber, C. G. (1960). Phoneme perception in lipreading. *Journal of Speech and Hearing Research*, 17, 212–222.

World Health Organization (WHO) (2001). *International Classification of Functioning, Disability, and Health*. Geneva, Switzerland: World Health Organization.

Wun, Y. T., Yam, C. C., & Shum, W. K. (1997). Impaired vision in the elderly: A preventable condition. *Family Practitioner*, 14, 289–292.

Wyant, J. (2007). Bluffing ...the (not so) social truth. *Volta Voices*, January/February, 32–34.

Yoshinaga-Itano, C. (1988). Speechreading instruction for children. *Volta Review*, 90, 241–260.

Yoshinaga-Itano, C., & Downey, D. M. (1996). Development of school-aged deaf, hard-of-hearing and normally hearing students' written language. *Volta Review*, 98, 3–7.

Yoshinaga-Itano, C., & Gravel, J. S. (2001). The evidence for universal newborn hearing screening. *American Journal of Audiology*, 10, 62–64.

Yoshingaga-Itano, C., Sedey, A., Coulter, D. K., & Mehl, A. L. (1998). Language of early and later identified children with hearing loss. *Pediatrics*, 102, 1161–1171.

Yoshinaga-Itano, C., Snyder, L. S., & Mayberry, R. (1996). How deaf and normally hearing students convey meaning within and between written sentences. *Volta Review*, 98, 9–38.

Young, A., & Tattersall, H. (2007). Universal newborn hearing screening and early identification of deafness: Parents' responses to knowing early and their expectations of child communication development. *Journal of Deaf Studies and Deaf Education*, 12, 209–220.

Yuen, K. C. P., Kam, A. C. S., & Lau, P. S. H. (2006). Comparative performance of an adaptive directional microphone system and a multichannel noise reduction system. *Journal of the American Academy of Audiology*, 17, 241–252.

Zimmerman-Phillips, S. (1997). *The Infant-Toddler Meaningful Auditory Integration Scale (IT-MAIS).* Retrieved 03/23/08 from http://www.BionicEar.com.

Zones, J., Estes, C., & Binney, E. (1987). Gender, public policy and the oldest old. *Aging Society*, 7, 275–302.

Zurif, E. B., Swinnery, D., Prather, P., Wingfield, A., & Brownell, H. (1995). The allocation of memory resources during sentence comprehension: Evidence from the elderly. *Journal of Psycholinguist Research*, 24,165–182.

Züst, H., & Tschopp, K. (1993). Influence of context on speech understanding ability using German sentence test materials. *Scandinavian Audiology*, 22, 251–255.

AUTHOR INDEX

A

Aberdden, J. S., 505, 755
Abrahamson, J. A., 321, 340, 457, 478, 754
Abrams, H., 17, 340, 691, 701
Adler, J., 481, 692
Aguilar, C., 503, 731
Ahlner, B. H., 342, 372, 695
Alcantara, J. I., 199, 235, 239, 692, 697
Alexander, G. C., 56, 109, 110, 295, 459, 461, 471, 702, 703
Allen, R. L., 130, 703
Allen, T. E., 633, 692
Allessie, H. M., 340, 515, 723
American Academy of Audiology (AAA), 21, 431, 693
American Speech-Language-Hearing Association (ASHA), 19, 20, 26–35, 426, 532, 693
Amos, N., 170, 699
Anderson, I., 130, 694
Anderson, K. L., 297, 307, 570, 620, 652, 694
Anderson, L. G., 74, 726
Andersson, G., 296, 694, 737
Andersson, U., 185, 213, 694
Andrews, R., 486, 715
Antia, S. D., 613, 614, 616, 618, 694, 719, 744
Arcaroli, J., 118, 726
Archbold, S. M., 568, 572, 733, 754
Arehart, K. H., 539, 694
Arensman, E., 496, 723

Arlinger, S., 185, 86, 296, 695, 718, 737
Arnold, P., 184, 695
Arts, H. A., 567, 702
Ashbaugh, C., 572, 721
Aslan, S., 269, 743
Auer, E. T., 186, 193, 198, 235, 238, 695, 697, 728
Axelsson, A., 405, 695

B

Backenroth, G. A. M., 342, 372, 695
Baguley, D. M., 406, 695
Baker, C., 74, 695
Baker, L. J., 453, 750
Baker, R. S., 398, 696
Bally, S. J., 192, 295, 296, 321, 323, 720
Bamford, J., 55, 696
Banks, W. A., 503, 695
Baran, J., 272, 701
Barber, C. G., 189, 756
Barcham, L. J., 297, 695
Barker, B., 633, 635, 743
Barley, M., 66, 185, 187, 718
Barney, H. L., 151
Barrager, D., 373, 745
Barry, J. G., 626, 697
Barth, C., 507, 732
Barton, G. R., 111, 727
Bauman, S. L., 206, 695
Baumgartner, W. D., 130, 694
Bayles, K. A., 400, 746
Baylock, R. L., 272, 342, 695

Bazargan, M., 398, 696
Bazargan, S. H., 398, 696
Beamer, S., 444, 745
Beattie, B. L., 503
Beck, P. H., 565, 696
Bell, Alexander Graham, 43, 223, 603
Beethoven, Ludwig Van, 6
Bench, J., 55, 696
Benguerel, A. P., 230, 735
Benitez, L., 73, 696
Bentler, R. A., 92, 107, 298, 300, 696
Berger, K. W., 190, 203, 696
Bergman, B., 499, 500, 696
Bergman, M., 239, 722
Bernstein, L. E., 186, 193, 198, 235, 238, 695, 695, 728
Berry, J. A., 456, 697
Bess, F. H., 511, 620, 697, 703
Bevan, K., 206, 720
Benyon, G., 340, 341, 696
Beyer, C. M., 17, 443, 474, 733
Biedenstein, J., 167, 730
Bierman, E. L., 486, 715
Bilger, R. C., 55, 697
Billermark, E., 296, 695
Binnie, C. A., 191, 236, 239, 697, 704
Binzer, S., 340, 378, 716
Birck, J. D., 74, 728
Birtles, G., 109, 295, 705
Blackwood, M. J., 487, 697
Blamey, P. J., 92, 199, 235, 626, 692, 697, 698, 733
Blanchfield, B. B., 511, 698

Blood, G. W., 264, 698
Blood, I. M., 264, 698
Bloom, S., 382, 698
Blumsak, J. T., 501, 698
Bochner, J., 56
Bode, D., 170, 698
Bodrova, E., 646, 698
Boettcher, F. A., 487, 698
Böheim, K., 130, 694
Boothroyd, A., 54, 55, 64, 65, 170, 185, 200, 698, 716, 738
Boppana, S., 543, 737
Borg, E., 372, 373, 698
Borrel-Carrio, F., 388, 698
Boswell, S., 410, 698
Boutin, L., 202, 710
Brackmann, D. E., 112, 726
Braida, L., 196, 199, 202, 699, 734
Brainerd, S. H., 298, 699
Brandt, F., 295, 296, 720
Brauckmann, Karl, 221
Brenner, C., 626, 746
Brewer, D., 340, 699
Brooks, B. M., 556, 722
Brooks, D. N., 296, 372, 699, 713
Brown, G. R., 455, 699
Brown, J., 296, 720
Brown, W., 444, 731
Brownell, H., 506, 757
Bruhn, M. E., 220
Bryant, M., 444, 731
Buckley, K., 170, 746
Budinger, A., 444, 731
Burk, M. H., 159, 170, 699
Burleson, D. F., 158
Burns, E., 617, 700
Busa, J., 580, 700

C

Caissie, R., 268, 269, 336, 700
Campbell, M. M., 336, 700
Campbell, R., 184, 186, 700, 729
Canadian Cochrane Network/Centre Affiliate Representatives, 21, 700
Capps, J., 506, 725
Carhart, R., 55, 647, 700, 746
Carney, A. E., 196, 701
Carrabba, L., 407, 727
Carrell, T., 171, 723, 747
Carson, A. J., 518, 735

Cascella, P. W., 547, 742
Cassels, L. A., 501, 717
Castle, D., 457, 700
Ceasar, L. G., 398, 700
Charest, M., 207, 710
Charlop, M., 580, 724
Chessman, M. G., 487, 701
Cherry, R., 223, 259, 701
Ching, T. Y., 130, 701
Chisolm, T. H., 17, 340, 341, 440, 692, 701
Choi, S. S., 202, 751
Christ, A., 176, 711
Christopherson, L. A., 487, 701
Chute, P. M., 630, 745
Cicchelli, M., 230, 735
Cienkowski, K. M., 196, 701
Ciocci, S., 272, 701
Clark, C., 232, 235, 361, 742
Clark, J. G., 72, 358, 360, 443, 702, 727
Cohen, M., 195, 199, 238, 711, 728, 733
Cohen, N., 512, 753
Cohen, R. D., 491, 744
Colbridge, C., 186, 741
Connor, C. M., 567, 572, 631, 633, 702
Coughlin, M., 487, 718
Coulter, D. K., 535, 756
Cowan, R. S. C., 199, 235, 692, 697
Cowie, R., 277, 278, 415, 702, 721
Cox, R. M., 22, 56, 108, 109, 110, 295, 459, 461, 471, 472, 702, 703
Craig, H. K., 572, 702
Craig, W. N., 65, 703
Crandell, C. C., 620, 703
Cray, J. W., 130, 703
Crimmins, E. M., 397, 715
Critz-Crosby, 625, 703
Crocker, S. R., 550, 721
Cruickshanks, K. J., 386, 401, 440, 703, 704, 754
Cuevas, C., 353, 744
Cummings, J., 629, 631, 713

D

Dagenais, P., 625, 703
Dalby, J. M., 158
Dalton, D., 440, 704

Dancer, J., 185, 237, 399, 456, 704, 717, 753
Daneman, M., 506, 735
Danhauer, J. L., 54, 72, 264, 698, 704, 730, 750
Daniloff, R., 628, 718
Dannermark, B., 361, 372, 698, 704
Danz, A. D., 236, 704
Davidson, L., 167, 730
Davies, E., 406, 695
Davis, A., 389, 405, 704
Davis, B. L., 624, 626, 752, 753
Davis, H., 55, 704, 716
Davis, J. M., 655, 706
De Filippo, C. L., 222, 235, 238, 239, 705
DeLavergne, R. W., 186, 741
Demorest, M. E., 109, 170, 186, 295, 298, 697, 705, 753
Dennis, K. C., 406, 715
Desai, M., 499, 705
Desbiens, C., 207, 710
DesGeorges, J., 655, 740
Devous, M., 170, 746
Di Francesca, S., 633, 705
Dillon, H., 103, 109, 295, 705
Dinon, D., 235, 237, 710
Dodd, B., 235, 237, 705
Doman, D., 567, 705
Donaldson, N., 363, 705
Dondorp, A. W., 340, 515, 723
Dorn, C., 232, 235, 742
Doucet, K., 209
Douglas-Cowie, E., 277, 278, 702
Dowell, R. C., 118, 130, 703, 727
Downey, D. M., 634, 756
Downs, M. P., 551, 733
Doyle, D., 170, 340, 724
Drinka, P., 494, 752
Driscoll, C., 547, 721
Dubno, J. R., 401, 487, 488, 706, 729
Dunbar, J. L., 511, 698
Durieux-Smith, A., 580, 708
Durlach, N., 202, 734
Durrant, J., 534, 743
Dworkin, M., 611, 706
Dye, C., 440, 706
Dykman, J., 404, 706

E

Edgerton, B. J., 54, 706
Edwards, C., 553, 706
Eggermont, J. J., 405, 706
Elfenbein, J., 338, 339, 341, 655, 706
Eliott, L., 54, 707
Elkayam, J., 372, 706
Ellis, A., 354, 707
Elman, R. J., 18, 707
El Nasser, H., 398, 706
Endicott, J., 503, 731
Engel, C., 485, 707
English, K. M., 358, 360, 361, 369, 372, 443, 538, 702, 707
Epstein, R. M., 388, 698
Erber, N. P., 54, 141, 167, 191, 192, 206, 207, 209, 258, 270, 279, 287, 303, 304, 306, 457, 707, 708, 725
Erdman, S. A., 64, 235, 236, 295, 298, 351, 440, 705, 754
Eriks-Brophy, A., 580, 612, 616, 708
Eriksson-Mangold, M., 296, 737
Erler, S. F., 402, 497, 708, 711
Ermann, M. G., 621, 741
Ertmer, D. J., 172, 173, 708
Espmark, A. K., 494, 708
Estabrooks, W., 578–79
Etymotic Research, 56, 63, 85, 708

F

Fairbanks, G., 297, 716
Feeley, J., 296, 720
Feldman, J. J., 511, 698
Ferguson, N. M., 517, 708
Fernandes, J., 410
Festen, J. M., 295, 723
Fiket, H. J., 92, 698
Firszt, J. B., 118, 571, 721, 753
Fitch, J. L., 203, 709
Fitzgibbons, P. J., 489, 712
Flanders, J., 658, 709
Flexer, C., 45, 125, 709
Flipsen, P., 547, 741
Flock, S., 630, 746
Folkins, J., 628, 749
Folstein, M. F., 503, 709
Folstein, S. E., 503, 709
Forner, L., 628, 709
Fountain, H., 194, 709

Fourcin, A. J., 200, 738
Fowler, K., 543, 737
Frankel, B. G., 298, 699
Frederick, E. A., 456, 697
Fredrickson, J. M., 104, 729
Fristoe, M., 642, 712
Frueh, F. X., 186, 741
Fryauf-Bertschy, H., 54, 572, 709, 750
Fu, Q.-J., 169, 709

G

Gabrel, C., 494, 709
Gagné, J. P., 202, 205, 207, 209, 235, 237, 239, 269, 270, 369, 437, 458, 513, 709, 710, 743
Gallagher, C., 494, 752
Gallaudet Research Institute, 548, 710
Galster, J., 92
Galusha, D., 387, 736
Galvin, J. J., 169, 709
Gantz, B. J., 116, 171, 633, 743, 747, 750
Gao, S., 628, 719
Garaham, M. B., 503, 710
Gardner, E., 630, 710
Garretson, C., 192, 321, 323, 720
Garrison, W., 56
Garstecki, D. C., 205, 402, 497, 708, 711
Gatehouse, S., 109, 110, 111, 296, 428, 434, 435, 484, 711
Gaustad, M. G., 613, 694
Geers, A. E., 17, 55, 65, 84, 171, 198, 567, 568, 626, 633, 644, 711, 716, 749
Geffner, D., 623, 725
Gellerstedt, L. C., 361, 704
Gentry, B., 185, 717
Gesi, A. T., 238, 711
Getty, L., 264, 268, 269, 296, 360, 362, 364, 365, 372, 437, 711, 716
Gfeller, K., 116, 131, 176, 632, 651, 711, 712, 740, 747
Gianni, P., 407, 727
Gibson, C. L., 269, 700
Gilbert-Bedia, E., 623, 750
Giles, E., 365, 447, 734

Gilmore, C., 56, 109, 110, 459, 702, 703
Ginis, J., 295, 705
Giolas, T. G., 297, 712
Gitles, T., 291, 712
Givens, G. D., 272, 712
Glennon, S. L., 338, 712
Glorig, A., 297, 716
Gold, M. A., 621, 741
Gold, S. L., 456, 697
Goldfield, A., 184, 736
Golding, M., 742
Golding-Meadow, S., 633, 712
Goldman, R., 642, 712
Goldstein, G., 614, 718
Goldstein, H., 580, 720
Golz, A., 547, 712
Gomolin, R., 512, 753
Goodale, C., 483, 712
Gordon-Salant, S., 489, 712
Gottermeier, L., 222, 232, 235, 238, 705, 742
Grant, K. W., 185, 205, 712
Gravel, J. S., 536, 756
Gray, J. A., 18, 21, 739
Grayden, D., 130, 550, 727, 736
Green, J., 630, 745
Green, W., 631, 712
Greenberg, J. H., 205, 713
Greenberg, S., 190, 713
Greenfeld, D., 272, 712
Gregory, M., 235, 237, 705
Grenette, W., 336, 700
Grice, H. P., 250, 713
Griffin, K., 486, 717
Griswold, E., 629, 631, 713

H

Hadjistavropoulos, T., 503
Hager, R. M., 18, 713
Hale, S., 505, 713
Hall, J. W., 535, 539, 713
Hallam, R. S., 296, 407, 713
Hallberg, L. R. M., 265, 296, 365, 372, 402, 713
Hambrecht, G., 206, 695
Hampton, D., 462, 714
Hanin, L., 55, 64, 65, 200, 205, 698
Hanratty, V., 486, 714
Hansen, V., 388, 746

Haras, N., 239, 722
Hardin-Jones, M. A., 655, 706
Harless, E., 440, 714
Harvey, M. A., 361, 714
Haskins, H., 55, 59, 714
Haycock, G. S., 628, 714
Hayes, D., 539, 714
Haynes, W., 605, 714
Hayward, M. D., 397, 715
Hazard, W. R., 486, 715
Hazell, J. W., 406, 695
He, W., 480, 481, 491, 715
Hecht, P., 259
Heermann, R., 571, 725
Heide, V., 458, 462, 463, 715
Helfer, K. S., 202, 402, 715
Helgeson, C. L., 205, 724
Heller, P. J., 610, 715
Helper, E. L., 109, 170, 753
Henkin, Y., 185, 722
Henry, A., 629, 728
Henry, J. A., 406, 453, 715
Henry, J. L., 455, 755
Hergils, A., 534, 716
Hergils, L., 534, 716
Hermann, B. S., 538, 716
Hétu, R., 264, 268, 269, 296, 360,
    362, 363, 364, 365, 372,
    412, 716
Heydebrand, G., 340, 362, 365, 373,
    378, 716
Hickson, L., 270, 279, 321, 340, 363,
    511, 516, 525, 567, 705, 716,
    725, 743
Hieber, S., 567, 702
High, W. S., 297, 716
Hill, F., 184, 695
Hill, M., 130, 701
Hirsh, I. J., 55, 79, 716, 741
Hixon, T., 628, 709
Hnath-Chisholm, T. E., 55, 64, 65,
    172, 185, 200, 340, 697, 716
Hodgson, W. R., 73, 754
Hogan, A., 275, 358, 365, 366, 371,
    447, 717, 734
Holbrook, A., 203, 709
Holgers, K. M., 407, 550, 717
Holmes, A. E., 170, 340, 516,
    723, 724
Honnell, S., 185, 717

Hood, J. B., 118, 571, 721
Hoover, B. M., 655, 735
Horii, Y., 628, 717, 718
Hornak, J., 369, 707
Horowitz, A., 501, 717
Houghton, M., 503, 710
Houle, C. O., 320, 717
House, J., 491, 717
Howarth, J., 624, 719
Hug, G. A., 297, 732
Hughes, E. K., 623, 753
Hull, R. H., 486, 717
Humes, L. E., 52, 159, 170, 458,
    485, 487, 489, 699, 701,
    717, 718
Hutton, C. L., 109, 718
Huttunen, K. H. 16, 718
Hyde, M. L., 428, 461, 718
Hygge, S., 185, 718

Idler, C., 259
Ijsseldijk, F. J., 206, 718
Illg, A., 571, 725
Incerti, P., 130, 701
Infante, A. A., 208, 235, 237,
    239, 742
Ishak, H., 195, 733
Israelite, N., 614, 616, 718
Itoh, M., 628, 718

Jackson, D. W., 651, 734
Jackson, P. L., 191
Jacobson, G. P., 297, 315, 732
Jacq, P., 626, 697
James, A., 295, 705
Jansson, G., 402, 714
Janota, J., 548, 719
Jastreboff, P. J., 407, 456, 718
Jaworski, A., 269, 297, 744
Jeffers, J., 66, 185, 187, 718
Jenkins, J. J., 205, 713
Jennings, M. B., 369, 710
Jensema, C., 567, 719
Jerger, J., 56, 185, 298, 719, 743
Jerger, S., 185, 729
Jerram, J. C., 439, 719
Jiménez-Sánchez, C., 616, 719
John, J., 624, 719

Johnson, C. D., 18, 560, 719
Johnson, C. E., 264, 704
Johnson, S. M., 301, 719
Joint Committee On Infant Hearing,
    536, 719
Jones, D. L., 628, 719
Jones, L., 363, 715
Jordan, T. R., 206, 208, 719
Jorgensen, B., 124, 719
Joseph, J. M., 538, 714
Jurma, W. E., 373, 516, 745
Juul, J., 550, 716

K

Kaderavek, J. N., 634, 733
Kaiser, A. R., 205, 720
Kam, A. C. S., 90, 92, 757
Kantrowitz, B., 504, 527, 720
Kaplan, G. A., 491, 744
Kaplan, H., 182, 295, 296, 321, 323,
    512, 720
Kapteyn, T. S., 295, 723
Karinen, P., 511, 753
Karlsen, B., 630, 710
Kashinath, S., 580, 581, 720
Kasten, R. N., 264, 704
Katz, D., 54, 707
Katz, S., 494, 720
Kei, J., 547, 721
Kelly L. A., 7, 736
Kelsay, D. R., 54, 333, 572, 709,
    749, 750
Kemper, S., 506, 724
Kentish, R. C., 550, 721
Keogh, T., 547, 721
Kerr, P. C., 269, 297, 415, 721
Kessels, R. P. C., 352, 721
Kiese-Himmel, C., 630, 721
Kiessling, J., 459, 484, 729
Kileny, P. R., 572, 721
Killion, M. C., 56, 721
Kinnefors, C., 186, 737
Kinze, C., 221
Kirchner, R., 500, 721
Kirk, K. I., 55, 59, 60, 79, 118,
    165, 205, 567, 571, 572, 626,
    630, 720, 721, 724, 729,
    745, 749
Kishon-Rabin, L., 185, 200, 239, 623,
    698, 722

Kitano, Y., 203, 722
Klein, B. E., 386, 440, 703, 704
Kluwin, T. N., 651, 722
Knutson, J. F., 131, 176, 360, 497, 711, 722
Koch, D., 572, 737
Kochkin, S. 14, 438, 439, 442, 443, 444, 722
Kochanek, K., 534, 743
Kozak, V. J., 556, 722
Kraaij, V., 496, 723
Krachmer, M. A., 633, 747
Kramer, S. E., 295, 298, 340, 515, 696, 723
Krantz, P., 580, 723
Kraus, N., 171, 723, 747
Kravitz, L., 537, 723
Kretschmer, L., 631, 644, 723
Kretschmer, R., 631, 644, 723
Kricos, P. B., 43, 141, 170, 191, 192, 193, 237, 340, 440, 489, 514, 516, 629, 723, 724, 725, 741
Kuhl, P. K., 184, 724
Kurtzer-White, E., 553, 726
Kynette, D., 506, 724

L

Lach, R., 624, 724
Lachs, L., 165, 205, 720, 724
Laipply, E., 185, 716
Lahar, C. J., 505, 755
Lalande, M., 268, 269, 363, 716
Lam, C. C., 499, 756
Lamb, S. H., 297, 712
Landis, K., 491, 717
Langer, E., 494, 752
Lansing, C. R., 188, 205, 360, 497, 722, 724
Larsby, B., 185, 718
Larson, E., 503, 751
Laski, K., 580, 724
Lau, P. S. H., 90, 92, 757
Lausberg, I., 459, 729
Lawlor, D. A., 486, 714
Lee, F. S., 401, 706
Lehiste, I., 54
Leigh, I. W., 614, 725
Lentzner, H., 499, 705
Leong, D. J., 646, 698

Leonard, J. S., 172, 173, 708
Lerman, J., 54, 623, 738
Leroux, T., 513, 743
Lesinski-Schiedar, A., 571, 725
Lesner, S., 191, 182, 193, 237, 513, 514, 725
Leung, J., 512, 725
Levine, L. M., 616, 694
Levitt, H., 623, 643, 725
Lewis, D. E., 655, 735
Lichtman, W., 537, 725
Lidestam, B., 213, 694
Light, J., 239, 728
Light, L., 506, 725
Lind, C., 270, 279, 304, 708, 725
Lindberg, P., 296, 694
Lindblade, D. D., 491, 502, 725
Ling, D., 239, 624, 627, 642, 724
Ling, L., 624, 724
Litovsky, R., 118, 726
Lloyd, J., 305, 726
Lombardi, L,, 505, 506, 755
Lonka, E., 235, 238, 726
Lovegrove, R., 109, 295, 705
Lowder, M., 116, 747
Lowe, D., 505, 506, 744
Luce, P. A., 59, 726
Lukomski, J., 614, 727
Luterman, D., 551, 553, 555, 726
Luxford, W. M., 112, 726
Lyman, R., 481, 726
Lynch, J., 631, 739
Lyxell, B., 185, 186, 187, 694, 726, 737

M

MacDonald, J., 195, 728
MacDuff, M., 580, 723
MacLeod, A., 64, 184, 727
MacSweeney, M., 186, 729
Mahendra, N., 400, 730
Mak, M., 130, 727
Marciano, E., 407, 727
Margolis, R. H., 352, 353, 727
Markides, A., 624, 628, 727
Markin, N. D., 652, 694
Marmor, M. E., 499, 564, 727
Marschark, M., 614, 633, 727
Marslen-Wilson, W. D., 205, 727
Martin, F. N., 72, 727

Martinez, C., 444, 745
Massaro, D., 195, 199, 209, 238, 239, 711, 728, 733, 744
Matthews, L. J., 401, 706
Mattys, S. L., 198, 728
Mauzé, E., 185, 340, 362, 378, 715, 728
Mayberry, R. I., 633, 634, 711, 756
McArdle, R., 17, 340, 692, 701
McCarthy, P., 43, 141, 724
McClannahan, L., 580, 723
McConkie, G. W., 188, 724
McConnell, F., 440, 714
McCracken, W., 551, 570, 728
McCullough, J. A., 74, 86, 728
McDonald, M., 491, 502
McDowd, J. M., 505, 728
McDuff, S., 437, 710
McFall, R. M., 301, 728
McGarr, N., 623, 625, 724, 728
McGee, T., 171, 723
McGuire, R., 482, 483, 728
McGukian, M., 629, 728
McGurk, H., 195, 729
McHugh, P. R., 503, 709
McKay, C., 550, 736
McKay, S., 651, 753
McKenna, L., 437, 550, 721, 729
McLean, J., 184, 736
Mehl, A. L., 535, 756
Mehr, M. A., 176, 711
Meikle, M., 455, 752
Meister, H., 459, 729
Melin, L., 296, 694
Mellon, N., 616, 729
Meltzoff, A. N., 184, 724
Mendel, L., 72, 369, 707, 730
Menn, L., 624, 753
Messina, C. M., 559, 729
Messina, J. J., 559, 729
Metz, D., 628, 729
Michaud, J., 205, 710
Miles, T. P., 397, 715
Miller, D. A., 104, 729
Miller, G. A., 57, 729
Miller, J. A., 503
Miller, J. D., 158
Mills, J. H., 487, 488, 729
Miskiel, L. W., 168, 169, 752
Mitchell, P., 485, 742

Miyamoto, R. T., 54, 567, 572, 630, 721, 729, 737, 745
Mize, J., 594, 729
Moeller, M. P., 487, 734
Mohammed, T., 186, 729
Monday, K. L., 207, 710
Monfils, B., 237, 753
Monranelli, D. S., 644, 736
Monsen, R., 624, 642, 729
Montgomery, A. A., 64, 170, 184, 191, 193, 235, 236, 730, 753
Montoya, L. A., 554, 736
Moog, J., 55, 167, 171, 644, 711, 730
Moore, B. C. J., 200, 738
Moran, D., 580, 730
Moran, M., 605, 714
Moriarty, M., 109, 734
Morley, J. E., 503, 695
Morrison, H. M., 626, 753
Moss, H. E., 205, 727
Most, T., 272, 730
Mowry, R. B., 517, 741
Moxley, A., 400, 401, 730
Mueller, H. G., 92, 107, 109, 300, 444, 696, 731, 734
Mulrow, C., 503, 731
Murdoch, B., 567, 705
Musiek, F. E., 733
Musselman, C., 651, 753
Myerson, J., 505, 713

N

National Center for Health Statistics, 499, 502, 731
National Council on Aging, 507, 511, 731
National Eye Institute (NEI), 501, 731
National Institutes of Health (NIH), 21, 532, 533, 732
National Institute on Deafness and Other Communication Disorders (NIDCD), 21, 732
National Mental Health Association, 486, 732
Navarra, J., 194, 754
Neely, K. K., 206, 732
Nekahm-Heis, D., 543, 754
Nerbonne, M. A., 312, 494, 517, 708, 740
Netzer, A., 547, 712

Neutzel, J. M., 55, 697
Newby, H. A., 50, 732
Newman, C. W., 297, 315, 732
Nicely, P. E., 57, 729
Nicholas, J., 17, 567, 711
Nicholas, M., 507, 732
Nicol, T. G., 171, 739
Nilsson, L. G., 185, 738
Nilsson, M. 55, 732
Niolopoulos, T. P., 568, 572, 733, 754
Nitchie, E. B., 64, 220
Nix, G. W., 564, 732
Noble, W., 110, 291, 711, 732
Noffsinger, D., 487, 733
Nondahl, D. M., 401, 407, 485, 755
Northern, J., 17, 443, 474, 551, 733
Novelli-Olmstead, T., 239
Nusbaum, N. J., 500, 733
Nussbaum, J. F., 494, 733

O

Oberg, M., 296, 695
Obler, L. K., 507, 732
Öhngren, G., 185, 738
O'Donoghue, G. M., 572, 733
Ohna, S. E., 613, 733
Olds, J., 580, 708
Olszewski, C., 131, 712
O'Neill, J. J., 205, 711
Orlando, N. A., 643, 744
Osberger, M. J., 54, 55, 59, 60, 79, 205, 572, 721, 737
Oticon, 618, 651, 733
Ouni, S., 195, 733
Overberg, P., 398, 706
Owens, E., 297, 712
Ower, J., 614, 718
Oyer, H., 170, 698

P

Paatsch, L. E., 626, 733
Pachuilo, M. L., 172, 173, 708
Pakulski, L. A., 634, 733
Pallarito, K., 608, 734
Palmer, C., 92, 109, 169, 300, 696, 731, 734, 745
Palmer, L., 56
Pang-Ching, G., 628, 737
Parkinson, A., 118, 726
Parsons, J., 235, 237, 710

Paul, P. V., 651, 734
Paynter, D. E., 646, 698
Peak, M., 440, 706
Pederson, K. E., 487, 734
Pedley, K., 365, 447, 734
Pelli, D., 500, 734
Peña, E. D., 73, 74, 752
Peterson, G. E., 54, 151
Peterson, R., 500, 721
Petitito, L., 564, 727
Philibert, I., 296, 716
Picheny, M. A., 202, 734
Pichora-Fuller, M. K., 230, 489, 490, 504, 505, 506, 518, 735
Pindzola, R., 605, 713
Pisoni, D. B., 55, 59, 60, 79, 165, 205, 572, 720, 721, 724, 726, 745
Pittman, A. L., 655, 735
Plant, G., 230, 235, 237, 329, 705, 735
Plath, P., 487, 735
Pollack, D., 140, 565, 735
Pollack, I., 184, 744
Poole, C., 340, 696
Poon, L. W., 505, 506, 744, 755
Popelka, G. R., 50, 535, 732
Pope, M. L., 54, 737
Potvin, M.-C., 209
Poulakis, Z., 623, 753
Power, D., 630, 739
Prather, P., 506, 757
Pratt, L., 499, 705
Pratt, S., 647, 735
Preece, J., 54, 64, 65, 199, 750
Preminger, J., 340, 260, 736
Prendergast, S. G., 7, 736
Primeau, R. L., 340, 736
Prince Market Research, 386, 736
Prosek, R., 170, 184, 193, 236, 730
Purdy, S. C., 271, 439, 719, 749

Q

Quigley, S., 630, 644, 735, 739

R

Rabinowitz, P. M., 387, 736
Rabinowitz, W. M., 55, 697
Rall, E., 554, 736
Rance, G., 550, 736

Raudenbush, S. W., 572, 702
Reeh, M., 630, 721
Rees, T., 503, 751
Refaie, A. E., 405, 704
Reich, G. E., 456, 736
Reisberg, D., 184, 736
Renshaw, 54, 737
Ricketts, T., 92
Riko, K., 428, 461, 718
Ringdahl, A., 296, 405, 459, 695, 737
Rivera, L., 543, 737
Riverin, L., 264, 363, 716
Robb, M., 628, 737
Robbins, A. M., 54, 572, 737, 745
Robinson, J. D., 494, 733
Robinson, K., 499, 705
Robson, J., 500, 734
Roenberg, W. M., 18, 21, 739
Rogers, C. R., 357, 737
Rojeski, T., 369, 707
Rönnberg, J., 185, 186, 187, 203, 694,
    718, 726, 737, 738
Rosen, S. M., 200, 738
Rosenbloom, S., 100, 391, 738
Rosenhall, U., 499, 500, 696
Rosenthal, U., 487, 734
Ross, M., 54, 353, 587, 623, 738
Rossiter, S., 407, 738
Rousey, C., 491, 738
Roush, J., 612, 738
Rubinstein, A., 170, 223, 701, 738
Rudman, H., 630, 710
Runge-Samuelson, C. L., 118, 753
Russell, K., 630, 739
Russo, N. M., 171, 739
Rychener, M., 131, 712

S

Sabes, J., 170, 745
Sackett, D. L., 18, 21, 739
Salthouse, T. A., 505, 739
Samar, V. J., 186, 739
Sandridge, S., 191, 192, 237, 725
Sarant, J. Z., 626, 733
Sass-Lehrer, M., 576, 739
Scarinci, N., 321, 340, 516, 716
Scarola, D., 17, 739
Schafer, D., 631, 739
Schafer, E. C., 130, 739
Schecter, M. A., 406, 715

Scherman, M. H., 494, 708
Schloss, P. J., 651, 739
Schmiedt, R. A., 487, 488, 729
Schneider, B., 489, 506, 735, 740
Schow, R. L., 312, 332, 494, 740
Schreibman, L., 580, 724
Schreuder, R., 633, 752
Schum, D. J., 202, 269, 270, 296,
    306, 450, 470, 740,750
Schum, R. L., 632, 711, 740
Schwartz, D., 170, 236, 730
Scott, A. O., 248, 740
Scudder, R. R., 272, 342, 695
Seaver, L., 655, 740
Sedey, A., 535, 756
Sedey, A. L., 17, 567, 711
Seitz, P. F., 112, 185, 205, 712, 741
Selekman, J., 537, 723
Sengupta, M., 480, 715
Sergeant, P., 208, 720
Serry, T. A., 626, 741
Seyfried, D. N., 629, 741
Shatner, W., 407, 741
Shaw, R. J., 505, 728
Shema, S. J., 491, 744
Shepherd, D., 186, 631, 712, 741
Shibuya, L., 586, 587, 741
Shriberg, L., 547, 741
Shultz, D., 517, 741
Shum, W. K., 499, 756
Siebein, G. W., 621, 741
Siegenthaler, B. M., 203, 722
Siemens Audiology Group, 141, 361,
    741
Silverman, S. R., 55, 61, 79, 704, 716
Sims, D. G., 186, 222, 232, 235, 238,
    705, 739, 741, 742
Sindhusake, D., 485, 742
Singh, G., 489, 504, 505, 735
Sininger, Y. S., 539, 742
Skinner, M., 378, 716
Slade, M. D., 387, 736
Smaldino, J., 297, 307, 620, 694,
    703
Small, L. H., 208, 235, 237,
    239, 742
Smith, C., 623, 742
Smith, M. A., 651, 739
Smith, R. J. H., 542, 544, 545, 742

Smith, S. L., 319, 742
Smurzynski, J., 534, 743
Snyder, L. S., 634, 756
Sobaski, C., 269, 270, 306, 750
Soli, S. D., 55, 732
Sommers, M., 70, 185, 196, 197, 199,
    211, 742, 749
Sonnenschein, E., 547, 742
Sorkin, D., 114, 743
Sorri, M., 511, 753
Southall, K., 513, 743
Souza, P. E., 489, 735
Speaks, C., 56, 73, 298, 696,
    719, 743
Spehar, B., 70, 185, 196, 197, 199,
    211, 742, 749
Spencer, L., 572, 582, 584, 623,
    626, 627, 630, 633, 635, 743,
    746, 750
Spens, K. E., 185, 694
Spinhoven, P., 496, 723
Spitzer, J. B., 297, 754
Springen, K., 504, 527, 720
Srinivasan, R. J., 203, 742
Stanton, J. F., 126, 743
Stark, P., 511, 743
Steele, B. R., 92, 698
Stelmacovich, P., 270, 655, 710, 743
Stephens, S. D., 269, 277, 297, 335,
    695, 744
Stevens, C., 407, 738
Stika, C. J., 353, 744
Stine, E. A., 505, 744, 755
Stinson, M. S., 613, 614, 694, 744
Stoel-Gammon, C., 624, 744
Stoker, R. G., 203, 722
Stout, G., 146, 744
Strauser, L., 170, 699
Strawbridge, W. J., 491, 744
Stuart, A., 130, 703
Suárez, M., 651, 653, 744
Subtelney, J. D., 643, 744
Suchman, A. L., 388, 698
Sullivan, J. A., 55, 732
Sumby, W. H., 184, 744
Summerfield, Q., 64, 111, 184,
    186, 727
Sunkyung, S., 202, 751
Sutherland, G., 452, 745
Svedlund, K., 407, 717

Svirsky, M. A., 567, 572, 628, 630, 719, 729, 737, 745
Sweetow, R., 169, 170, 373, 453, 457, 745
Swinney, D., 506, 757

T

Taitelbaum, R., 623, 722
Takahashi, G., 444, 745
Talley, L., 487, 718
Tambas, K., 403
Tannen, D., 252, 746
Task Force on Newborn Infant Hearing, 537, 746
Tattersall, H., 551, 570, 728, 756
Taylor, B., 63, 388, 746
Taylor, K. S., 372, 516, 746
Teresi, J. A., 501, 717
Tharpe, A. M., 92
Thibodeau, L. M., 130, 739
Thielke, H., 547, 741
Thomas, A. J., 496, 746
Thompson, T., 494, 733
Thomson, V., 539, 694
Thornton, A. R., 538, 715
Thornton, F., 340, 696
Tillman, T. W., 55, 746
Tobey, E., 170, 567, 626, 746
Tobi, H., 295, 723
Tobin, Y., 623, 722
Tomblin, J. B., 623, 626, 630, 633, 635, 750
Tomoeda, C. K., 400, 747
Toner, J., 111, 727
Torres, E., 651, 744
Trammell, J. L., 56, 298, 719, 743
Tremblay, K. L., 171, 747
Trybus, R., 567, 633, 719
Trychin, S., 302, 318, 353, 371, 372, 747
Tschopp, K., 205, 757
Tun, P. A., 506, 757
Tucker, P. E., 186, 235, 238, 697
Tugby, K. G., 205, 710
Tuokko, H., 503
Turner, C., 116, 747
Tweed, T. S., 386, 703
Tye-Murray, N., 54, 64, 65, 70, 84, 169, 171, 185, 196, 197, 198, 199, 211, 232, 259, 269, 270, 271, 272, 306, 322, 333, 340, 341, 362, 378, 450, 470, 568, 572, 623, 625, 626, 627, 628, 747–750
Tyler, R. S., 54, 64, 65, 171, 199, 453, 572, 708, 750, 751

U

Uchanski, R. 202, 751
Uhlmann, R., 503, 751
Umberson, D., 491, 717
Underwood, N., 657, 658, 751
Urbantschitsch, V., 141, 169, 751
U.S. Government Printing Office, 221

V

van Bon, W., 633, 752
Van Camp, G., 542, 544, 545, 742
VanderBrink, R. H. S., 297, 751
van Halen, S., 205, 727
Van Hecke, M., 393, 752
Vega-Barachowitz, C., 400, 730
Velkoff, V. A., 480, 715
Ventry, I., 297, 298, 311, 440, 515, 752, 754
Vergara, K. C., 168, 169, 752
Vermeulen, A. M., 633, 752
Vernon, J. A., 455, 752
Villchur, E., 56, 721
Voeks, S., 494, 752
Von Hapsburg, D., 73, 74, 624, 752
Vonlanthen, A., 102, 752
Vouloumanos, A., 194, 754
Vuorialho, A., 511, 753

W

Wackym, P. A., 118, 753
Wake, M., 623, 753
Walden, B. E., 64, 109, 170, 184, 185, 193, 235, 236, 298, 712, 730, 753
Walker, G., 407, 738
Wallace, V., 624, 753
Waller, J. A., 503, 710
Wallis, D., 651, 753
Waltzman, S., 117, 512, 753
Wang, N., 512, 725
Warner-Czyz, A. D., 626, 753

Warren, S. F., 581, 753
Warren, Y., 237, 754
Watson, C. S., 158
Watson, L. M., 568, 754
Wayner, D. S., 321, 446, 457, 476, 754
Weichold, V., 543, 754
Weikum, W. M., 194, 754
Weinstein, B. E., 297, 298, 311, 315, 440, 515, 732, 754
Weisleder, P., 73, 754
Westermann, S. T., 547, 712
West, R. L., 319, 742
White, K. R., 532, 534, 754
Whitehead, B., 628, 729
Whitehead, R., 628, 643, 729, 744, 754
Whitman, T., 580, 730
Wigley, H., 594, 729
Wilbur, R. B., 644, 736
Wilde, O., 253
Wiley, T. L., 401, 755
Wilhite, G., 301, 719
Wilkins, A., 500, 734
Williams, D. R., 398, 700
Willott, J. F., 486, 489, 755
Wilson, P. H., 455, 755
Wilson, R. H., 74, 86, 487, 728, 733
Wilzl-Mueller, K., 543, 754
Windel, J., 146, 744
Wingfield, A., 505, 506, 507, 744, 755, 757
Witt, S., 131, 176, 240, 269, 270, 272, 306, 322, 711, 750, 757
Woods, D. L., 170, 756
Woods, J., 580, 720
Woodward, M. F., 189, 756
Woodworth, G., 171, 271, 572, 623, 627, 749, 750
World Health Organization (WHO), 431, 756
Worrall, L., 321, 340, 363, 516, 525, 705, 716
Wright, F., 371, 744
Wun, Y. T., 499, 756
Wyant, J., 267, 754
Wylie, K. M., 269, 710
Wynne, M. K., 272, 342, 695

Y

Yang, Y., 397, 715
Yeagle, J., 512, 725
Ying, E. A., 630, 721
Yoder, P. J., 581, 753
Yoshinaga-Itano, C., 231, 536, 539, 623, 624, 634, 694, 753, 756

Young, A., 551, 570, 614, 727, 728, 756
Yovetich, W., 270, 710
Yuen, K. C. P., 90, 92, 757
Yund, E. W., 170, 756

Z

Zecker, S. G., 171, 739
Zimmermann, G., 628, 750

Zimmerman-Phillips, S., 570, 757
Zöger, S., 407, 717
Zurif, E. B., 506, 757
Züst, H., 205, 757
Zwolan, T. A., 572, 633, 702, 721

SUBJECT INDEX

A

AAA. *See* American Academy of Audiology
A-B-C-D-E model of counseling, 356
Acknowledgement gestures, 256
Acceptance, 417, 555
Acknowledgement of hearing loss, 264
Acoupedic approach to communication, 565
Acoustic feedback cancellation, 90
Acoustic lexical neighborhoods, 59, 196. *See also* lexical neighborhoods
Acquired hearing loss, 12
Active Communication Education (ACE) program, 516, 525
Activity limitations, 4–6, 108, 431–34, 484
Acute otitis media, 547
ADA. *See* Americans with Disabilities Act
Adaptive communication strategies, 256–59
Adjacency pairs, 271
Adjustment to hearing loss, 415
ADA. *See* Alzheimer's disease
ADM. *See* Automatic directional microphone
Adults with hearing loss, 15, 386–426
    assessment phase of aural rehabilitation, 428–34
    auditory training benefits, 170
    case study, 418

characteristics of adult-onset hearing loss, 389–91
cochlear implant candidacy, 117
handout for speechreading training class, 223
patient-centered approach to rehabilitation, 388
patient characteristics and rehabilitation design, 391–412, 428–38
phases of adjustment, 412–18
prevalence of hearing loss, 386–88
self-help and professional organizations, 477
speech characteristics, 628
Adventitious hearing loss, 623
Affective approach to counseling, 357–59
Aided thresholds, 44
Air-bone gap, 44
Air conduction, 44
ALD. *See* assistive listening devices
ALGO (automated ABR screening device), 538
Altered speech, 68
Alzheimer's disease (AD), 503
Ambient noise, 120
American Academy of Audiology (AAA), 21
American National Standards Institute (ANSI), 11, 44
American Sign Language (ASL), 562–6

American Speech-Language Hearing Association (ASHA)
    evidence-based practice, advocating, 18–19
    knowledge and skills for audiologists and speech-language pathologists, 10
    knowledge and skills for audiologists providing aural rehabilitation, 26–31
Americans with Disabilities Act (ADA), 15, 126, 414
American Tinnitus Association (ATA), 456
Amplifier, hearing aid, 91
Analytic auditory training, 147, 150–59, 515
Analytic speechreading training, 224–28
Anoxia, 542
Anticipatory communication strategies, 258
Apgar score, 536
Apple Tree Language Curriculum, 649
Appropriate format accommodations, 617
Appropriate speaking behaviors, 334
Arthritis, 502
Articulation
    clarity of, 67
    manner of, 155–58
    place of, 154
    testing in children, 642

ASHA. *See* American Speech-Language Hearing Association

ASL. *See* American Sign Language

Assessment, hearing and speech recognition, 41–86
difficulties with speech recognition assessment, 69–73
hearing impairment, 431
multicultural issues, 73
patient variables, 52
purpose of speech recognition testing, 51
speech audiometry, 49
stimuli units, 54–69
test battery approach for speech recognition, 75
test procedures for speech recognition, 62–69

Assertive conversational style, 274, 275

Assertiveness training, 371

Assistive listening devices (ALDs), 120–29
adult aural rehabilitation program, 449–52
assessment of need or interest in, 470
children with hearing loss, 618–20
checklist for systems, 470
frequency modulation (FM) systems, 121, 619
hard-wired systems, 127
infrared systems, 124
manufacturers and contact information, 137
older adults, 502, 512–14
other types of HAT, 127
situations appropriate for use, 120
wireless systems, 121–27

Asymmetrical hearing loss, 11

ATA. *See* American Tinnitus Association

Attention
communication strategies training, 326
older adults, 505

Audio boot, 97, 123

Audiograms, 11, 43–48, 488

Audiological terms, Spanish and English, 423–25

Audiologic rehabilitation, 8

Audiologists, 9
knowledge and skills for aural rehabilitation, 26–31
role of, 606–8

Audiometry, 49
behavioral/observational (BOA), 540
conditioned play audiometry (CPA), 540
pure tone, 43–49
speech, 49
sound field testing, 50
test environment, 50
visual reinforcement audiometry (VRA), 540

Audition-only testing, 62

Audition-plus-vision testing, 63

Auditory brain stem response (ABR), 538

Auditory enhancement, 63

Auditory neuropathy/dys-synchrony, 550

Auditory-verbal approach to communication, 565

Audiovisual integration, 195–200
models of, 195–98
quantifying, 199

Auditory enhancement. *See* speechreading enhancement

Auditory information, role in speech acquisition, 627

Auditory lexical neighborhoods. *See* lexical neighborhoods

Auditory processing, age-related decline, 487

Auditory skill level, 142–47

Auditory training, 140–82
adults with cochlear implants, 448
analytic training objectives, 150–59
benefits of, 169–72
candidacy for, 142
case studies, 172–75
design principles, 142–50
formal and informal, 161–65
history of, 140
interweaving with aural rehabilitation components, 165

programs, 166–69
synthetic training objectives, 159–61

Aural habilitation, 8

Aural/oral language, 171, 564–68, 602, 632

Aural rehabilitation, 2, 7–10
combining with auditory training, 165
components of a typical program, 7
costs and cost-effectiveness, 17
evidence-based practice (EBP), 18–23
providers of, 9
service needs, 14–17
settings for, 8–9

Aural rehabilitation for adults, 15, 428–478
assessment, 428–438
assisted listening devices, 449–52
case study, 462
cochlear implants, 446–49
development of objectives, 436–38
follow-up, 461
hearing aids, 438–46
hearing impairment diagnosis, 431
hearing-related difficulties, 431–34
individual factors, 434
information counseling, 435
orientation sessions, 446
outcomes assessment, 458–61
telephone training, 457
tinnitus intervention, 452–57

Aural rehabilitation for children, 14, 531–598. *See also* children with hearing loss
case study, 586
cochlear implants, 571–75
communication modes, 562–68
early-intervention programs, 576–80
federal law on early intervention, 557–60
hearing aids, 568–71
support and instruction for parents, 580–85

Aural rehabilitation for older adults, 15, 480–527
  activity and participation limitations, 484
  audiological testing, 485
  case study, 519
  in institutional settings, 517–20
  life situation factors, 490–8
  listening devices, 507–17
  model of plan, 483
  otologic health evaluation, 485
  other services, 514
  presbycusis, 486
  physical and cognitive variables, 498–507
Autosomal dominant, 545
Autosomal recessive, 545
Automatic directional microphones (ADMs), 92
Automatic gain control (AGC), 93, 95

B
Babbling, 624
Baby boomers, 387, 482, 485
Background noise, 63, 121, 620
Batteries in hearing aids, 91
Behavioral approach to counseling, 356
Behavioral/observational audiometry (BOA), 539, 540
Behind-the-ear (BTE) hearing aids, 89, 96, 97, 99, 123, 588
Benefits assessment, 107–10, 459
Bilateral hearing loss, 12
Bilingual, 73, 74
Bilingual/bicultural model, 564
Binaural amplification, 103
Binaural advantage, 103, 118
Bluffing, 263–67, 268
BOA. See behavioral/observational audiometry
Body hearing aids, 98
Bone conduction, 44, 98
Bone conduction hearing aid, 98
Brain plasticity, 171
BTE. See behind-the-ear hearing aids.

C
Canonical babbling, 624
CAPD. See central auditory processing disorder

Carrier phrase, 74, 158, 185
Cataracts, 50
CAT scans. See computerized axial tomography scans
Causation of hearing loss, 13
CAVET, See Children's Audiovisual Enhancement Test
CC. See closed captioning
CDT. See continuous discourse tracking
Center-based programs, 576
Central auditory processing disorder (CAPD), 548–50
Children's Audiovisual Enhancement Test (CAVET), 65, 75, 84
Children with hearing loss, 600–655
  amplification and ALDs, 618–20
  auditory training benefits assessment, 171–75
  aural rehabilitation strategy, 601
  beginnings of U.S. education for, 602
  case studies, 655–57
  causes of hearing loss, 541–48
  classroom acoustics, 620–22
  classroom placement, 613–18
  cochlear implant candidacy, 227
  communication strategies training, 336–40, 341
  early intervention and aural rehabilitation strategy, 557–76
  early intervention programs, 576–80
  holistic approach to speechreading training, 231
  identifying and quantifying, 538–41
  individualized education plan (IEP), 604–6
  listening devices, 568–75
  mild or moderate losses, 654
  multidisciplinary team for IEP, 606–12
  other services, 651
  parent counseling, 551–56
  psychosocial issues, 361, 651–54
  repair strategy use, 272
  school placement, 612
  speech and language evaluation, 637–46

speech and language therapy, 646–50
speech, language, and literacy development, 622–36
tinnitus, 550
CIC. See completely-in-the-canal hearing aids
CICI. See completely implantable cochlear implants
CID Everyday Sentence Test, 61, 79–83
Citation indexes for evidence-based practice, 37
Clarification, 359
Class handouts for speechreading, 222
Classrooms
  acoustics, 620–22
  placement, children with hearing loss, 613–18
Clear speech, 202, 336
Client Oriented Scale of Improvement (COSI), 434, 466, 469
Clinical significance, 21, 72
Clock-time orientation, 400
Closed captioning (CC), 126
Closed-ended questions, 298
Closed-set tests, 66
CMV. See cytomegalovirus
Cochlear implant mapping, 447, 448
Cochlear implant team, 446
Cochlear implants, adults, 64, 111–119, 673
  for adults, 446–49
  auditory training case studies, 172–75
  aural rehabilitation, 447
  candidacy for, 116–18, 448
  case study, 130
  components, 112–116
  experimental designs, 116
  follow-up, 447
  formal evaluation, 447
  fitting and mapping, 447, 448
  history of development, 111
  for older adults, 511
  manufacturers and contact information, 137
  process of, 118, 447
  surgery, 447

Cochlear implants, children, 571–76
  aural rehabilitation, 575
  benefits of early implantation, 571
  case studies, 172–75
  fitting, 574
  follow-up visits, 575
  formal evaluation, 574
  preliminary counseling, 573
  initial contact, 573
  reading achievement in
      children, 633
  language acquisition in
      children, 630
  speech of children using, 625–28
  surgery, 574
  vocabulary acquisition, 631
Code of ethics, oral interpreters, 213
Coenrollment model, 616
Cognitive abilities
  affected by aging in older adults,
      504
  unaffected by aging in older
      adults, 506
Cognitive approach to counseling,
    354–56
Comfortable loudness level, 43, 49,
    106
Communication behaviors, 276–80,
    299–301
Communication breakdowns, 259–73,
    287, 305, 339. *See also* repair
    strategies for communication
Communication modes, 53, 562–68
Communication strategies, 248
  case study, 279
  conversation, 248–54
  conversational styles and behav-
      iors, 273–79
  facilitative, 255–59
  repair, 259–73
Communication strategies training,
    248, 318–348
  attention, focusing, 326
  benefits of, 340–43
  for children, 337–40
  continuous discourse tracking,
      327
  formal instruction, 322
  for frequent communication
      partners, 333–36

guided learning, 323
issues in program development,
    320
model for training, 322
modeling, 324
older adults, 501, 515
real-world practice, 329
role-playing, 325
self-efficacy, 319
short-term training, 330–32
videotaped scenario analysis, 326
Complementary signals (speechread-
    ing), 221–23
Completely implantable cochlear im-
    plants (CICI), 112
Completely-in-the-canal (CIC) hearing
    aids, 98, 102
Comprehension level of auditory skill,
    146
Compression, 93
Computed axial tomography (CAT)
    scans, 544
Computerized instruction
  auditory training, 169
  speechreading training, 232–35
Conditioned play audiometry (CPA),
    540
Conductive hearing loss, 13, 44,
    545–47
Configuration of hearing loss, 11
Confirmation repair strategy, 272
Congenital hearing loss, 12
Congruence with self, 358
Consonants
  auditory training objectives,
      154–58, 181
  classification system for phoneme
      feature analysis, 58
  consonant-vowel-consonant
      (CVC), 59, 73
  lipreading, 189, 192
  phoneme confusion errors, 57
  speechreading training objectives,
      226–28
Constructive communication
    strategies, 256
Construct validity, 72, 290
Contained classrooms, 613
Content validity, 72
Content (language), 630

Context
  contextual information, 61
  linguistic context and speech
      recognition, 205
Continuous discourse tracking (CDT),
    230, 327
Contralateral routing of signal
    (CROS), 653
Conversation, 248–54
  behaviors, 276–79
  case study, couple conversing, 279
  hand gestures, 251
  involving person with hearing
      loss, 251–54
  pragmatics, children with hearing
      loss, 631
  rules of, 248–50
  styles, 273–75
Conversational fluency, 2, 287–90
  case study, 307
  defining factors, 287
  daily logs self-monitoring
      procedure, 299–301
  general considerations for
      evaluating, 288–90
  group discussion assessment
      procedure, 301–3
  interview assessments, 290–94
  questionnaire assessments,
      294–99, 312
  structured communication
      interactions, 303
  unstructured communication
      interactions, 305
Conversational rules, 248–50
Conversation Made Easy program,
    232–34
Cooperative spirit in conversation, 265
Corner audiogram, 45
COSI (Client Oriented Scale of
    Improvements), 434, 466, 469
Cost-effectiveness and costs, 17
Costs
  hearing aid selection and, 105
  hearing aids, out-of-pocket, 440
  hearing loss adjustment, 417
Counseling, 350–60. *See also*
    psychosocial support
  benefits of, 351
  informational, 351, 352, 435

parent counseling, 551–56
personal adjustment, 352, 353–59
pre-implant, for adult cochlear
implant, 447
pre-implant, for child cochlear
implant, 573
targeting for particular concerns,
359
tinnitus management, 455
Critical period, 533, 587
CROS. *See* contralateral routing of
signal
Cued speech, 565
Cultural and linguistic competence,
400, 426
Culture, 397, 399
Cycling, 169
Cytomegalovirus (CMV), 542, 543

D

DAI. *See* direct audio input
Daily logs, as assessment, 299–301,
460
Deaf culture, 12, 408–11, 551
Degree of hearing loss, 10–13, 104,
652–55
Delayed-onset hereditary hearing
loss, 545
Dementia, 502
Denial, 416, 553
Desensitization, 356
Difficulty level in auditory training,
148–50
Digital signal processing (DSP), 90, 93
Direct audio input (DAI), 89, 97,
122, 123
Directional microphones, 92
Disability, 2, 288–90, 313, 341
Dissonance theory, 415
Dominating conversational
behaviors, 278
Drill activity, 220, 221
DSP. *See* digital signal processing),
90, 93
Dyalog, 305, 306

E

Early Hearing Detection and Intervention (EHDI), 534–37
Earmolds, 96, 99, 100, 101, 424

Ear protection, 424, 433
EBP. *See* evidence-based practice
Educational audiologists, 607, 619
Education for All Handicapped Children Act (1975), 557, 612
Education. *See also* school-age children
with hearing loss
acronyms used for children's
needs, 665
classroom acoustics, 620–22
classroom placement, children
with hearing loss, 613–18
guidelines for classroom teachers,
664
individualized education plan
(IEP), 604–6
Individuals with Disabilities Education Act (IDEA), 558, 604,
655–57, 678
school placement, 612
Efficacy of speechreading training,
235–39
Elicitation techniques, 305
Emotional issues, 211. *See also* counseling; psychosocial support
older adults with untreated hearing loss, 507
Environment
classroom acoustics, 620–22
communication environment for
older adults, 501
constructive communication
strategies, 256
effects on speechreading, 205–10
speech recognition testing, 50
Equivalent lists, 59
Ethnicity, race, and culture, 397–400
Event-time orientation, 400
Evidence-based practice (EBP), 18–23
citation indexes, 37
decision-making case study, 22
electronic databases, 37
five-step approach to, 21
journals for consultation, 36
levels of evidence, 20
Evoked potential, 538
Executive Order 13166, 400
Expanded speech, 68
Expectations, 432, 439–41
Explicit categorization, 352

Expressive language, 629
Expressive repair strategies, 267,
337–340
Extended communication repair, 262

F

F1 *See* first formant
F2 *See* second formant
Facilitative communication strategies,
254–59
adaptive strategies, 256
anticipatory strategies, 258
constructive strategies for the
environment, 256
maladaptive strategies, 257
message-tailoring strategies, 256
Facilitative language techniques, 58
False-negative responses, 53
False-positive responses, 535
Familial deafness, 544
Families, 15–17
family support services, 596–98
parental counseling, 551–56
participation in aural rehabilita-
tion with older adults, 515
relationships with older adult
members, 491
support and instruction for
parents, 580–85
FAPE. *See* free and appropriate public
education
Favorable seating for speech
reading, 207
Features of articulation, 154–58
Filtered speech, 68
Fingerspelling, 562–64
First formant (F1), 151, 153
Flat audiogram, 46
Flat hearing loss, 11
Fluctuating hearing loss, 12
FM. *See* frequency modulation;
frequency modulation systems
FM boot, 123
FM trainer, 121, 123, 124
Formal auditory training, 148,
161–63
Formal communication strategies
training, 322, 323
Formal speechreading training
objectives, 223–31

Formants, vowel articulation, 57, 151–54, 224–226
Form (language), 629
Free and appropriate public education (FAPE), 557
Frequency, 44–48
Frequency modulation (FM) systems, 121
    boot, 123
    checking, 664
    sound amplification system, 619
    wireless assistive listening devices, 121–25
Frequent communication partners, 4–6, 15–17, 108
    communication strategies training, 333–36
    miscommunication with older adults, 494
    psychosocial support for, 362–64
Frequency of usage (words), 59, 198, 204
Full-on gain, 106
Functional gain, 94
Functional magnetic resonance imaging (fMRI), 184

G

Gain/frequency response, 106
Gain, 92–95
Gender effects on aural rehabilitation, 401
Gender of the talker and speechreading difficulty, 203
Generous listening, 291–94
Genetic causes of sensorineural hearing loss, 544–47
Genetic counseling, 544
Genetics, terminology, 595
Gestures in conversation, 251
Glaucoma, 500
Grief, 553
Goals, 150, 168
Grounding (in conversations), 253
Group aural rehabilitation program rules, 347
Group discussions, 301–3
Guided learning, 323–29
Guilt, 554

H

HAE. *See* hearing aid evaluation.
Hand gestures, 251
Handicap, 3, 314–16
Handouts for speechreading class, 222
HAO. *See* hearing aid orientation.
Hard of hearing, 12
Hard-wired ALDs, 121, 123, 127
Head shadow, 103
Health-related quality of life (HRQoL), 440
Hearing aids, 88–111, 438–46
    binaural versus monaural fitting, 103
    candidacy for, 438
    checking, 663
    for children, 568–71
    components and features, 91–97
    electroacoustic properties, 106
    evaluation for adults, 442
    fitting and orientation, 442
    follow-up orientation sessions, 446, 474–76
    history of development, 88–91
    manufacturers and contact information, 136
    older adults, 502, 509–11
    orientation, 110, 473
    outcome assessment, 472
    satisfaction assessment, 471
    selecting and assessing benefits, 107–110, 568, 570
    styles, 97–111
    use pattern, establishing, 444–46
Hearing aid evaluation (HAE), 438, 441, 442, 473
Hearing aid orientation (HAO), 110, 442, 443, 446
Hearing aid use pattern, 108, 444–46
Hearing assistance technology (HAT), 127
Hearing conservation, 387, 433
Hearing culture, 408
Hearing Handicap Inventory for the Elderly (HHIE), 311
Hearing impairment, 3. *See also* hearing loss/disability
Hearing Loss Association of America (HLAA), 462, 477
Hearing loss/disability

adjustment to, 412–18
age-related (presbycusis), 486
assessment, 431
categories of, 10
changes in perception of, 341
comments on, by older adults, 490
conversational fluency and, 288–90
degree of, 10–13, 104, 652–55
disability assessment questions, 313
genetic causes of, 544–47
group discussion assessment procedure, 301–3
Hearing Handicap Inventory for the Elderly (HHIE), 311
hearing-related difficulties, 431–35
handicap assessment questions, 314
Hearing Handicap Inventory for Adults (HHIA), 315
identifying and quantifying in children, 538–41
interview assessment procedure, 290–94
questionnaire assessment procedure, 294–99
Self-Assessment of Communication (SAC), 312
self-help and professional organizations, 477
self-monitoring through daily logs, 299–301
simple questions for diagnosing, 59
untreated, 440
Hearing protection, 387, 433
Hearing-related difficulties, 431–35
Hearing-related disability, 2, 3–6, 288–90, 313
Hearing-related stress, 360–62
Hearing threshold, 43, 45, 49, 63, 69
Hereditary sensorineural hearing loss, 544–47
HHIA. *See* Hearing Handicap Inventory for Adults
HHIE. *See* Hearing Handicap Inventory for the Elderly

High conversational fluency, 388
High-frequency hearing loss, 11
HLAA. *See* Hearing Loss Association of America
Holistic approach to speechreading, 231
Home-based programs, 576
Home, school, and vocational communication difficulties, 403
Homophenes, 189, 191–93
HRQoL. *See* health-related quality of life
Hybrid devices, 116

I

IADLs. *See* Instrumental Activities of Daily Living
ICF-WHO. *See* International Classification of Functioning, Disability, and Health
IDEA. *See* Individuals with Disabilities Education Act
Identification, 145, 14
Idiopathic hearing loss, 541
IEP. *See* individualized education plan
IFSP. *See* individualized family service plan
Impairment, 3, 12
Inclusion, 613–16
Independence, older adults, 497
Individualized education plan (IEP), 604–6
Individualized family service plan (IFSP), 560–62
Individuals with Disabilities Education Act (IDEA), 558, 604, 655–57
Induction loop systems, 126
Infants and toddlers with hearing loss, 14, 532–598. *See also* children with hearing loss
  babies identified with hearing loss, 533
  newborn screening, 534–41
Informal training, 148, 163–65
Informational counseling, 351, 352, 429, 435
Infrared systems, 121, 124
Insert earphone, 44
Insertion gain, 92
In-service, 517

International Classification of Functioning, Disability, and Health (ICF-WHO), 3–6, 431
Institutional settings, aural rehabilitation, 517
Instructional facilitative communication strategies, 254, 323, 327
Instrumental Activities of Daily Living (IADLs), 494
Insurance coverage of aural rehabilitation, 17
Intelligibility of speech, 624, 638–43
Interactive communication behaviors, 276
Interdisciplinary teams, 600, 606–12
Internal components, cochlear implants, 112
International Outcome Inventory-Hearing Aids (IOI-HA), 461, 472
In-the-canal (ITC) hearing aids, 89, 97, 101, 102, 440, 498
In-the-ear (ITE) hearing aids, 89, 97, 101, 440, 588
Interleaved pulsatile stimulation, 114
Interpreters, 399, 611
Interviews, as assessment, 290–94, 432
IOI-HA, *See* International Outcome Inventory-Hearing Aids
ITC. *See* in-the-canal hearing aids
ITE. *See* in-the-ear hearing aids
Itinerant teachers, 611, 613, 617, 656

J

Jena method, 221
Journals for evidence-based practice, 36

K

Keying, 251
Kinesthetic forms and sensations, 221

L

Labeling, 489, 582
Language development, 629–32, 643, 648–50
Learning effect, 69–71
Least restrictive environment (LRE), 558, 559, 655
LEP. *See* limited English proficiency
Levels of evidence, 20

Lexical neighborhoods, 59, 79, 196–98, 208
Lexical Neighborhood Test, 79
Life factors, 394–96
  evaluation for older adults, 490–8
Life stages and impact of hearing loss, 392–94
Limited English proficiency (LEP), 400
Limited set, 66
Linear amplification, 93
Linguistic competence, 400, 423–426
Linked adjacency pairs, 271
Lipreading, 184, 223. *See also* speechreading
Listening behaviors, 291–94, 336
Listening check, 663
Listening devices. *See also* assistive listening devices; cochlear implants; hearing aids
  children with hearing loss, 568–80
  older adults with hearing loss, 507–17
  sources for information, 136–38
Literacy development, 632–36
Live-voice testing, 67
Loudness balancing, 119
Loudness comfort level, 119
Loudness discomfort level (LDL), 106
Loudness summation, 103
Loudspeaker azimuth, 50
Low conversational fluency, 288
LRE. *See* Least restrictive environment
Luminance, speechreading and, 209

M

Macular degeneration, 500
Mainstream classrooms, 616–18, 645, 651, 652
Mainstreaming, 613
Maladaptive communication strategies, 256, 257
Managed care, 18
Manner of articulation, 155–58
Manual alphabet, 562–64
Manually coded English, 564, 581
Mapping, cochlear implants, 119
Masker, 407, 455
Masking, 121, 122, 390
Matrix test format, 70

Maximum comfort level (MCL), 119
Maximum power output (MPO), 93, 106
MCL. *See* most comfortable loudness
Mean length turn (MLT) ratio, 287
Medicaid, 17
Medicare, 17
Medical home, 561
Mental health problem, 496
Message-tailoring communication facilitation strategies, 256
Metacommunication, 256
Microphones in hearing aids, 91, 92
Middle ear implants, 102–04
Mimetic forms and sensations, 221
Mixed hearing loss, 13, 545–48
MLT, *See* mean length turn
Modeling, 324
Monolingual, 73
Most comfortable loudness (MCL), 43, 49
Motivation in adults to use hearing aids, 441
MPO. *See* maximum power output
Mueller-Walle method, 220
Multiband compression, 95
Multichannel cochlear implants, 114
Multicultural issues in speech recognition testing, 73
Multidisciplinary teams, 600, 606–12
Multiple memory hearing aids, 90
Multisensory approach to communication, 565
Music, listening for cochlear implant users, 130, 176

N

NAM. *See* Neighborhood Activation Model, 196–98
Nasality, 57, 58
Naturalistic methods of language instruction, 650
Neckloop wireless ALDs, 123, 127
Neighborhood Activation Model (NAM), 196–98
Newborn nursery, 534
Newborn screening, 534–41
Nitchie method, 221
No Child Left Behind Act, 558, 644
Noise

background noise in speech recognition tests, 63
in classrooms, 620–22
sources common to communication settings, 210
Noise-induced hearing loss, 387
Noise notch, 386
Noise reduction, 90
Nongenetic causes of sensorineural hearing loss, 542
Noninteractive conversational behavior, 277
Nonspecific repair strategies, 259, 269, 270, 272
Nonsense syllables, 57, 58
Nonsyndromic hearing loss, 545
Nursing homes, 494, 517

O

OAEs. *See* otoacoustic emissions
Objectives, 683
    auditory training, 150–60
    formulating for adult aural rehabilitation, 437
Occlusion effect, 102, 104
Occupational hearing loss, 487
Older adults with hearing loss, 15. *See also* aural rehabilitation, older adults
    conversations with, 253
    Hearing Handicap Inventory for the Elderly (HHIE), 311
Omnidirectional microphones, 92
On-off control, 96
Onset of hearing loss, 12
Open-ended questions, 298
Open-set tests, 66
Oral interpreters, 212, 613
Oralism, 602, 603, 632
Oral transliteration, 212
Organized messages, 204
Orientation service, hearing aids, 110
Otitis media, 13, 106, 547–48
Otoacoustic emissions (OAEs), 539
Ototoxic drugs, 13, 543
Outcomes assessment, 18
    aural rehabilitation program for adults, 458–61
    aural rehabilitation for older adults, 516
Output limiting, 94, 95

P

Parallel talk, 582
Parameterization of hearing loss, 10–14
Parent advocacy in IEP process, 657
Parental support and instruction, 580–86
Parent-support group, 562, 580
Parent counseling, 551–56
Parent's guide to hearing and language milestones, 593
Part B, Public Law PL 105–17 (IDEA), 608
Part C, Public Law PL 108–446, 558
Participation restrictions, 4–6, 431–34, 484
Passive-aggressive conversational style, 274
Passive conversational style, 273
Patient-centered orientation, 388
    nonauditory needs assessment, 434
Patient variables
    in adults with hearing loss, 434
    in older adults with hearing loss, 495–98
    in speech recognition testing, 52
Pattern perception, 145
Peak-clipping, 93
Perilingual hearing loss, 12
Perinatal, 542
Personal adjustment counseling, 353–59
Personal FM trainer, 121, 123, 124
Phonetically balanced (PB) words, 59
Pitch ranking, 119
Place of articulation, 57, 58, 154, 156–58, 161, 171, 173
Plasticity, 171
Play audiometry, 539–41
Postlingual hearing loss, 12, 13, 117
Postnatal, 542
Pragmatics, 631
Preamplifier stage in hearing aids, 93
Predicament, 461
Prelingual hearing loss, 12, 142, 172–74
Prenatal, 542
Prescription procedures, 107

Prevalence of hearing loss, 14, 386, 389
Probe microphone, 107
Problem identification-exploration-resolution, 365–71
Processing speed, 504
Processing strategy, 90, 113–15
Programmable hearing aids, 89, 97, 138
Psychological factors, 406, 416
Psychological well-being and aural rehabilitation, 402
Psychologists, role in evaluating children, 610
Psychosocial adjustment to hearing loss, 416
Psychosocial support, 275, 350, 360–71
   assertiveness training, 371
   case study, 373
   children with hearing loss, 651–54
   frequent communication partners, 362–64
   intervention paradigm, 364
   persons with hearing loss, 360–62
   problem-solving model, 365–71
   related research, 372
   St. Louis Psychosocial Hearing Rehabilitation Workshop, 378–82
Psychotherapy, 367. *See also* psychosocial support
Public Law 94–142 (1975), 557

Q

Quest?AR, 304
Questionnaires, as assessment, 294–99, 453
QuickSIN, 56, 63, 85

R

Race, ethnicity, and culture, 397–400
Randomized controlled trials, 19
Rapidity of speech, 189, 190
Rational Emotive Behavior Therapy (REBT), 354–356
Reactive procedure (self monitoring), 301
Reading, children with hearing loss, 633, 644–46

Real-ear measures, 108
Real-time closed captioning, 126, 414
Real-world practice, 585
REBT. *See* Rational Emotive Behavior Therapy
Receivers, 95
Receptive language, 629
Receptive repair strategy, 259, 305
Recorded stimuli, 67, 208, 234
Referential communication, 304
Reflection, in counseling, 359
Reinforcement, 162
Relaxation techniques, 358
Relay systems, 129
Release time, 95
Reliability, in testing, 72
Reluctance to admit hearing loss, 265
Remote control, hearing aids, 97
Repair strategies for communications, 259–73, 329, 333, 335
   bluffing, 263–67, 268
   consequences of using, 269–71
   expressive strategies, 267, 337–340
   individuals likely to use them, 271
   nonspecific strategies, 269
   research on use by children, 272
   research related to usage, 267
   stages of communication breakdown, 260
   training for children, 337–40
   topic shading, 268
Request for information repair strategy, 272
Resource rooms, 613
Response formats, speech recognition testing, 66
Reverberation, 121, 620
Retinitis pigmentosa, 545
Role-play, 318, 321, 323, 325
Room conditions and speechreading, 208–10
Rules of conversation, 248–50

S

SAC. *See* Self-Assessment of Communication
St. Louis Psychosocial Hearing Rehabilitation Workshop, 378–82

St. Louis University Mental Status Examination (SLUMS), 503
Sales orientation to rehabilitation, 388
Satisfaction assessment, 108, 461, 471
School-age children with hearing loss, 15, 600–665. *See also* children with hearing loss
   acronynms used, 665
   amplification and ALDs, 618–20
   case study, IDEA(s) for all, 655–57
   classroom acoustics, 620–22
   classroom placement, 613–18
   individualized education plan (IEP), 604–6
   mild or moderate hearing loss, 654
   multidisciplinary team implementing the IEP, 606–12
   other services, 651
   psychosocial issues, 651–54
   school placement, 612
   speech and language evaluation, 637–46
   speech and language therapy, 646–50
   speech, language, and literacy development, 622–36
Screenings, 28, 33, 35, 497, 498, 500, 534–541
SDT. *See* speech detection threshold
Second formant (F2), 151, 153
Seeing Essential English (SEE 1), 564
SEE 11 (Signing Exact English), 564
Segmental errors, 622, 625
Segmentals, speech testing, 641
Self-Assessment of Communication (SAC), 312
Self-concept, 498
Self-contained classroom, 612, 613, 614, 617, 621
Self-efficacy, 319, 342
Self-help and professional organizations for adults with hearing loss, 477
Self-image, 350, 651
Self-stigma, 264
Self-sufficiency and independence, 497
Self-talk, 582
Semantics, 200, 629, 645, 650

Sender, 259, 267, 585
Sentence stimuli, speech recognition testing 60
  CID Everyday Sentence Test, 61, 79–83
  Quick SIN test, 85
Service coordinator, 561
Shock, 553
Signal processing, 90, 93
Signal-to-noise (S/N) ratio, 63, 85
Signed English, 564
Significance of hearing-related difficulties, 432
Signing Exact English (SEE 11), 564
Sign language interpreters, 411
Sign language, 562–64
Simultaneous communication, 184, 475, 564, 567, 568
Situation-specific behaviors, 372
SLP. *See* speech-language pathologists
SL. *See* sensation level
SNHL. *See* sensorineural hearing loss
Social factors, 397–400
Social relationships, older adults, 491–94, 508
Social skills development in children, 651–54
Social stigma, 264
Socioeconomic status, 396
Sound awareness, 145, 146
Sound discrimination, 145, 146
Sound field, 121
Sound-field (FM) amplification, 125, 619
Sound-field (FM) system, 121–23, 125
Sound field testing, 50
Sound visibility, 189, 191–93
Spanish audiological terms, 423–25
Spanish Picture-Identification Test, 74, 86
Sparse (lexical) neighborhood, 59
Speaking behaviors training for frequent communication partners, 334
Specific repair strategies, 269
Speech and language assessment, children
  language skills, 643
  reading skills, 644–46
  speech skills, 638–43

Speech audiometry, 59
  speech reception threshold, 49, 541
  speech recognition testing, 41–86
Speech characteristics, assessment for children 622–29
Speech detection threshold (SDT), 49
Speech, language, and literacy development
  auditory information, role in speech acquisition, 627
  children with cochlear implants, 625, 626
  language, 629–32
  literacy, 632–36
  speech characteristics, children with hearing loss 622–29
Speech-language pathologists (SLP), 9
  knowledge and skills for aural rehabilitation services, 31–35
  role of, 608–10
Speech perception training for older adults, 501
Speech processor, 113
Speechreading, 184–218
  analytic training objectives, 224–28
  by babies, 194
  candidacy for training, 220
  case study, 213, 240
  combining with auditory training, 165
  for communication, 184
  computerized instruction, 232–35
  defined, 184
  developing skills, 222–24
  difficulty of, factors influencing, 188–94
  efficacy of training, 235–41
  enhancement of, 63–65
  environment and communication situation, 205–10
  factors affecting, 200
  familiarity with the speaker, 203
  gender of the talker, 203
  holistic approach to training children, 231
  linguistic context and, 205
  masking hearing loss, 66
  message of the talker, 204

  older adults and, 501
  oral interpreters, 212
  process of, 187, 195–200
  residual hearing, importance of, 200
  speechreader characteristics, 185–87, 210–12
  synthetic training objectives, 228–31
  talker effects, 193, 201–03
  topical cues, 205
  traditional training methods, 220–22
Speechreading enhancement, 63–65
Speech reception threshold (SRT), 49, 541
Speech recognition, 42
  decline in older adults, 487–89, 504
  testing, 41–86
Speech therapy, 646–48
SRT. *See* speech reception threshold
Stages of life, 392–94
Stimuli units, speech recognition testing
  auditory training, 147
  live-voice versus recorded materials, 67
  phonemes, 57
  phrases and sentences, 60
  selection of, 61
  synthesized and altered speech, 68
  words, 59
Stop consonants, 155
Stress effects, 189, 191
Stress, hearing-related, 360–62
Structured communication interactions, 290, 303
Sudden hearing loss, 14
Suprasegmental errors, 622, 626
Suprasegmentals, 159, 643
Syndrome, 545–47
Syntax, 200, 252, 564, 629, 643, 645, 649
Synthesized speech, 68
Synthetic training, 147, 159–61, 175
Synthetic sentences, 73
Synthetic speechreading training objectives, 228–31